Human Mobility, Spatiotemporal Context, and Environmental Health

Human Mobility, Spatiotemporal Context, and Environmental Health

Recent Advances in Approaches and Methods

Special Issue Editor

Mei-Po Kwan

MDPI • Basel • Beijing • Wuhan • Barcelona • Belgrade

MDPI

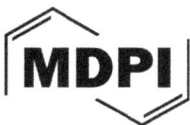

Special Issue Editor
Mei-Po Kwan
University of Illinois at Urbana-Champaign
USA

Editorial Office
MDPI
St. Alban-Anlage 66
4052 Basel, Switzerland

This is a reprint of articles from the Special Issue published online in the open access journal *International Journal of Environmental Research and Public Health* (ISSN 1660-4601) from 2018 to 2019 (available at: https://www.mdpi.com/journal/ijerph/special_issues/Human_Mobility_Spatiotemporal_Context)

For citation purposes, cite each article independently as indicated on the article page online and as indicated below:

LastName, A.A.; LastName, B.B.; LastName, C.C. Article Title. *Journal Name* **Year**, *Article Number*, Page Range.

ISBN 978-3-03921-183-8 (Pbk)
ISBN 978-3-03921-184-5 (PDF)

Contents

About the Special Issue Editor

Mei-Po Kwan Professor of Geography and Resource Management of the Chinese University of Hong Kong. She had served as an editor of Annals of the American Association of Geographers for 12 years and is editor of the book series entitled SAGE Advances in Geographic Information Science and Technology. She is an associate editor of Travel Behaviour and Society, and serves on the editorial boards of Journal of Transport Geography, Applied Geography, International Journal of Geographical Information Science, and Geographical Analysis. Kwan is Fellow of the U.K. Academy of Social Sciences, the American Association for the Advancement of Science, and the John Simon Guggenheim Memorial Foundation. She has received many prestigious honors and awards, including the Distinguished Scholarship Honors from the American Association of Geographers and the Alan Hay Award from the Transport Geography Research Group of the Royal Geographical Society with the Institute of British Geographers. Kwan has published 38 edited or co-edited volumes and 210 peer-reviewed journal articles and book chapters. She has delivered over 200 keynote addresses and invited lectures in about 20 countries. Her research interests include environmental health, sustainable cities, human mobility, urban/social issues in cities, and GIScience. She has made ground-breaking contributions to these areas. Her recent collaborative projects include the development of a unified cyberinfrastructure framework for scalable spatiotemporal data analytics, the development of a Geospatial Virtual Data Enclave (GVDE) for sharing and analyzing confidential geospatial data, and examination of the health risks of female sex workers, adolescent and adult participation in high-risk drug use, individual exposure to air pollution and noise, and environmental influences on physical activity.

Preface to "Human Mobility, Spatiotemporal Context, and Environmental Health"

Environmental health researchers have long recognized the importance of geographic context for understanding the effects of different environmental factors on human health. While geographic context and neighborhood effects are fundamental constructs for assessing people's exposure to contextual or environmental influences, they still tend to be largely conceptualized in static spatial terms, which ignores the fact that people move around in their daily life and come under the influence of many different neighborhood contexts outside their residential neighborhoods. Past studies also tend to ignore the role of human mobility at various spatial and temporal scales (e.g., daily travel, migratory movements, and movements over the life course) in various health issues. They tend to ignore the temporality of exposures that shape people's exposure to environmental influences and subjective wellbeing—such as the duration, frequency, and recency of exposure, as well as people's residential history and cumulative exposure over the life course.

Recent studies, however, have started to incorporate human mobility, non-residential neighborhoods, and the temporality of exposures through the collection and use of data from GPS, accelerometers, mobile phones, various types of sensors, and social media. Innovative approaches and methods have also emerged. This Special Issue aims to showcase studies that use new approaches, methods, and data to examine the role of various forms of human mobility, non-residential contexts, and the temporality of exposures on human health behaviors and outcomes. It includes 21 articles that cover a wide range of topics, including individual exposure to air pollution, exposure and access to green spaces, spatial access to healthcare services, environmental influences on physical activity, food environmental and diet behavior, exposure to noise and its impact on mental health, and broader methodological issues such as the uncertain geographic context problem (UGCoP) and the neighborhood effect averaging problem (NEAP). The editor would like to thank all the authors for their excellent contributions and the competent support and professionalism of the IJERPH editorial staff.

Mei-Po Kwan
Special Issue Editor

International Journal of
*Environmental Research
and Public Health*

MDPI

Article

The Uncertain Geographic Context Problem in the Analysis of the Relationships between Obesity and the Built Environment in Guangzhou

Pengxiang Zhao [1], Mei-Po Kwan [2,3] and Suhong Zhou [4,5,*]

[1] Department of Land Surveying and Geo-Informatics, the Hong Kong Polytechnic University, Hong Kong, China; peng.x.zhao@polyu.edu.hk
[2] Department of Geography and Geographic Information Science, University of Illinois at Urbana-Champaign, Natural History Building, MC-150, 1301 W Green Street, Urbana, IL 61801, USA; mpk654@gmail.com
[3] Department of Human Geography and Spatial Planning, Faculty of Geosciences, Utrecht University, P.O. Box 80125, 3508 TC Utrecht, The Netherlands
[4] School of Geography and Planning, Sun Yat-sen University, Guangzhou 510275, China
[5] Guangdong Key Laboratory for Urbanization and Geo-simulation, Guangzhou 510275, China
* Correspondence: eeszsh@mail.sysu.edu.cn

Received: 28 December 2017; Accepted: 5 February 2018; Published: 10 February 2018

Abstract: Traditionally, static units of analysis such as administrative units are used when studying obesity. However, using these fixed contextual units ignores environmental influences experienced by individuals in areas beyond their residential neighborhood and may render the results unreliable. This problem has been articulated as the uncertain geographic context problem (UGCoP). This study investigates the UGCoP through exploring the relationships between the built environment and obesity based on individuals' activity space. First, a survey was conducted to collect individuals' daily activity and weight information in Guangzhou in January 2016. Then, the data were used to calculate and compare the values of several built environment variables based on seven activity space delineations, including home buffers, workplace buffers (WPB), fitness place buffers (FPB), the standard deviational ellipse at two standard deviations (SDE2), the weighted standard deviational ellipse at two standard deviations (WSDE2), the minimum convex polygon (MCP), and road network buffers (RNB). Lastly, we conducted comparative analysis and regression analysis based on different activity space measures. The results indicate that significant differences exist between variables obtained with different activity space delineations. Further, regression analyses show that the activity space delineations used in the analysis have a significant influence on the results concerning the relationships between the built environment and obesity. The study sheds light on the UGCoP in analyzing the relationships between obesity and the built environment.

Keywords: obesity; built environment; activity space; regression analysis; UGCoP

1. Introduction

Much health and geographic research has examined how the physical and social environment affects people's health. As a major risk factor for a series of health problems, including heart disease, stroke, cardiovascular disease, diabetes, sleep apnea, osteoarthritis, and some cancers, obesity has become a major public health concern worldwide [1,2]. Excessive energy intake and a lack of physical activity have been identified as major risk factor for obesity at the individual level [3]. In this context, disparities in obesity prevalence can be attributed to people's food environment and built environment. In past studies, the food environment is often regarded as part of the built environment. Recent extensive studies indicate that the built environment has a potential influence on obesity [4–7]. For instance, Li et al., examined the relationships between weight, and physical and social environments, using multi-level regression analysis based on social survey data [8]. Townshend and Lake investigated how the built environment influences physical activity and dietary behaviors [9].

The built environment is broadly defined as human-made facilities and infrastructure used to support human activity, including roads, public transportation, buildings, restaurants, supermarkets, and other amenities, which influence obesity-related behaviors [10,11]. Many studies have examined the relationships between the built environment and obesity [11–14]. However, a fundamental methodological issue in research on this relationship at the individual level remains: different delineations of geographic context may lead to different values of the contextual variables, and may thus influence the results concerning the relationships between the contextual variables and the health behavior or outcome being studied.

In most of the previous studies on obesity, the influence of the built environment on obesity was examined using geographic context based on people's residential neighborhoods or administrative units, such as census tracks or postcode areas. For instance, Frank et al. used a 1 km network distance buffer around each participant's place of residence to develop objective measures of land use mix, residential density, and street connectivity [15]. Statistical analysis was conducted to test the impacts of specific measures on obesity. The results indicated that land use mix has the strongest association with obesity. Rutt and Coleman examined the relationship between land use mix and body mass index (BMI), in which a 0.25-mile radius around each person's residence is defined as neighborhood, to assess transportation and other variables [16]. Eventually, a positive relationship was found between land use mix and BMI. Gordon-Larsen et al. investigated the availability of physical activity and recreational facilities in an 8.05 km (approximate 5 m) buffer area around each participant's residence [17]. The results indicated that increasing the availability of physical activity and recreational facilities is conducive to lower people's body weight at the population level. Some studies also employed administrative areas, like census units and postcode areas, to delineate neighborhood [4,7,18–20]. For example, Wen and Kowaleski-Jones explored the relationship between the built environment and obesity risk based on census tracts in the United States. The results indicate that attributes of the built environment significantly correlate with obesity risk [20]. Xu et al. examined the associations between built environment factors and individual odds of overweight and obesity at both zip code and county levels [7]. Cobb et al. examined the relationship between local food environments and obesity based on administrative units. The results indicate that density measures based on administrative units are more likely to find expected associations than buffers of less than one mile around individual addresses [21]. Sun et al. examined the influences of the built environment on individual BMI at the county level. It is found that population density and accessibility of facilities are positively related to individual BMI [22].

In summary, a common practice in previous studies has been to use static areas, such as census tracts, postcode areas, or buffer areas around people's residence as contextual units to study the relationship between the built environment and obesity. However, as several researchers in this area have argued in recent years [23–26], it is inappropriate to use the residential neighborhood or buffers around people's home location to represent the actual area that exerts contextual influences on people's health, since individuals move around in their daily life, and are thus exposed to other neighborhoods outside of their residential neighborhood. Thus, how to identify and delineate geographic units that capture individuals' daily activities and represent their true context is a fundamental challenge in health research on obesity. This challenge has been recently articulated as the uncertain geographic context problem (UGCoP), which is the problem that analytical results can be different for different delineations of contextual units, even if other factors are the same, due to the spatial and temporal uncertainty of the true geographic context [27,28]. Therefore, given that residential neighborhoods may mischaracterize built environment variables for different individuals, this paper seeks to advance our understanding of how different contextual units used to derive environmental variables may affect results in obesity research. It examines the uncertain geographic context problem through analyzing the relationship between the built environment and obesity. Individuals' residences, workplaces, and primary physical activity locations are simultaneously taken into account while constructing their activity spaces. The focus of this work is to delineate context units using different activity space measures and to examine the relationship between the corresponding built environment variables and obesity for individuals.

2. Contextual Uncertainties in Health Research

2.1. Neighborhood Effect on Obesity and Physical Activity

In the past 20 years or so, relations between health and place have been observed for a variety of health behaviors and outcomes at various spatial scales [24,29–34]. For instance, Cummins et al. identified several neighborhood features associated with fair to very bad self-rated health (independent of individual factors, such as gender, age, and social class), including poor quality of the physical residential environment, high unemployment, and lower access to private transport [35]. Arcury et al. showed the importance of geographic and spatial behavior factors in rural health care utilization [36]. Based on 40 studies that investigated the associations between neighborhood social environments and coronary heart disease (CHD), Chaix concluded that individuals in at least one population subgroup (e.g., gender, ethnicity) in neighborhoods with deprived socioeconomic positions have an increased coronary heart disease risk, even after controlling for individual-level factors [37]. To conclude, many neighborhood factors exert important contextual influence that directly or indirectly shape health behaviors and outcomes. These factors include physical features of the environment (e.g., walkability, green spaces), the availability and quality of food and other amenities (e.g., grocery stores, health services), the general attractiveness and perceived quality of the neighborhood (e.g., safety, crime), and the level of social organization and support of the local community [38].

Physical activity or obesity is one of the research focuses in health research. There is also considerable research to date that examines the relationship between neighborhood context and physical activity or obesity [39–43]. Many studies used neighborhood disadvantage as a proxy for exposure to, or availability of healthy food options [38]. For instance, Robert and Reither found that increased census tract level disadvantage is associated with higher body mass index (BMI) for women, after taking into account individual-level characteristics such as age, race, individual socioeconomic status (SES), and physical activity [44]. However, results for men indicate no association between BMI and either individual SES or community disadvantage. Using census blocks and block groups as neighborhoods, Boardman et al. found that neighborhoods characterized by high proportions of black residents have a greater prevalence of obesity than areas in which the majority of the residents are white [40]. The association between neighborhood racial composition and obesity, however, is completely attenuated after including statistical controls for the poverty rate and obesity prevalence of respondents' neighborhoods. Brown et al., observed no direct association between neighborhood type and BMI. However, household heads of single-family dwellings in neighborhoods where respondents made more utilitarian trips by walking or bicycling have lower BMI [45]. Black and Macinko reviewed 37 studies that examined neighborhood determinants of obesity and concluded that the influence of neighborhood-level factors appears mixed [38]. While these studies consistently found that decreased neighborhood-level economic and social resources are associated with high obesity rates, the associations between neighborhood income inequality and racial composition with obesity are mixed. The mixed results, as the authors argued, may be partly due to the different definitions of the neighborhood. For instance, neighborhoods in these studies have been variously delimited based on census tracts, zip code areas, socially and historically defined geographic areas, administrative units, metropolitan statistical areas, and counties. However, these definitions may not adequately operationalize the true geographic context which people are exposed to and interact with. While these studies used administrative areas as contextual units (largely due to the fact that available data on environmental variables are based on these areas), the authors of these studies emphasized that future studies need to provide better justification on how neighborhoods are defined, in order to improve study comparability and clarify the meaning of different neighborhood boundaries and measures. Specifically, the causally relevant contextual area for a particular individual might deviate significantly from any administrative unit. Various neighborhood definitions may lead to different built environment measures and further influence the final results. Therefore, it is necessary to define contextual areas based on the locations of individuals' daily activities, to take into account the influence of non-residential neighborhoods on their health behaviors or outcomes.

Similarly, in a study that also considered where subjects shop for groceries, Inagami et al. found that people have higher BMI if they reside in disadvantaged areas and in areas where the average person frequents grocery stores located in more disadvantaged neighborhoods [46]. The study observed that where people shop for groceries and distance traveled to grocery stores are independently associated with BMI. The authors suggested that exposure to grocery stores mediate and suppress the association of residential neighborhoods with BMI, and this may explain why previous studies did not find consistent associations between residential disadvantage and BMI: because they did not account for the shopping behavior of its residents. In a related study, Inagami et al. found that while residence in disadvantaged neighborhoods was associated with worse self-rated health, individuals with greater exposure to less disadvantaged non-residential neighborhoods in their daily activities have better self-rated health [47]. Both studies indicate that exposure to sociogeographic environments, besides where one lives, may modify the impact of the residential neighborhood on health in important ways. As the studies highlight, a person's activity space is not limited to the residential neighborhood, and it better represents the individual's environmental and social exposures that are crucial in influencing health outcomes. An important implication is that we need to look beyond the advantage or disadvantage of people's residential neighborhood (or home census tract) to take into account the advantage or disadvantage of other neighborhoods that may have an impact, either positive or negative, on their health behaviors or outcomes. In particular, instead of stressing that advantage or disadvantage in people's non-residential neighborhoods may affect their health, this paper emphasizes that people's activity places (which include both their residential and non-residential neighborhoods) may also influence their health.

2.2. Delineations of Neighborhood Units

As this discussion reveals, neighborhoods in past studies are delineated based on a variety of zones or administrative units, such as census tracts, census block groups, metropolitan statistical areas, or counties [37,38]. Berke et al., for instance, derived objective measures such as land use, land slope, vehicular traffic, and public transit data using neighborhoods delimited with 1 km or 3 km circular zones (buffers) around each respondent's home [39]. Frank et al., on the other hand, derived objective measures of urban form such as land use mix and residential density, based on neighborhoods delineated with a 1 km road network-based buffer around each participant's place of residence [48]. For Brownson et al., a neighborhood is defined as a half-mile radius or a 10 min walk from the respondent's home for some variables, and as a 10-mile radius or a 20 min drive from the respondent's home for several other variables [49].

A possible reason for the mixed results of past studies may thus be the different definitions of neighborhood they used [38]. In addition, these definitions may not adequately operationalize the space where people live and undertake their daily activities and travel. A presupposition of these studies is that the neighborhood of residence or a residence-based buffer area delimited by various means is the most relevant area affecting health behaviors and outcomes, and that neighborhood effects largely operate through interactions among residents of the same neighborhood unit. Another presupposition underlying these delimitations of neighborhood is that individuals who live in the same neighborhood experience the same level of contextual influences, regardless of where they actually live or where they undertake their daily activities and trips.

Health behaviors and outcomes, however, are related not only to variables derived based on the neighborhood of residence, but also to relevant factors and processes across neighborhoods [29].

The most important determinants of people's exposure to neighborhood effects or contextual influences are where and how much time they spend while engaged in their daily activities [25,37,50]. People's activities (and thus exposure to contextual influences) do not take place at one time point and wholly within any static, administrative neighborhood unit. Residential location is only one of the locations where people spend their time, and for most people, the residential neighborhood does not capture the majority of their activities or the locations of these activities [25]. The action space or activity space of individuals is not limited to the residential neighborhood, but may better represent an individual's environmental and social exposures that affect health behaviors and outcomes [46,47]. Further, exposure to contextual or socioeconomic influences besides where one lives may modify the impact of the residential neighborhood on health in important ways, rendering results among different studies inconsistent.

In light of this, important characteristics of people's use of and movement across space and time (known as activity space) should also be taken into account when examining the contextual determinants of health behaviors and outcomes [26,38]. These include (1) how much time people actually spend in their residential communities; (2) where else they go, how much time they spend there, and what activities they are involved in when they travel outside of their neighborhoods; (3) what types of areas other residents or peers travel to, and how prevalent and time-extensive these extra-community activities are; and (4) what types of non-residents regularly spend time within the borders of a given local area, and what activities they are engaged in while there [50].

This paper seeks to expand conventional notions of neighborhood effects in health research to a broader understanding of sociogeographic context that takes into account where people actually undertake their daily activities. This new concept of context is, in turn, based on the notion of activity space, which is the area containing all locations that an individual has direct contact as a result of his or her daily activities [51]. Because where and when people spend their time differs from individual to individual, the paper argues that this new notion of sociogeographic context will allow us to more accurately evaluate the role of various contextual influences on health behaviors and outcomes for each individual. Since an individual's activity space can be defined or delineated using different methods, it is important to examine how sociogeographic context, defined and operationalized differently, may influence the analytical results.

Specifically, this study compares the effects of contextual variables derived from seven different delineations of neighborhood: (1) an individual's home buffer; (2) an individual's workplace buffer; (3) an individual's fitness place buffer; (4) neighborhoods delimited using the standard deviational ellipse; and (5) neighborhoods delimited with the weighted standard deviational ellipse; (6) neighborhoods delimited with the minimum convex polygon; and (7) neighborhoods delimited with road network buffers. In this study, buffers based on an individual's home, workplace, and fitness place refer to areas around the person's home, workplace, and fitness place, generated using a specific buffer distance (note that all buffer radii are set to 1 km). Using these seven delineations of neighborhood units, the study moves beyond the neighborhood of residence, and considers the activities and trips that individuals undertake in their daily lives when evaluating people's exposure to contextual influences. To explore how different definitions of the neighborhood may affect neighborhood effects on health outcomes, the study evaluates the effect of socioeconomic advantage (or disadvantage), derived based on these seven delineations of the neighborhood, on people's body mass index (BMI).

3. Study Area and Data

The study area of this research is located within the city of Guangzhou, which is the capital of Guangdong Province in China and one of the country's major cities. The city had a population of approximately 12.7 million in 2010. Its total area is 7434.4 square kilometers. In this study, the peripheral zone outside the beltway in Guangzhou (as shown in Figure 1) is selected as the study area, which includes the central, transition, and marginal districts [52,53]. This area is chosen based on its history, location, and housing types (e.g., traditional self-built housing, welfare housing, *danwei* compounds, mixed residential areas, commercial housing, and urban villages). It includes seven urban districts: Liwan, Panyu, Tianhe, Haizhu, Huangpu, Baiyun, and Yuexiu.

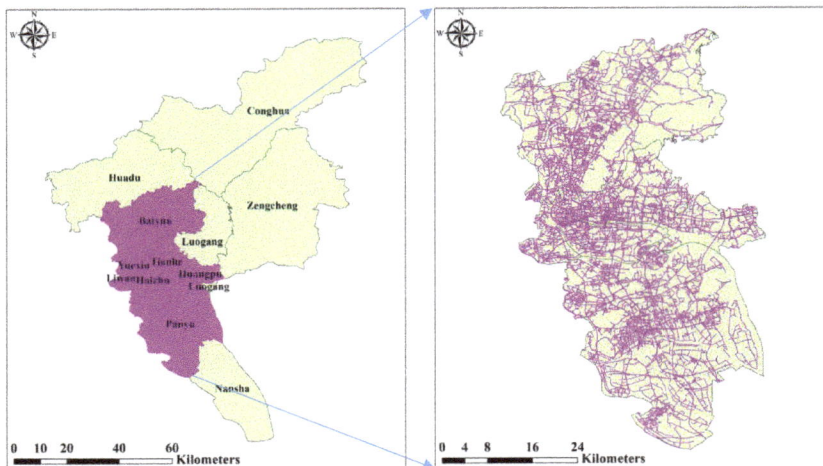

Figure 1. The administrative units of Guangzhou city and study area.

As the main urban areas in Guangzhou, these seven districts have different population density and resident income. For example, census data show that the population density of Yuexiu district is 33,920 per square kilometer, while the population density of Huangpu district is 1856 per square kilometer in 2015 the same year. Areas of higher population density tend to have a higher proportion of the population that use active transportation, as destinations in these areas are closer together and can often be reached by walking or bicycling [54]. More importantly, these highly urbanized districts often account for higher proportions of public facilities (e.g., schools, hospitals, and shopping malls) when compared to other areas such as suburbs. However, differences also exist among these districts. For instance, the main urban zones have approximately 80% of the large and medium-sized medical institutions in the city, of which 50% of the ministerial, provincial, and municipal medical institutions are located in Yuexiu district. These urban characteristics of the study area may affect the participants' physical activity and body weight. Geographic data of the study area, including road networks data and points of interest (POI) data in 2015, are used in the study to calculate the built environment variables.

4. Methods

This study seeks to examine how various built environment variables derived with different delineations of contextual areas affect their influence on people's body weight. It uses body weight (implemented with the body mass index) as the health outcome or dependent variable. It uses five built environment variables as the contextual influences or independent variables: residential density, land use mix, street density, fast food restaurants density, and transit stations density. Various delineations of contextual areas are implemented. These are the standard deviational ellipse (SDE), the weighted standard deviational ellipse (WSDE), the minimum convex polygon (MCP), the road network buffer (RNB), the workplace buffer (WPB), and the fitness place buffer (FPB), which are compared with the residential buffer (note that all buffer radii are set to 1 km). Through delineating individuals' contextual areas using various activity spaces, we examine how built environment variables derived with different activity spaces may influence the association between physical activity and body weight. Participants' weight status in this study is assessed by the body mass index (BMI), which is calculated based on height and weight of actual measurement provided in the survey data: BMI = weight(kg)/(height (m))^2. According to Flegal et al. [55], an adult of 20 years old or older, who has a BMI between 25.0 and 29.9, is considered overweight, and a BMI of 30 or higher is defined as obese.

4.1. Social Survey

The original individual-level data used in the study were collected from survey questionnaires based on a random sample of households in Guangzhou in January 2016. The survey sought to examine residential and employment change, as well as health and medical care of the city's residents. Information collected from the participants includes personal information (including weight and height), residential and employment change, personal fitness, lifestyle habits, health care, and community environment. Thirty-six communities in 11 neighborhoods with the size of approximately 1 km^2 were selected from all of the administrative districts in Guangzhou. The detailed selection process is described in the literature [53]. A total of 1029 returned questionnaires were valid and usable.

Note that the numbers of respondents' activity locations recorded in the survey are different. There are 1029 homes, 1011 workplaces, and 784 fitness places. In addition, the fitness places where moderate-to-vigorous physical activities were performed for several respondents are the same as their home location or their other recorded fitness locations. In this study, since constructing several activity space measures (e.g., standard deviational ellipse and minimum convex polygon) require three or more activity places, we only include the respondents whose residential, workplace, and fitness places are not the same place, to ensure that the possibility of deriving all activity space measures. Eventually, 403 respondents meet this condition and were included in the analysis.

Table 1 summarizes the socioeconomic characteristics of the participants, whose gender, age, education, income, and marital status are described. The proportions are closely balanced between men and women. More than 75% of the participants are under the age of 50, in which juveniles under 18 are excluded. The majority of the residents' level of education is high school or below. Income is divided into five levels, in which participants with income less than 15,000 Yuan account for 60%. Marriage is summarized as single, married, and divorced status, in which married status occupies the major proportion.

Table 1. Individual's socioeconomic characteristics.

Socioeconomic Variables		Number of Participants	Percentage
Gender (G)	Men	203	50.4%
	Women	200	49.6%
Age (A)	18–29	91	22.6%
	30–40	110	27.3%
	41–50	114	28.3%
	51–65	46	11.4%
	65+	42	10.4%
Education (E)	High school or below	165	40.9%
	Technical school	59	14.6%
	Junior college	103	25.6%
	College or high	76	18.9%
Income (I)	Less than ¥ 15,000	245	60.8%
	¥ 15,000 to less than ¥ 20,000	98	24.3%
	¥ 20,000 to less than ¥ 30,000	46	11.4%
	¥ 30,000 to less than ¥ 50,000	9	2.2%
	¥ 50,000 or more	5	1.3%
Marriage (M)	Single	78	19.4%
	Married	323	80.1%
	Divorced	2	0.5%

4.2. Built Environment Variables

As mentioned above, insufficient physical activity and excessive energy intake contributes to individual's excessive body weight and may lead to obesity. In this study, built environment variables are delineated based on these two aspects, namely, neighborhood walkability, and fast food outlets. Numerous studies have indicated that better walkability tends to associate with higher levels of physical activity, and easy access to fast food outlets usually enhance extra calorie intake. For instance, if individuals' residences are close to activity destinations, such as public transit stations or to areas with higher street density, they tend to undertake more walking or bicycling. Neighborhood walkability is often conceptualized via the three Ds: density, design, and diversity [4,56]. Density provides a large collection of people, which can be measured by population or residential density. Design and diversity are often measured by street density and mixed land use, respectively. Transit station density can be used to measure accessibility. In this paper, five built environment variables closely associated with individual's body weight are selected as the contextual variables: residential density, land use mix, street density, fast food restaurant density, and transit station density.

Residential density (RD) is commonly defined as the density of residences within an individual's 1 km home buffer [34,48]. Areas with greater residential density are normally considered more walkable than areas with lower residential density. In addition, if an area has a higher residential density, it is often more mixed and interconnected and more likely to promote physical activity [48]. In this study, RD is defined as the density of residences within a participant's activity space.

Land use mix (LUM) can be calculated using a variation of entropy index, where the proportion of land use types, including commercial, residential, office, and entertainment in an area, are taken into account [41,48,57]. In this study, the area is a participant's activity space. The values of land use mix range from 0 to 1, which measures how evenly the proportion of commercial, residential, office, and entertainment area is distributed within each area. The values 0 and 1 correspond to a single land use environment and one with the greatest land use heterogeneity, respectively. Previous studies have shown that physical activity can also be facilitated by higher land use mix, since it provides a variety of destinations within walking distance, such as restaurants, parks, and transit stations. Therefore, land use mix tends to encourage more walking. The formula for land use mix is shown as follows:

$$H = -1 \left(\sum_{i=1}^{n} p_i * \ln(p_i) \right) / \ln(n) \tag{1}$$

where H is the land use mix score, p_i is the proportion of land use i among all land use classes, and n is the number of land use types.

Street density (SD) is calculated as road or street length (in kilometer) divided by land area within 500 m and 1000 m buffers, which can be used to measure neighborhood design characteristics and reflect road network connectivity [58]. It has also been shown that street density is closely related to physical activity. Higher density of street networks and more densely-connected street networks represent shorter distances between destinations, which is conducive to walking trips [59]. In this study, we define street density (SD) as the total length of the street or road segments within a participant's activity space divided by the area of the activity space.

Fast food restaurant density (FFRD) is the number of fast food restaurants within a participant's activity space divided by the area of the activity space. Here, fast food restaurants are defined as food outlets that prepare and serve mass-produced food very quickly, and they include both Western and Chinese style fast food outlets. A growing number of studies indicated that food consumption tied to fast food restaurants is more likely to enhance higher caloric intake. FFRD reflects the accessibility of high-energy diets to a certain extent. If fast food restaurants are located near an individual's home, he/she tends to consume more high-energy meals. It has also been found that better access to fast food is closely associated with a higher likelihood of obesity [60].

Transit station density (TSD) refers to the number of transit stations per square kilometer in an area. In this study, this area is the area of a participant's activity space. As the primary mode of access to transit, walking is also closely related to transit station density, and more use of transit often corresponds to more walking when compared to driving. Past research indicates that participants in areas with high transit station density are more likely to use transit than those located within the same distance from transit stations in areas with low transit station density [61].

4.3. Delineating Individuals' Contextual Areas Using Activity Space

As discussed above, traditional contextual units, such as census tracts or postcode areas, may not accurately represent individuals' activity spaces, since they ignore individual's mobility, spatial habits, and travel environment [27,28,62]. In this study, activity space is used to delineate individuals' contextual units. It is the area within which an individual undertakes or travels to his/her actual daily activities [62,63]. Activity space can be expressed as a two-dimensional area that covers the spatial distribution of the locations an individual visited. Several factors determine the geometry, size, and structure of an individual's activity space. These include the home location, the location of the workplace, the locations of regular activities, and the daily movements between these locations and activities. Therefore, activity spaces are often delineated by many activity locations of an individual, or based on individual's actual travel trajectory when detailed movement data are available.

In this paper, the survey data mainly contain participants' three activity destinations: home, workplace, and a fitness place (the primary location where the participant undertakes physical activity). Note that while each participant may perform several physical activities, only the location for their primary physical activity (called the fitness place in this study) is included in this analysis. The activity space measures for this study are thus constructed based on these three places. Although the activity spaces delineated in this study may not fully represent the participants' actual activity spaces due to this data limitation, they are still more accurate when compared to conventional delineations of contextual units based only on the home or working place location, since they not only consider both of these locations but also take the primary location of physical activity into account.

Considering that different activity spaces may yield different results, this paper presents four different activity space delineations, including the standard deviational ellipse, the weighted standard deviational ellipse, the minimum convex polygon, and road network buffer. They are used to study the relationship between environmental variables and participants' BMI, and they are also compared with the results based on participant's home buffers, workplace buffers, and fitness place buffers.

4.3.1. The Standard Deviational Ellipse

The standard deviational ellipse (SDE) measures the spatial distribution of activity destinations and can be calculated using the CRIMESTAT spatial statistics package [64]. The long axis and short axis of the SDE correspond to the direction of maximum dispersion and minimum dispersion, respectively, among the points. The SDE has been used to measure individuals' travel behaviors in urban environments [63,65]. It has been implemented as one standard deviational ellipse (SDE1) and/or two standard deviational ellipse (SDE2), which cover approximately 68% and 95% of all activity points, respectively (if all points have equal weights). As shown in Figure 2a, activity space of a single respondent is represented with standard deviational ellipses, including SDE1 and SDE2.

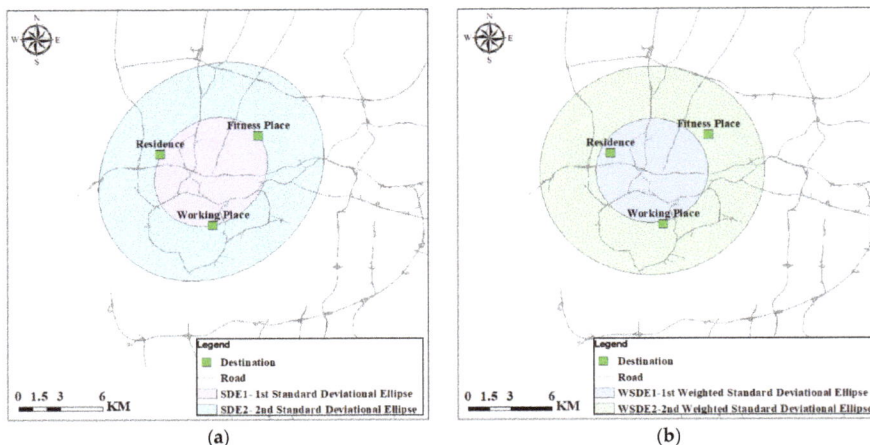

Figure 2. Examples of the standard deviational ellipse and weighted standard deviational ellipse. (**a**) Standard deviational ellipse; and (**b**) weighted standard deviational ellipse.

Generally speaking, the numbers of times per year an individual visits different destination are different. We further construct the weighted standard deviational ellipse based on visit frequencies in this study. Activity destinations are weighted based on the number of times per year the destinations are visited by the individual. Since the survey data only include the visit frequency of fitness places, the visited frequencies of home and workplace are set based on the following assumptions. The weighted value is set to 365 for the residence, assuming that individuals go home every day. Working places are weighted by the value 260 (5 times for 52 weeks), assuming that individuals work five times per week. For fitness place, weighted values are determined based on the data provided by participants in the survey. Here, we use the respondent in Figure 2a as an example to explicate the construction of weighted standard deviational ellipse (WSDE). The visit frequencies to the residence, workplace and fitness place are 365, 260, 208 respectively. The weighted standard deviational ellipse can be obtained on the basis of these frequencies, as displayed in Figure 2b. Considering that SDE1 just covers 68% of activity points and only three activity points are used to construct the standard deviational ellipse, several participants' activity space may not be constructed using SDE1. Therefore, this study selects SDE2 and WSDE2 to delineate activity space.

4.3.2. The Minimum Convex Polygon

The minimum convex polygon (MCP) is the smallest convex polygon that covers a set of points [63]. The MCP is straightforward to construct using ArcGIS 10.1 ArcToolbox, which can be used to identify the contexts related to individual's BMI. Since only three destinations are included in the survey, the MCPs constructed in this study are triangles. As shown in Figure 3, the activity space of a single respondent is represented by the MCP, which covers the respondent's residence, workplace, and fitness place.

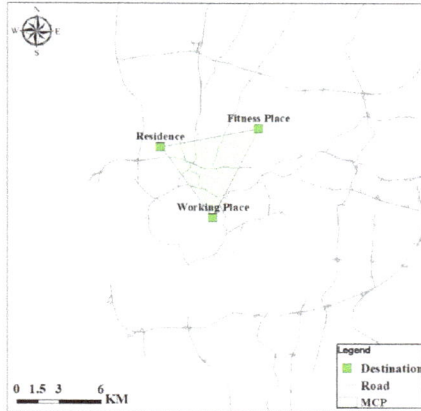

Figure 3. Example of the minimum convex polygon.

4.3.3. The Road Network Buffer

The road network buffer (RNB) is constructed based on the roads used by an individual to travel among the home, workplace, and other activity locations [62]. First, the shortest paths between respondents' residence and the other two destinations are calculated using the ArcGIS Network Analyst Extension. Then, a buffer is obtained around the shortest paths. However, two limitations exist in the construction of the RNB. The first limitation is that the quality of the RNB is closely related to the road network data. The second limitation is that the shortest paths between home and other destinations are not necessarily the respondent's actual routes. The selection of buffer size is also crucial for constructing the RNB. Previous studies indicated that 1 km buffers are appropriate [48,62]. In this paper, we also choose 1 km as the buffer size for constructing the RNB. Figure 4 displays the RNB for the same respondent in Figures 2 and 3. It indicates that the shape, area, and extent of RNB are different from SDE and MCP.

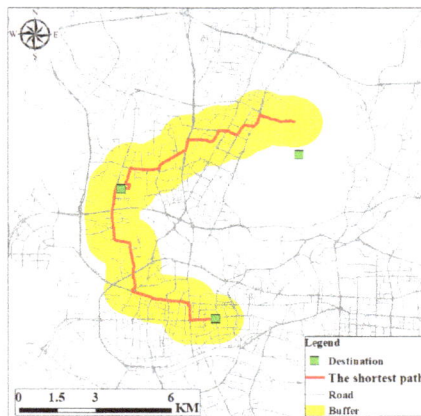

Figure 4. Example of road network buffer.

4.4. Statistical Analysis

The statistical analysis of different activity space measures has two main objectives. The first is to compare the contextual variables obtained with different activity space delineations in order to examine whether they are significantly different. A 1-km buffer area is created around each participant's home location. Paired sample *t*-tests are utilized to examine whether significant differences exist between activity space based contextual variables, and those obtained using the home buffers. Second, regression analysis is conducted using multivariate linear regression, which takes the built environment variables and individual variables as the independent variables, and BMI as the dependent variable. The purpose is to analyze the effect of environmental and sociodemographic variables on participants' BMI. Previous related studies also demonstrate that age has close associations with obesity [66]. The model is as follows:

$$\begin{aligned} BMI = \quad & \beta_0 + \beta_1 RD + \beta_2 LUM + \beta_3 SD + \beta_4 FFRD + \beta_5 TSD \\ & + \beta_6 G + \beta_7 A + \beta_8 E + \beta_9 I + \beta_{10} M + \varepsilon \end{aligned} \qquad (2)$$

The independent variables of the model are explained in Table 2.

Table 2. Explanations of the abbreviations for the independent variables.

Abbreviations	Independent Variables
RD	Residential density
LUM	Land use mix
SD	Street density
FFRD	Fast food restaurant density
TSD	Transit station density
G	Gender
A	Age
E	Education
I	Income
M	Marriage

5. Analysis

5.1. Comparative Analysis of Activity Space Measures

We compare the activity space measures with the home buffer, working place buffer, and fitness place buffer, respectively, with respect to two aspects: attributes of various delineations of activity space, and values of the contextual variables derived with them. First, areas of the activity space are compared in order to understand the differences between the measures (see Table 3). Since the buffer sizes of each respondent's home buffer are identical, the home buffers, workplace buffers, and fitness place buffers have the same mean, median, and maximum area (3.14 km^2). Among the various contextual areas, the home buffers, working place buffers, and fitness place buffers have the smallest mean area (3.14 km^2) and the smallest maximum area (3.14 km^2), while SDE2 has the largest mean area (43.96 km^2) and the largest maximum area (1135.75 km^2). The MCP has the smallest median area (1.38 km^2), while RNB has the largest median area (23.68 km^2). Compared with SDE2, WSDE2 has lower mean, median, and maximum area, respectively.

Table 3. Area of activity space measures.

Activity Space	Mean Area (km²)	Median Area (km²)	Maximum Area (km²)
Home Buffers	3.14	3.14	3.14
WPB	3.14	3.14	3.14
FPB	3.14	3.14	3.14
SDE2	43.96	13.18	1135.75
WSDE2	30.98	9.71	576.77
MCP	4.59	1.38	117.34
RNB	26.06	23.68	108.48

(Home Buffers = buffers around home; WPB = buffers around workplace; FPB = buffers around the fitness place; SDE2 = standard deviational ellipse at two standard deviations; WSDE2 = weighted standard deviational ellipse at two standard deviations; MCP = minimum convex polygon; RNB = road network buffer).

Further, we analyze the range, median, and interquartile range of the built environment variables based on different activity measures. Figure 5 shows the distribution of the environmental variables derived with different activity space delineations using boxplots. It indicates that the built environment measures have various distribution characteristics due to different shapes and sizes of the contextual areas. For instance, the values of RD derived with road network buffers have a range of 0–50, while those of WSDE2 have a range between 0 and 100.

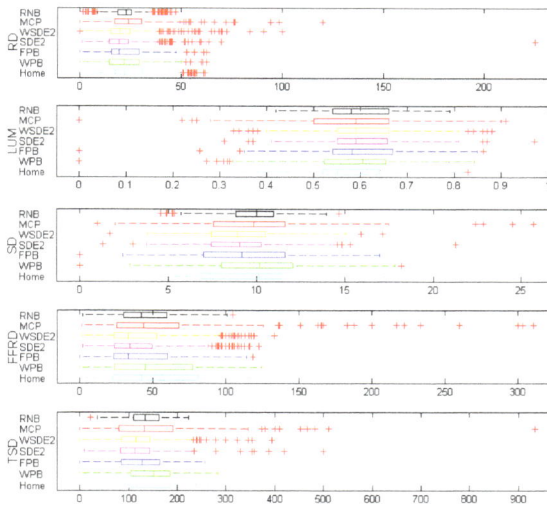

Figure 5. Distribution of normalized built environment measures. Boxes represent the interquartile range, whiskers represent the range of values, and crosses represent the outliers.

Next, we performed paired sample *t*-tests to examine whether significant differences are evident in the built environment variables obtained from different activity space delineations, and from the home buffers. Table 4 summarizes the significance of paired sample *t*-test for built environment variables between the activity space measures for the 403 participants. A significance level of 0.05 is used to judge whether two measures are significantly different. As shown in Table 4, significant differences exist for the built environment variables for most of the pairs of contextual areas. However, there are also several pairs of contextual areas with no significant differences for the built environment variables. For instance, there are no significant differences for residential density (RD) between measures derived with the following ten pairs of contextual areas: WPB and FPB, WPB and SDE2, WPB and WSDE2, WPB and RNB, FPB and SDE2, FPB and WSDE2, FPB and RNB, WSDE2 and SDE2, WSDE2 and RNB, and MCP and the home buffers. For land use mix (LUM), significant differences are non-existent between measures derived with WPB and home buffers, FPB and MCP, WSDE2 and SDE2. Significant differences are non-existent for street density (SD) between measures derived with the following five pairs of contextual areas: FPB and SDE2, FPB and WSDE2, WSDE2 and SDE2, MCP and RNB, and MCP and the home buffers. For fast food restaurant density (FFRD), significant differences exist for measures derived with the following five pairs of contextual areas: WPB and home buffers, FPB and RNB, WPB and MCP, WSDE2 and SDE2, and MCP and the home buffers. Lastly, significant differences exist for transit station density (TSD) between measures derived with the following six pairs of contextual areas: WPB and home buffers, WPB and MCP, FPB and SDE2, WSDE2 and SDE2, MCP and the home buffers, and RNB and the home buffers. In addition, all pairs of the built environment variables derived with WSDE2 and SDE2 have no significant difference. Four of the five built environment variables derived with MCP and the home buffers are not significantly different. These differences may affect research findings concerning the influence of environmental variables on people's BMI. We explore this possibility in what follows.

Table 4. Significance of paired sample *t*-test for built environment variables between the activity space measures.

		Home	WPB	FPB	SDE2	WSDE2	MCP	RNB
	Home		0.003 *	0.000 *	0.000 *	0.000 *	0.563	0.000 *
	WPB	0.003 *		0.767	0.208	0.869	0.000 *	0.302
	FPB	0.000 *	0.767		0.316	0.863	0.000 *	0.084
RD	SDE2	0.000 *	0.208	0.316		0.185	0.000 *	0.010 *
	WSDE2	0.000 *	0.869	0.863	0.185		0.000 *	0.146
	MCP	0.563	0.000 *	0.000 *	0.000 *	0.000 *		0.001 *
	RNB	0.000 *	0.302	0.084	0.010 *	0.146	0.001 *	
	Home		0.746	0.005 *	0.000 *	0.000 *	0.000 *	0.001 *
	WPB	0.746		0.041 *	0.001 *	0.002 *	0.008 *	0.025 *
	FPB	0.005 *	0.041 *		0.000 *	0.000 *	0.503	0.000 *
LUM	SDE2	0.000 *	0.001 *	0.000 *		0.396	0.000 *	0.002 *
	WSDE2	0.000 *	0.002 *	0.000 *	0.396		0.000 *	0.013 *
	MCP	0.000 *	0.008 *	0.503	0.000 *	0.000 *		0.000 *
	RNB	0.001 *	0.025 *	0.000 *	0.002 *	0.013 *	0.000 *	
	Home		0.003 *	0.000 *	0.000 *	0.000 *	0.447	0.025 *
	WPB	0.003 *		0.000 *	0.000 *	0.000 *	0.031 *	0.011 *
	FPB	0.000 *	0.000 *		0.822	0.794	0.000 *	0.000 *
SD	SDE2	0.000 *	0.000 *	0.822		0.930	0.000 *	0.000 *
	WSDE2	0.000 *	0.000 *	0.794	0.930		0.000 *	0.000 *
	MCP	0.447	0.031 *	0.000 *	0.000 *	0.000 *		0.421
	RNB	0.025 *	0.011 *	0.000 *	0.000 *	0.000 *	0.421	
	Home		0.974	0.001 *	0.000 *	0.000 *	0.171	0.000 *
	WPB	0.974		0.004 *	0.000 *	0.000 *	0.211	0.000 *
	FPB	0.001 *	0.004 *		0.001 *	0.009 *	0.000 *	0.442
FFRD	SDE2	0.000 *	0.000 *	0.001 *		0.064	0.000 *	0.000 *
	WSDE2	0.000 *	0.000 *	0.009 *	0.064		0.000 *	0.000 *
	MCP	0.171	0.211	0.000 *	0.000 *	0.000 *		0.000 *
	RNB	0.000 *	0.000 *	0.422	0.000 *	0.000 *	0.000 *	
	Home		0.262	0.000 *	0.000 *	0.000 *	0.201	0.073
	WPB	0.262		0.000 *	0.000 *	0.000 *	0.733	0.001 *
	FPB	0.000 *	0.000 *		0.094	0.019 *	0.000 *	0.000 *
TSD	SDE2	0.000 *	0.000 *	0.094		0.240	0.000 *	0.000 *
	WSDE2	0.000 *	0.000 *	0.019 *	0.240		0.000 *	0.000 *
	MCP	0.201	0.733	0.000 *	0.000 *	0.000 *		0.025 *
	RNB	0.073	0.001 *	0.000 *	0.000 *	0.000 *	0.025 *	

* Significance level at $p < 0.05$.

5.2. Regression Analysis of Obesity

In this section, regression analysis is conducted to explore how built environment variables derived with different contextual areas influence participants' BMI. In order to further demonstrate whether individuals' activity space influences the results, we also compare the regression analysis results based on the home buffers, WPB, and FPB with that of other activity space measures.

Table 5 summarizes the results of the regression analysis based on different activity space measures, including home buffers, WPB, FPB, SDE2, WSDE2, MCP, and RNB. Coefficients with an asterisk mean that the corresponding independent variables are significant in the regression models. The regression results indicate that the selection of activity space measures may influence which built environment variables have significant effects on obesity. On the one hand, different variables may be significant in models using variables derived with different contextual areas. For instance, significant built environment variables are street density, fast food restaurant density, and transit station density in the model using environmental variables derived with home buffers, while significant built environment variables for models that used variables derived with SDE2 and RNB are land use mix and transit station density, respectively. Built environment variables are not significant in the models that used variables based on WSDE2 and MCP. The regression coefficients reflect the relationships between the variables and participants' BMI. For the model that used environmental variables derived with home buffers, the coefficients of SD, FFRD, TSD (−0.183, 0.305, and −0.330) indicate that street density and transit station density are negatively associated with BMI, while fast food restaurant density is positively related with BMI.

Table 5. Results of multiple linear regression based on different activity space measures.

	Multiple Linear Regression Models						
	Home Buffer (R^2 = 0.218) Coefficient	WPB (R^2 = 0.178) Coefficient	FPB (R^2 = 0.184) Coefficient	SDE2 (R^2 = 0.183) Coefficient	WSDE2 (R^2 = 0.182) Coefficient	MCP (R^2 = 0.176) Coefficient	RNB (R^2 = 0.188) Coefficient
NRD	0.135	−0.026	0.155 *	−0.09	0.007	0.009	0.091
LUM	−0.07	−0.062	−0.002	0.123 *	0.088	0.07	−0.066
SD	−0.183 *	0.056	0.012	−0.032	−0.058	−0.034	0.002
FFRD	0.305 *	0.024	−0.127	0.069	0.053	0.021	0.238
TSD	−0.33 *	−0.082	0.005	−0.013	−0.02	0.014	−0.315 *
G	−0.06	−0.064	−0.061	−0.056	−0.063	−0.067	−0.079
A	0.301 *	0.233 *	0.272 *	0.269 *	0.268 *	0.258 *	0.264 *
E	−0.085	−0.112	−0.090	−0.101	−0.106	−0.096	−0.116
I	−0.152 *	−0.117 *	−0.136 *	−0.138 *	−0.147 *	−0.127 *	−0.141 *
M	0.107 *	0.145 *	0.138 *	0.128 *	0.128 *	0.129 *	0.131 *

* Coefficient significant at $p < 0.05$.

In contrast, the demographic variables of age, income, and marital status are significant for all the models. Further, their relationships with participants' BMI are consistent for all of the seven regression models. Higher income is associated with lower BMI, and being older and being married are associated with higher BMI. On the other hand, values of the adjusted R^2 are different for the regression models, as shown in Table 4. The different R^2 values represent the different explanatory power of these models. For instance, the adjusted R^2 (0.202) of the model that used variables derived with home buffers indicates the variables explain 20.2% of the variance of the dependent variable (BMI). We also calculate the variance inflation factor (VIF) values of each variable for all models, which are all far less than 10. This suggests that there is no multi-collinearity among the independent variables. In addition, we assess the significance of each regression model using the F test. The results indicate that all the models are significant at the 0.05 significant level. In other words, there is a significant linear relationship between the dependent variable and the independent variables.

6. Discussion

Overall, the research findings highlight the existence of the uncertain geographic context problem when examining the relationships between the built environment and obesity. In other words, whether an environmental variable has a significant influence on participants' BMI depends on the contextual areas used to derive it. The aim of this study is not to determine which activity space delineation should be used, but to apply the concept of activity space to illustrate the uncertain geographic context problem through analyzing the relationships between a set of built environment variables and obesity. After all, people are not fixed to a single location in their daily life, and it is inadequate to delineate their activity space with any fixed location [62]. The results indicate that the selection of activity space measures influence whether an environmental variable affects obesity. A few previous studies also demonstrated the effect of geographic context on health. For example, Boone-Heinonen et al. analyzed the impact of buffer sizes on moderate and vigorous physical activity (MVPA) and found that the measures within buffers with different radii had different relationships with MVPA [67]. James et al. studied the effects of buffer size and shape on associations between the built environment and people's energy balance, and demonstrated that the scale and shape of buffers influenced the results [59]. The results of these studies indicate the importance of the uncertain geographic context problem in health research and illustrate this problem by delineating geographic context using various activity spaces.

Our analysis examines the associations between built environment variables and obesity for different activity space measures. Although the coefficients of the built environment variables based on participants' home buffers are slightly higher than those based on other neighborhood or activity space delineations, it does not indicate that built environment variables based on home buffers are the best measures for analyzing the impact of the built environment on obesity. Specifically, the home buffers model is not suitable for delineating all the environmental variables. It is worth noting that since the environmental variables of street density (SD) and fast food restaurant density (FFRD) have a significant effect on participants' BMI for the home buffers model, but do not have a significant effect on participants' BMI for other activity space delineations. For instance, FPB and SDE2 are suitable to analyze the influence of residential density (RD) and land use mix (LUM) on obesity, respectively. The results support conclusions made by other related studies that perhaps there is no one "best" single measure for depicting people's activity space based on a small number of activity places [59,62,65,68]. For the higher coefficient of the home buffer model, it is possible that the residential neighborhood may be the most influential environment in which participants' daily activities are conducted, and much of their environmental exposures are experienced. For instance, high density of road network and bus stops around people's residences are more likely to encourage residents to give up traveling by motor vehicles. Besides, large numbers of fast food restaurants around people's residences may attract them to select fast food.

In addition, we also compare the effects of contextual variables derived from seven activity space measures, including home buffers, WPB, FPB, SDE2, WSDE2, MCP, and RNB. However, four of these measures, namely SDE2, WSDE2, MCP, and RNB, combine home, workplace, and fitness place into one large activity space, which may not be able to differentiate the activities that people undertake in these areas. The activity spaces based on each of these areas separately may facilitate us to compare the impact of the different built environments of different areas on people's health. The results from Tables 4 and 5 demonstrate that there are some significant differences in the relationships between built environment variables and obesity based on activity spaces that centered on one area, and on activity spaces that combined three areas (residence, workplace, and fitness place).

7. Conclusions

The objective of this study is to examine the uncertain geographic context problem when analyzing the associations between obesity and the built environment. The uncertain geographic context problem emphasizes that the impact of the precise geographic delineations of contextual units or the deviation of the contextual units from the actual geographic context on analytical results. However, previous studies mainly focused on analyzing the associations between obesity and built environment variables based on static geographic units [5,7,20]. Little attention has been paid to accurately capturing individuals' exposure to environmental influences when studying obesity. As far as we know, this study is one of the first to examine associations between obesity and built environment variables via delineating individuals' actual activity space.

Using survey and GIS data of Guangzhou, five built environment variables are computed: residential density, land use mix, street density, fast food restaurant density, and transit station density. These variables are derived using seven different contextual areas, including home buffers, WPB, CPB, SDE2, WSDE2, MCP, and RNB. In addition, sociodemographic variables such as gender, age, education, income, and marital status are included. Different activity space delineations are compared, and the results show that differences between activity space sizes are evident. In addition, we compare the built environment variables obtained with different activity space measures using paired sample *t*-tests. The test results indicate that significant differences exist between several activity space based built environment variables. On the other hand, we analyze associations between obesity and the built environment and individuals' sociodemographic variables based on different activity space measures using multivariate linear regression models. It is found that individuals' activity space delineations have a significant influence on analytical results. The relationships between obesity and the built environment are influenced by the contextual areas used to derive the environmental variables. Finally, it is noteworthy that age, income, and marital status play an important role in obesity in all models.

In conclusion, the UGCoP as a fundamental problem in health research calls for continuous concerns on its confounding effects and mitigation. The present study sheds light on the UGCoP in analyzing the relationships between obesity and the built environment. Nevertheless, two limitations of this research need to be acknowledged. First, only the home, workplace, and primary physical activity location for each participant are used to delineate individual activity space in this study due to data limitation. Using more complete activity–travel data of subjects (e.g., collected with GPS) may be helpful in more accurately representing participants' activity space. Second, previous studies indicate that demographic variables are important moderators of the relationships between obesity and environmental variables. This study only considers a small number of respondents' sociodemographic characteristics as control variables. Future research is warranted to investigate how other demographic variables may influence analytical results.

Acknowledgments: This research was supported by two grants from the National Natural Science Foundation of China (41522104 and 41529101) and a grant from the Natural Science Foundation of Guangdong Province, China (2017A030313228). In addition, Mei-Po Kwan was supported by a John Simon Guggenheim Memorial Foundation Fellowship.

Author Contributions: P.Z., M.-P.K. and S.Z. conceived and designed the experiments in this paper. P.Z. performed the experiments and wrote the paper with M.-P.K. together. S.Z. contributed to result analysis and revising the paper.

Conflicts of Interest: The authors declare no conflicts of interest.

References

1. Zhang, X.; Hua, L.; Holt, J.B. Modeling spatial accessibility to parks: A national study. *Int. J. Health Geogr.* **2011**, *10*, 1–14. [CrossRef] [PubMed]

2. Ahima, R.S.; Lazar, M.A. The health risk of obesity—Better metrics imperative. *Science* **2013**, *341*, 856–858. [CrossRef] [PubMed]

3. Lau, D.C.; Douketis, J.D.; Morrison, K.M.; Hramiak, I.M.; Sharma, A.M. 2006 Canadian clinical practice guidelines on the management and prevention of obesity in adults and children. *Can. Med. Assoc. J.* **2007**, *176*, 1–13. [CrossRef] [PubMed]

4. Yamada, I.; Brown, B.B.; Smith, K.R.; Zick, C.D.; Kowaleski-Jones, L.; Fan, J.X. Mixed Land Use and Obesity: An Empirical Comparison of Alternative Land Use Measures and Geographic Scales. *Prof. Geogr.* **2012**, *64*, 157–177. [CrossRef] [PubMed]

5. Wang, F.; Wen, M.; Xu, Y. Population-Adjusted Street Connectivity, Urbanicity and Risk of Obesity in the U.S. *Appl. Geogr.* **2013**, *41*, 1–14. [CrossRef] [PubMed]

6. Xu, Y.; Wang, L. GIS-based analysis of obesity and the built environment in the US. *Cartogr. Geogr. Inf. Sci.* **2014**, *42*, 9–21. [CrossRef]

7. Xu, Y.; Ming, W.; Wang, F. Multilevel built environment features and individual odds of overweight and obesity in Utah. *Appl. Geogr.* **2015**, *60*, 197–203. [CrossRef] [PubMed]

8. Li, Y.; Carter, W.M.; Robinson, L.E. Social environmental disparities on children's psychosocial stress, physical activity and weight status in Eastern Alabama counties. *Appl. Geogr.* **2016**, *76*, 106–114. [CrossRef]

9. Townshend, T.; Lake, A. Obesogenic environments: Current evidence of the built and food environments. *Perspect. Public Health* **2017**, *137*, 38–44. [CrossRef] [PubMed]

10. Davis, R.; Cook, D.; Cohen, L. A community resilience approach to reducing ethnic and racial disparities in health. *Am. J. Public Health* **2005**, *95*, 2168–2173. [CrossRef] [PubMed]

11. Xu, Y.; Wang, F. Built environment and obesity by urbanicity in the U.S. *Health Place* **2015**, *34*, 19–29. [CrossRef] [PubMed]

12. Feng, J.; Glass, T.A.; Curriero, F.C.; Stewart, W.F.; Schwartz, B.S. The built environment and obesity: A systematic review of the epidemiologic evidence. *Health Place* **2010**, *16*, 175–190. [CrossRef] [PubMed]

13. Durand, C.P.; Andalib, M.; Dunton, G.F.; Wolch, J.; Pentz, M.A. A systematic review of built environment factors related to physical activity and obesity risk: Implications for smart growth urban planning. *Obes. Rev.* **2011**, *12*, E173–E182. [CrossRef] [PubMed]

14. Ferdinand, A.O.; Sen, B.; Rahurkar, S.; Engler, S.; Menachemi, N. The relationship between built environments and physical activity: A systematic review. *Am. J. Public Health* **2012**, *102*, E7–E13. [CrossRef] [PubMed]

15. Frank, L.D.; Andresen, M.A.; Schmid, T.L. Obesity relationships with community design, physical activity, and time spent in cars. *Am. J. Prev. Med.* **2004**, *27*, 87–96. [CrossRef] [PubMed]

16. Rutt, C.D.; Coleman, K.J. Examining the relationships among built environment, physical activity, and body mass index in El Paso, TX. *Prev. Med.* **2005**, *40*, 831–841. [CrossRef] [PubMed]

17. Gordon-Larsen, P.; Nelson, M.C.; Page, P.; Popkin, B.M. Inequality in the built environment underlies key health disparities in physical activity and obesity. *Pediatrics* **2006**, *117*, 417–424. [CrossRef] [PubMed]

18. Smith, K.R.; Brown, B.B.; Yamada, I.; Kowaleski-Jones, L.; Zick, C.D.; Fan, J.X. Walkability and body mass index: Density, design, and new diversity measures. *Am. J. Prev. Med.* **2008**, *35*, 237–244. [CrossRef] [PubMed]

19. Zick, C.D.; Smith, K.R.; Fan, J.X.; Brown, B.B.; Yamada, I.; Kowaleski-Jones, L. Running to the store? The relationship between neighborhood environments and the risk of obesity. *Soc. Sci. Med.* **2009**, *69*, 1493–1500. [CrossRef] [PubMed]

20. Wen, M.; Kowaleski-Jones, L. The built environment and risk of obesity in the United States: Racial-ethnic disparities. *Health Place* **2012**, *18*, 1314–1322. [CrossRef] [PubMed]

21. Cobb, L.K.; Appel, L.J.; Franco, M.; Jones-Smith, J.C.; Nur, A.; Anderson, C.A. The relationship of the local food environment with obesity: A systematic review of methods, study quality, and results. *Obesity* **2015**, *23*, 1331–1344. [CrossRef] [PubMed]

22. Sun, B.; Yan, H.; Zhang, T. Built environmental impacts on individual mode choice and BMI: Evidence from China. *J. Transp. Geogr.* **2017**, *63*, 11–21. [CrossRef]

23. Cook, T.D. The case for studying multiple contexts simultaneously. *Addiction* **2003**, *98* (Suppl. 1), 151–155. [CrossRef] [PubMed]

24. Cummins, S. Commentary: Investigating neighbourhood effects on health—Avoiding the 'local trap'. *Int. J. Epidemiol.* **2007**, *36*, 355–357. [CrossRef] [PubMed]

25. Matthews, S.A. The salience of neighborhood: Some lessons from sociology. *Am. J. Prev. Med.* **2008**, *34*, 257–259. [CrossRef] [PubMed]

26. Kwan, M.-P. From place-based to people-based exposure measures. *Soc. Sci. Med.* **2009**, *69*, 1311–1313. [CrossRef] [PubMed]

27. Kwan, M.-P. The uncertain geographic context problem. *Ann. Assoc. Am. Geogr.* **2012**, *102*, 958–968. [CrossRef]

28. Kwan, M.-P. How GIS can help address the uncertain geographic context problem in social science research. *Ann. GIS* **2012**, *18*, 245–255. [CrossRef]

29. Bernard, P.; Charafeddine, R.; Frohlich, K.L.; Daniel, M.; Kestens, Y.; Potvin, L. Health inequalities and place: A theoretical conception of neighbourhood. *Soc. Sci. Med.* **2007**, *65*, 1839–1852. [CrossRef] [PubMed]

30. Jones, K.; Moon, G. Medical geography: Taking space seriously. *Prog. Hum. Geogr.* **1993**, *17*, 515–524. [CrossRef]

31. Kearns, R.A. Place and health: Towards a reformed medical geography. *Prof. Geogr.* **1993**, *45*, 139–147. [CrossRef]

32. Macintyre, S.; Ellaway, A. Ecological approaches: Rediscovering the role of the physical and social environment. *Soc. Epidemiol.* **2000**, *9*, 332–348.

33. Macintyre, S.; Ellaway, A.; Cummins, S. Place effects on health: How can we conceptualise, operationalise and measure them? *Soc. Sci. Med.* **2002**, *55*, 125–139. [CrossRef]

34. Sallis, J.F.; Cerin, E.; Conway, T.L.; Adams, M.A.; Frank, L.D.; Pratt, M.; Salvo, D.; Schipperijn, J.; Smith, G.; Cain, K.L.; et al. Physical activity in relation to urban environments in 14 cities worldwide: A cross-sectional study. *Lancet* **2016**, *387*, 2207–2217. [CrossRef]

35. Cummins, S.; Stafford, M.; Macintyre, S.; Marmot, M.; Ellaway, A. Neighbourhood environment and its association with self-rated health: Evidence from Scotland and England. *J. Epidemiol. Community Health* **2005**, *59*, 207–213. [CrossRef] [PubMed]

36. Arcury, T.A.; Gesler, W.M.; Preisser, J.S.; Sherman, J.; Spencer, J.; Perin, J. The effects of geography and spatial behavior on health care utilization among the residents of a rural region. *Health Serv. Res.* **2005**, *40*, 135–156. [CrossRef] [PubMed]

37. Chaix, B. Geographic life environments and coronary heart disease: A literature review, theoretical contributions, methodological updates, and a research agenda. *Public Health* **2009**, *30*, 81–105. [CrossRef] [PubMed]

38. Black, J.L.; Macinko, J. Neighborhoods and obesity. *Nutr. Rev.* **2008**, *66*, 2–20. [CrossRef] [PubMed]

39. Berke, E.M.; Koepsell, T.D.; Moudon, A.V.; Hoskins, R.E.; Larson, E.B. Association of the built environment with physical activity and obesity in older persons. *Am. J. Public Health* **2007**, *97*, 486–492. [CrossRef] [PubMed]

40. Boardman, J.D.; Saint Onge, J.M.; Rogers, R.G.; Denney, J.T. Race differentials in obesity: The impact of place. *J. Health Soc. Behav.* **2005**, *46*, 229–243. [CrossRef] [PubMed]

41. Frank, L.D.; Saelens, B.E.; Powell, K.E.; Chapman, J.E. Stepping toward Causation: Do Built Environments or Neighborhood and Travel Preferences Explain Physical Activity, Driving, and Obesity? *Soc. Sci. Med.* **2007**, *65*, 1898–1914. [CrossRef] [PubMed]

42. Grafova, I.B.; Freedman, V.A.; Kumar, R.; Rogowski, J. Neighborhoods and obesity in later life. *Am. J. Public Health* **2008**, *98*, 2065–2071. [CrossRef] [PubMed]

43. Rundle, A.; Field, S.; Park, Y.; Freeman, L.; Weiss, C.C.; Neckerman, K. Personal and neighborhood socioeconomic status and indices of neighborhood walk-ability predict body mass index in New York City. *Soc. Sci. Med.* **2008**, *67*, 1951–1958. [CrossRef] [PubMed]

44. Robert, S.A.; Reither, E.N. A multilevel analysis of race, community disadvantage, and body mass index among adults in the US. *Soc. Sci. Med.* **2004**, *59*, 2421–2434. [CrossRef] [PubMed]

45. Brown, A.L.; Khattak, A.J.; Rodriguez, D.A. Neighbourhood Types, Travel and Body Mass: A Study of New Urbanist and Suburban Neighbourhoods in the US. *Urban Stud.* **2008**, *45*, 963–988. [CrossRef]

46. Inagami, S.; Cohen, D.A.; Finch, B.K.; Asch, S.M. You are where you shop: Grocery store locations, weight, and neighborhoods. *Am. J. Prev. Med.* **2006**, *31*, 10–17. [CrossRef] [PubMed]

47. Inagami, S.; Cohen, D.A.; Finch, B.K. Non-residential neighborhood exposures suppress neighborhood effects on self-rated health. *Soc. Sci. Med.* **2007**, *65*, 1779–1791. [CrossRef] [PubMed]

48. Frank, L.D.; Schmid, T.L.; Sallis, J.F.; Chapman, J.; Saelens, B.E. Linking objectively measured physical activity with objectively measured urban form: Findings from SMARTRAQ. *Am. J. Prev. Med.* **2005**, *28*, 117–125. [CrossRef] [PubMed]

49. Brownson, R.C.; Chang, J.J.; Eyler, A.A.; Ainsworth, B.E.; Kirtland, K.A.; Saelens, B.E.; Sallis, J.F. Measuring the environment for friendliness toward physical activity: A comparison of the reliability of 3 questionnaires. *Am. J. Public Health* **2004**, *94*, 473–483. [CrossRef] [PubMed]

50. Kwan, M.P.; Peterson, R.D.; Browning, C.R.; Burrington, L.A.; Calder, C.A.; Krivo, L.J. Reconceptualizing sociogeographic context for the study of drug use, abuse, and addiction. In *Geography and Drug Addiction*; Springer: Dordrecht, the Netherlands, 2008; pp. 437–446.

51. Golledge, R.G.; Stimson, R.J. *Spatial Behavior: A Geographical Perspective*; Guilford: New York, NY, USA, 1997.

52. Zhou, S.; Liu, Y. The Situation and Transition of Jobs-housing Relocation in Guangzhou, China. *Acta Geogr. Sin.* **2010**, *65*, 191–201.

53. Zhou, S.; Deng, L.; Kwan, M.P.; Yan, R. Social and spatial differentiation of high and low income groups' out-of-home activities in Guangzhou, China. *Cities* **2015**, *45*, 81–90. [CrossRef]

54. Sallis, J.F.; Floyd, M.F.; Rodríguez, D.A.; Saelens, B.E. Role of built environments in physical activity, obesity, and cardiovascular disease. *Circulation* **2012**, *125*, 729–737. [CrossRef] [PubMed]

55. Flegal, K.M.; Carroll, M.D.; Ogden, C.L.; Curtin, L.R. Prevalence and Trends in Obesity among US Adults, 1999–2008. *J. Am. Med. Assoc.* **2010**, *303*, 235–241. [CrossRef] [PubMed]

56. Cervero, R.; Kockelman, K. Travel demand and the 3Ds: Density, diversity, and design. *Transp. Res. Part D* **1997**, *2*, 199–219. [CrossRef]

57. Christian, H.E.; Bull, F.C.; Middleton, N.J.; Knuiman, M.W.; Divitini, M.L.; Hooper, P.; Amarasinghe, A.; Giles-Corti, B. How important is the land use mix measure in understanding walking behaviour? Results from the RESIDE study. *Int. J. Behav. Nutr. Phys. Act.* **2011**, *8*, 69–72. [CrossRef] [PubMed]

58. Cervero, R.; Sarmiento, O.L.; Jacoby, E.; Gomez, L.F.; Neiman, A. Influences of built environments on walking and cycling: Lessons from Bogotá. *Int. J. Sustain. Transp.* **2009**, *3*, 203–226. [CrossRef]

59. James, P.; Berrigan, D.; Hart, J.E.; Hipp, J.A.; Hoehner, C.M.; Kerr, J.; Major, J.M.; Oka, M.; Laden, F. Effects of buffer size and shape on associations between the built environment and energy balance. *Health Place* **2014**, *27*, 162–170. [CrossRef] [PubMed]

60. Chen, X.; Kwan, M.P. Contextual uncertainties, human mobility, and perceived food environment: The uncertain geographic context problem in food access research. *Am. J. Public Health* **2015**, *105*, 1734–1737. [CrossRef] [PubMed]

61. Frank, L.D. Land Use and Transportation Interaction Implications on Public Health and Quality of Life. *J. Plan. Educ. Res.* **2000**, *20*, 6–22. [CrossRef]

62. Sherman, J.E.; Spencer, J.; Preisser, J.S.; Gesler, W.M.; Arcury, T.A. A suite of methods for representing activity space in a healthcare accessibility study. *Int. J. Health Geogr.* **2005**, *4*. [CrossRef] [PubMed]

63. Rainham, D.; Mcdowell, I.; Krewski, D.; Sawada, M. Conceptualizing the healthscape: Contributions of time geography, location technologies and spatial ecology to place and health research. *Soc. Sci. Med.* **2010**, *70*, 668–676. [CrossRef] [PubMed]

64. Levine, N. *CrimeStat III: A Spatial Statistics Program for the Analysis of Crime Incident Locations (Version 3.0)*; Ned Levine & Associates: Houston, TX, USA; National Institute of Justice: Washington, DC, USA, 2004.

65. Zenk, S.N.; Schulz, A.J.; Matthews, S.A.; Odoms-Young, A.; Wilbur, J.; Wegrzyn, L.; Gibbs, K.; Braunschweig, C.; Stokes, C. Activity space environment and dietary and physical activity behaviors: A pilot study. *Health Place* **2011**, *17*, 1150–1161. [CrossRef] [PubMed]

66. Ball, K.; Lamb, K.; Travaglini, N.; Ellaway, A. Street connectivity and obesity in Glasgow, Scotland: Impact of age, sex and socioeconomic position. *Health Place* **2012**, *18*, 1307–1313. [CrossRef] [PubMed]

67. Boone-Heinonen, J.; Popkin, B.M.; Song, Y.; Gordon-Larsen, P. What neighborhood area captures built environment features related to adolescent physical activity? *Health Place* **2010**, *16*, 1280–1286. [CrossRef] [PubMed]

68. Boruff, B.J.; Nathan, A.; Nijënstein, S. Using GPS technology to (re)-examine operational definitions of 'neighbourhood' in place-based health research. *Int. J. Health Geogr.* **2012**, *11*. [CrossRef] [PubMed]

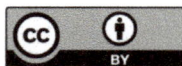

International Journal of
*Environmental Research
and Public Health*

MDPI

Article

Using Individual GPS Trajectories to Explore Foodscape Exposure: A Case Study in Beijing Metropolitan Area

Qiujun Wei, Jiangfeng She *, Shuhua Zhang and Jinsong Ma

Jiangsu Provincial Key Laboratory of Geographic Information Science and Technology,
School of Geographic and Oceanographic Sciences, Nanjing University, Nanjing 210023, China;
qiujun@smail.nju.edu.cn (Q.W.); zhangshuhua11@mails.ucas.ac.cn (S.Z.); majs@nju.edu.cn (J.M.)
* Correspondence: gisjf@nju.edu.cn; Tel.: +86-25-8968-1296

Received: 13 January 2018; Accepted: 25 February 2018; Published: 27 February 2018

Abstract: With the growing interest in studying the characteristics of people's access to the food environment and its influence upon individual health, there has been a focus on assessing individual food exposure based on GPS trajectories. However, existing studies have largely focused on the overall activity space using short-period trajectories, which ignores the complexity of human movements and the heterogeneity of the spaces that are experienced by the individual over daily life schedules. In this study, we propose a novel framework to extract the exposure areas consisting of the localized activity spaces around daily life centers and non-motorized commuting routes from long-term GPS trajectories. The newly proposed framework is individual-specific and can incorporate the internal heterogeneity of individual activities (spatial extent, stay duration, and timing) in different places as well as the dynamics of the context. A pilot study of the GeoLife dataset suggests that there are significant variations in the magnitude as well as the composition of the food environment in different parts of the individual exposure area, and residential environment is not representative of the overall foodscape exposure.

Keywords: foodscape exposure; activity space; commuting route; space-time kernel density estimation; time-weighted exposure; Beijing

1. Introduction

The relationship between the built environment and individual health has long been of interest to the public and researchers [1]. Within nutritional and epidemiological research, substantial focus has been placed on uncovering the spatial inequalities of the food environment ("foodscape") and measuring their effects on personal health outcomes as well as eating behaviors such as obesity, body weight, body mass index (BMI), and food consumption [2–6]. Historically, most studies characterized the food environment solely based on the residential neighborhood including administrative units and residence-based buffers [7]. Such choices were primarily due to the availability of censuses and surveys data that can be easily used to estimate the population health [8]. However, the spatial extent of a neighborhood was individual-specific, and the artificially designated neighborhood often failed to coincide with the observations [9,10]. Indeed, people are not bound to their neighborhoods: they move around to perform their routine activities and may encounter different types and levels of resources in their activity locations [11].

The popularity of location-aware devices, geo-sensor networks, and web-based mapping tools enables us to objectively collect detailed data on human movement, which is a favorable step towards the refined assessment of environmental exposure accounting for daily mobility [12]. Recently, a growing body of studies have used GPS-based travel surveys to measure the food exposure and have made great progress in re-examining the effects of non-residential contexts in foodscape exposure [13–15]. For example, Christian et al. (2012) compared neighborhood-based food exposure with activity-based food exposure and found that 83.4% of the participants encountered very different food environment in their daily travels compared with the residential neighborhoods [16]. Conventionally, the majority of the current literature have generally used the short-termed GPS data and adopted the overall activity space—the subset of all the locations within which an individual has direct contact as a result of his or her day-to-day activities—to conceptualize the environment experienced by the individuals [17]. They employed exhaustive GPS logging points and generated a uniform geospatial boundary in the form of standard deviation ellipse (SDE), daily path area (DPA), kernel density surface or minimum convex polygon (MCP) to represent the exposure area [18–20]. However, this approach has some limitations.

The widely-used overall activity space ignores the internal heterogeneity of its component places and the complexity of daily movement [21,22]. Basically, human activities are multi-centered [23]. The daily life centers (also termed anchor points) are usually composed of the places where people organize their daily activities (e.g., home) and to which people are relatively obligated to go (e.g., workplace) [24]. Each anchor point serves an aspect of daily life for the individual (e.g., dwelling, working, schooling, and recreation) and in turn the activities around these places have different spatial patterns and temporal rhythms such as the spatial extent people move around, the activity duration and the timing of these activities, which are very relevant to quantify the individual exposure [8]. Nevertheless, the uniform spatial delimitation of the overall activity space usually involves a considerable part of unexperienced areas that the participant rarely visits and would indirectly give rise to the overestimation of individual exposure [25]. Moreover, this uncertainty is particularly evident in the short-period GPS studies, wherein the observation window of a few days could hardly capture the relevant geographic contexts that an individual encounter and may import some occasional travels in this period [26,27]. To address this issue, a promising solution is to differentiate GPS data based on the characteristics of the activities practiced at different places and reconstruct the multiple contexts from the long-term GPS data [28]. Despite the advance in theory, little progress has been made in practice to incorporate the spatial extent and temporal patterns of the individual activities into the foodscape exposure assessment in a multi-context environment from GPS data [29].

The overall activity space also ignores the heterogeneity of the transportation modes of individual commuting behavior [30]. To date, numerous GPS-based studies have simply utilized all the traveling paths to model the exposure areas and failed to account for the transportation modes [20,31,32]. However, people within high-speed vehicles or underground transport tend to isolate themselves from the outside environment, and therefore have less opportunity to access food outlets without the vehicle stopping and them getting out [30]. To this end, it will be more reasonable for researchers to investigate the individual foodscape exposure along the commuting journeys based on the non-motorized trips rather than the entire paths [24,30].

In this paper, we proposed investigating individual foodscape exposure from the long-term GPS trajectories using a novel framework to incorporate the localized activity spaces around the daily life centers (residence, workplace and other major places) and non-motorized commuting routes across these places (Figure 2). To address this issue, we first integrated the density-based spatial clustering of applications with noise (DBSCAN) and the space-time kernel density estimation (ST-KDE) to identify clusters of frequently visited places [33,34]. A supervised machine-learning method, namely, the stochastic gradient descent (SGD) classification, was later used to extract the non-motorized segments [35]. Then, the clusters of frequently visited places and non-motorized commuting routes were used to construct the exposure areas. Finally, a case study in the Beijing metropolitan area was conducted to explore the characteristics of food environment exposure around the residence, workplace, other major places, and along the commuting journeys from a long-time perspective.

2. Study Dataset

The study area consisted of the urban area and three suburb districts with dense residential communities or industrial parks (Huilongguan, Dongxiaokou and Yizhuang) in Beijing, with an area over 1473 km^2 (Figure 1). The GPS dataset was part of the GeoLife project by Microsoft Research Asia (MSRA) in Beijing [36]. The preliminary dataset contained 17,621 GPS trajectories collected by 182 volunteers from a period of over five years (from April 2007 to August 2012). In the data collection program, a great portion of participants ($n = 107$) remained living in the study area, while some of the others only stayed in Beijing for a few months and then migrated from/to other cities later. The GPS loggers used in the project were handheld GPS receivers including Magellan Explorist 210/300, G-Rays 2 and QSTARZ BTQ-1000P. In general, the sampling rate of the GPS loggers was two seconds and the positioning accuracy was more than three meters. In this dataset, a GPS trajectory was a time-stamped sequence of GPS points $p_i = (x_i, y_i, t_i)$, where x_i, y_i and t_i represented the latitude, longitude and time-stamp, respectively. Typically, each trajectory recorded one complete trip of individual movement in the outdoor space, such as going to work, going home or leisure activities, and a considerable part of the trajectories were annotated with transportation modes by the participants (9813 tracks from 73 users).

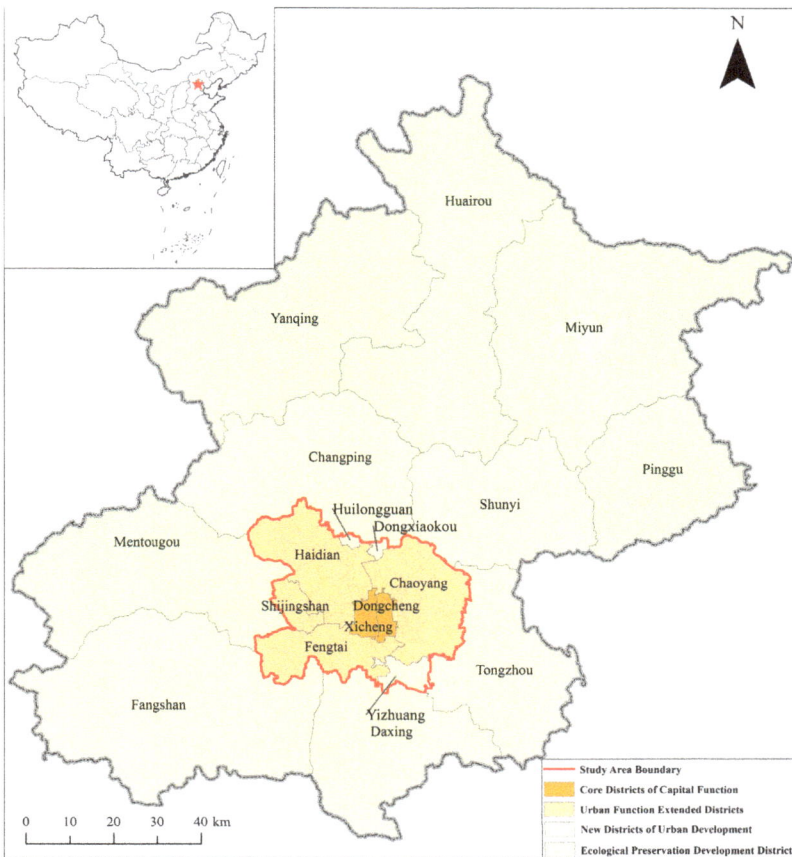

Figure 1. The study area consists of the urban area and three suburb districts with dense residential communities or industrial parks (Huilongguan, Dongxiaokou, and Yizhuang).

The points of interest (POIs) dataset were obtained from the AutoNavi Map, a Chinese navigation and location-based service provider. The dataset was collected in 2012 and was the only POI data available to us, which contained various types (22 groups, 728 classes) of POIs, such as the commercial facilities, hospitals, schools, and residential communities in Beijing. After online validations of the POIs, we classified the food services into five categories for exposure estimation, namely, convenience stores, fast food outlets, supermarkets, restaurants, and vegetable and fruit stores based on the Standard Industrial Code (SIC). Furthermore, the road and public transport datasets were supplied from the Beijing Municipal Commission of Transportation [37].

3. Methodology

As shown in Figure 2, the proposed framework was composed of four phases, namely, the data pre-processing phase, significant places extraction phase, non-motorized commuting paths extraction, and exposure area construction phase.

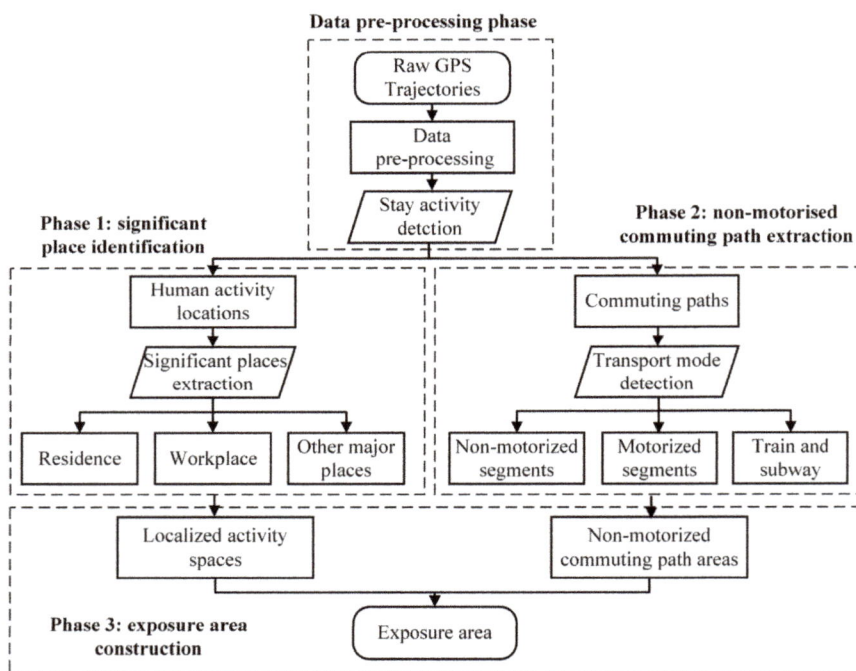

Figure 2. The methodology flowchart.

3.1. Identification of Significant Places

Several criteria were developed to reduce the spatial drift and data insufficiency in the pre-processing stage. GPS trajectories or points that satisfied the following criteria were removed: (1) GPS points further than 500 m from their consecutive points; (2) GPS trajectories with less than one minutes traveling time; and, (3) GPS points located outside the study area.

3.1.1. Step 1: Extraction of Activity Locations

As a single GPS point has no semantic information, we first extracted human activity from the GPS trajectories, which was defined as a meaningful location where people spent their time [38].

As illustrated in Figure 3, two situations should be considered to extract human activities: one case was that an individual roamed around a geospatial region for a certain period like visiting a park; and the other situation was that a user stayed at a fixed location exceeding a time threshold, like entering a building [39]. Furthermore, it should be noted that for the latter case, there were some random movements in the GPS records due to the inaccuracy of the GPS loggers even if the participant did not move [40]. Therefore, a human activity could be detected if the sub-trajectory from point p_m to point p_n satisfied the following constraints:

$$Dist(p_m, p_n) < D_{max} \text{ \&\& } Td(p_m, p_n) > T_{min} \tag{1}$$

where $Dist(p_m, p_n)$ refers to the Euclidean distance between p_m and p_n. $Td(p_m, p_n)$ refers to the timespan of the sub-trajectory. D_{max} and T_{min} are the two tuning parameters corresponding to the spatial range and dwelling time, respectively. In this study, we followed previous studies to use a distance threshold of 200 m and a time threshold of 20 min [41,42]. The centroid of the sub-trajectory—interpreted as a human activity—was used to represent the activity location [41]. In addition, the origins and destinations (ODs) of travels over one hour were also obtained due to their significance in mining individual activity patterns. As the individual stay activities are not bound to the street, in this stage, we did not match the activity locations to the street network.

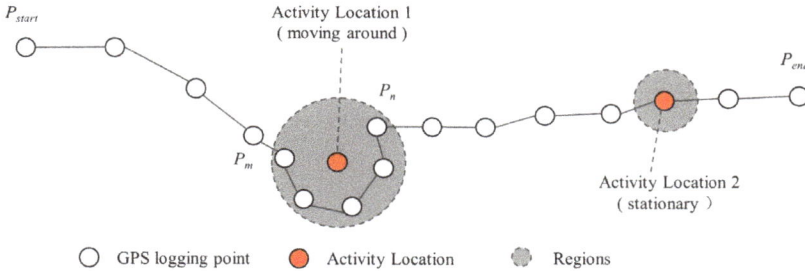

Figure 3. Extracting activity locations from GPS trajectory.

3.1.2. Step 2: Detection of Significant Place Candidates

In the next step, ST-KDE was integrated with DBSCAN to identify individual significant places according to the space-time proximity of the activity locations. By extending two-dimensional (2D) kernel density estimation to the three-dimensional (3D) form that accounts for time dimension, ST-KDE provides an efficient way to interpret the space-time patterns of point events and lifts our ability to reveal the spatio-temporal hotspots [43]. In this study, the input was the activity locations obtained in Step 1, and the output was a raster volume where each space-time cube $C(x, y, t)$ was assigned a density estimation. For each cube, the space-time density $\hat{f}(x, y, t)$ was estimated using the following formula:

$$\hat{f}(x, y, t) = \frac{1}{n b_s^2 b_t} \sum_{i=1}^{n} k_s \left(\frac{x - x_i}{h_s}, \frac{y - y_i}{h_s} \right) k_t \left(\frac{t - t_i}{h_t} \right) \tag{2}$$

where n is the number of the activity locations. h_s and h_t are the spatial and temporal bandwidths, respectively. k_s and k_t are the space and time kernel functions to determine the weight of point $P_i(x_i, y_i, t_i)$ according to its space-time distance to the cube centroid $P(x, y, t)$. In particular, the Epanecknikov kernel was utilized as a result of its good fitness to geographic phenomenon [44]. The space-time K-function algorithm proposed by Delmelle et al. (2011) was adopted to find the optimal bandwidths, and a pair of bandwidth (200 m, 1 day) was applied [45]. Figure 4a shows an example of ST-KDE cube based on user #065's activity locations.

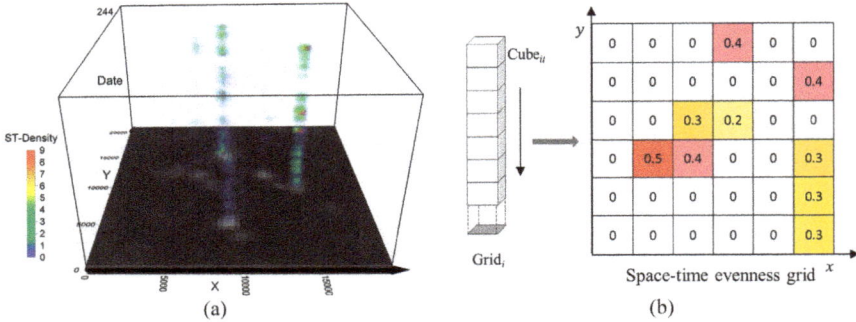

Figure 4. (**a**) An example of space-time kernel density estimation (ST-KDE) cube based on activity locations of #user 065. The base of the cube was the cumulative density by summing space-time density on each layer together. (**b**) Schematic diagram of compressing the space-time density cube into the space-time evenness grid.

To identify significant places from the long-term GPS dataset, we proposed a space-time evenness index (STEI) to measure the spatio-temporal dispersion of the activity locations by compressing the human activity intensities into a continuous surface (Figure 4b). For each cell $Grid_i$, we got the STEI value by calculating the coefficient of variation (CV) of all of the space-time density with the same spatial base. The formulas are:

$$\overline{STD_i} = \frac{\sum_{t=1}^{T} STD_{it}}{T} \tag{3}$$

$$\delta_i = \sqrt{\frac{\sum_{t=1}^{T} \left(\overline{STD_i} - STD_{it}\right)^2}{T}} \tag{4}$$

$$STEI_i = \frac{\delta_i}{\overline{STD_i}} \tag{5}$$

where $\overline{STD_i}$ refers to the mean of cumulative space-time density on $Grid_i$ within the observed period T, and STD_{it} refers to the space-time density for $Cube_i$ on day t. $STEI_i$ refers to the variation of activity intensity on $Grid_i$, whereas the small value of STEI indicated an even temporal distribution of day-to-day activities, and a large value of STEI appeared when there existed only explosive visits in a short period of time. Therefore, the indicator could be employed to approximately detect the significant places from a long-time perspective. As the output of STEI was raster-based, which may give rise to the inaccuracy in detecting the significant place candidates, the hotspot areas were first extracted from the STEI surface and DBSCAN was further used to incorporate the evidence from space, as well as refining the spatial precision. Finally, the activity clusters intersected with or bounded by the hotspot areas in the space-time evenness surface were considered as the candidates of significant places. Figure 5 shows an example of the identification of significant places by combining the space-time evenness grid with the clustering result.

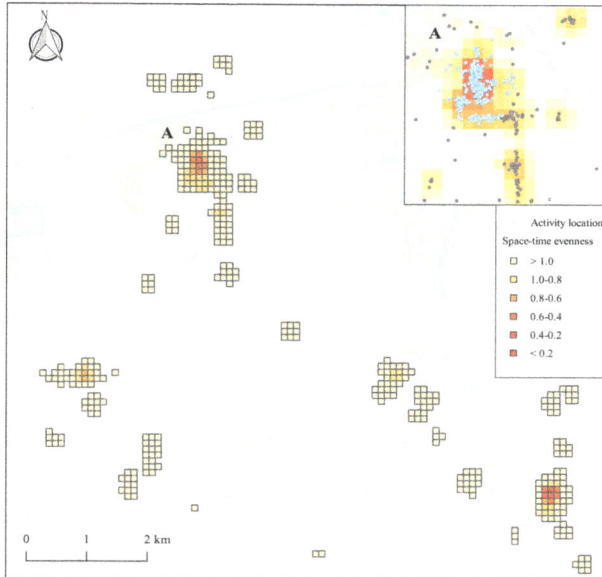

Figure 5. An example of space-time evenness grids. The dark color suggests uniform activity distribution across time and light color means intermittent occurrence of activities. Cluster A is a candidate of significant places.

3.1.3. Step 3: Labeling of Significant Places

To label the significant place candidates with semantic tags (e.g., residence and workplace), we first ranked the candidates of significant places by the frequency of reoccurrence and stay duration, then the use of places across the day were compared. The place where the individual spent the night (8:00 p.m.–6:00 a.m.) in most cases was marked as the residence and the workplace was identified when activities in a particular region demonstrated a dense distribution in working/school hours (8:00 a.m.–12:00 a.m. and 2:00 p.m.–6:00 p.m.) [46–48]. In short-period GPS studies, this method may introduce theoretically possible issues of people who work nightshift or those who had strong social ties to stay overnight with other families or friends [49]. To resolve the former issue, we compared the candidate of residences and workplaces with related POIs. For the latter issue, our method was based on the evidence from long-period observations and could filter out places that the participant had visited sparsely. Theoretically, some participants may spend most of their nighttime at others for a long period. In that case, these places played the role of home and were regarded as the residences. The candidate places except for the residences and workplaces were matched to the POIs dataset to determine their attributes, and these places were collectively termed as other major places.

3.2. Extraction of Non-Motorized Routes

GPS trajectories across the significant places were split into segments to extract the non-motorized commuting routes. Typically, a new segment was created if the time difference between two consecutive points was greater than five minutes [50]. To detect the transportation modes, the support vector machine (SVM) classification, which is a common approach to infer transportation modes from raw GPS trajectories, was adopted [51]. In this study, a linear kernel was chosen as the basis for the hyperplanes due to its short training time and feature transformation computation simplicity [52,53]. The SGD classifier, an efficient implementation based on a linear SVM, was then used to extract the non-motorized segments [35]. For each segment, four kinds of features, namely, speed, bearing change, distance, and duration were employed to construct the classifier [54]. The feature extraction of speed and bearing change was based on the cumulative statistics of the constituent GPS points rather than the features of the segment as the mean, minimum and maximum of these variables fail to reflect the actual distribution in many cases [49]. For instance, to obtain the speed features, a cumulative histogram was created to record the speed distributions (cumulative speed and the amount of time spent at them) and the speed where the cumulative value surpassed 10% to 90% of time were extracted.

To train the classifier, the user-annotated transportation modes were aggregated into four categories: airplane, train, motorized mode and non-motorized mode based on the similarity of the movement features. The train label included data marked as the train and subway. The motorized mode was a combination of taxi, bus, and car. The non-motorized mode was composed of walk, run and bike. To validate the accuracy of the classification, one half of the annotated segments were randomly selected as the training samples and the others were used as the validation data. The results showed that the classification precision of non-motorized trips was up to 93%, which was a quite high value when compared with similar studies and could meet the study requirements [55]. Once the classifier was validated, we used it to classify the remaining dataset. Some post-processing steps were further employed to adjust the isolated segments surrounded by tracks labeled with different transportation modes and merge adjacent segments with the same transportation mode. Moreover, the motorized and non-motorized commuting paths across the significant places were matched to the road network using Graphhopper, respectively.

3.3. Construction of Exposure Area

Before describing the construction method of the exposure area, we have to define the localized activity spaces and the non-motorized path areas that are mentioned in this paper. In light of the overall activity space, the localized activity spaces (residential space, workspace and other major spaces) were defined as "the subset of locations visited by an individual over a given period, corresponding to her/his exhaustive spatial footprint around the anchor points (residence, workplace and other major places)". This definition has been implicitly proposed by Chaix et al. (2012) to assess individual mobility patterns [24]. The non-motorized path areas were defined as "the subset of locations with which individuals have direct contact as the result of day-to-day non-motorized commuting behaviors" with reference to the daily (potential) path area [20,56].

To model the localized activity spaces, three kinds of geometry were created based on the notion of activity space and home range, such as network-based street buffer (NSB), SDE, and MCP [57]. NSB were created using the three most widely-used radii (200 m, 500 m and 1000 m) around the anchor points [58]. SDE and MCP were generated entirely based on the distribution of the activity location clusters marked as the residences, workplaces, and other major places. To determine a proper geographic representation for localized activity spaces, we evaluated the representativeness of these definitions in terms of the ability to capture clustered activities, the ability to filter out unclustered activities and the geometric area. Results indicated that MCP was superior to NSB and SDE in characterizing individual activities in the local scale (see Table S1 and Figure S1 in Supplementary Materials) and was used in later analysis. Furthermore, a 50 m buffer was further employed for the non-motorized trips to represent the participants' exposure area along their commuting routes, as it could capture the food outlets that were accessible along the street [32]. The exposure area is composed of the residential space, workspace, other major spaces, and the non-motorized commuting path areas. Each part of the exposure area (e.g., residential space) has its spatio-temporal characteristics, such as the spatial extent, duration, and timing of individual activities.

3.4. Food Environmental Exposure Evaluation

To evaluate the foodscape exposure, the count of food outlets, the Physical Food Environment Indicator (PFEI) [59] and the diversity of average densities index (DADI) [60] were adopted to evaluate individual exposure to the food environment. PFEI is defined as the proportion of fast-food restaurants, convenience stores and small food stores (merged into convenience stores in this study) to all outlets in a certain region [59]. As fast-food restaurants and convenience stores are commonly classified as unhealthy (less healthy) outlets, PFEI reflects the healthiness of local food environment [61]. The value of the PFEI ranges from 0 to 1 and the higher the PFEI, the less healthy the food environment. The DADI is defined in the entropy form and is often used to calculate the diversity of local food services:

$$DADI = -\sum_{i=1}^{n} p_i \times \frac{ln(p_i)}{ln(n)} \tag{6}$$

where n is the number of the food store categories in the area. p_i refers to the ratio of the i-th category food outlets. The value of DADI ranges from 0 to 1, where a higher level of the DADI indicated a more diverse foodscape.

To incorporate the temporal dimension into the food exposure assessment, a time-weighted contextual measure was introduced based on the stay duration an individual spent in multiple contexts (residential spaces, workspaces, other major spaces and the commuting path areas) [62]. The following formula was used to derive the time-weighted exposure measures:

$$TWE_i = \sum_{j=1}^{n} D_{ij} \times W_j \tag{7}$$

where TWE_i is the aggregated exposure to food services of the *i*-th category in multiple contexts. D_{ij} refers to the count of food outlets of the *i*-th category in the *j*-th place. W_j refers to the time weight for the *j*-th place, which is calculated as the ratio of the stay duration in the *j*-th place to the average stay duration in multiple contexts. Note that the time weight was determined strictly based on evidence from the entire observation, rather than a fragmentary period or empirical assumptions. The temporal constraints of food acquisition were further taken into account by matching the timing of individual activities and the opening hours of the food outlets. Only food outlets in their operating time when the individual activities took place were included in the assessment of food exposure.

4. Results

4.1. Description of the Study Sample

As shown in Table 1, the study samples (*n* = 107) were composed of full-time employees, government staff, college students and research fellows [36,41]. Young people were the main GPS data contributors and the average age of the participants was 24. The majority were between 22 and 30 years old, accounting for 75% of study samples, and people younger than 22 and older than 30 contributed 16% and 9% of the data, respectively. The participants were gender balanced and their education background ranged from undergraduate students to PhD holders.

As shown in Figure 6, most of the participants' localized activity spaces were distributed in the northern part of Beijing, especially in the area that is encompassed by the North 2nd Ring Road and North 5th Ring Road. Moreover, there were evident separations between the spatial distributions of different types of localized activity spaces. The residential spaces distributed dispersedly and the majority were situated in the outer zones (outside the 3rd Ring Road). A considerable number of participants had their residential spaces located in the new districts of urban development. In contrast, the workspaces were mainly aggregated in the industrial parks and office zones such as Zhongguancun and Yizhuang. Furthermore, the places where the individual regularly visited besides working and living were either close to their residences or workplaces, and a small part of isolated places arose at the commercial centers, like the Beijing Central Business District (Guomao), Wangjing and Sanlitun. These findings were consistent with related studies [41].

Table 1. Descriptive statistics of sample characteristics ($n = 107$).

Characteristic	Percentage	n
Age		
$\geq$30	9%	10
26–29	30%	32
22–25	45%	48
$\leq$22	16%	17
Gender		
Male	54%	58
Female	46%	49
Career		
MSRA employees	18%	19
Employees of other companies	14%	15
Government staff	10%	11
College students and Researchers	58%	62

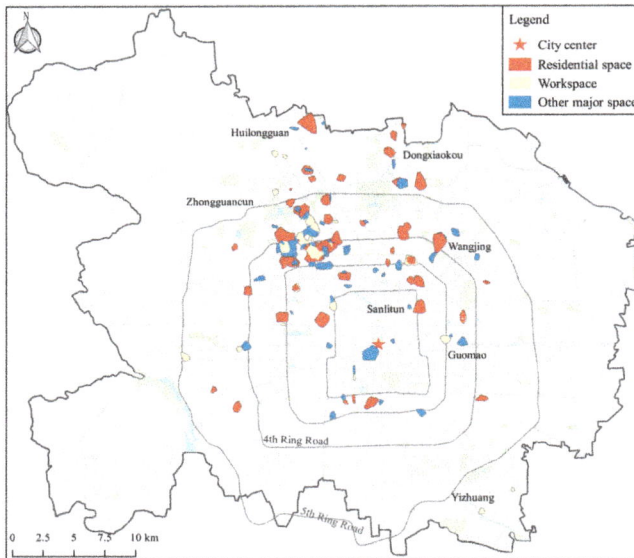

Figure 6. The aggregated distribution of the participants' localized activity spaces ($n = 107$).

4.2. Analysis of Foodscape Exposure in Multiple Context

Table 2 shows the characteristics of the food outlet numbers among each part the exposure areas. In general, there were significant differences among the magnitude of food exposure in the residential spaces, workspaces, other major spaces, and the commuting path areas. The number of all the food outlets along the commuting routes (147.5) was 93% higher than that of the residence spaces (76.3), and the food outlet numbers in workspaces (54.0) and other major spaces (41.5) were lower than that of the residence spaces at percentages of 29% and 46%, respectively. This tendency was also tenable when taking the categories of food outlets into consideration. However, the gap of foodscape exposure among the localized activity spaces varied by food outlet types. For example, the greatest variations of food outlets numbers that the participants were exposed to around their homes and workplaces were found in restaurants and fast food outlets. As for the commuting routes and residential space, convenience stores, and vegetable and fruit stores dominated the differences.

Table 2. Descriptive statistics of food outlets counts in residential space, workspaces, other major spaces, and commuting path areas ($n = 107$).

Category		RS	WS	Difference at WS	OMS	Difference at OMS	DPA [a]	Difference at DPA [a]
All outlets	Mean (SD)	76.3 (139.2)	54.0 (53.1)	−29% *	41.5 (47.3)	−46% *	147.5 (372.9)	+93%
	Range	292	282		245		379	
Convenience stores	Mean (SD)	6.5 (10.7)	5.2 (5.3)	−21% *	3.8 (3.9)	−42% *	15.3 (43.8)	+136% *
	Range	74	24		20		159	
Fast food outlets	Mean (SD)	14.9 (29.9)	10.4 (11.5)	−30%	7.5 (9.9)	−50%	25.2 (62.4)	+69%
	Range	116	65		67		114	
Supermarket	Mean (SD)	2.9 (5.0)	2.6 (2.4)	−19%	2.3 (2.6)	−30% *	5.2 (13.1)	+80% *
	Range	29	9		12		73	
Restaurants	Mean (SD)	43.0 (75.6)	29.5 (28.6)	−32%	22.9 (26.3)	−47%	82.9 (208.0)	+93%
	Range	198	139		131		427	
Vegetable and fruit stores	Mean (SD)	9.0 (20.9)	6.7 (8.2)	−25% *	5.0 (7.0)	−44% *	18.9 (48.6)	+110% *
	Range	41	45		32		104	

Note: * Significant difference (ANOVA, $p < 0.05$) between the food outlets numbers in residential space and other localized activity spaces. [a] Food exposure of DPA were defined as the sum of food outlets counted along the non-motorized commuting path areas. Abbreviations: RS-residential space, WS-workspace, OMS-other major space, DPA-non-motorized commuting path area.

Figure 7 shows the variations of PFEI, DADI, and the percentage of food outlet numbers in different spaces. On average, the lowest level of PFEI was found in the residential spaces and the commuting path areas (0.14), indicating that the participants encountered the healthiest foodscape around home and along the commuting paths, except the few participants who lived near the 2nd Ring Road. When compared with the residential spaces and the commuting path areas, the workspaces had a greater level of PFEI (0.16) and the largest PFEI was observed in other major spaces (0.21).

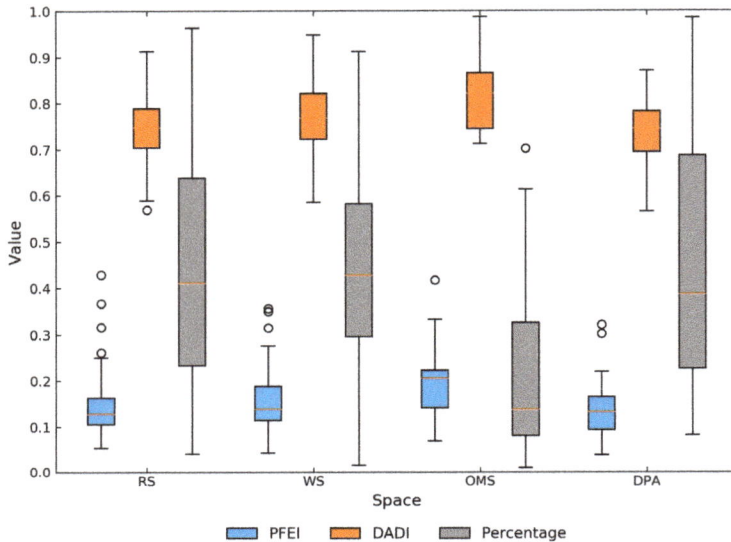

Figure 7. The PFEI, DADI, and Percentage of food outlet numbers in different spaces. (Abbreviations: RS-residential space, WS-workspace, OMS-other major space, DPA-non-motorized commuting path area).

In addition, the diversity of the food environment in different spaces demonstrated similar patterns with PFEI: the largest DADI was found in other major spaces (0.82), followed by the workspaces (0.77), commuting path areas (0.75), and residential spaces (0.74). Furthermore, the percentage of food outlets in different parts of the exposure area demonstrated a broad range of variations (0.2–0.7), suggesting that there were great variations in the contribution of food exposure in different spaces. However, on the whole, the commuting path areas, residential spaces and workplaces made up the largest part of the foodscape in the participants' daily life, and the ratio of food outlets in other major spaces was quite small.

Table 3 shows the correlation coefficients of food outlet numbers in the residential spaces related with the workspaces, other major spaces and commuting areas, using the Spearman-Rank analysis method. No significant correlations of food exposure between these places were observed, except for the convenience stores in the residential spaces and workspaces, where the relationship was weak (0.33). This result indicated that the foodscape in the residential spaces could hardly characterize the overall environment.

Table 3. Correlation of food outlet counts in residential space (RS), workspace (WS), other major space (OMS), and the non-motorized commuting path area (DPA) (*n* = 107).

Food Outlet Type	RS × WS	RS × OMS	RS × DPA
Convenience stores	−0.02	0.33 **	0.10
Fast food outlets	0.10	0.09	0.01
Supermarket	−0.10	0.21	0.08
Restaurants	0.11	0.04	−0.04
Vegetable & fruit stores	−0.10	−0.05	−0.05
All food outlets	0.06	0.07	−0.02

Note: ** $p < 0.01$.

4.3. Analysis of Overall Foodscape Exposure

Figure 8 shows the time distribution of individual daily activities in different spaces. There were three activity peaks in the residential spaces during the day, namely, 7:00 a.m.–9:00 a.m., 12:00 p.m.–1:00 p.m., and 5:00 p.m.–8:00 p.m. Additionally, a less activity peak was found near midnight (10:00 p.m.–1:00 a.m.), which implied that the participants were more likely to interact with the food outlets around the residences during these periods. The workspace shared similar activity patterns with the residential space, but its magnitude was relatively smaller, except during rush hours (8:00 a.m.–10:00 a.m.). The leisure activities were flourishing during the valley period of home and work-related activities (10:00 a.m.–11:00 a.m. and 4:00 p.m.–5:00 p.m.).

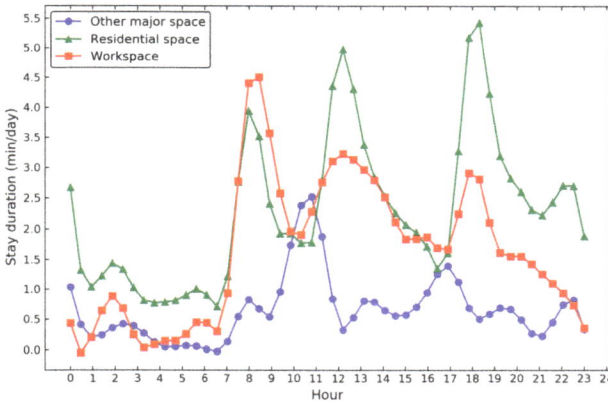

Figure 8. The timing of daily activities and average stay duration in different spaces per day (*n* = 107).

Figure 9 shows the average food outlets numbers of the overall foodscape exposure. The classic exposure, or Classic-E, was the average of the food outlets numbers in the residential spaces, workspaces, other major spaces and non-motorized commuting path areas for each of the participants. The time-weighted exposure, or TW-E, was calculated as the cumulative sum of the product of the food outlets numbers in each space and the proportion of stay duration. The time-weighted exposure with temporal constraint, or TWE-TC, was the extension of TW-E by incorporating the timing of the activities and the opening hours of nearby food outlets.

On average, the participants were exposed to 6.19 convenience stores, 11.75 fast food outlets, 2.49 supermarkets, 35.98 restaurants, and 7.99 vegetable and fruit stores in the spatial dimension. Taking the stay duration and temporal constraints into consideration, the number of food outlets changed disproportionately. A typical case was the supermarkets and restaurants based on the criteria of TW-E and TWE-TC, the number of restaurants declined from 56.60 to 44.17 when we matched the timing of individual activities and the opening status of restaurants the participants went by, whereas the number of supermarkets barely changed.

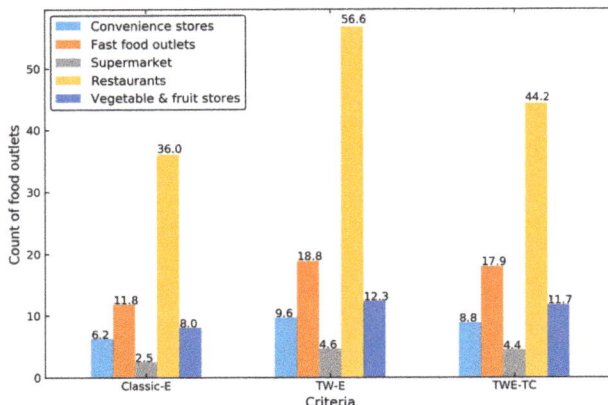

Figure 9. Average food outlet counts of the overall foodscape using Classic-E, TW-E, and TWE-TC, stratified by food outlet types.

Figure 10 shows the density curves of the food outlets numbers in the overall environment by type, based on TWE-TC. The majority of the participants were exposed to a small number of supermarkets, convenience stores, vegetable and fruit stores, and the overall exposure to over 16 outlets of these types was rare. When compared with other kinds of food outlets, the restaurant distribution was broader and shifted to the right, indicating that there were great variations in the number of accessible restaurants among the participants. On the other hand, although numerous participants held wide-range exposure areas that contained a considerable number of food outlets that seemed to be accessible, the majority only witnessed a few food outlets when taking the stay duration and temporal constraints into consideration (Figure 6).

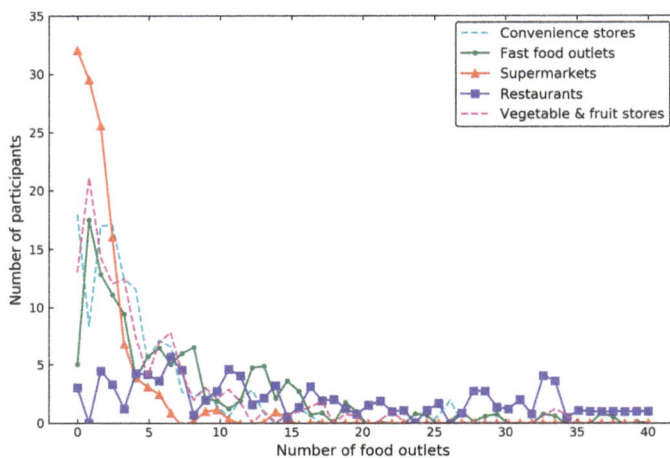

Figure 10. The overall food outlet distributions by food outlet types based on TWE-TC.

5. Discussion

5.1. Main Findings

As the pilot study showed, there were considerable variations in the magnitude of food outlets between the residential environment (residential space) and the non-residential environment (workspace, other major spaces and the commuting path areas) from the perspective of space (Table 2). When compared with non-residential context, the residential environment only contributed a small part to the overall foodscape exposure, more specifically, the food outlets numbers in the residential space were even smaller than that along the non-motorized commuting routes. In addition, the composition of the food outlets varied by spaces (Figure 7). In general, the percentage of fast food restaurants and convenience stores was the lowest in the residential space and the non-motorized commuting path areas. Other major spaces encountered the highest ratio of these two kind food outlets, followed by the workspace. Similar patterns were also found in the diversity of food outlets. Nevertheless, the quantity of food outlets in the residential space and other non-residential areas were poorly correlated. These findings indicated that the foodscape exposure was heterogeneous in different spaces and the foodscape exposure in the residential environment could hardly represent the overall foodscape that people encountered while engaged in their routine activities [7,11]. Perhaps this could explain why neighborhood effects based on the residences were often weak and even insignificant [63]. A different finding from prior neighborhood-based literature was the difference of the quantity of food outlets between the residence and workplace, where the number of food outlets in the workspace was greater than that in the residential space [64,65]. This was partly because the participants' localized activity spaces were individual-specific and the size of workspaces was smaller than that of the residential spaces in many cases (see Table S2 in Supplementary Materials), while in the literature, the same sized neighborhoods were assigned to the home and workplace [8].

The variations of foodscape exposure in different spaces may be related to the jobs-housing separations in the area [66]. The demographic census in 2013 showed that 51.1% of the resident population in Beijing were gathered outside the 5th Ring Road, whereas 70% of the residents were employed inside the 4th Ring Road [67]. Similar patterns were found here: as shown in Figure 6, numerous participants lived in the outer areas and worked in core areas. Additionally, the structure of foodscape in these places varied greatly. For example, other major spaces where the participants conducted their leisure activities were mainly distributed in the major business centers of the city and the commercial streets, so that the variety of the food outlets and the proportion of fast food restaurants were comparatively higher. In contrast, the residential spaces were mainly located near the residential communities and the proportion of fast food restaurants was smaller. Moreover, the jobs-housing separations gave rise to the long-distance commuting journeys and indirectly provided the opportunity for individuals to interact with the foodscape outside their residences and workplaces.

Taking stay duration and temporal constraints into consideration, most of the participants were exposed to only a small number of food outlets during their routine activities. Restaurants were the main difference in the overall foodscape exposure in the study sample. Although the participants encountered a larger number of food outlets along the commuting routes, the commuting time was shorter when compared with their stay durations in the residential spaces and workspaces, so that their contribution decreased correspondingly (see Table S2 in Supplementary Materials). These findings suggested that relying solely on the spatial dimension would likely lead to the mischaracterization of the overall foodscape exposure and therefore attenuated the associations between exposures and health outcomes [22]. In addition, when incorporating the timing of individual activities and the operating hours of the food services, the number of food outlets that were accessible changed disproportionately by type. On average, the number of restaurants and vegetable and fruit stores decreased by 22% and 8%, respectively, while the number of supermarkets only declined by 4%. This phenomenon was probably related to the way of the individual life and the regularity of the business. For example, if a full-time worker started off early in the morning and returned home late in the evening, he/she might need to purchase food on the way to work or home. In this period, many restaurants did not operate (especially for those that did not provide breakfast or closed early in the evening), whilst most supermarkets were open, thereby shaping the foodscape dynamically.

5.2. Strengths and Limitations

One major highlight of the proposed framework was that the proposed exposure area could capture the non-residential environment experienced by the individuals during their daily movement. The size of the exposure area was individual-specific and was determined by the distribution of individual daily activities. This differs from conventional place-based methods where the exposure area was mostly defined as a static neighborhood [7]. In this study, the proposed framework constructed the exposure area by integrating the local activity spaces (e.g., residential spaces and workspaces) and the commuting path areas. Furthermore, the commuting path areas were created entirely based on non-motorized commuting routes rather than the entire trips that involved a mix of transportation modes. This is a step toward the refinement of measuring the foodscape exposure and may potentially reduce the uncertainty of modeling the interaction between the individual and the food environment along the commuting paths [28].

Another strength of the proposed framework was that it enabled us to incorporate the space-time heterogeneity (spatial extent, stay duration, and timing) of individual behaviors in different spaces and the dynamics of the surrounding food environment. This is particularly important as the contextual exposure varies by places and time, whilst individual activities around different daily life centers (e.g., home and workplace) had various space-time patterns (Figure 8). Moreover, the adoption of long-term GPS data was superior to the short-period data in understanding the persistence of human activity patterns over time, and helped to differentiate the significant places visited at a high frequency and journeys from those that were rarely visited. This is a further exploration on addressing the uncertain geographic context problem (UGCoP) caused by the overall activity space, where the frequency, duration and temporality of individual daily activities were overlooked [27,68].

There were, however, several limitations in this study that can be attributed to the data quality and study design. First of all, the proposed method was procedure-oriented, and in some phases, parameters were needed (e.g., the space-time thresholds to define a human activity, the parameter to define activity clusters and the distance to define the commuting path areas). Although there have been numerous approaches specializing in the parameter selections that can be inferred to, simple combinations of these methods designed for different purposes may not always find the appropriate parameters, which would more or less bring about uncertainty in the construction of the exposure area.

Secondly, the adoption of stay duration in measuring multiple contexts of food exposure also needs reconsideration. Although the use of time-weighted exposure measure was commonsense in environmental studies, using the cumulative sum of food outlets numbers multiplied by the time-weight to measure the overall exposure remains to be verified [62]. More studies to further our understanding of the relationship between cumulative foodscape exposure and the stay duration are expected.

Another limitation to this study was related to the data quality of the dataset. The small samples limited the power to reveal the differences of foodscape among different spaces, and the restricted demographic scopes of the sample limited the generalizability of the findings. For example, due to the clustering of the participants in space, overlaps of the residential spaces and workspaces were found in the study sample, and therefore raised concerns about the spatial autocorrelations. The introduction of geographically weighted regression and spatial econometric approaches may resolve this issue. Nevertheless, as the POI dataset in 2012 was the only data accessible, information about the food outlets (e.g., operating status and opening hours) were not in step with individual activities timely. All of these issues should be considered in the next step.

6. Conclusions

This study explored the use of long-term GPS data in investigating individual foodscape exposure. To derive the exposure area, a novel framework based on the space-time proximity of individual physical activities was proposed to extract the localized activity spaces around daily life centers and the non-motorized commuting routes. When compared with conventional methods, the newly proposed exposure areas were individual-specific and could incorporate the internal heterogeneity of individual activities (spatial extent, stay duration, and timing) and the dynamic of the context. The pilot study in Beijing suggested that there were significant variations in the magnitude as well as the composition of food outlets in the exposure area, and the cumulative foodscape exposure far outweighed the food exposure that experienced by the individual in the residential space alone. Furthermore, restaurants were the main differences of the overall foodscape exposure among the participants. In the future, we will improve the robustness of the proposed method and implement our framework into a dynamic model for more researchers to use. Spatio-temporal clustering and other classification methods will be involved in processing the long-term GPS datasets. In addition, if data are available, much deeper research will be conducted to reveal the relationship between public health and the foodscape exposure accounting for the internal heterogeneity of individual movements and the temporal dynamics of the food environment.

Supplementary Materials: The following are available in the http://www.mdpi.com/1660-4601/15/3/405/s1. Figure S1: Results of different representation methods of localized activity spaces. Table S1: A summary evaluation of representativeness of the localized activity spaces. Table S2: Spatial extent, average stay duration, and frequency of stay activities around the anchor places and along the commuting routes (n = 107).

Acknowledgments: This research was supported by the National Natural Science Foundation of China under Grant No. 41371365 and the State Key Program of the National Natural Science of China (Grant No. 41230751).

Author Contributions: Jiangfeng She conceived the experiment and edited the manuscript; Qiujun Wei performed the task of data processing and coding, analyzed the results, and wrote the manuscript. Shuhua Zhang and Jinsong Ma were involved in the analysis process and partially contributed to the data processing work.

Conflicts of Interest: The authors declare no conflict of interest.

References

1. Kwan, M.-P. Geographies of health. *Ann. Assoc. Am. Geogr.* **2012**, *102*, 891–892. [CrossRef]
2. Berke, E.M.; Koepsell, T.D.; Moudon, A.V.; Hoskins, R.E.; Larson, E.B. Association of the built environment with physical activity and obesity in older persons. *Am. J. Public Health* **2007**, *97*, 486–492. [CrossRef] [PubMed]
3. Dubowitz, T.; Zenk, S.N.; Ghosh-Dastidar, B.; Cohen, D.A.; Beckman, R.; Hunter, G.; Steiner, E.D.; Collins, R.L. Healthy food access for urban food desert residents: Examination of the food environment, food purchasing practices, diet and BMI. *Public Health Nutr.* **2015**, *18*, 2220–2230. [CrossRef] [PubMed]
4. Inagami, S.; Cohen, D.A.; Brown, A.F.; Asch, S.M. Body mass index, neighborhood fast food and restaurant concentration, and car ownership. *J. Urban Health* **2009**, *86*, 683–695. [CrossRef] [PubMed]
5. Pearce, J.; Hiscock, R.; Blakely, T.; Witten, K. The contextual effects of neighbourhood access to supermarkets and convenience stores on individual fruit and vegetable consumption. *J. Epidemiol. Community Health* **2008**, *62*, 198–201. [CrossRef] [PubMed]
6. Laska, M.N.; Hearst, M.O.; Forsyth, A.; Pasch, K.E.; Lytle, L. Neighbourhood food environments: Are they associated with adolescent dietary intake, food purchases and weight status? *Public Health Nutr.* **2010**, *13*, 1757–1763. [CrossRef] [PubMed]
7. Kwan, M.P. From place-based to people-based exposure measures. *Soc. Sci. Med.* **2009**, *69*, 1311–1313. [CrossRef] [PubMed]
8. Perchoux, C.; Chaix, B.; Cummins, S.; Kestens, Y. Conceptualization and measurement of environmental exposure in epidemiology: Accounting for activity space related to daily mobility. *Health Place* **2013**, *21*, 86–93. [CrossRef] [PubMed]
9. Basta, L.A.; Richmond, T.S.; Wiebe, D.J. Neighborhoods, daily activities, and measuring health risks experienced in urban environments. *Soc. Sci. Med.* **2010**, *71*, 1943–1950. [CrossRef] [PubMed]

10. Troped, P.J.; Wilson, J.S.; Matthews, C.E.; Cromley, E.K.; Melly, S.J. The built environment and location-based physical activity. *Am. J. Prev. Med.* **2010**, *38*, 429–438. [CrossRef] [PubMed]

11. Shareck, M.; Kestens, Y.; Frohlich, K.L. Moving beyond the residential neighborhood to explore social inequalities in exposure to area-level disadvantage: Results from the interdisciplinary study on inequalities in smoking. *Soc. Sci. Med.* **2014**, *108*, 106–114. [CrossRef] [PubMed]

12. Richardson, D.B.; Volkow, N.D.; Kwan, M.P.; Kaplan, R.M.; Goodchild, M.F.; Croyle, R.T. Medicine. Spatial turn in health research. *Science* **2013**, *339*, 1390–1392. [CrossRef] [PubMed]

13. Boruff, B.J.; Nathan, A.; Nijënstein, S. Using GPS technology to (re)-examine operational definitions of 'neighbourhood' in place-based health research. *Int. J. Health Geogr.* **2012**, *11*, 22. [CrossRef] [PubMed]

14. Kestens, Y.; Lebel, A.; Chaix, B.; Clary, C.; Daniel, M.; Pampalon, R.; Theriault, M.; Subramanian, S.V.P. Association between activity space exposure to food establishments and individual risk of overweight. *PLoS ONE* **2012**, *7*, e41418.

15. Shearer, C.; Rainham, D.; Blanchard, C.; Dummer, T.; Lyons, R.; Kirk, S. Measuring food availability and accessibility among adolescents: Moving beyond the neighbourhood boundary. *Soc. Sci. Med.* **2015**, *133*, 322–330. [CrossRef] [PubMed]

16. Christian, W.J. Using geospatial technologies to explore activity-based retail food environments. *Spat. Spatio-Temporal Epidemiol.* **2012**, *3*, 287–295. [CrossRef] [PubMed]

17. Cetateanu, A.; Jones, A. How can GPS technology help us better understand exposure to the food environment? A systematic review. *SSM Popul. Health* **2016**, *2*, 196–205. [CrossRef] [PubMed]

18. Gustafson, A.; Christian, J.W.; Lewis, S.; Moore, K.; Jilcott, S. Food venue choice, consumer food environment, but not food venue availability within daily travel patterns are associated with dietary intake among adults, Lexington Kentucky 2011. *Nutr. J.* **2013**, *12*, 17. [CrossRef] [PubMed]

19. Rainham, D.; McDowell, I.; Krewski, D.; Sawada, M. Conceptualizing the healthscape: Contributions of time geography, location technologies and spatial ecology to place and health research. *Soc. Sci. Med.* **2010**, *70*, 668–676. [CrossRef] [PubMed]

20. Zenk, S.N.; Schulz, A.J.; Matthews, S.A.; Odoms-Young, A.; Wilbur, J.; Wegrzyn, L.; Gibbs, K.; Braunschweig, C.; Stokes, C. Activity space environment and dietary and physical activity behaviors: A pilot study. *Health Place* **2011**, *17*, 1150–1161. [CrossRef] [PubMed]

21. Matthews, S.A.; Yang, T.C. Spatial polygamy and contextual exposures (spaces): Promoting activity space approaches in research on place and health. *Am. Behav. Sci.* **2013**, *57*, 1057–1081. [CrossRef] [PubMed]

22. Kwan, M.-P. Beyond space (as we knew it): Toward temporally integrated geographies of segregation, health, and accessibility. *Ann. Assoc. Am. Geogr.* **2013**, *103*, 1078–1086. [CrossRef]

23. Axhausen, K.W.; Zimmermann, A.; Schönfelder, S.; Rindsfüser, G.; Haupt, T. Observing the rhythms of daily life: A six-week travel diary. *Transportation* **2002**, *29*, 95–124. [CrossRef]

24. Chaix, B.; Kestens, Y.; Perchoux, C.; Karusisi, N.; Merlo, J.; Labadi, K. An interactive mapping tool to assess individual mobility patterns in neighborhood studies. *Am. J. Prev. Med.* **2012**, *43*, 440–450. [CrossRef] [PubMed]

25. Holliday, K.M.; Howard, A.G.; Emch, M.; Rodriguez, D.A.; Evenson, K.R. Are buffers around home representative of physical activity spaces among adults? *Health Place* **2017**, *45*, 181–188. [CrossRef] [PubMed]

26. Chaix, B.; Meline, J.; Duncan, S.; Merrien, C.; Karusisi, N.; Perchoux, C.; Lewin, A.; Labadi, K.; Kestens, Y. GPS tracking in neighborhood and health studies: A step forward for environmental exposure assessment, a step backward for causal inference? *Health Place* **2013**, *21*, 46–51. [CrossRef] [PubMed]

27. Kwan, M.-P. The uncertain geographic context problem. *Ann. Assoc. Am. Geogr.* **2012**, *102*, 958–968. [CrossRef]

28. Matthews, S.A. Uncertain geographic context problem. In *International Encyclopedia of Geography: People, the Earth, Environment and Technology*; John Wiley & Sons, Ltd.: Hoboken, NJ, USA, 2016.

29. Chen, X.; Kwan, M.-P. Contextual uncertainties, human mobility, and perceived food environment: The uncertain geographic context problem in food access research. *Am. J. Public Health* **2015**, *105*, 1734–1737. [CrossRef] [PubMed]

30. Cetateanu, A.; Luca, B.-A.; Popescu, A.A.; Page, A.; Cooper, A.; Jones, A. A novel methodology for identifying environmental exposures using GPS data. *Int. J. Geogr. Inf. Sci.* **2016**, *30*, 1944–1960. [CrossRef]

31. Lipperman-Kreda, S.; Morrison, C.; Grube, J.W.; Gaidus, A. Youth activity spaces and daily exposure to tobacco outlets. *Health Place* **2015**, *34*, 30–33. [CrossRef] [PubMed]

32. Lyseen, A.K.; Hansen, H.S.; Harder, H.; Jensen, A.S.; Mikkelsen, B.E. Defining neighbourhoods as a measure of exposure to the food environment. *Int. J. Environ. Res. Public Health* **2015**, *12*, 8504–8525. [CrossRef] [PubMed]

33. Ester, M.; Kriegel, H.-P.; Sander, J.; Xu, X. Density-based spatial clustering of applications with noise. In Proceedings of the International Conference on Knowledge Discovery and Data Mining, Portland, OR, USA, 2–4 August 1996.

34. Brunsdon, C.; Corcoran, J.; Higgs, G. Visualising space and time in crime patterns: A comparison of methods. *Comput. Environ. Urban Syst.* **2007**, *31*, 52–75. [CrossRef]

35. Stochastic Gradient Descent Classifier. Available online: http://scikit-learn.org/stable/modules/generated/sklearn.linear_model.SGDClassifier.html (accessed on 9 August 2017).

36. Zheng, Y.; Xie, X.; Ma, W.Y. Geolife: A collaborative social networking service among user, location and trajectory. *IEEE Data Eng. Bull.* **2010**, *33*, 32–39.

37. Bus Routes and Stops Datasets of Beijing. Available online: http://www.bjdata.gov.cn/ (accessed on 9 August 2017).

38. Ashbrook, D.; Starner, T. Using GPS to learn significant locations and predict movement across multiple users. *Persnol Ubiquitous Comput.* **2003**, *7*, 275–286. [CrossRef]

39. Zhou, C.; Frankowski, D.; Ludford, P.; Shekhar, S.; Terveen, L. Discovering personally meaningful places. *ACM Trans. Inf. Syst.* **2007**, *25*, 12. [CrossRef]

40. Bhattacharya, T.; Kulik, L.; Bailey, J. Automatically recognizing places of interest from unreliable GPS data using spatio-temporal density estimation and line intersections. *Pervasive Mob. Comput.* **2015**, *19*, 86–107. [CrossRef]

41. Zheng, Y.; Zhang, L.; Xie, X.; Ma, W.-Y. Mining interesting locations and travel sequences from GPS trajectories. In Proceedings of the 18th International Conference on World Wide Web, Madrid, Spain, 20–24 April 2009; ACM: New York, NY, USA, 2009; pp. 791–800.

42. Huang, W.; Li, S.; Liu, X.; Ban, Y. Predicting human mobility with activity changes. *Int. J. Geogr. Inf. Sci.* **2015**, *29*, 1569–1587. [CrossRef]

43. Lee, J.; Gong, J.; Li, S. Exploring spatiotemporal clusters based on extended kernel estimation methods. *Int. J. Geogr. Inf. Sci.* **2017**, *31*, 1154–1177.

44. Nakaya, T.; Yano, K. Visualising crime clusters in a space-time cube: An exploratory data-analysis approach using space-time kernel density estimation and scan statistics. *Trans. GIS* **2010**, *14*, 223–239. [CrossRef]

45. Delmelle, E.; Delmelle, E.C.; Casas, I.; Barto, T. H.E.L.P: A GIS-based health exploratory analysis tool for practitioners. *Appl. Spat. Anal. Policy* **2011**, *4*, 113–137. [CrossRef]

46. Cao, X.; Cong, G.; Jensen, C.S. Mining significant semantic locations from GPS data. *Proc. VLDB Endow.* **2010**, *3*, 1009–1020. [CrossRef]

47. Andrienko, G.L.; Andrienko, N.V.; Fuchs, G.; Raimond, A.-M.O.; Symanzik, J.; Ziemlicki, C. Extracting semantics of individual places from movement data by analyzing temporal patterns of visits. In Proceedings of the First ACM SIGSPATIAL International Workshop on Computational Models of Place, Orlando, FL, USA, 5–8 November 2013; pp. 9–15.

48. Falcone, D.; Mascolo, C.; Comito, C.; Talia, D.; Crowcroft, J. What is this place? Inferring place categories through user patterns identification in geo-tagged tweets. In Proceedings of the 2014 6th International Conference on Mobile Computing, Applications and Services (MobiCASE), Austin, TX, USA, 6–7 November 2014; pp. 10–19.

49. Siła-Nowicka, K.; Vandrol, J.; Oshan, T.; Long, J.A.; Demšar, U.; Fotheringham, A.S. Analysis of human mobility patterns from GPS trajectories and contextual information. *Int. J. Geogr. Inf. Sci.* **2015**, *30*, 881–906. [CrossRef]

50. Gong, L.; Morikawa, T.; Yamamoto, T.; Sato, H. Deriving personal trip data from GPS data: A literature review on the existing methodologies. *Proced. Soc. Behav. Sci.* **2014**, *138*, 557–565. [CrossRef]

51. Prelipcean, A.C.; Gidófalvi, G.; Susilo, Y.O. Transportation mode detection—An in-depth review of applicability and reliability. *Transp. Rev.* **2017**, *37*, 442–464. [CrossRef]

52. Reddy, S.; Mun, M.; Burke, J.; Estrin, D.; Hansen, M.; Srivastava, M. Using mobile phones to determine transportation modes. *ACM Trans. Sens. Netw. (TOSN)* **2010**, *6*, 13. [CrossRef]

53. Zheng, Y.; Liu, L.; Wang, L.; Xie, X. Learning transportation mode from raw GPS data for geographic applications on the web. In Proceedings of the 17th International Conference on World Wide Web, Beijing, China, 21–25 April 2008; ACM: New York, NY, USA, 2008; pp. 247–256.

54. Bolbol, A.; Cheng, T.; Tsapakis, I.; Haworth, J. Inferring hybrid transportation modes from sparse GPS data using a moving window SVM classification. *Comput. Environ. Urban Syst.* **2012**, *36*, 526–537. [CrossRef]

55. Stenneth, L.; Wolfson, O.; Yu, P.S.; Xu, B. Transportation mode detection using mobile phones and GIS information. In Proceedings of the 19th ACM SIGSPATIAL International Conference on Advances in Geographic Information Systems, Chicago, IL, USA, 1–4 November 2011; ACM: New York, NY, USA, 2011; pp. 54–63.

56. Kwan, M.P. Gender and individual access to urban opportunities: A study using space—Time measures. *Prof. Geogr.* **1999**, *51*, 210–227. [CrossRef]

57. Patterson, Z.; Farber, S. Potential path areas and activity spaces in application: A review. *Transp. Rev.* **2015**, *35*, 679–700. [CrossRef]

58. Perchoux, C.; Chaix, B.; Brondeel, R.; Kestens, Y. Residential buffer, perceived neighborhood, and individual activity space: New refinements in the definition of exposure areas—The record cohort study. *Health Place* **2016**, *40*, 116–122. [CrossRef] [PubMed]

59. Truong, K.; Fernandes, M.; An, R.; Shier, V.; Sturm, R. Measuring the physical food environment and its relationship with obesity: Evidence from California. *Public Health* **2010**, *124*, 115–118. [CrossRef] [PubMed]

60. Kestens, Y.; Lebel, A.; Daniel, M.; Theriault, M.; Pampalon, R. Using experienced activity spaces to measure foodscape exposure. *Health Place* **2010**, *16*, 1094–1103. [CrossRef] [PubMed]

61. Ahalya, M.; Jane, Y.P.; Éric, R.; Marc, L.; Tina, M.; Leia, M.M. Geographic retail food environment measures for use in public health. *Health Promot. Chronic Dis. Prev. Can. Res. Policy Pract.* **2017**, *37*, 357–362.

62. Sharp, G.; Denney, J.T.; Kimbro, R.T. Multiple contexts of exposure: Activity spaces, residential neighborhoods, and self-rated health. *Soc. Sci. Med.* **2015**, *146*, 204–213. [CrossRef] [PubMed]

63. Cobb, L.K.; Appel, L.J.; Franco, M.; Jones-Smith, J.C.; Nur, A.; Anderson, C.A. The relationship of the local food environment with obesity: A systematic review of methods, study quality, and results. *Obesity* **2015**, *23*, 1331–1344. [CrossRef] [PubMed]

64. Burgoine, T.; Monsivais, P. Characterising food environment exposure at home, at work, and along commuting journeys using data on adults in the UK. *Int. J. Behav. Nutr. Phys. Act.* **2013**, *10*, 85. [CrossRef] [PubMed]

65. Jeffery, R.W.; Baxter, J.; McGuire, M.; Linde, J. Are fast food restaurants an environmental risk factor for obesity? *Int. J. Behav. Nutr. Phys. Act.* **2006**, *3*, 2. [CrossRef] [PubMed]

66. Bin, M. The spatial organization of the separation between jobs and residential locations in Beijing. *Acta Geogr. Sin.* **2009**, *64*, 1457–1466.

67. Beijing Municipal Statistics Bulletin of National Economy and Social Development in 2013. Available online: http://www.bjstats.gov.cn/ (accessed on 9 August 2017).

68. Kwan, M.-P. How GIS can help address the uncertain geographic context problem in social science research. *Ann. GIS* **2012**, *18*, 245–255. [CrossRef]

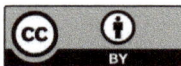

International Journal of
*Environmental Research
and Public Health*

MDPI

Article

Cycling for Transportation in Sao Paulo City: Associations with Bike Paths, Train and Subway Stations

Alex Antonio Florindo [1,2,*], Ligia Vizeu Barrozo [3], Gavin Turrell [4],
João Paulo dos Anjos Souza Barbosa [2], William Cabral-Miranda [3], Chester Luiz Galvão Cesar [5]
and Moisés Goldbaum [6]

[1] School of Arts, Sciences and Humanities, University of Sao Paulo, Sao Paulo City 03828-000, Brazil
[2] Graduate Program in Nutrition in Public Health, Department of Nutrition, School of Public Health, University of Sao Paulo, Sao Paulo City 01246-904, Brazil; jpdosanjos@usp.br
[3] Department of Geography, School of Philosophy, Literature and Human Sciences, University of Sao Paulo, Sao Paulo City 05508-080, Brazil; lija@usp.br (L.V.B.); williamcabral@usp.br (W.C.-M.)
[4] Institute for Health and Ageing, Australian Catholic University, Melbourne, VIC 3065, Australia; gavin.turrell@acu.edu.au
[5] Department of Epidemiology, School of Public Health, University of Sao Paulo, Sao Paulo City 01246-904, Brazil; clcesar@usp.br
[6] Department of Preventive Medicine, School of Medicine, University of Sao Paulo, Sao Paulo City 01246-903, Brazil; mgoldbau@usp.br
* Correspondence: aflorind@usp.br; Tel.: +55-11-3091-8157

Received: 8 December 2017; Accepted: 2 March 2018; Published: 21 March 2018

Abstract: Cities that support cycling for transportation reap many public health benefits. However, the prevalence of this mode of transportation is low in Latin American countries and the association with facilities such as bike paths and train/subway stations have not been clarified. We conducted a cross-sectional analysis of the relationship between bike paths, train/subway stations and cycling for transportation in adults from the city of Sao Paulo. We used data from the Sao Paulo Health Survey (n = 3145). Cycling for transportation was evaluated by a questionnaire and bike paths and train/subway stations were geocoded using the geographic coordinates of the adults' residential addresses in 1500-m buffers. We used multilevel logistic regression, taking account of clustering by census tract and households. The prevalence of cycling for transportation was low (5.1%), and was more prevalent in males, singles, those active in leisure time, and in people with bicycle ownership in their family. Cycling for transportation was associated with bike paths up to a distance of 500 m from residences (OR (Odds Ratio) = 2.54, 95% CI (Confidence interval) 1.16–5.54) and with the presence of train/subway stations for distances >500 m from residences (OR = 2.07, 95% CI 1.10–3.86). These results are important to support policies to improve cycling for transportation in megacities such as Sao Paulo.

Keywords: cycling for transportation; bike paths; train stations; subway stations; adults; Brazil

---

1. Introduction

Cities that promote and support cycling for transportation reap many public health benefits for their populations, such as reduced risk for chronic disease, lower rates of overweight and obesity, fewer traffic accidents and injuries, and lower levels of air pollution [1–5]. However, increasing the population prevalence of cycling for transportation is a big challenge for many countries. In Latin American cities, for example, less than 10% of the adult population use a bicycle for transport [6].

This contrasts with European countries such as the Netherlands and Denmark, where more than 25% of transport-related trips are undertaken by bicycle [7].

Cycling for transportation is most prevalent in men and in people of middle-age and young adults [3,8–14]. Studies from high-income countries show that built and social environments as well as associated policies are very important in terms of increasing the use of the bicycle for transportation purposes. Two reviews showed that bike paths, a safe riding environment, integration of the bicycle with other forms of transportation, bike parking, bicycle ownership, and interventions based on education and mass media are important factors for increasing the use of this mode of transportation [15,16]. Empirical studies show that access to bike paths close to residences is associated with cycling for transportation [8,10–12,17–19]. However, knowledge of the factors that explain the use of cycling in Latin American countries is limited. For example, a review of cycling for transportation in Curitiba (Brazil), Santiago (Chile), and Bogota (Colombia) recommended that policy-makers increase bike path availability and accessibility as a way of promoting active transportation [6]. However, a study conducted in Curitiba found no significant association between the presence of bike paths in 500-m buffers with cycling for transportation [20]. This is important because some megacities in upper-middle income countries such as Brazil and Colombia are increasing the length of bike paths to promote and support cycling. Sao Paulo (Southeastern, Brazil) is a good example, because this city has more than 400 km of bike paths. In addition, 4.7 million people use the subway daily for transportation on weekdays [21]. In this case, it is important to investigate if bike paths and train or subway stations in Sao Paulo are associated with cycling for transportation. Therefore, the aims of this study were: (1) to identify the profile of adults that use cycling for transportation in Sao Paulo city; (2) to assess whether the presence of train or subway stations is associated with cycling for transportation; (3) to examine if the distance of bike paths from residences is associated with cycling for transportation; and (4) to assess if the mix of the presence of train or subway stations and the distance of bike paths from residences is associated with cycling for transportation.

2. Material and Methods

2.1. Sao Paulo Health Survey

Sao Paulo had a population of 12,038,175 inhabitants living in 1521.11 km^2 in 2017. The city is divided in 96 districts, 32 administrations, concentrates 11% of gross national product from Brazil, and is one of the 10 most populated cities in world. Sao Paulo currently has 468 km of bike paths, 80.4 km of subway, and 71 stations (Figure 1) [21,22].

The sample for the Sao Paulo Health Survey included 3145 adults (aged 18 years or more) who were interviewed in their homes and had their residential addresses' geocoded. The Sao Paulo Health Survey is a cross-sectional study based on a representative sample of adults who lived in Sao Paulo city in 2014 and 2015. Details about the sampling and geocoding process are described elsewhere [23].

The Ethics Committee of the School of Arts, Sciences, and Humanities at the University of Sao Paulo approved this study (process number 55846116.6.0000.5390).

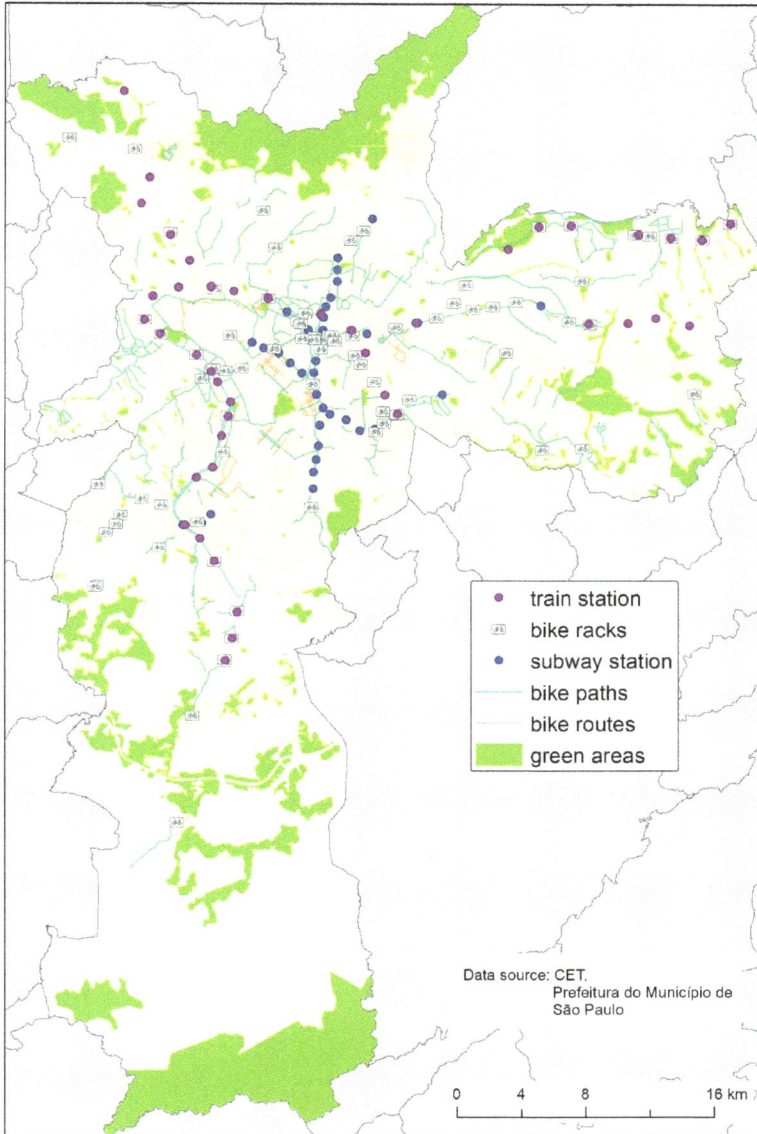

Figure 1. Map of bike paths, bike lanes, bike racks, train and subway stations in Sao Paulo, 2017.

2.2. Outcome Variable

The outcome was cycling for transportation measured using the International Physical Activity Questionnaire (IPAQ) long version. The IPAQ has been validated and used in the Brazilian adult population [24], and this module was standardized to capture the frequency (times per week) and duration (minutes per day) of cycling for transportation. In this study we focus only on the binary outcome: the use of a bicycle for transportation in a normal week (yes or no).

2.3. Covariates

The covariates used in this study were: sex (men, women), age (18–29 years, 30–39 years, 40–49 years, 50–59 years, and 60 years or older), education (incomplete elementary school, elementary to incomplete high school, complete high school, undergraduate incomplete to complete), marital status (married/de facto, single, divorced/separated/widowed), physical activity in leisure-time measured using the IPAQ long ($\geq$150 min per week, <150 min per week), body mass index based on self-reported height and weight ($\geq$30 kg/m^2, <30 kg/m^2), smoking (yes or no), self-report of health (good/very good/excellent, regular/bad/very bad), employment situation (work: yes or no), car or motorcycle ownership (yes or no), bicycle ownership (yes or no), and length of living in the residence (up to 1 year, between 1 and 5 years, >5 years).

2.4. Built Environment Variables

We used a georeferenced street dataset from Sao Paulo to obtain bike paths as well as train and subway stations [22]. We used a Geographic Information System to delineate radial buffers of 1500 m based on the geographic coordinates of the adults' residential addresses. This distance is based on the distance that people can access within 15 min of walking [25]. We used Arc Map software (version 10.3, Redlands, CA, USA).

Within each buffer we recorded: (1) the presence or absence of train or subway stations; (2) the distance of bike paths from the participants' residences.

2.5. Statistical Analysis

We calculated the prevalence ratio for cycling for transportation according to social, demographics, health, and work characteristics. We used Poisson regression and complex sample design according to the census tract (primary unit of sample) in five health areas in Sao Paulo (strata), and the sample weight. This weight took into account the design effect, post-stratification by sex and age, and the non-response rate. For these analyses we used Stata (version SE 12.1, StataCorp, College Station, TX, USA).

To examine the relationship between the built environment and cycling for transportation, we conducted multilevel logistic regression. We used three independent variables: (1) the presence of train or subway stations; (2) the distance of bike paths from residences; and (3) the mix of the presence of train or subway stations and the distance of bike paths from residences. We used the distance of up to 500 m and above 500 m from participants' residences to compare with places without facilities [23]. The modeling was undertaken in two stages: Model 1 took into account clustering by census tract and household, and was adjusted for sex and age; Model 2 used all variables in Model 1 plus adjustment for education, the time that people lived at the same residence, and the area of residence (North, Midwest, Southeast, South, East).

For multilevel analyses of this article, we had 34 missing data points and we worked with $n = 3111$ people in 2224 residences and 149 census tracts. All analyses were undertaken using the xtmelogit command in Stata (version SE 12.1, StataCorp).

3. Results

The overall prevalence of cycling for transportation was 5.1% (95% CI 4.0–6.2). The prevalence ratio was high for males, singles, those active in leisure time, and for people with bicycle ownership in their family (Table 1).

Table 1. Descriptive characteristics and prevalence ratio for cycling for transportation in adults from Sao Paulo, 2015.

Variables	Sample Characteristics (%) *	Prevalence Ratio (95 %CI) **
Sex (*n* = 3145)		
Female	53.5	1.00
Male	46.5	**4.59 (2.82–7.46)** [#]
Age group (*n* = 3145)		
18–29 years	24.5	1.00
30–39 years	22.8	1.18 (0.74–1.89)
40–49 years	18.7	1.37 (0.76–2.45)
50–59 years	15.8	0.66 (0.33–1.34)
60 years or older	18.2	0.63 (0.29–1.41)
Education (*n* = 3145)		
Incomplete elementary school	17.4	1.00
Elementary to incomplete high school	24.0	0.93 (0.50–1.75)
Complete high school	29.0	0.89 (0.49–1.59)
Undergraduate incomplete to complete	29.6	1.00 (0.51–1.98)
Marital Status (*n* = 3136)		
Married or de facto	56.9	1.00
Single	28.3	**1.64 (1.04–2.59)** [#]
Divorced, separated, or widowed	14.8	1.33 (0.74–2.36)
Physical activity in leisure time (*n* = 3141)		
<150 min per week	78.0	1.00
≥150 min per week	22.0	**1.59 (1.11–2.28)** [#]
Obesity (*n* = 3077)		
Body mass index ≥ 30 kg/m^2	79.0	1.00
Body mass index < 30 kg/m^2	21.0	1.28 (0.73–2.24)
Smoking (*n* = 3142)		
No	82.6	1.00
Yes	17.4	1.10 (0.68–1.79)
Self-report of health (*n* = 3141)		
Regular/bad/very bad	27.2	1.00
Good/very good/excellent	72.8	1.22 (0.81–1.84)
Employees (*n* = 3100)		
No	34.9	1.00
Yes	65.1	1.50 (0.99–2.27)
Car or motorcycle ownership (*n* = 3145)		
No	42.8	1.00
Yes	57.2	0.77 (0.52–1.15)
Bicycle ownership (*n* = 3052)		
No	68.3	1.00
Yes	31.7	**4.48 (2.95–6.79)** [#]
Time in the same residence (*n* = 3111)		
Up to 1 year	12.4	1.00
Between 1 and 5 years	21.0	0.90 (0.49–1.67)
More than 5 years	66.6	0.73 (0.42–1.28)

CI: confidence interval; * Weighted percentage; ** Adjusted by all variables in Table 1; [#] $p < 0.05$.

Bicycle ownership in families was more prevalent according to educational level (p-trend < 0.001). The prevalence ratio was 1.15 (95% CI 1.09–1.23) for people that had incomplete undergraduate studies than people had only incomplete elementary school (Figure 2).

Just under one-third of people had bike paths or train or subway stations within 500 m of their residence (Table 2). Only a quarter of people had train or subway stations within 1500-m buffers (Table 2).

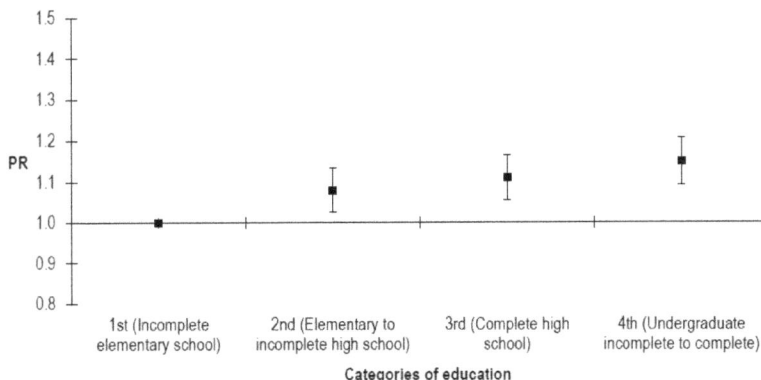

Figure 2. Prevalence ratio (PR) for bicycle ownership according to education and adjusted by age and sex.

Table 2. Distribution of facilities according to participants' residence.

Facilities in 1500-m Buffers	% of People with Bike Paths *	% of People with Train/Subway Stations **	% of People with Bike Paths and Train/Subway Stations in the Same Buffers ***
None	30.9	70.9	80.8
Up to 500 m	29.3	4.7	4.4
Bewteen 500 m and 1500 m	39.8	24.4	14.8

* Distance from the participants' residence; ** only the presence (yes or not); *** According to distances between bike paths from residences and the presence of train or subway stations in these distances.

After adjusting for the covariates, the odds of cycling for transportation were 154% higher if there was a bike path within 500 m of a person's residence (Table 3).

Table 3. Results of the multilevel model for the association between cycling for transportation with bike paths and train or subway stations.

Bike Paths	Model 1 OR (95% CI) *	Model 2 OR (95% CI) **
Bike paths only		
None	1	1
Up to 500 m	2.11 (1.04–4.27) [#]	2.54 (1.16–5.54) [#]
Between 500 m and 1500 m	1.14 (0.59–2.21)	1.62 (0.78–3.36)
Train or subway stations only		
None	1	1
Up to 500 m	1.30 (0.36–4.61)	1.26 (0.33–4.74)
Between 500 m and 1500 m	1.87 (1.01–3.45) [#]	2.07 (1.10–3.86) [#]
Bike paths and train or subway stations ***		
None	1	1
Up to 500 m	0.78 (0.20–3.04)	0.72 (0.17–3.00)
Between 500 m and 1500 m	0.88 (0.41–1.88)	1.15 (0.54–2.48)

OR: Odds ratio; CI: confidence interval; * Model 1: adjusted by sex, age; ** Model 2: adjusted by variables in Model 1 plus education, place where people lived in Sao Paulo, and the length of time that they lived in the same residence; *** in the same buffers; [#] $p < 0.05$.

The presence of train or subway stations was associated with cycling for transportation in distances above 500 m from residences: for people living in buffers with these facilities the odds of cycling for transport were 107% higher, independent of sex, age, education, places where people live, and length of time living in the same residence (Table 3).

There was no association found between cycling for transport with the mix of train or subway station and bike paths in the same buffers (Table 3).

4. Discussion

This study showed that the presence of bike paths within 500 m of residences and the presence of train or subway stations within 1500 m of residences were associated with the prevalence of cycling for transportation in adults living in Sao Paulo. However, the prevalence of cycling for transportation was generally low, although it was higher in males, singles, those active in leisure time, and in people with bicycle ownership in their family.

An international review showed that most of the studies found a positive significant association between bike paths and cycling in high-income countries [15]. Dill and Carr found that with a greater amount of bike paths, the prevalence of commuting by bicycle was higher in 35 cities in the United States [19]. A study conducted in Brisbane, Australia, showed that people living in neighborhoods with more kilometers of bike paths had a significantly greater likelihood of cycling for transport [26]. Bike paths are very important to cycling in high-income countries, and in the Netherlands and Germany the investment to improve these facilities paths started in the 1970s [7]. However, in Latin American countries, these actions and facilities have been implemented more recently, with the wider creation of bike paths in Sao Paulo beginning in 2014. The discussion now is about possible effects of these facilities on the use of cycling for commuting. We found a significant likelihood of cycling for transportation for people who lived in residences within 500 m of bike paths. However, other studies conducted in Brazil found results different from those reported here. Hino et al. did not find a significant association between the presence or the length of bike paths and cycling for transport in adults who lived in Curitiba, south of Brazil [20]. A review that discussed transport and health in Chile, Brazil, and Colombia, however, recommended the adoption of bike paths to improve cycle commuting in cities in Latin American countries [6]. We need more cross-sectional and longitudinal studies in Latin American cities and in other megacities from upper- and middle-income countries to verify the contribution of bike paths because many factors may influence the use of the bicycle for transportation purposes.

We did not find a significant association between cycling for transportation and bike paths at distances greater than 500 m from residences. A study conducted with adults from Arlington, USA, showed that for each increase of 0.25 miles (~400 m) in the distance from residences to trails and bike paths, the likelihood of cycling decreases [11]. Another study conducted with adults from King County, Washington, USA, showed that people who lived in places that had bike paths or trails within 0.5 m of their residence (~800 m) had a significant likelihood of commuting by bicycle [8]. In cities like Sao Paulo, it can be very difficult to access bike paths located long distances from residences because there exist many barriers such vehicle traffic and streets on which it is dangerous to cycle. Some areas of Sao Paulo also present steep hills, which may discourage cycling. In addition, studies show that safety perception is associated with cycle commuting in different populations [12,15,27], and the presence of bike paths in neighborhoods is associated with a better safety perception of bicycle use [28].

We found a significant likelihood of cycling for transportation associated with the presence of train or subway stations, but only for distances greater than 500 m from residences. In addition, there was no association found between cycling for transport and the mix of bike paths and train or subway stations in the same buffers. The odds ratio was not improved with the inclusion of train and subway stations in the models of bike paths within 500 m of residences, which were significant to the increased prevalence of cycling for transportation. We had a low number of train and subway stations located within 500 m of residences (<5%) as well as a low incidence of bike paths and train or subway stations in the same buffers where people lived (<5% within 500 m and <15% above 500 m). Probably as a consequence of this, we did not find a significant association with these factors. We did not find other studies that examined the relationship between the presence of train and subway stations in different buffer sizes and cycle commuting. However, a study conducted with adults from Brisbane, Australia, found that people who perceived transport destinations to be within 20 min of walking from their residences had a significant likelihood of cycling for transportation [29].

In addition, other facilities are important to increase cycling for transportation. Winters et al. showed that not only bike paths were important for cycling for transport, but also hills, destinations, and connectivity [30]. The authors examined the bike score that was based on bike paths, hills, and destinations in census tracts and showed that this score was positively associated with the cycling commuting in 24 cities in the USA and Canada. A study conducted in Stockholm, Sweden, showed that factors such as aesthetics, greenery, car traffic, and noise were important factors affecting bikeability [31]. However, in Curitiba, Brazil, Hino et al. showed an inverse association between land use mix and cycling for transportation in adults [20]. Therefore, we not only need to increase the number of bike paths, but also better integrate cycling facilities with train and subway stations [15]. For example, people cannot transport bicycles in the subway in Sao Paulo during weekdays until 8:30 pm., there are a only few bicycle parking locations in operation [21], and the bike-share system has been found to be unstable and insufficient for the city in last two years.

Another important question is about bicycle ownership, which was found to be more likely in people with better education. A study conducted with adults who lived in Seattle, Baltimore, and Washington, USA, showed that bicycle ownership was positively associated with education level [12]. Sá et al. showed a significant decrease in the prevalence of cycling in Sao Paulo between 2007 to 2012 in low-income adults as well as an increase of cycling prevalence in high-income adults in the same period [3]. We showed that the prevalence of cycling for transportation was more common in people who had bicycle ownership in their family. These results are important because they show that we need more policies to improve the population's capacity to purchase bicycles in Brazil and improve bicycle-share programs with low costs.

We found a low prevalence of cycling for transportation in the adult population in Sao Paulo (~5%). Surveys conducted with adults who lived in three cities from Brazil showed that the prevalence of cycling for transport varied between 8.8% in Vitoria (Southeast) to 16.6% in Recife (Northeast), and 13.3% for the total population [32]. A trend-study conducted with adults from Sao Paulo showed that there was an increased number of cyclists from 1997 (3.9 per 1000 people) to 2007 (6.3 per 1000 people) but a decrease in 2012 (5.4 per 1000 people) [3]. Compared with European countries that are cycling-friendly such as the Netherlands, where 27% of trips are made by bicycle, Brazil is very far from achieving widespread cycling for transportation [7]. Only in Rio Claro (a small city in Sao Paulo State) did a survey find 28.3% transport cycling prevalence. The authors argued that this city is ideal for cyclists because it is a small city with a flat topography with many kilometers of bike paths and bike lanes. Moreover, this city has poor public transportation with few services that are expensive for the population [14].

The prevalence of cycling for transportation was higher in males and singles that are generally younger adults. This profile is similar to studies conducted in Brazil, Australia, Canada, and the United States [8,9,11,32–34]. Another interesting finding was that cyclists were more active in leisure time. These results are consistent with the literature, which showed that cycling for transportation is a healthy activity. Studies have shown that active transportation and cycling for transportation contribute to increased physical activity and life expectancy and are associated with lower odds of obesity, hypertension, and high triglycerides [4,5,35]. In addition, a study published by Tainio et al. showed that the benefits of cycling in Sao Paulo overcome the risks of air pollution exposure [36]. Therefore, these results are important because an increase in cycling for transportation can contribute to increasing physical activity, for health promotion, and for disease prevention.

In addition, we think that increasing the prevalence of cycling for transportation is much more complex than merely building bike paths or train/subway stations. We need intervention programs such as media campaigns and educational programs in communities and schools [15]. For example, surveys conducted with Colombian adults in Bogota showed that people who participated in the community-based "Ciclovia Program" were significantly more likely to cycle for transportation [37]. Another study conducted in Cali, Colombia, showed that adults' participation in the "Ciclovia Program" was associated positively with the presence of a "Ciclovia corridor", which are streets closed for cars and open for walking or cycling on weekends and public holidays [38]. The longitudinal study "Cycling Connecting Communities" conducted with adults in Sydney, Australia, based on a social marketing framework and behavior change theories, found that after two years people who received the intervention had a significant likelihood of using bike paths [28]. In addition, other variables are associated with cycling for transportation such as self-efficacy, physical activity habit, attitude, and social support [29,38]. Finally, we need better facilities in subways and train stations, such as permission to travel with bicycles, bicycle parking, and bicycle-share programs across the cities.

This study has a number of limitations. Firstly, as the study was cross-sectional we cannot be sure if interviews were conducted after the implementation of bike paths, because the interviews were conducted from August 2014 to December to 2015, during which time many kilometers of bike paths were built in Sao Paulo. A longitudinal analysis like that conducted in England [39] may provide better evidence about the possible influences of bike paths on bicycle use for people living in Sao Paulo. Secondly, we worked with radial buffers that may introduce measurement error [40]. Future analysis with network buffers around residences should be compared with radial buffers. Thirdly, we did not control for self-selection in the neighborhood [41]; people who are cyclists may choose to live in neighborhoods with better bike paths and subway or train station facilities.

5. Conclusions

An increase in cycling for transportation can contribute to improved physical activity, reduced cardiovascular and respiratory disease, reduced air pollution, and improved public health and well-being in big cities [1,2,4,5,35,42]. We showed that bike paths close to residences (within 500 m) as well as access to train or subway stations (1500-m buffers) are factors that can increase cycling for transportation in Sao Paulo. However, the prevalence of cycling for transportation is low in Sao Paulo city (5.1%) and increasing this activity is not an easy task because active transport has multiple determinants. We need an increase in bike paths and a better integration of cycling with train and subway stations, including better and more secure facilities such as bike parking in addition to bicycle transportation in subway and train stations. Moreover, people need more opportunities to own a bicycle, a more extensively developed bike-share program, and community-based interventions to demonstrate the opportunities and benefits of this type of transportation for different populations.

Acknowledgments: Alex Antonio Florindo received an international scholarship from Sao Paulo Research Foundation (FAPESP) (grant 2014/12681-1) to develop this study and is receiving a research fellowship from the Brazilian National Council for Scientific and Technological Development (CNPq) (grant 306635/2016-0). Acknowledgments to The University of Melbourne for the reception of the international visit of Alex Antonio Florindo to develop this project in the Melbourne School of Population and Global Health. Acknowledgments to Professor Billie Giles-Corti for his support of the work in Melbourne School of Population and Global Health. Acknowledgments to ISA Study Group (Marilisa Berti de Azevedo Barros, PhD, University of Campinas, Maria Cecília Goi Porto Alves, PhD, Health of Institute, Sao Paulo, and Regina Mara Fisberg, PhD, University of Sao Paulo). The Sao Paulo Municipal Health Department (no grant number) and Sao Paulo Research Foundation (FAPESP) (grant 41 2012/22113-9) supported this ISA study in Sao Paulo.

Author Contributions: Alex Antonio Florindo conceptualized the idea, analyzed the data, and led the writing. Ligia Vizeu Barrozo and William Cabral-Miranda geocoded the residential address and open spaces data and took the measures in GIS. Gavin Turrell and João Paulo dos Anjos Souza Barbosa helped with statistical analysis. Chester Luiz Galvão Cesar and Moisés Goldbaum coordinated and supervised data collected from the ISA survey in Sao Paulo. All authors contributed significantly to the critical revision and drafting of the article.

Conflicts of Interest: All authors declare no conflict of interest.

References

1. Giles-Corti, B.; Vernez-Moudon, A.; Reis, R.; Turrell, G.; Dannenberg, A.L.; Badland, H.; Foster, S.; Lowe, M.; Sallis, J.F.; Stevenson, M.; et al. City planning and population health: A global challenge. *Lancet* **2016**, *388*, 2912–2924. [CrossRef]
2. Stevenson, M.; Thompson, J.; de Sa, T.H.; Ewing, R.; Mohan, D.; McClure, R.; Roberts, I.; Tiwari, G.; Giles-Corti, B.; Sun, X.; et al. Land use, transport, and population health: Estimating the health benefits of compact cities. *Lancet* **2016**, *388*, 2925–2935. [CrossRef]
3. Sa, T.H.; Duran, A.C.; Tainio, M.; Monteiro, C.A.; Woodcock, J. Cycling in Sao Paulo, Brazil (1997–2012): Correlates, time trends and health consequences. *Prev. Med. Rep.* **2016**, *4*, 540–545. [CrossRef] [PubMed]
4. Rojas-Rueda, D.; de Nazelle, A.; Teixido, O.; Nieuwenhuijsen, M.J. Replacing car trips by increasing bike and public transport in the greater Barcelona metropolitan area: A health impact assessment study. *Environ. Int.* **2012**, *49*, 100–109. [CrossRef] [PubMed]
5. Berger, A.T.; Qian, X.L.; Pereira, M.A. Associations between bicycling for transportation and cardiometabolic risk factors among Minneapolis-Saint Paul area commuters: A cross-sectional study in working-age adults. *Am. J. Health Promot.* **2017**, *32*, 631–637. [CrossRef] [PubMed]
6. Becerra, J.M.; Reis, R.S.; Frank, L.D.; Ramirez-Marrero, F.A.; Welle, B.; Arriaga Cordero, E.; Mendez Paz, F.; Crespo, C.; Dujon, V.; Jacoby, E.; et al. Transport and health: A look at three Latin American cities. *Cad. Saude Publica* **2013**, *29*, 654–666. [CrossRef] [PubMed]
7. Martens, K. The bicycle as a feedering mode: Experiences from three European countries. *Transp. Res.* **2004**, *9*, 281–294. [CrossRef]
8. Moudon, A.V.; Lee, C.; Cheadle, A.D.; Collier, C.W.; Johnson, D.; Schmid, T.; Weather, R.D. Cycling and the built environment, a US perspective. *Transp. Res. Part D* **2005**, *10*, 245–261. [CrossRef]
9. Rissel, C.; Merom, D.; Bauman, A.; Garrard, J.; Wen, L.M.; New, C. Current cycling, bicycle path use, and willingness to cycle more–findings from a community survey of cycling in southwest Sydney, Australia. *J. Phys. Act. Health* **2010**, *7*, 267–272. [CrossRef] [PubMed]
10. Titze, S.; Giles-Corti, B.; Knuiman, M.W.; Pikora, T.J.; Timperio, A.; Bull, F.C.; van Niel, K. Associations between intrapersonal and neighborhood environmental characteristics and cycling for transport and recreation in adults: Baseline results from the RESIDE study. *J. Phys. Act. Health* **2010**, *7*, 423–431. [CrossRef] [PubMed]
11. Troped, P.J.; Saunders, R.P.; Pate, R.R.; Reininger, B.; Ureda, J.R.; Thompson, S.J. Associations between self-reported and objective physical environmental factors and use of a community rail-trail. *Prev. Med.* **2001**, *32*, 191–200. [CrossRef] [PubMed]
12. Sallis, J.F.; Conway, T.L.; Dillon, L.I.; Frank, L.D.; Adams, M.A.; Cain, K.L.; Saelens, B.E. Environmental and demographic correlates of bicycling. *Prev. Med.* **2013**, *57*, 456–460. [CrossRef] [PubMed]
13. Kienteka, M.; Reis, R.S.; Rech, C.R. Personal and behavioral factors associated with bicycling in adults from Curitiba, Parana State, Brazil. *Cad. Saude Publica* **2014**, *30*, 79–87. [CrossRef] [PubMed]
14. Teixeira, I.P.; Nakamura, P.M.; Smirmaul, B.P.C.; Fernandes, R.A.; Kokubun, E. Fatores associados ao uso de bicicleta como meio de transporte em uma cidade de médio porte. *Rev. Bras. Atividade Fis. Saude* **2013**, *18*, 698–710. (In Portuguese) [CrossRef]
15. Pucher, J.; Dill, J.; Handy, S. Infrastructure, programs, and policies to increase bicycling: An international review. *Prev. Med.* **2010**, *50* (Suppl. S1), S106–S125. [CrossRef] [PubMed]
16. Fraser, S.D.; Lock, K. Cycling for transport and public health: A systematic review of the effect of the environment on cycling. *Eur. J. Public Health* **2011**, *21*, 738–743. [CrossRef] [PubMed]
17. Dill, J. Bicycling for transportation and health: The role of infrastructure. *J. Public Health Policy* **2009**, *30* (Suppl. S1), S95–S110. [CrossRef] [PubMed]
18. Garrard, J.; Rose, G.; Lo, S.K. Promoting transportation cycling for women: The role of bicycle infrastructure. *Prev. Med.* **2008**, *46*, 55–59. [CrossRef] [PubMed]
19. Dill, J.; Carr, T. Bicycle commuting and facilities in major U.S. cities: If you build them, commuters will use them—Another look. In *82 TRB Annual Meeting*; Transportation Research Board: Washington, DC, USA, 2003; pp. 1–9.
20. Hino, A.A.; Reis, R.S.; Sarmiento, O.L.; Parra, D.C.; Brownson, R.C. Built environment and physical activity for transportation in adults from Curitiba, Brazil. *J. Urban Health* **2014**, *91*, 446–462. [CrossRef] [PubMed]

21. State of Sao Paulo. Companhia do Metropolitano de Sao Paulo. Subway Stations in Sao Paulo City. Available online: http://www.metro.sp.gov.br/ (accessed on 7 February 2018). (In Portuguese)

22. Municipality of Sao Paulo. Geosampa. Bike Paths in Sao Paulo City. Available online: http://geosampa. prefeitura.sp.gov.br/PaginasPublicas/_SBC.aspx (accessed on 1 July 2016). (In Portuguese)

23. Florindo, A.A.; Barrozo, L.V.; Miranda, W.C.; Rodrigues, E.Q.; Turrell, G.; Goldbaum, M.; Cesar, C.L.G.; Giles-Corti, B. Open Spaces and Walking in Leisure Time in Brazilian Adults. *Int. J. Environ. Res. Public Health* **2017**, *14*, 553. [CrossRef] [PubMed]

24. Hallal, P.C.; Gomez, L.F.; Parra, D.C.; Lobelo, F.; Mosquera, J.; Florindo, A.A.; Reis, R.S.; Pratt, M.; Sarmiento, O.L. Lessons learned after 10 years of IPAQ use in Brazil and Colombia. *J. Phys. Act. Health* **2010**, *7* (Suppl. S2), S259–S264. [CrossRef] [PubMed]

25. McCormack, G.R.; Giles-Corti, B.; Bulsara, M. The relationship between destination proximity, destination mix and physical activity behaviors. *Prev. Med.* **2008**, *46*, 33–40. [CrossRef] [PubMed]

26. Heesch, K.C.; Giles-Corti, B.; Turrell, G. Cycling for transport and recreation: Associations with the socio-economic, natural and built environment. *Health Place* **2015**, *36*, 152–161. [CrossRef] [PubMed]

27. Guell, C.; Panter, J.; Ogilvie, D. Walking and cycling to work despite reporting an unsupportive environment: Insights from a mixed-method exploration of counterintuitive findings. *BMC Public Health* **2013**, *13*, 497. [CrossRef] [PubMed]

28. Rissel, C.E.; New, C.; Wen, L.M.; Merom, D.; Bauman, A.E.; Garrard, J. The effectiveness of community-based cycling promotion: Findings from the Cycling Connecting Communities project in Sydney, Australia. *Int. J. Behav. Nutr. Phys. Act.* **2010**, *7*, 8. [CrossRef] [PubMed]

29. Heesch, K.C.; Giles-Corti, B.; Turrell, G. Cycling for transport and recreation: Associations with socio-economic position, environmental perceptions, and psychological disposition. *Prev. Med.* **2014**, *63*, 29–35. [CrossRef] [PubMed]

30. Winters, M.; Teschke, K.; Brauer, M.; Fuller, D. Bike Score (R): Associations between urban bikeability and cycling behavior in 24 cities. *Int. J. Behav. Nutr. Phys. Act.* **2016**, *13*, 18. [CrossRef] [PubMed]

31. Wahlgren, L.; Schantz, P. Exploring bikeability in a suburban metropolitan area using the Active Commuting Route Environment Scale (ACRES). *Int. J. Environ. Res. Public Health* **2014**, *11*, 8276–8300. [CrossRef] [PubMed]

32. Reis, R.S.; Hino, A.A.; Parra, D.C.; Hallal, P.C.; Brownson, R.C. Bicycling and walking for transportation in three Brazilian cities. *Am. J. Prev. Med.* **2013**, *44*, e9–e17. [CrossRef] [PubMed]

33. Winters, M.; Teschke, K. Route preferences among adults in the near market for bicycling: Findings of the cycling in cities study. *Am. J. Health Promot.* **2010**, *25*, 40–47. [CrossRef] [PubMed]

34. Rachele, J.N.; Kavanagh, A.M.; Badland, H.; Giles-Corti, B.; Washington, S.; Turrell, G. Associations between individual socioeconomic position, neighbourhood disadvantage and transport mode: Baseline results from the HABITAT multilevel study. *J. Epidemiol. Community Health* **2015**, *69*, 1217–1223. [CrossRef] [PubMed]

35. Mueller, N.; Rojas-Rueda, D.; Cole-Hunter, T.; de Nazelle, A.; Dons, E.; Gerike, R.; Gotschi, T.; Int Panis, L.; Kahlmeier, S.; Nieuwenhuijsen, M. Health impact assessment of active transportation: A systematic review. *Prev. Med.* **2015**, *76*, 103–114. [CrossRef] [PubMed]

36. Tainio, M.; de Nazelle, A.J.; Gotschi, T.; Kahlmeier, S.; Rojas-Rueda, D.; Nieuwenhuijsen, M.J.; de Sa, T.H.; Kelly, P.; Woodcock, J. Can air pollution negate the health benefits of cycling and walking? *Prev. Med.* **2016**, *87*, 233–236. [CrossRef] [PubMed]

37. Torres, A.; Sarmiento, O.L.; Stauber, C.; Zarama, R. The Ciclovia and Cicloruta programs: Promising interventions to promote physical activity and social capital in Bogota, Colombia. *Am. J. Public Health* **2013**, *103*, e23–e30. [CrossRef] [PubMed]

38. Gomez, L.F.; Mosquera, J.; Gomez, O.L.; Moreno, J.; Pinzon, J.D.; Jacoby, E.; Cepeda, M.; Parra, D.C. Social conditions and urban environment associated with participation in the Ciclovia program among adults from Cali, Colombia. *Cad. Saude Publica* **2015**, *31* (Suppl. S1), 257–266. [PubMed]

39. Goodman, A.; Sahlqvist, S.; Ogilvie, D.; iConnect, C. New walking and cycling routes and increased physical activity: One- and 2-year findings from the UK iConnect Study. *Am. J. Public Health* **2014**, *104*, e38–e46. [CrossRef] [PubMed]

40. Oliver, L.N.; Schuurman, N.; Hall, A.W. Comparing circular and network buffers to examine the influence of land use on walking for leisure and errands. *Int. J. Health Geogr.* **2007**, *6*, 41. [CrossRef] [PubMed]

41. Giles-Corti, B.; Bull, F.; Knuiman, M.; McCormack, G.; Van Niel, K.; Timperio, A.; Christian, H.; Foster, S.; Divitini, M.; Middleton, N.; et al. The influence of urban design on neighbourhood walking following residential relocation: Longitudinal results from the RESIDE study. *Soc. Sci. Med.* **2013**, *77*, 20–30. [CrossRef] [PubMed]

42. Goenka, S.; Andersen, L.B. Urban design and transport to promote healthy lives. *Lancet* **2016**, *388*, 2851–2853. [CrossRef]

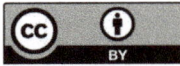

International Journal of
Environmental Research and Public Health

MDPI

Article

Estimating Vehicle Fuel Consumption and Emissions Using GPS Big Data

Zihan Kan [1], Luliang Tang [1,*], Mei-Po Kwan [2,3] and Xia Zhang [4]

[1] State Key Laboratory of Information Engineering in Surveying, Mapping and Remote Sensing, Wuhan University, 129 Luoyu Road, Wuhan 430079, China; kzh@whu.edu.cn
[2] Department of Geography & Geographic Information Science, University of Illinois at Urbana-Champaign, 1301 W Green Street, Urbana, IL 61801, USA; mpk654@gmail.com
[3] Department of Human Geography and Spatial Planning, Faculty of Geosciences, Utrecht University, P.O. Box 80125, 3508 TC Utrecht, The Netherlands
[4] School of Urban Design, Wuhan University, Wuhan 430070, China; xiazhang@whu.edu.cn
* Correspondence: tll@whu.edu.cn; Tel.: +86-027-6877-9788

Received: 14 February 2018; Accepted: 20 March 2018; Published: 21 March 2018

Abstract: The energy consumption and emissions from vehicles adversely affect human health and urban sustainability. Analysis of GPS big data collected from vehicles can provide useful insights about the quantity and distribution of such energy consumption and emissions. Previous studies, which estimated fuel consumption/emissions from traffic based on GPS sampled data, have not sufficiently considered vehicle activities and may have led to erroneous estimations. By adopting the analytical construct of the space-time path in time geography, this study proposes methods that more accurately estimate and visualize vehicle energy consumption/emissions based on analysis of vehicles' mobile activities (*MA*) and stationary activities (*SA*). First, we build space-time paths of individual vehicles, extract moving parameters, and identify *MA* and *SA* from each space-time path segment (STPS). Then we present an N-Dimensional framework for estimating and visualizing fuel consumption/emissions. For each STPS, fuel consumption, hot emissions, and cold start emissions are estimated based on activity type, i.e., *MA*, *SA* with engine-on and *SA* with engine-off. In the case study, fuel consumption and emissions of a single vehicle and a road network are estimated and visualized with GPS data. The estimation accuracy of the proposed approach is 88.6%. We also analyze the types of activities that produced fuel consumption on each road segment to explore the patterns and mechanisms of fuel consumption in the study area. The results not only show the effectiveness of the proposed approaches in estimating fuel consumption/emissions but also indicate their advantages for uncovering the relationships between fuel consumption and vehicles' activities in road networks.

Keywords: fuel consumption; emissions estimation; GPS trace; big data

---

1. Introduction

As urbanization accelerates, transport-related environmental issues deteriorate. The report of Intergovernmental Panel on Climate Change (IPCC) shows that 20–30% of total greenhouse gases (GHGs) are released from urban transportation operation including passenger and freight transportation [1]. Estimating and visualizing fuel consumption and emissions from transportation provide an understanding of the energy cost and air pollution caused by travel or transportation. However, previous studies often estimated fuel consumption/emissions without considering vehicles' activities and thus might lead to erroneous estimations. Therefore, this study proposes approaches that estimate and visualize vehicles' fuel consumption/emissions accurately by considering vehicles' mobile and stationary activities in a space-time-integrated framework with vehicles' GPS trajectories data.

Traditional ways to estimate air pollution rely on air pollution monitoring stations that are located at specific sites throughout a city. Data collected by these monitoring stations can be further used to evaluate the status of atmosphere according to clean air standards and historical information. While these data are more reliable, monitoring stations are expensive to set up and maintain [2], and thus there are usually a very limited number of monitoring stations in a particular city. For the emissions and fuel consumption from the transportation sector, although it is recognized that vehicular emissions and fuel consumption play a significant role in air pollution and energy consumption, the exact volume and spatial distribution of pollution/fuel consumption of vehicles remain unknown. As the exact volume emissions and fuel consumption can only be measured with professional equipment installed on individual vehicles, such measurement can hardly be implemented in practice. Therefore, emissions and fuel consumption estimation approaches have been widely investigated in past decades.

At early stages, some researchers estimated fuel consumption/emissions from aggregate fuel-used data at a large spatiotemporal scale [3]. However, these studies only provided a rough estimation due to a lack of information about vehicle technology and moving parameters. In past decades, energy/emission estimation models, such as the U.S. EPA's MOBILE and MOVES models, European Commission's COPERT model, California's EMFAC and IVE model, have been extensively developed [4–8]. In these models, vehicle technology data and moving parameters are necessary for estimating fuel consumption/emissions. In order to collect these data and estimate fuel consumption/emissions with the estimation models, surveys and sensors that are installed in some segments of a road such as loop detectors [9] and video cameras [10] have been used in the literature. However, details of vehicles' driving parameters are absent in survey data and loop detector data. Large-scale survey data can only provide vehicle technology and rough driving speeds in a city or a nation, and loop detector data only contains traffic information collected at specific locations on roads that are not representative enough for the driving parameters over larger road segments. Therefore, survey data and loop detector data can only be employed to estimate fuel consumption/emissions at a coarse spatial resolution, or as a supplement to other estimation approaches.

The rapid development of data collection, storage, and networking have created an environment with big data infiltrating many aspects of society and technology. As an important component of big data, GPS trajectory data are widely used due to their large coverage, good continuity, low cost, as well as rich information about vehicles' movements. Vehicle trajectories contain rich information about vehicles' driving modes and traffic states, which could be used to fit emission models to obtain more accurate emissions estimations. Early studies used vehicle trajectory data to estimate macroscopic pollutant emissions at the city scale [11]. In recent years, some researchers proposed emissions estimation methods that used GPS tracks of vehicles [2,12–15]. These methods quantified fuel consumption and emissions using emission models based on the premise that the amount of pollution emitted by a vehicle mainly depends on load and moving parameters [16]. For example, Sun et al. [13] and Shang et al. [14] reconstructed traffic volume from GPS data so that traffic-related emissions can be estimated based on the trajectories of sampled vehicles and the developed estimation model.

Among all kinds of vehicles' trajectory data, taxis trajectory data have become a popular data source for traffic monitoring and fuel consumption/emissions estimation, as taxis are important part of urban transportation systems and account for a large share of urban traffic flows. Gühnemann et al. [11] estimated traffic NOx emissions using GPS data from a fleet of taxis using an average speed-dependent estimation model. Based on the COPERT model, Shang et al. [14] analyzed the patterns of fuel consumption/emissions in Beijing using taxi GPS trajectory data. Luo et al. [17] analyzed the spatial-temporal patterns of taxis' fuel consumption/emissions as well as the relationships between taxis' travel patterns and fuel consumption/emissions. These studies estimated fuel consumption/emissions with low-sampling GPS data of 30–60 seconds. They adopted macroscopic estimation models that take variables such as vehicle category constitution, fuel parameters, emission legislation, and average speed of vehicles into consideration but did not need detailed parameters of vehicles' driving modes such as accelerations in the estimation.

In order to distinguish the different driving modes of vehicles (acceleration, deceleration, idling and cruising) and estimate the fuel consumption/emissions of vehicles in a more fine-grained way, some researchers adopted high-resolution GPS data and microscopic estimation models in their work. Nikoleris et al. [18] proposed a detailed estimation of fuel consumption and emissions using aircraft position data. Engine emissions inventories which provide fuel flows and emission indices as a function of engine thrust were used in their study. Zhao et al. [15] estimated CO_2 emissions using taxi GPS data and analyzed the relationships between CO_2 emissions and trip purposes. The estimations in their study was based on a microscopic model that considers instantaneous driving modes of vehicles, whereas the GPS data in their study were sampled at 60 s, indicating that the data could not reflect vehicles' instantaneous condition. Sun et al. [13] estimated emissions of vehicles under different driving modes (e.g., acceleration, idle, cruise and deceleration) with variables of second-by-second speed profiles. Nyhan et al. [2] estimated taxi emissions in Singapore based on the microscopic emission model proposed by Osorio and Nanduri [19], in which instantaneous speed, instantaneous acceleration, vehicle type and fuel type are all needed in the estimation. High-frequency GPS data (less than 5 s) were used in the study to obtain the instantaneous moving parameters. Although the parameters of the driving modes of vehicles contained in high-resolution GPS data result in more-accurate estimations, high-frequency GPS data are not used in many studies due to the additional cost in data collection and storage, as well as the complexity and computational inefficiency in estimation. Despite the lower-resolution of macroscopic models, the analytical structural information they provide can contribute to enhancing the computational efficiency of fuel consumption/emissions estimations [19].

While driving mode parameters such as acceleration and deceleration can be obtained with high-resolution GPS data, existing studies estimating fuel consumption/emissions with GPS trajectory data lack analysis of vehicles' stationary activities. In a movement path, an activity conducted by a vehicle from one location to another location is a mobile activity (*MA*), and an activity conducted in a fixed location is a stationary activity (*SA*). An *SA* of a vehicle may occur under conditions of engine-on or engine-off. For an *SA* with engine-on, vehicles consume fuel and release emissions. Estimating factors of fuel consumption/emissions of *SA*s with engine-on are different with *MA*s. For an *SA* with engine-off, vehicles do not consume fuel or release emissions. However, additional cold start emissions are released when a vehicle restarts. Previous studies did not analyze different types of *SA*s in vehicle trajectories. As a result, hot emissions generated when the vehicle's engine is running and cold start emissions released during the engine's warming-up phase cannot be distinguished. Research results show that about 20% of the total emissions from vehicles are cold start emissions [20]. Therefore, the distinction between hot emissions and cold start emissions is important due to the substantial differences in vehicular emission performance during those two phases, and a different approach is required to estimate over-emissions during the engine's warming-up period.

Table 1 illustrates the characteristics of data and models in the aforementioned studies and this study. For each study, Table 1 lists the resolution of GPS trajectory data, the emissions model used in each study, whether driving modes and stationary activities are considered, and whether hot emissions and cold start emissions are distinguished. For the emission models in the table, the basic variables of emissions and fuel consumption estimation include vehicle category, fuel type and travel speed of vehicles. While parameters of road condition such as road type and slope are available in the COPERT model that is used in studies [14,17], and the CMEM model used in study [13], such parameters have not been widely used for estimating emissions and fuel consumption in practice due to the lack of data. This study estimates vehicles' consumption/emissions based on the COPERT model, which is a typical mathematical model. Based on distinguishing vehicle categories, fuel types and other parameters, the COPERT model determines the emission of different pollutants and consumption by performing regression analysis for speeds of vehicles and volume of emissions/consumption. As the operating conditions and engine technologies of the test vehicles in the COPERT model are similar to that of the experiments in this study, the estimated emissions/consumption are considered closer to the true value. The key estimation parameters in the COPERT model include constitution of fleet, average speed, average mileage, fuel parameters, load and slope, among which the default value of average mileage is provided in case that the parameter is absent in estimation. Therefore, based on the determination of all the parameters in the COPERT model, the emissions/consumption factors are modeled as functions of average speed of vehicles. In contrast, the microscopic estimation models in studies [2,13,18] can simulate the instantaneous moving conditions of vehicles and hence generate more accurate estimations. In that case, instantaneous acceleration is a better parameter to model the engines' thrust compared with instantaneous speed and average speed. The parameters of vehicle engines such as type, age or other performance parameters are very important in some microscopic models such as the CMEM model (in study [13]) which investigate the physical relationships between the instantaneous operating states of vehicles and instantaneous emissions/consumption. These estimation models can simulate the emissions/consumption accurately while they have not been widely used in large-scale emission/consumption estimations as engine parameters are hard to acquire.

Table 1. Data and models in recent studies.

Models	Resolution of GPS Data		Emission Model		Driving Modes Analysis	Stationary Activity Analysis	Hot/Cold Start Emissions Estimation
	High	Low	Macro	Micro			
Gühnemann et al. [11]		√	√				
Shang et al. [14]		√	√				
Luo et al. [17]		√	√				
Zhao et al. [15]		√		√			
Sun et al. [13]	√			√	√		
Nikoleris et al. [18]	√			√	√		
Nyhan et al. [2]	√			√	√		
This study		√	√			√	√

Table 1 shows that recent studies that used low-resolution GPS data included average moving parameters such as average speed into macroscopic estimation models to estimate fuel consumption/emissions of a road segment. However, it is difficult to identify driving modes such as acceleration, idling, deceleration and cruising in these studies due to the low resolution of the data. While research conducted with high-resolution GPS data includes driving mode analysis, stationary activities analysis is absent in these studies. As a result, different phases of emissions over a particular driving cycle are not distinguished in recent studies with both low-resolution and high-resolution data. Therefore, the purpose of this article is to estimate vehicles' fuel consumption/emissions more accurately by taking into account vehicles' activity types.

In order to differentiate cold start emissions and hot emissions in a vehicle's driving cycle, *MAs*, *SAs* with engine-on and *SAs* with engine-off need to be analyzed first. In this study, we analyze different types of vehicle activities based on the space-time path of individual vehicles. The space-time path was developed by Hägerstrand [21] and his colleagues at Lund University as a component of the time-geographic framework, which is a powerful approach for analyzing movement patterns of individuals in space and time. Originally, time geography was used mainly to investigate the movement and activity-travel patterns of humans [22–26]. It was later applied to transportation networks [27–29]. One of the core problems in time geography is to visually represent different elements through a 3-D space-time framework [23,30]. A space-time path portrays the trajectory of an object in a 3-D orthogonal system consisting of two spatial dimensions (a plane) and a vertical temporal dimension. Not only people's activity patterns [23,24,31,32] but also moving parameters in one's trajectory [25] can be represented by space-time paths.

This study proposes approaches that accurately estimate and visualize vehicles' energy consumption/emissions based on analysis of vehicles' mobile activities (*MA*) and stationary activities (*SA*). Different phases of emissions over a particular driving cycle, i.e., hot emissions and cold start emissions are estimated based on activity analysis. In the case study, fuel consumption and emissions of a single vehicle and a road network are estimated and visualized with GPS trajectory data. We also analyze the types of activities that produced fuel consumption on each road segment to explore the patterns and mechanisms of fuel consumption in the study area. To our best knowledge, this is the first study to estimate different phases of taxi emissions with GPS trajectory data and the first study to distinguish stationary and moving activities in fuel consumption/emissions estimation.

2. Materials and Methods

2.1. Data

This study first estimates fuel consumption and emissions for an experimental vehicle and verify the estimating accuracy of fuel consumption, then estimates fuel consumption and emissions for an experimental area with taxis' GPS trace data.

2.1.1. A Single Trajectory with Real Fuel Consumption

We first estimate the fuel consumption and emissions for a gasoline vehicle with its GPS trajectories. The GPS trajectory data were collected from an experimental vehicle of our project team, and its real fuel consumption was recorded during the time period of experiment (from 23 March to 25 March 2016) to validate the estimation methods. The GPS data have an approximate sampling interval of 10 s, a minimum sampling interval of 6 s, a maximum sampling interval of 16 s, an average sampling interval of 10.56 s and a standard deviation of the sampling interval of 0.52 s. A description of the data is shown in Table 2, where "VID" represents the vehicle's ID, "Time" denotes the sampling timestamp when a record was generated, "Longitude" and "Latitude" are the geographic location of the vehicle at the timestamp. In order to estimate the fuel consumption and emissions more accurately, the temperatures are needed, which are 12 °C, 9 °C and 10 °C on 23–25 March, respectively.

Table 2. Description of GPS data of a gasoline experimental vehicle from 23 March to 25 March 2016.

VID	Time	Longitude	Latitude
1	2016-03-23 8:00:00	114.3550441	30.5604297
1	2016-03-23 8:00:09	114.3550441	30.5604297
1	2016-03-23 8:00:20	114.3549372	30.5601104
1	2016-03-25 17:59:50	114.35481	30.559673
1	2015-03-25 18:00:01	114.3550441	30.5604297

We recorded the real fuel consumption for verifying the estimating accuracy of the proposed approach. The detailed information of the vehicle model, fuel, and real fuel consumption are shown in Table 3. The GPS data and space-time paths of the vehicle are shown in Figure 1.

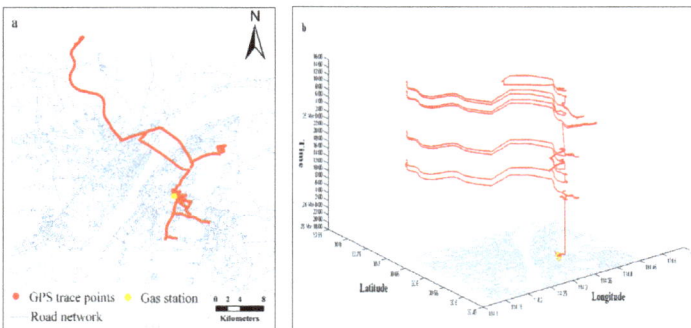

Figure 1. The vehicle's GPS trace and space-time path. (**a**) Shows the GPS traces of the vehicle and (**b**) Describes the space-time path built from GPS trace.

Table 3. Vehicle and fuel parameters of the experimental vehicle and real fuel consumption.

Vehicle Parameter	Model	Year	Engine Capacity
	Buick Park Avenue	2009	3.0 L
Fuel Parameter	Gasoline label Number	Density	
	No. 97	0.737 g/mL	
Real Fuel Consumption	40.66 kg		

2.1.2. The Experimental Network Area and Taxi GPS Dataset

Second, we use GPS data to estimate the fuel consumption an emissions for an experimental area in Wuhan, China. The GPS data were obtained from the Wuhan Transportation Bureau, which were collected from 6658 taxis operating in the urban area of Wuhan on 6 May 2015 (Friday). The taxis account for about 44% of all the taxis in the urban area.

The taxi GPS trajectories were sampled at an approximate time interval of 60 s (the minimum sampling interval is 11 s, the maximum sampling interval is 121 s, the average sampling interval is 62.9 s and the standard deviation of the sampling interval is 20.5 s), with a position accuracy of approximately 15 m. A description of the taxi GPS data is shown in Table 4, where "VID" stands for the taxi's ID, "Time" is the sampling time when a record was generated, "Longitude" and "Latitude" are the geographic location of the taxi, and "Direction" represents the taxi's driving direction, "Speed" provides the instantaneous velocity (km/h), "Status" represents the taxi's passenger status (1 denotes an occupied status and 0 indicates a vacant status). The temperature on 6 May 2015 is 21.5 °C. The road network in the study area is shown in Figure 2, in which the road names are abbreviated.

Table 4. Description of GPS data of taxi GPS data in Wuhan, on 6 May 2015.

VID	Time	Longitude	Latitude	Direction	Speed	Status
1001	2015-05-06 00:00:00	114.260889	30.583315	265	20	0
1001	2015-05-06 00:01:01	114.260765	30.583395	190	40	0
1001	2015-05-06 00:02:00	114.260765	30.583415	188	19	0
1002	2015-05-06 08:01:02	114.26122	30.583289	120	10	1
1002	2015-05-06 08:02:00	114.26089	30.583322	30	29	1

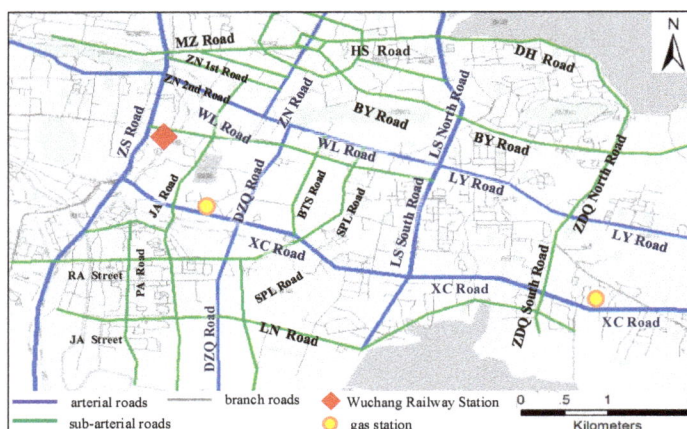

Figure 2. Road network in the experimental area.

2.2. Methods

This section describes fuel consumption/emissions estimation based on space-time path segment (STPS). We present an N-dimensional framework for estimating and visualizing fuel consumption/emissions of both an individual vehicle and a network area. Hot emissions and cold start emissions of each STPS are also distinguished based on activity types.

2.2.1. Building Space-Time Path and Extracting Moving Parameters

Based on the vehicles' GPS data, this study first builds space-time paths for individual vehicles according to the locations and timestamp of each GPS track point. A space-time path depicts the movements of individuals in both space and time. Each space-time path comprises a series of space-time path segments (STPS), which are the line segments between consecutive track points. In this section, we build space-time path of an individual vehicle and extract moving parameters of each STPS. The space-time path of an individual in space-time coordinate is as Figure 3 shows.

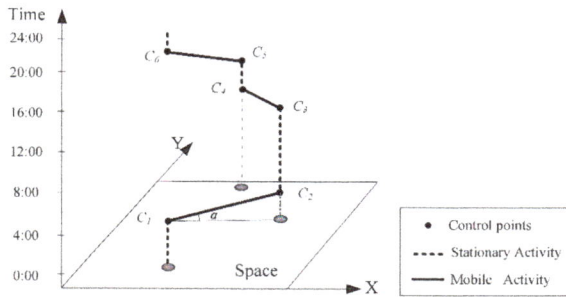

Figure 3. 3-D Space–time coordinate and individual space-time path.

In Figure 3, the space-time path P^m for an individual m consists of a sequence of control points and a corresponding sequence of STPSs connecting the control points [33]. The control points are a finite list of observations in chronological order, normally collected by location sensors such as GPS devices. Each control point, c_i, consists of a tuple:

$$c_i = <Loc_i, t_i> \tag{1}$$

where Loc_i is the location and t_i the time stamp. The STPS s_i between adjacent control points c_i and c_{i+1} is a straight line segment:

$$s_i = <c_i, c_{i+1}> \tag{2}$$

It is assumed that the individual is moving at a constant speed in each STPS [33], based on which the speed of the STPS s_i is:

$$v_i = \frac{\|s_i\|}{t_{i+1} - t_i} \tag{3}$$

where $\|s_i\|$ is the length of STPS s_i. If the instantaneous velocity of each control point v' is recorded, average acceleration a_i of an STPS s_i can be calculated by:

$$a_i = \frac{v'_{i+1} - v'_i}{t_{i+1} - t_i} \tag{4}$$

In time geography, each STPS represents at least one activity, which consists of two adjacent GPS track points. As is shown in Figure 3, an activity conducted from one location to another location is a mobile activity (*MA*), depicted by a tilted line segment (the solid line in Figure 3), and an activity conducted at a fixed location is a stationary activity (*SA*), depicted by a vertical line segment (dashed line in Figure 3). In this article, *MA* and *SA* can be defined by:

$$MA = \{(Loc(S), T_S), (Loc(E), T_E), \mid\mid Loc(E) - Loc(S)\mid \geq \delta\} \tag{5}$$

$$SA = \{(Loc(S), T_S), (Loc(E), T_E), \mid\mid Loc(E) - Loc(S)\mid < \delta\} \tag{6}$$

where $Loc(S)$ and $Loc(E)$ are locations of start and end points of activities, T_S and T_E the start and end times. In Equations (5) and (6), $Loc(S)$, $Loc(E)$, T_S and T_E can be obtained through the coordinates and timestamp of the adjacent GPS track points. Besides, the threshold δ can be set according to the GPS positional error (approximately 15 meters in this study). For each activity, if the distance between the adjacent GPS track points is smaller than δ, there is a stationary activity (*SA*); if the distance between the adjacent GPS track points is larger than δ, there is a mobile activity (*MA*). The value of δ would impact the classification of activity and the estimation of cold start emissions because cold start emissions are closely related to vehicles' stop behaviors. Setting the value of δ too high would lead to misidentifications of *MAs* as *SAs*, resulting in overestimations of cold start emissions. Setting the value of δ too low would lead to misidentifications of *SAs* as *MAs*, resulting in underestimations of cold start emissions.

2.2.2. An N-Dimensional Representation for Fuel Consumption/Emissions Based on Space-Time Path

Based on individual space-time path, we present an N-dimensional representation for visually estimating fuel consumption/emissions and representing different multi-dimensional information based on STPS. Each STPS contains multi-dimensional information of individuals including space and time, fuel consumption/emissions, moving parameters (e.g., speed, acceleration) and other individual attributes (e.g., human or vehicle, age, gender). Therefore, in the N-dimensional representation describing N attributes of individuals, a space-time path consisting of *M* STPS can be described as a M×N matrix, as Equation (7) shows:

$$P = \begin{bmatrix} S_1.Time & S_1.Location & S_1.speed & \dots & S_1.consumption & S_1.emissions \\ S_2.Time & S_2.Location & S_2.speed & \dots & S_2.consumption & S_2.emissions \\ \dots & \dots & \dots & & \dots & \dots \\ S_M.Time & S_M.Location & S_M.speed & \dots & S_M.consumption & S_M.emissions \end{bmatrix}_{M \times N} \tag{7}$$

The visualizing framework of the N-Dimensional model is shown in Figure 4, where each STPS is attached with different dimensions of information represented by rectangles with different colors.

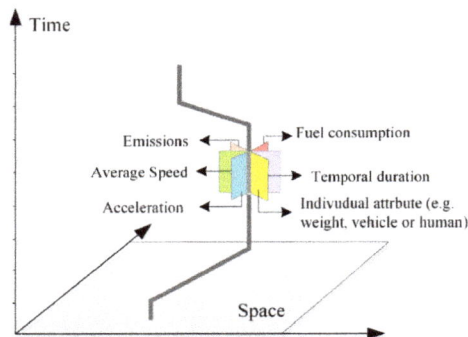

Figure 4. N-dimensional model of individual space-time path.

The N-dimensional representation of moving parameters is shown in Figure 5. In the representation, different dimensional information of each STPS is represented by attached rectangles with different colors. In the representation of acceleration, there is no speed but acceleration for STPSs 4 and 6 because they are SAs with engine-on, and there are no speed and acceleration dimensions for STPSs 1 and 8 because they are SAs with engine-off.

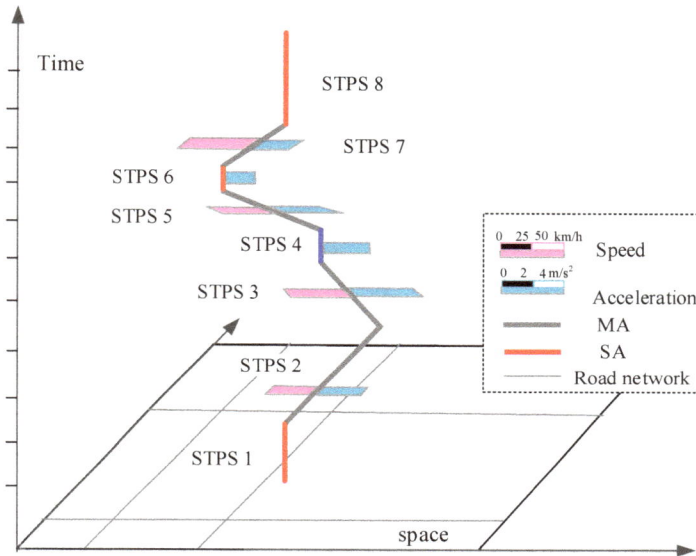

Figure 5. N-Dimensional representation of moving parameters.

2.2.3. Estimating Fuel Consumption/Emissions Based on Individual Space-Time Path

In this section, we estimate fuel consumption and emissions on an STPS basis. Hot emissions and cold start emissions of each STPS are also distinguished based on the determination of vehicles' activity types.

Firstly, we determine the operating conditions of vehicles. Section 2.2.1 demonstrates that each STPS represents either a mobile activity (*MA*) or a stationary activity (*SA*). For an *MA* STPS, fuel consumption and emissions can be estimated according to moving parameters such as average speed. While operating conditions of *SA* STPS need to be further distinguished in fuel consumption/emissions estimation, as an *SA* may happen with the engine-on or with engine-off. In both situations, the average speeds of an STPS are zero. However, for *SAs* with engine-off, vehicles do not consume fuel or release emissions, but for *SAs* with engine-on, vehicles need to consume fuel and thus release emissions to keep the engines running. Therefore, this article infers vehicles' operating conditions from stay time of an *SA* and GPS sampling frequency, as Figure 6 shows. Figure 6a represents a *SA* with engine-on, in which the locations of the vehicle is recorded at a sampled frequency during the stay time. Figure 6b depicts an *SA* with engine-off, in which there are no GPS points recorded during the stay time of the *SA*.

Secondly, we estimate fuel consumption and emissions of *MAs* based on COPERT model [4]. This article adopts COPERT model in the estimation of *MAs* because the vehicles that the data are collected from in the case study follow European-3 emission standard. We estimate the consumption and emissions from average speeds and lengths of each STPS. We first estimate fuel consumption for each STPS, then estimate hot emissions and cold start emissions for each STPS.

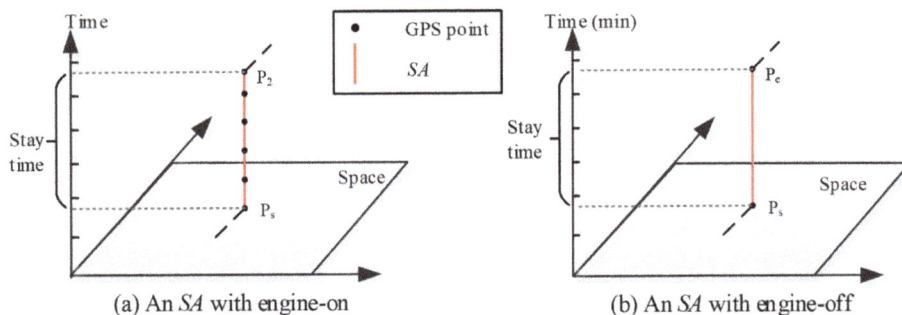

Figure 6. Vehicles' *SA* with (**a**) Engine-on and (**b**) Engine-off.

- Fuel Consumption Estimation

In COPERT model, the fuel consumption for *MAs* of gasoline passenger cars with a capacity of 1.4 L–2.0 L is estimated according to Equation (8), where *FC* is the fuel consumption factor (g/km) of each STPS, and *V* is the average speed of each STPS:

$$FC_{MA} = (217 + 0.253V + 0.00965V^2)/(1 + 0.096V - 0.000421V^2) \tag{8}$$

Because COPERT model doesn't contain the emissions factor of *SAs* with engine-on, the fuel consumption for *SAs* with engine-on is estimated based on four-mode elemental fuel model [34,35], as Equation (9) shows, where the unit for *FC* is milliliters, and *T* is stay time(seconds) of an *SA*:

$$FC_{SA} = 0.361*T \tag{9}$$

Therefore, fuel consumption (FC) for the space-time path of a vehicle that includes fuel consumption for both *MAs* and *SAs* with engine-on can be calculated based on Equations (8) and (9):

$$FC = FC_{MA}*Dist + FC_{SA}*\sigma \tag{10}$$

where *Dist* is the driving distance for a vehicle and δ is the density of the fuel. For gasoline, σ = 0.77 g/mL.

- Emissions Estimation

For *SAs* with engine-off, there are no emissions. For other activities, the total emissions are composed of three components, which are:

$$E_{TOTAL} = E_{HOT} + E_{COLD} + E_{EVAP} \tag{11}$$

In Equation (11), E_{TOTAL} is total emissions of a certain pollutant. E_{HOT} refers to the emissions under the condition of thermal stability of the engine. E_{COLD} is the emission during starting process of the engine. E_{EVAP} is the emission caused by temperature changes. This study estimates hot emissions and cold start emissions because of their prominence in the total emissions.

Figure 7 illustrates hot and cold start emissions as a function of time after a vehicle restart with its engine and catalyst reaching ambient temperature. Cold start emissions are initially high but decrease as the temperatures of engine and catalyst increase, followed by a stable phase when the normal operational temperatures have been reached. The duration of the first cold-start phase is signified by t_{cold}, and the emission during cold-start phase is given by E_{cold}, as shaded area shows. Whereas hot emission rate keeps stable with time, and the emission during thermally stable operation is given by E_{hot}.

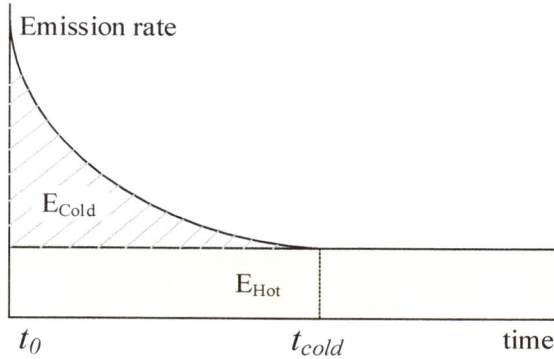

Figure 7. Hot and cold start emissions with time.

(1)   Hot Emission

Hot emissions for *MAs* are determined by the average-speed-dependent baseline emission factor and vehicle's mileage correction and fuel effect correction. Generally, the hot emission factors after legislation Euro-1 is represented by Equation (12):

$$EF_{MA} = (a + cV + eV^2)/(1 + bV + dV^2) \tag{12}$$

where EF_{MA} is the hot emission factor for an *MA*, denoted by the mass per kilometer (g/km), V the average speed, and a-e parameters in emission determination. For example, for gasoline passenger cars with a capacity of 1.4 L–2.0 L under Euro-3 standards, the parameters a-e for CO, NO_x and Hydrocarbon are shown in Table 5.

Table 5. Parameters of emission factors for different pollutants in COPERT model.

Pollutants	a	b	c	d	e
CO	71.7	35.4	11.4	−0.248	0
NO_x	9.29×10^{-2}	-1.22×10^{-2}	-1.49×10^{-3}	3.97×10^{-5}	6.53×10^{-6}
Hydrocarbon	5.57×10^{-2}	3.65×10^{-2}	-1.1×10^{-3}	-1.88×10^{-4}	1.25×10^{-5}

For *SAs* with engine-on, the emissions is estimated as Equation (13) shows [34,35], where the unit for *EF* is milliliters, and *T* is stay time(seconds) of an *SA* for CO, NOx and Hydrocarbon, α equals to 13.889, 0.566 and 2.222, respectively:

$$EF_{SA} = \alpha^*T \tag{13}$$

In this way, emissions for the space-time path of a vehicle that includes fuel consumption for both *MAs* and *SAs* with engine-on can be calculated based on Equations (12) and (13) and as shown in Equation (14), where *Dist* is the driving distance for a vehicle and δ is the density of the fuel. For gasoline, σ =0.77 g/mL:

$$EF = EF_{MA}^*Dist + EF_{SA}^*\sigma \tag{14}$$

(2)   Cold Start Emissions

Cold start emissions are produced when a vehicle restarts and depend on parameters such as engine and catalyst temperature when the vehicle restart, ambient temperature, moving speed, and distance of the new trip. The parameter of engine/catalyst temperature when a vehicle starts is important in the cold start emission estimation but is hard to obtain. However, the engine/catalyst temperature can be inferred according to ambient temperature and the vehicle's parking time with engine-off. Therefore, we adopt a method which models cold start emissions as a function of ambient temperature T, average speed V, traveled distance d and parking duration t [36]. The parking duration is the stay time of SAs with engine-off in this study.

In the model, the cold start emission (gram) per start can be calculated by:

$$E_{cold}(T, V, \delta, t) = f(T, V)*h(\varsigma)*g(t) \qquad (15)$$

where ς is dimensionless distance. The functions $f(T, V)$, $h(\delta)$ and $g(t)$ for CO, HC and NOx are given in Table 6.

Table 6. Functions for cold start emissions estimation per start.

Pollutants	$f(T, V)$	$h(\varsigma)$	$g(t)$
CO	$4.291 - 0.176*T + 0.012V$	$(1 - e^{-7.288\delta})/(1 - e^{-7.288})$	(1) $4.614 \times 10^{-3} t - 2.302 \times 10^{-6} t^2 - 2.966 \times 10^{-9} t^3$ ($t \le 720$ min) (2) 1 ($t > 720$ min)
HC	$9.093 - 0.459*T + 0.054V$	$(1 - e^{-8.624\delta})/(1 - e^{-8.624})$	(1) $7.641 \times 10^{-3} t^{-2} - 2.639 \times 10^{-5} t^2 + 3.128 \times 10^{-8} t^3$ ($t \le 240$ min) (2) $0.625 + 5.208 \times 10^{-4} t$ ($240 \le t \le 720$ min) (3) 1 ($t > 720$ min)
NOx	$0.808 - 0.005*T + 0.015V$	$(1 - e^{-0.739\delta})/(1 - e^{-0.739})$	(1) $7.141 \times 10^{-3} t + 1.568 \times 10^{-3} t^2 - 3.204 \times 10^{-5} t^3 + 1.594 \times 10^{-7} t^4$ ($t \le 50$ min) (2) $1.290 - 4.030 \times 10^{-4} t$ ($50 \le t \le 720$ min) (3) 1 ($t > 720$ min)

Finally, fuel consumption (FC) and different kinds of emissions can be estimated according to the Equations (8)–(15). Based on the estimation, we represent multi-dimensional information of each STPS using the proposed N-dimensional model, as Figure 8 shows.

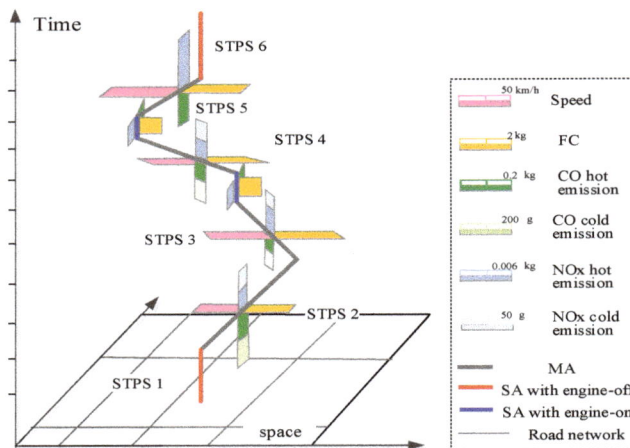

Figure 8. Representation of multi-dimensional information in N-Dimensional framework.

In Figure 8, speed, fuel consumption, CO and NOx emissions of each STPS are represented by attached rectangles with different colors. STPSs representing MAs and SAs with engine-on are attached with fuel consumption and emissions, but there is no fuel consumption or emissions on SAs with engine-off. In the space-time path, the rectangles for cold start emissions are only attached in STPSs

2–4, because cold start emissions are released after a vehicle's stop with engine-off and restart, and last for a period. After the engine has got its normal operating temperature, there are only hot emissions.

2.2.4. Estimating Fuel Consumption/Emissions for Road Network

After get the fuel consumption and emissions for individual space-time path, we estimate fuel consumption/emissions for road network based on STPS. For a time interval [ts, te], fuel consumption/emissions volume for a road is estimated according to Equation (16):

$$Vol_j^k(ts, te) = \sum_{i=1}^{N} \int_{ts}^{te} [EF_i^k(v) \cdot (P_i(t) \cap R_j)] dt \tag{16}$$

where k is the category of fuel consumption/emissions, j is the jth road in the study area, $Vol_j^k(ts, te)$ is the fuel consumption/emissions volume for a road j in a time period [ts, te]. N denotes the number of space-time paths in the experimental area. $P_i(t)$ is the space-time path of an individual i, because the locations of an individual are considered as a function of time. $EF_i^k(v)$ is the fuel consumption/emission factor (kg/km) for a fuel consumption/emission k and a space-time path i. $P_i(t) \cap R_j$ represent the intersection of a space-time path i and road j. $EF_i^k(v) \cdot (P_i(t) \cap R_j)$ indicates the volume of fuel consumption/emissions k of an individual i on road j at time instant t. Therefore, Equation (16) represents the volume of fuel consumption/emissions k for a road in a time interval [ts, te].

Figure 9 illustrates the visual estimation and representation of fuel consumption/emissions for a single road and road network. STPSs during the time interval [ts, te] and matched to Road j are firstly identified. Then for each STPS, we estimate fuel consumption/emissions, and lastly we add up the fuel consumption/emissions of all STPSs to obtain fuel consumption/emissions for each road in the road network area.

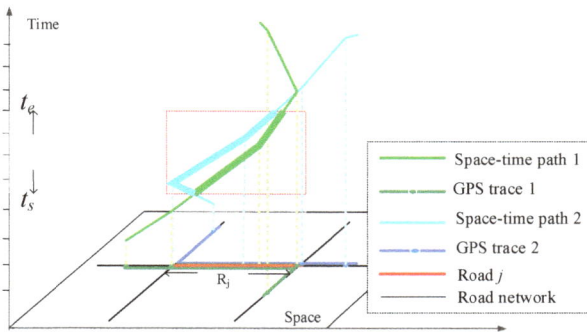

Figure 9. Fuel consumption/emissions estimation for road network.

3. Results

3.1. Estimating Fuel Consumption and Emissions for a Single Trace

First, we determine the activity types (*SA* or *MA*), calculate the average speed of each STPS, and get 3975 *MAs* and 2528 *SAs*. Then we analyze the running condition for each *SA* and obtain 357 *SAs* with engine-on and 2171 *SAs* with engine-off. After that, fuel consumption of *MAs* and *SAs* with engine-on are estimated based on the COPERT model. As a result, fuel consumption of the whole space-time path is calculated based on the fuel consumption of *MAs* and *SAs* with engine-on. The estimation results are compared with the estimated result from the average speed of the vehicle's trajectories [11] and results from the average speed between adjacent GPS points [13], as shown in Table 7.

Table 7 shows the comparison results of three estimating approaches using GPS trajectories for estimating fuel consumption of the experimental vehicle. The first approach [11] uses the average speed of a whole trajectory and the total travel distance for estimating fuel consumption. This approach overestimates the fuel consumption (57.25 kg) because it takes all types of activities in a trajectory into estimation including *SA*s with engine-off, which actually produce no fuel consumption or emissions.

Table 7. Comparison of fuel consumption estimation results of average speed based approach and STPS-based approach in this article.

Estimating Approaches	Average Speed (km/h)	Fuel Consumption Factor (g/km)	Travel Distance (km)	Fuel Consumption Estimated (kg)	Real Fuel Consumption (kg)	Accuracy
Average speed of a vehicle [11]	22.23	116.64		57.25		71.02%
Average speed of trace points [13]	Depend on GPS trace points		490.84	31.79	40.66	78.2%
Proposed STPS-based approach	Depend on each STPS			45.31		88.6%

As a result, the first approach gets a relatively low accuracy of 71.02%. In the second approach [13], speed and distance of each pair of adjacent GPS points are calculated, according to which fuel consumption is estimated. The second approach takes the changes of speeds in the trajectory into consideration, and hence gets a better result than the first approach with an accuracy of 78.2%. However, the activity types are not distinguished in the second approach. For example, a parked vehicle (with engine-off) or an idling vehicle (with engine-on) both have speeds of zero, but they have different fuel consumptions. The second approach takes all types of activities with speed of zero as *SA*s with engine-off and with no fuel consumption. The estimating result shows that it underestimates the fuel consumption because of undifferentiated estimation of activity types. In contrast, the STPS-based approach in this study estimates fuel consumption based on activity types of each STPS. We calculate the speed and distance of each STPS, determine the activity types of each STPS (*MA*, *SA* with engine-on or *SA* with engine-off), and estimate the fuel consumption of each *MA* and *SA* with engine-on. The estimation results illustrate that accuracy is significantly improved (88.6%) when compared with the other two estimation approaches (71.02% and 78.2%), which indicates that the STPS-based approach this study develops can better restore the running condition of vehicles.

Nevertheless, there is also a gap between the estimations of this study and the real value. There are probably two reasons for the error. First, since any estimation model cannot fully simulate all the emission/consumption-related factors—such as the continuous conditions of vehicle engines, road conditions, ambient environments, and driving behaviours—all estimation models can only estimate the results as close to the real value as possible rather than generate completely accurate estimations. Second, this study estimates emission/fuel consumption based on the COPERT model, which is a mathematical model that determines the emission of different pollutants and consumption by performing regression analysis for speeds of different types of vehicles and the volume of emissions/consumption. Because the COPERT model takes the average speed as the key parameter in estimation without simulating the instantaneous conditions of vehicles, the estimated results would have errors when compared to the real values. For example, within the time period of a sampling interval, a vehicle may maintain a constant speed or it may accelerate then decelerate. In both cases the average speeds are the same but the emissions and fuel consumption are different. Therefore, using high-resolution data with small sampling intervals can reduce the error because fine sampling can reduce the uncertainty of vehicles' driving modes within the sampling interval. Since the instantaneous parameters are not available in many practical cases, this study develops an estimating method that can be applied to large-scale GPS datasets and can be used to estimate emissions/fuel consumption more accurately than other average-speed-based methods by considering different types of activities.

Figure 10 shows the N-dimensional representation of a part of space-time path of the experimental vehicle's trace. Two *SA*s are identified in the space-time path. The first *SA* (the blue line) is an *SA* with engine-on, so fuel consumption and emissions are estimated for it. Whereas the second *SA* (the red line) is an *SA* with engine-off, so there is no fuel consumption and emissions. In addition, from Section 2.2.3 we know that cold start emissions are produced after a vehicle's engine shuts down and restart. Therefore, cold start emissions are estimated for the STPS after the *SA* with engine-off, according to Equation (15).

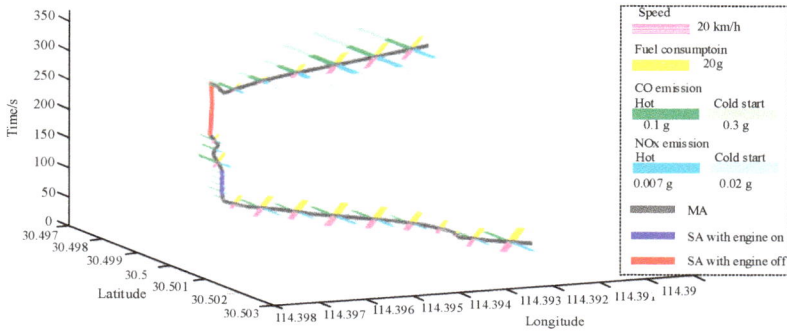

Figure 10. N-dimensional representation of a part of space-time path in a single trace.

3.2. Estimating and Analyzing Fuel Consumption/Emissions for a Network Area

Using the taxi GPS dataset, we firstly match the GPS points to the road network, and build space-time paths for all traces according to the recorded timestamps and locations. With the GPS points matched to the road network, we can restore the routes of the taxis and obtain more accurate distances and speeds. Then *MA*s, *SA*s with engine-on and *SA*s with engine-off are distinguished based on average speed and stay time of each STPS. As a result, fuel consumption, hot emissions and cold start emissions of each STPS are estimated based on Equations (8)–(15). In this study, the fuel consumption and emissions for vehicles of both 1.4–2.0 L and 3.0 L are estimated based on the COPERT model, in which there are different sets of parameters for different vehicle types. Since the average speed is the key parameter in the estimation, the model is applicable to different types of vehicles. Finally, the whole fuel consumption, CO and NOx emissions for each road and for different time periods are obtained. Figure 11a–c shows the visualization results of fuel consumption/emissions estimation in the study area during periods of 2:00–4:00, 8:00–10:00, 14:00–16:00 and 20:00–22:00.

Obvious spatial and temporal patterns of fuel consumption and emissions are recognized with the big data analysis, as Figure 11 shows. First, the volume of fuel consumption is far more than CO and NOx emissions, and NOx emissions are the least. During 2:00–4:00, the volumes of fuel consumption, CO and NOx emissions are relatively low because of low traffic volume. Fuel consumption and CO emissions concentrate on sub-arterial roads such as SPL Road (Shipailing Road), branch roads in the residential area in the southwest of the study area and east segment of XC Road (Xiongchu Road), while elevated levels of NOx emissions are identified in expressways and arterial roads, such as LY Road (Luoyu Road), a west segment of XC Road (near the gas station), LS south Road (Luoshi South Road) and ZS Road (Zhongshan Road).

During morning rush hours 8:00–10:00, fuel consumption and emissions increase across the study area. Elevated levels of fuel consumption and CO emissions shift from sub-arterial roads and branch roads to arterial roads and expressways such as LY Road, WL Road (Wuluo Road) and ZS Road. Besides, the high traffic volumes in morning rush hours and congestions in arterial roads lead to concentrations of CO and NOx emissions at the intersection of LY Road and LS South Road, and the intersection of ZN Road (Zhongnan Road) and WL Road. Elevated levels of NOx emissions remain on the same roads while the ranges have expanded.

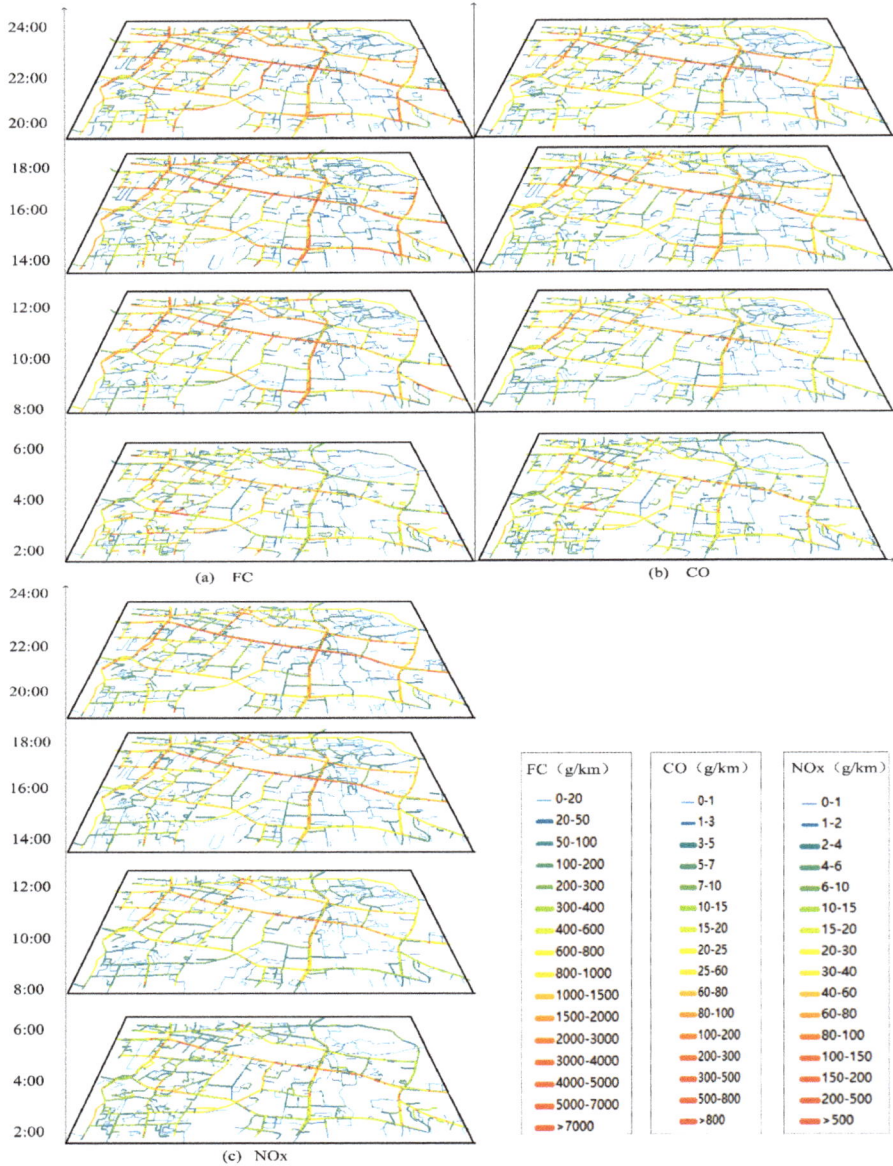

Figure 11. Space-time visualization of fuel consumption/emissions estimation. (**a**) Fuel Consumption, (**b**) is CO emission and (**c**) is NOx emission.

During 14:00–16:00, CO emissions and fuel consumption increase in roads of low grade compared with that in 8:00–10:00. During evening hours 20:00–22:00, sub-arterial roads and branch roads in residential areas in the southwest of the study area further decrease compared with that in daytime. Because the number of taxis increase after evening rush hours, elevated levels of fuel consumption and emissions are identified in arterial roads such as WL Road, LY Road, intersection of LY Road and LS South Road, intersection of ZN Road and WL Road, ZS Road, Wuchang Railway Station and east segment of XC Road.

3.3. Analyzing Activity Types Producing Fuel Consumption and Emissions in the Study Area

The visualization results in Figure 11 demonstrate that the proposed approach can discover the space-time distributions of fuel consumption and emissions intuitively and effectively. Furthermore, Figure 11 shows that not only arterial roads but also some of the small roads in residential areas such as southwest of the study area present high volume of fuel consumption and emissions, which is against our experience. From the analysis above, we know that both MAs and SAs with engine-on contribute to the fuel consumption and emissions. Therefore, we analyze and distinguish the types of fuel consumption and emissions of each road, and explore the patterns and mechanisms of fuel consumption/emissions in the study area. Figure 12 shows the percentages of fuel consumption/emissions produced by SAs with engine-on in the study area.

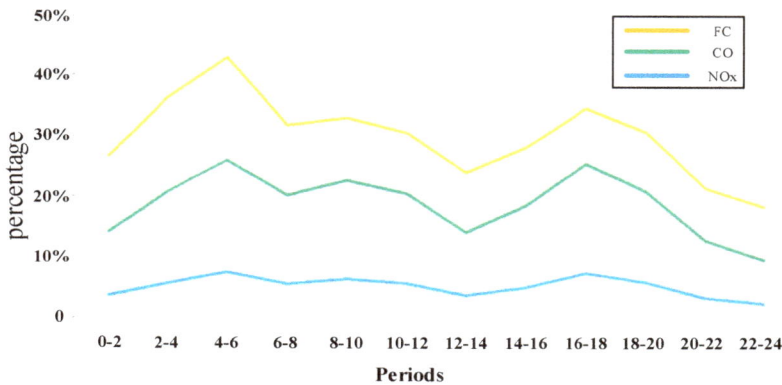

Figure 12. Percentages of fuel consumption/emissions of SAs with engine-on.

In Figure 12, the percentages of fuel consumption and emissions from SAs with engine-on in the 12 periods present a bimodal distribution. The first peak value appears during 4:00–6:00, in which fuel consumption, CO and NOx emissions of SAs with engine-on constitute for 42%, 25% and 5% of the whole fuel consumption and emissions in the study area. The other peak values are in evening peak hours (16:00–18:00), in which fuel consumption, CO and NOx emissions of SAs with engine-on constitute for 35%, 25% and 6% of the whole fuel consumption and emissions. The second peak value of fuel consumption is lower than the first peak values, and are nearly equal to the percentages in morning peak hours (8:00–10:00). Figure 12 also illustrates that SAs with engine-on have the strongest influence on fuel consumption compared with CO and NOx emissions. A large percentage of fuel consumption produced by SAs with engine-on on a road shows that speeds of taxis on the road approach to zero, implying there are traffic congestions or other stop behaviors with engine-on of taxis. In order to uncover the spatial-temporal distribution of fuel consumption produced by SAs with engine-on, we identify the roads where more than 70% of fuel consumption are produced by SAs with engine-on in the study area. Because the fuel consumption from the identified roads are mostly produced by vehicles under idling conditions, we name these identified roads as idle roads.

Space-time distributions of fuel consumption and idle roads in the study area shown in Figure 13, where the grey-shaded roads are idle roads.

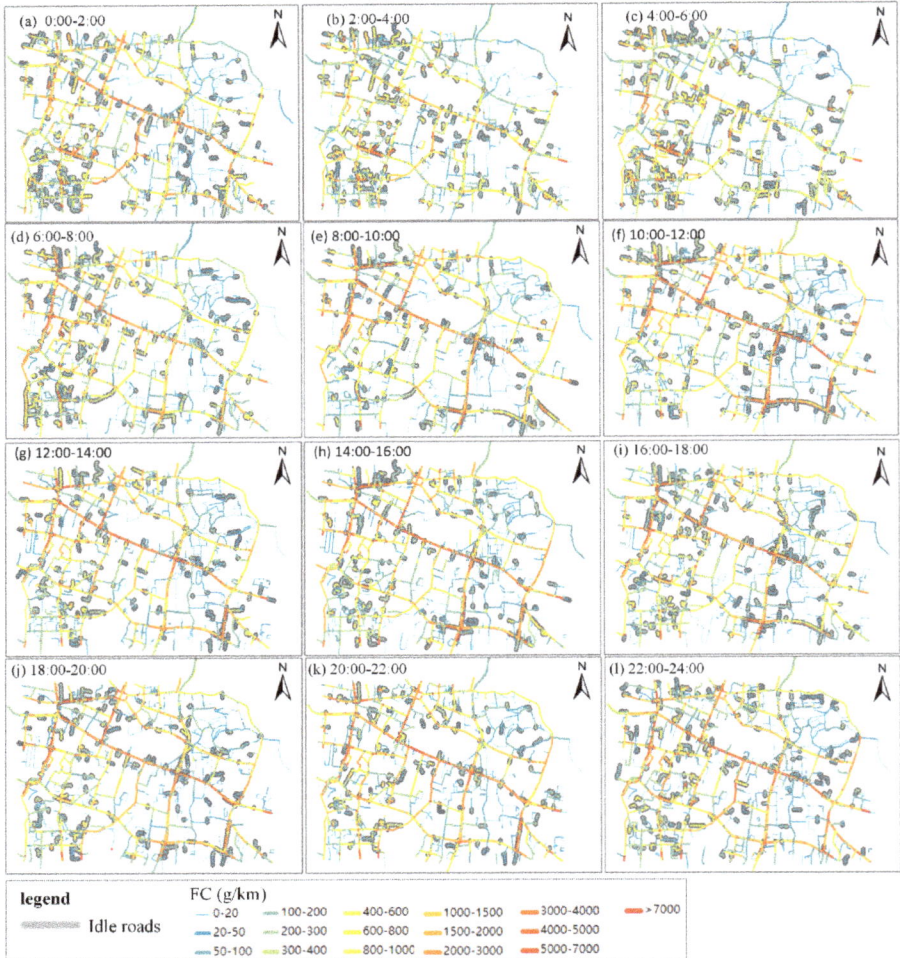

Figure 13. Space-time distribution of fuel consumption and idle roads in the study area in different period. (a) is 0:00–2:00, (b) is 2:00–4:00, (c) is 4:00–6:00, (d) is 6:00–8:00, (e) is 8:00–10:00, (f) is 10:00–12:00, (g) is 12:00–14:00, (h) is 14:00–16:00, (i) is 16:00–18:00, (j) is 18:00–20:00, (k) is 20:00–22:00, (l) is 22:00–24:00.

Figure 13 uncovers the space-time distribution patterns of idle roads and fuel consumption in the study area. In general, hot spots of idle roads tend to appear in arterial roads in the daytime while tend to appear in branch roads and residential areas at night and early-morning. In addition, the middle of ZS Road is identified as a hotspot of idle segments across a day because railway station locates in ZS Road. Taxis could stop or hover idly around railway station for waiting or picking-up/dropping-off passengers around the railway station, producing high idle fuel consumptions.

More specifically, during periods 0:00–6:00, there are fuel consumptions in non-idle arterial roads such as LY road, LS roads, indicating that the fuel consumptions in these arterial roads are produced from taxis' normal running. Clusters of idle roads are identified in branches of arterial roads such as branches of LY Road, branch roads in the residential area in the southwest of the study area, and gas station in the west of XC Road. These branch roads have relatively higher fuel consumption than other roads in the period, indicating the fuel consumption in the periods are mainly caused by taxis' hovering and refueling activities.

During morning rush hours (period 4, 6:00–8:00), idle roads distribute more balanced compared with last periods. Fuel consumptions in arterial roads such as LN Road, ZS Road increase significantly, and idle roads in branch roads and gas stations decrease. During 6 a.m.–4 p.m., idle roads in branch roads in residential area decrease, while idle roads appear in arterial roads and intersections, such as LY Road, XC Road, LS Road, intersection of ZDQ Road (Zhuodaoquan Road) and XC Road, intersection of LS Road and LY Road, and intersection of LY Road and ZN Road. The characteristics of idle roads in daytime reflect that increasing traffic volumes in daytime lead to traffic congestions in arterial roads and intersections, bringing high idle fuel consumptions.

During evening rush hours (16:00–18:00), idle roads in branch roads and gas stations further decrease. In comparison, idle roads in arterial roads and sub-arterial roads increase, such as LY Road, WL Road, BY Road (Bayi Road) and MZ Road (Minzhu Road). Besides, idle range in XC Road expand. After 18:00, clusters of idle segments in arterial roads spread to sub-arterial roads, branch roads and gas stations.

4. Discussion

In this case study, we illustrate the effectiveness of the proposed methodology, which may be replicated in other cities throughout the world. Useful insights about fuel consumption/emissions estimation are uncovered through activity analysis with big data. First, we recorded the fuel consumption of an experimental vehicle (3.0 L) for verifying the estimating accuracy of the proposed approach. Estimation accuracy is significantly improved by considering activity types when compared with previous studies. Second, spatial-temporal distribution of fuel consumption/ emissions of taxis (1.4–2.0 L) in a network area shows that elevated levels of fuel consumption and emissions are identified on arterial roads with high traffic volume during the day and evening hours but on small roads in the early morning. We then explore the patterns and mechanisms of fuel consumption/emissions in the study area by analyzing the types of fuel consumption and emissions of each road. Our results indicate that the spatial-temporal patterns of fuel consumption of taxis are highly related to their activities, especially idling stops, which have a notable impact on fuel consumption. A major crisis is the "congestion" due to the number of vehicles on road, which is more severe during the rush hours. Besides, taxis' idling stops (SAs with engine-on) that lead to high volumes of fuel consumption include not only traffic congestions but also non-service stop activities such as refueling or waiting for passengers. Hence, encouraging taxis to turn their engines off during their non-service stop activities in the elevated areas of idle roads can help to reduce the fuel consumption. Therefore, studying the patterns of taxis' activities provide an understanding of the volumes and constitution of fuel consumption/emissions in urban traffic, and may bring solutions to the problem of fuel consumption.

In the case study, we validate the estimation methods with an experimental vehicle of 3.0 L capacity, while the accuracy of fuel consumption estimation in the experiment of a large area is unavailable because the real value of fuel consumption and emissions of the taxis (1.4–2.0 L) can hardly be obtained. For the same reason, many existing studies that estimate emissions/fuel consumption using GPS data only present the estimation results without quantitatively assessing their validity [2,10–17]. Although this study only validates the accuracy of fuel consumption estimation of 3.0 L gasoline vehicle, the estimations for the 3.0 L gasoline vehicle and 1.4–2.0 L gasoline vehicles are both based on the COPERT model using the same estimation principle and processing. Furthermore, the purpose of this study is to improve the estimations of fuel consumption and emissions by considering different types of activities. In both cases the fuel consumption and emissions are estimated in the same way, as a result, the validity of the 3.0 L vehicle is considered representative in this study.

While previous studies have not identified *MAs* and *SAs* in vehicles' traces, the analysis in this study illustrates that in addition to different types of activities, modes of *SAs* also have a great impact on the fuel consumption/emissions produced during and after *SAs*. First, during *SAs* with engine-off, vehicles do not consume fuel or release emissions, but during *SAs* with engine-on, vehicles need to consume fuel and thus release emissions to keep the engines running. Second, because cold start emissions are produced when a vehicle restarts, they are closely related to the modes of *SA*. After an *SA* with engine-on, no cold start emissions are released, but after an *SA* with engine-off during which the temperature of the vehicle's engine has decreased, cold start emissions are produced until the temperature of the engine has reached the stable temperature. Without analyzing the modes of *SAs*, cold start emissions in a vehicle's trajectory cannot be estimated, which would lead to underestimations of fuel consumption/emissions since cold start emissions are many times higher than hot emissions. By comparison, this study identified *MAs*, *SAs* with engine-on and *SAs* with engine-off. Fuel consumption, hot emissions and cold start emissions are estimated according to different activity types, thus producing a more fine-grained and more precise estimation.

Lastly, besides bringing about deep insights about mechanisms of traffic fuel consumption/emissions, activity analysis with GPS big data also improves the accuracy of fuel consumption/emissions estimation. Compared with previous studies such as researches [14] and [17], we improved the accuracy and detailed level of fuel consumption/emissions estimation in two aspects. First, researches [14] and [17] divide the study areas into grids for analyzing the spatial distributions of emissions. In that way, moving parameters of vehicles are calculated based on Euclidean distances between GPS records, which leads to bias in the estimation of fuel consumption/emissions because vehicles actually move on the road network and run network distances rather than Euclidean distances. Moreover, emissions and fuel consumption are also visualized in units of planar spatial grids. Since a grid may contain several roads in the study area, patterns of fuel consumption/emissions in different roads cannot be distinguished. In contrast, we estimate and visualize fuel consumption/emissions based on road segments. With GPS trace matched to the road, we can restore the routes of vehicles and obtain more accurate moving parameters of vehicles from network distance, which is a critical factor in fuel consumption/emissions estimation.

5. Conclusions

The widespread spatial big data such as GPS data has brought fuel consumption/emissions estimation to a new perspective. While many researchers focus on the possibilities to understand the spatial-temporal distribution of fuel consumption/emissions with such big data, inadequate attention is paid to the estimation accuracy, which is the basis for uncovering the fuel consumption/emissions patterns. Emissions and fuel consumption are complex processes, related to factors including fuel parameters, vehicle model, and weather. In addition, fuel consumption/emissions are significantly affected by vehicles' activities. Existing studies do not take the activity types of vehicles into consideration in estimation. Therefore, this study proposes approaches for estimating fuel consumption/emissions based on analysis of different types of activities in vehicles' space-time paths. In our approach, we firstly build space-time paths of individual vehicles and extract moving parameters of each STPS. Then we present an N-dimensional representation approach for estimating and visualizing fuel consumption/emissions of both individual vehicle and a network area. In the case study, fuel consumption and emissions of a single vehicle and a road network area are estimated and visualized with GPS trace data. The estimating result illustrates that the estimating accuracy is significantly improved (88.6%) compared with the other two estimating approaches (71.02% and 78.2%) that do not distinguish activity types in estimation. The results indicate that the STPS based approach this study developed can estimate fuel consumption more accurately. In conclusion, the contributions of this article are mainly in the following aspects.

First, we present an N-dimensional representation framework for estimating and visualizing fuel consumption/emissions. Quantities and distribution patterns of fuel consumption/emissions can be explored under the framework.

Second, we determine different types of activities from space-time paths and identify mobile activities (*MA*s), stationary activities (*SA*s) with engine-on and with engine-off. Fuel consumption, hot emissions, and cold start emissions are estimated according to different activity types, thus producing a more fine-grained and more precise estimation.

Finally, based on the determination of different types of activities, we further analyzed the constituents of fuel consumption of each road, that is, what percentage of the whole fuel consumption do *MA*s and *SA*s with engine-on contribute. As a result, patterns and mechanisms of fuel consumption in the study area can be uncovered.

The limitations of this study include: (1) this study provides a methodology that estimates fuel consumption/emissions based on activity types. The study area is considered sufficient for evaluating the effectiveness of the proposed method, while citywide distribution patterns of fuel consumption/emissions are not reflected in this study. (2) The spatiotemporal patterns of fuel consumption/emissions during a day are uncovered in this study, while the differences between workdays and weekends are not included. (3) This study mainly puts effort on analyzing *SA*s in taxis' GPS traces, but patterns of vehicles' *MA*s are not analyzed in-depth. Future studies include estimating fuel consumption/emissions in a larger scale and a larger time span and studying approaches to reduce fuel consumption/emissions of taxis by adjusting their activity patterns, including *SA* patterns and *MA* patterns.

Acknowledgments: This work was supported by the grants from National Key Research and Development Plan of China (2017YFB0503604, 2016YFE0200400), the grants from the National Natural Science Foundation of China (41671442, 41571430, 41529101, 41271442), and the Joint Foundation of Ministry of Education of China (6141A02022341). In addition, Mei-Po Kwan was supported by a John Simon Guggenheim Memorial Foundation Fellowship.

Author Contributions: Z.K., L.T. and X.Z. conceived and designed the experiments; Z.K. performed the experiments and analyzed the data; Z.K. wrote the paper with M.-P.K., who also contributed to revising and refining the paper.

Conflicts of Interest: The authors declare no conflict of interest.

References

1. Intergovernmental Panel on Climate Change (IPCC). The Fifth Assessment Report of IPCC. 2013. Available online: http://www.ipcc.ch/pdf/assessment-report/ar5/wg3/ipcc_wg3_ar5_chapter8.pdf (accessed on 1 March 2017).

2. Nyhan, M.; Sobolevsky, S.; Kang, C.; Robinson, P.; Corti, A.; Szell, M.; Streets, D.; Lu, Z.; Britter, R. Predicting vehicular emissions in high spatial resolution using pervasively measured transportation data and microscopic emissions model. *Atmos. Environ.* **2016**, *140*, 352–363. [CrossRef]

3. Cai, H.; Xie, S.D. Estimation of vehicular emission inventories in China from 1980 to 2005. *Atmos. Environ.* **2007**, *41*, 8963–8979. [CrossRef]

4. Ntziachristos, L.; Samaras, Z.; Eggleston, S.; Samaras, Z. COPERT III. In *Computer Programme to Calculate Emissions from Road Transport, Methodology and Emission Factors (Version 2.1)*; European Energy Agency (EEA): Copenhagen, Denmark, 2000.

5. Sharma, P.; Khare, M. Modeling of vehicular exhausts—A review. *Transp. Res. D Transp. Environ.* **2001**, *6*, 179–198. [CrossRef]

6. Rakha, H.; Ahn, K.; Trani, A. Comparison of MOBILE5a, MOBILE6, VT-MICRO, and CMEM models for estimating hot-stabilized light-duty gasoline vehicle emissions. *Can. J. Civ. Eng.* **2003**, *30*, 1010–1021. [CrossRef]

7. Abo-Qudais, S.; Abuqdais, H. Performance evaluation of vehicles emissions prediction models. *Clean Technol. Environ. Policy.* **2005**, *7*, 279–284. [CrossRef]

8. U.S. Environmental Protection Agency. *Motor Vehicle Emission Simulator (MOVES) 2010: User Guide*; Report No. EPA-420-B-09-041; Environmental Protection Agency: Ann Arbor, MI, USA, 2010.

9. Chang, X.; Chen, B.; Li, Q.; Cui, X.; Tang, L.; Liu, C. Estimating real-time traffic carbon dioxide emissions based on intelligent transportation system technologies. *IEEE Trans. Intell. Transp. Syst.* **2013**, *14*, 469–479. [CrossRef]

10. Yang, Q.; Boriboonsomsin, K.; Barth, M. Arterial roadway energy/emissions estimation using modal-based trajectory reconstruction. In Proceedings of the 2011 14th International IEEE Conference on Intelligent Transportation System (ITSC 2011), Piscataway, NJ, USA, 5–7 October 2011; pp. 809–814.

11. Gühnemann, A.; Schäfer, R.; Thiessenhusen, K.; Wagner, P. *Monitoring Traffic and Emissions by Floating Car Data*; DLR—German Aerospace Centre Institute of Transport Research Rutherfordstr: Berlin, German, 2004.

12. Kouridis, C.; Gkatzoflias, D.; Kioutsioukis, I.; Ntziachristos, L.; Pastorello, C.; Dilara, P. Uncertainty estimates and guidance for road transport emission calculations. *Publ. Off. Eur. Un. EUR* **2010**. [CrossRef]

13. Sun, Z.; Hao, P.; Ban, X.J.; Yang, D. Trajectory-based vehicle energy/emissions estimation for signalized arterials using mobile sensing data. *Transp. Res. Part. D Transp. Environ.* **2015**, *34*, 27–40. [CrossRef]

14. Shang, J.; Zheng, Y.; Tong, W.; Chang, E.; Yu, Y. Inferring gas consumption and pollution emission of vehicles throughout a city. In Proceedings of the 20th ACM SIGKDD International Conference on Knowledge Discovery and Data Mining, New York, NY, USA, 24–27 August 2014; pp. 1027–1036. [CrossRef]

15. Zhao, P.; Kwan, M.P.; Qin, K. Uncovering the spatiotemporal patterns of CO_2 emissions by taxis based on individuals' daily travel. *J. Transp. Geogr.* **2017**, *62*, 122–135. [CrossRef]

16. Çağrı, K.; Bektaş, T.; Jabali, O.; Laporte, G. The fleet size and mix pollution-routing problem. *Transp. Res. B Meth.* **2014**, *70*, 239–254. [CrossRef]

17. Luo, X.; Dong, L.; Dou, Y.; Zhang, N.; Ren, J.; Li, Y.; Sun, L.; Yao, S. Analysis on spatial-temporal features of taxis' emissions from big data informed travel patterns: A case of Shanghai, China. *J. Clean. Prod.* **2017**, *142*, 926–935. [CrossRef]

18. Nikoleris, T.; Gupta, G.; Kistler, M. Detailed estimation of fuel consumption and emissions during aircraft taxi operations at Dallas/Fort Worth International Airport. *Transp. Res. Part D Transp. Environ.* **2011**, *16*, 302–308. [CrossRef]

19. Osorio, C.; Nanduri, K. Urban transportation emissions mitigation: Coupling high-resolution vehicular emissions and traffic models for traffic signal optimization. *Transp. Res. Part B Meth.* **2015**, *81*, 520–538. [CrossRef]

20. Wang, H.; Chen, C.; Huang, C.; Fu, L. On-road vehicle emission inventory and its uncertainty analysis for Shanghai, China. *Sci. Total Environ.* **2008**, *398*, 60–67. [CrossRef] [PubMed]

21. Hägerstrand, T. What about people in regional science? In *Papers of the Regional Science Association*; Springer: Berlin, Germany, 1970; Volume 24, pp. 6–21. [CrossRef]

22. Kwan, M.-P. Gender, the home-work link, and space-time patterns of non-employment activities. *Econ. Geogr.* **1999**, *75*, 370–394. [CrossRef]

23. Kwan, M.-P. Interactive geovisualization of activity-travel patterns using three-dimensional geographical information systems: A methodological exploration with a large data set. *Transp. Res. Part C Emerg. Technol.* **2000**, *8*, 185–203. [CrossRef]

24. Buliung, R.N.; Kanaroglou, P.S. A GIS toolkit for exploring geographies of household activity/travel behavior. *J. Transp. Geogr.* **2006**, *14*, 35–51. [CrossRef]

25. Shaw, S.L.; Yu, H.; Bombom, L.S. A space-time GIS approach to exploring large individual-based spatiotemporal datasets. *Trans. GIS* **2008**, *12*, 425–441. [CrossRef]

26. Yin, L.; Shaw, S.-L. Exploring space–time paths in physical and social closeness spaces: A space–time GIS approach. *Int. J. Geogr. Inf. Sci.* **2015**, *29*, 742–761. [CrossRef]

27. Miller, H.J. Modelling accessibility using space-time prism concepts within geographical information systems. *Int. J. Geogr. Inf. Syst.* **1991**, *5*, 287–301. [CrossRef]

28. Neutens, T.; Van de Weghe, N.; Witlox, F.; De Maeyer, P. A three-dimensional network-based space—Time prism. *J. Geogr. Syst.* **2008**, *10*, 89–107. [CrossRef]

29. Downs, J.A.; Horner, M.W. Probabilistic potential path trees for visualizing and analyzing vehicle tracking data. *J. Transp. Geogr.* **2012**, *23*, 72–80. [CrossRef]

30. Chai, Y. *Space-Time Structure of Chinese Cities*; Peking University Press: Beijing, China, 2002; pp. 10–11.

31. Kwan, M.-P. GIS Methods in Time-Geographic Research: Geocomputation and Geovisualization of Human Activity Patterns. *Geogr. Ann. Ser. B* **2004**, *86*, 267–280. [CrossRef]
32. Yu, H. Visualizing and analyzing activities in an integrated space-time environment: Temporal geographic information system design and implementation. *Transp. Res. Rec.* **2008**, *2024*, 54–62. [CrossRef]
33. Miller, H.J. A Measurement Theory for Time Geography. *Geogr. Anal.* **2005**, *37*, 17–45. [CrossRef]
34. Demir, E.; Bektaş, T.; Laporte, G. A comparative analysis of several vehicle emission models for road freight transportation. *Transp. Res. D Transp. Environ.* **2011**, *16*, 347–357. [CrossRef]
35. Akçelk, R.; Smit, R.; Besley, M. Calibrating Fuel Consumption and Emission Models for Modern Vehicles. In Proceedings of the IPENZ Transportation Group Conference, New Zealand, Oceania, 18–21 March 2012. Available online: http://www.sidrasolutions.com/cms_data/contents/sidra/folders/resources/articles/articles/~contents/8kr2vybbfm8vpnls/akcelik_fuel-emissionmodels-ipenz2012-.pdf (accessed on 2 March 2017).
36. Andre, J.M.; Joumard, R. Modeling of cold start excess emissions for passenger cars. In *INRETS Report LTE0509*; Laboratoire Transports et Environment; INRETS: Bron cedex, France, 2005.

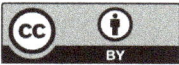

International Journal of
Environmental Research and Public Health

MDPI

Article

Real-Time Estimation of Population Exposure to PM$_{2.5}$ Using Mobile- and Station-Based Big Data

Bin Chen [1,2], Yimeng Song [3], Tingting Jiang [1], Ziyue Chen [4], Bo Huang [3,*] and Bing Xu [1,4,5,*]

[1] Ministry of Education Key Laboratory for Earth System Modelling, Department of Earth System Science,
    Tsinghua University, Beijing 100084, China; bin.chen792@gmail.com (B.C.); ecnu_jtt@163.com (T.J.)
[2] Department of Land, Air and Water Resources, University of California, Davis, CA 95616, USA
[3] Department of Geography and Resource Management, The Chinese University of Hong Kong, Shatin,
    Hong Kong, China; yimengsong@link.cuhk.edu.hk
[4] State Key Laboratory of Remote Sensing Science, College of Global Change and Earth System Science,
    Beijing Normal University, Beijing 100875, China; zychen@bnu.edu.cn
[5] Department of Geography, University of Utah, 260 S. Central Campus Dr., Salt Lake City, UT 84112, USA
*   Correspondence: bohuang@cuhk.edu.hk (B.H.); bingxu@tsinghua.edu.cn (B.X.);
    Tel.: +852-3943-6536 (B.H.); +86-10-6279-3906 (B.X.)

Received: 5 March 2018; Accepted: 16 March 2018; Published: 23 March 2018

Abstract: Extremely high fine particulate matter (PM$_{2.5}$) concentration has been a topic of special concern in recent years because of its important and sensitive relation with health risks. However, many previous PM$_{2.5}$ exposure assessments have practical limitations, due to the assumption that population distribution or air pollution levels are spatially stationary and temporally constant and people move within regions of generally the same air quality throughout a day or other time periods. To deal with this challenge, we propose a novel method to achieve the real-time estimation of population exposure to PM$_{2.5}$ in China by integrating mobile-phone locating-request (MPL) big data and station-based PM$_{2.5}$ observations. Nationwide experiments show that the proposed method can yield the estimation of population exposure to PM$_{2.5}$ concentrations and cumulative inhaled PM$_{2.5}$ masses with a 3-h updating frequency. Compared with the census-based method, it introduced the dynamics of population distribution into the exposure estimation, thereby providing an improved way to better assess the population exposure to PM$_{2.5}$ at different temporal scales. Additionally, the proposed method and dataset can be easily extended to estimate other ambient pollutant exposures such as PM$_{10}$, O$_3$, SO$_2$, and NO$_2$, and may hold potential utilities in supporting the environmental exposure assessment and related policy-driven environmental actions.

Keywords: air pollution exposure; human mobility; mobile phone data; dynamic assessment

1. Introduction

Air pollutants, especially fine particulate matters such as PM$_{2.5}$ (particles with an aerodynamic diameter less than 2.5 µm), have been the focus of increasing public concern because of its strong relation with health risks [1,2]. Numerous epidemiologic studies have established robust associations between long-term exposure to PM$_{2.5}$ and premature mortality associated with various health conditions—such as heart disease, cardiovascular and respiratory diseases, and lung cancer—that substantially reduce life expectancy [2–7]. With the unprecedented economic development and urbanization over the past three decades, the severe and widespread PM$_{2.5}$ pollution has been one of the biggest health threats in China [8,9]. The Ministry of Environmental Protection reported that only eight of the 74 monitored cities meet China's ambient air quality standards (annual mean: 35 µg/m^3; and 24-h mean: 75 µg/m^3) in 2014 [10], and the number of cities was only three in 2013 [11]. The country environmental analysis report from the Asian Development Bank shows that only <1% of

500 largest cities in China could meet the air quality guidance [12] (annual mean: 10 µg/m³; and 24-h mean: 25 µg/m³) suggested by the World Health Organization (WHO) [13].

Numerous studies have attempted to estimate ground $PM_{2.5}$ concentration levels over the past decade. As ground monitoring stations provide temporally continuous records of air pollutant concentrations, the most straightforward method applied in previous researches is using the station-based $PM_{2.5}$ observations directly to interpolate point- or surface-based $PM_{2.5}$ concentration levels [14,15], thereby offering the near real-time estimations of $PM_{2.5}$ pollution levels from local to regional scales. However, these stations are always limited in number and unevenly distributed, resulting in potential biases from interpolating local point-based measurements to surface-based estimations at a large spatial scale. Fortunately, the satellite-derived atmospheric aerosol optical depth (AOD) [16–18] has greatly advanced our understanding of spatially- and temporally- explicit changes of $PM_{2.5}$ concentrations at both regional and global scales. Over the past decade, a number of pioneering works have been devoted to quantifying the relationship between satellite-based AOD retrievals and ground-measured $PM_{2.5}$ concentrations. Here we categorize them into three major groups, (i) the chemical transport models. This type of models is based on characteristics of the vertical distribution and dispersal of aerosols, and it can further integrate aerosols' components and the effects of other pollutants to predict ground-level $PM_{2.5}$ concentrations. For example, Liu et al. [19] coupled the global atmospheric chemistry model (GEOS-CHEM) with AOD retrieved by the Multiangle Imaging Spectroradiometer (MISR) to map annual mean ground-level $PM_{2.5}$ concentrations over the contiguous United States. By simulating factors that affect the relation between AOD and $PM_{2.5}$, van Donkelaar et al. [17] estimated a global field of surface $PM_{2.5}$ concentrations with the AOD retrieved from both the Moderate-resolution Imaging Spectroradiometer (MODIS) and MISR observations. (ii) The semi-empirical models. This type of models is generally based on the modeling of the AOD-$PM_{2.5}$ relationships by incorporating environmental factors. For example, several semi-empirical models have been developed ranging from simple linear relationships to complex nonlinear relationships involving meteorological and geographic variables [20,21]. (iii) The statistical regression models. This type of models is based on statistical regressions by regarding ground-based $PM_{2.5}$ measurements as the dependent variables, and the satellite-based AOD retrievals and other factors including topography, land cover/use types, humidity, temperature, wind speed, wind direction, vertical visibility, and the height of boundary layer, etc., as the independent variables [22–27]. Despite the integration of satellite- and station-based observations has proven to be useful in improving the retrieval accuracy of $PM_{2.5}$ concentrations, the available datasets are still with a coarse temporal resolution from daily, to monthly or yearly scales, rather than depicting the spatiotemporal variation of $PM_{2.5}$ concentrations within a day.

Another critical issue relating to the estimation of population exposure to $PM_{2.5}$ pollutants is that most of existing exposure assessments always regard population as static, without considering the temporal dynamics of population distribution [14,28]. Currently, demographic data based on administrative units are the most widely used data source for estimating air pollution exposure risks. It provides accurate population census information over a certain time period based on the smallest administrative unit (i.e., census block) and often includes kinds of socio-economic attributes such as age, gender, education, and income. However, such kind of data has limitations for estimating the real-time exposure risks to air pollutants since it just regards population as a homogeneous entity for each census block without diving into the spatial heterogeneity of population distribution. More importantly, it does not consider spatiotemporal dynamics of the human mobility due to the very low updating frequency. In contrast, recent studies have demonstrated the necessity of considering spatiotemporal variability of air pollution and human mobility in exposure assessments [14,29–31]. That is because, first, air pollution concentrations are not only spatially varied but also changing across temporal scales from minutes to hours, and second, population exposure to air pollutants is actually determined by both the specific location and how much time spent on that location, rather than the assumption that people move within regions of generally the same air quality throughout a day or other time periods.

Thus, how to obtain real-time estimations of population exposure to $PM_{2.5}$ concentrations is urgently needed for instant or short-time assessments (e.g., hourly or short-term $PM_{2.5}$ concentrations are more relevant to vulnerable population groups than the daily or monthly concentrations on average [14]) and cumulative exposure effects (the aggregation of short-term assessments is more robust than the monthly or annual average).

Addressing these ubiquitous challenges, more information on human space-time location is required. Some of previous studies have tried to use surveying data, such as travel questionnaire surveys, personal GPS or smart sensor based devices [14,31,32] to delineate how an individual move in the city during his/her daily life. For example, Lu and Fang [32] used the GPS-equipped portable air sensor to measure air pollutant intakes in individual's immediate surroundings and space-time movement trajectories in Huston, Texas. However, their high expenses and limited samples within local areas barricade the data availability. The alternative approaches are to use mathematical models to simulate population mobility patterns, such as gravity model [33] and radiation model [34]. This kind of methods allow us to draw more quantitative conclusions from a larger population size, but their results are only valid for situations with similar initial parameters in the simulation process [29]. Recently, Park and Kwan [14] simulated 80 possible daily movement trajectories based on daily trip distribution data from the Congestion Management Program Report to reflect the actual commuting tendency of Los Angeles (USA) county residents, and estimated exposure risks by considering the interactions between air pollution and individuals' location. However, such kind of studies are still constrained to limited spatial and temporal scales. With the rapid growth of mobile internet, especially the location-based services of applications (apps) in the smartphones, it makes us possible to access direct spatiotemporal records of human activities [35,36]. Additionally, the high correlation between the mobile-phone locating-request records and the spatiotemporal characteristics of human activities has been revealed by many studies [37–39]. A growing number of studies have started to use mobile phone data in the field of environmental exposure assessments [29,30,40]. For example, Dewulf et al. [29] collected mobile phone data of approximately five million mobile users in Belgium to calculate the daily exposure to NO_2. Gariazzo et al. [30] conducted a dynamic city-wide air pollution (NO_2, O_3, and $PM_{2.5}$) exposure assessment by using time resolved population distributions derived from mobile phone traffic data, and modelled air pollutants concentrations. Yu et al. [40] combined cell phone location data from 9886 SIMcard IDs in Shenzhen, China to assess the misclassification errors in air pollution exposure estimation. Although all these pioneering studies highlight the promising advantages of incorporating population dynamics in estimating air pollution exposure, the available datasets are still limited to sample sizes and spatiotemporal scales due to the cost and time for collecting fine-resolution data, data privacy and confidentiality issues, and computational complexities [41].

To investigate the nationwide $PM_{2.5}$ concentration risks for population in China, spatially explicit and temporally continuous studies are needed to detect hotspots, estimate vulnerability, and assess population exposure at finer temporal scales. In this paper, we propose a novel approach to achieve the real-time estimation of population exposure to $PM_{2.5}$ by integrating mobile-phone locating-request (MPL) big data and station-based $PM_{2.5}$ observations. Compared with previous studies regarding ambient pollution exposure assessments, it has the following highlights. First, the proposed method introduces the dynamics of population distribution into the nationwide exposure estimation, thereby providing an improved way to better assess the actual exposure risk to $PM_{2.5}$ at different temporal scales. Second, to the best of our knowledge, it is the first time to provide the real-time estimation of nationwide population exposure to $PM_{2.5}$ at pixel-based level (~1.2 km) in China. Third, the proposed method and dataset can be easily extended to estimate other ambient pollutant exposures such as PM_{10}, O_3, SO_2, and NO_2, and may hold potential utilities in supporting the environmental exposure assessments and related policy-driven environmental actions.

2. Materials and Methods

2.1. Ground-Station PM$_{2.5}$ Measurements

Hourly ground-station PM$_{2.5}$ measurements from 1 March to 31 March 2016 were collected from the official website of the China Environmental Monitoring Center (http://113.108.142.147:20035/emcpublish/). According to the Chinese National Ambient Air Quality Standard (CNAAQS), the station-based PM$_{2.5}$ data in China were obtained using the tapered element oscillating microbalance method (TEOM) or the beta-attenuation method, combined with the periodic calibration. In this study, we used a total of 1465 monitoring stations (Figure 1) that have been established in all provinces for monitoring ambient air quality.

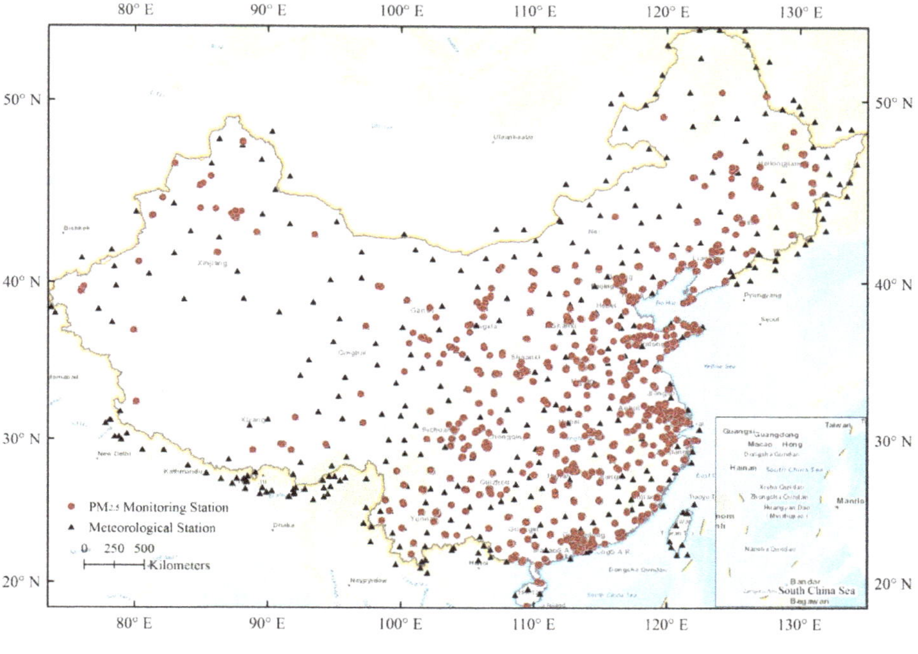

Figure 1. Spatial distribution of nationwide monitoring stations for PM$_{2.5}$ concentrations (red dots) and meteorological stations (black triangles) in China.

2.2. Ground-Station Meteorological Measurements

Ground-station meteorological variables, including air temperature (AT), surface wind speed (WS), and horizontal visibility (VIS) were used from Global Telecommunication System (GTS) established by World Meteorological Organization (https://rda.ucar.edu/datasets/ds461.0/). In this study, the 3-h measurements (from 2:00 a.m. to 23:00 p.m. local time) from 411 stations in China and 128 stations within the 0.01-degree buffer zones around the boundary of China (Figure 1) were collected from 1 March to 31 March 2016.

2.3. Mobile Phone Locating-Request Big Data

By retrieving real-time locating requests from mobile phone users' activities in apps, the mobile phone locating-request (MPL) data was used in this study to monitor human movement. The MPL data are from Tencent big data platform in China, which is one of the largest Internet service providers both nationwide and worldwide. All of the MPL data are produced by active smartphone users using apps, which have been enabled to report real-time locations from the mobile devices. Due to the widespread usage of Tencent apps (e.g., WeChat, QQ, Tencent Map, etc.) and their location-based services, the daily locating records have reached 36 billion from more than 450 million users globally in 2016 [42]. Thus, the MPL big data can be represented as an indicator to characterize human activities and population distribution in a fine spatiotemporal scale. The Tencent MPL dataset used in this study was collected from 1 March to 31 March 2016 via the application program interface (API) from the Tencent big data platform (http://heat.qq.com). The original Tencent MPL dataset was recorded by aggregating the real-time locations of active apps users every five minutes within a mesh grid at a spatial resolution of 30 arc-second (~1.2 km). All the information regarding users' identities and privacies were removed in this publicly available dataset.

2.4. Population Census Data

The latest city-level population census of China in 2014 obtained from the national scientific data sharing platform for population and health (http://www.ncmi.cn/) was used in this study. This dataset was established and maintained by infectious disease network reporting system, and it was derived based on population census released by the State Statistics Bureau. It collected all population census including permanent resident and registered resident at the county level by gender and age group since 2004.

2.5. Estimation of Spatiotemporal Continuous $PM_{2.5}$ Concentrations

Due to the difference in geographic locations between $PM_{2.5}$ monitoring stations and meteorological stations, all datasets were processed to be consistent in spatial and temporal domains. The meteorological variables were first interpolated by ordinary Kriging method [43] to obtain data that covering the entire study area with a spatial resolution of 30 arc-second (~1.2 km). To mitigate the interpolation biases, we averaged all meteorological observations with a 30 arc-second search radius around each $PM_{2.5}$ monitoring station, and then assigned the result to the corresponding $PM_{2.5}$ monitoring station. In addition, the widely used Geographically Weighted Regression (GWR) model [44] with adaptive Gaussian bandwidth was adopted to build the statistical relationship between meteorological variables and $PM_{2.5}$ concentrations. Specifically, we grouped all variables within a month into 8 time points (i.e., from 2:00 a.m., 5:00 a.m., . . . , 23:00 p.m.), and then developed 8 GWR models for each time point in this study as follows:

$$PM_{2.5,i,t} = \beta_{0,i,t} + \beta_{1,i,t}VIS_{i,t} + \beta_{2,i,t}AT_{i,t} + \beta_{3,i,t}WS_{i,t} \tag{1}$$

where $PM_{2.5,i,t}$ denotes the $PM_{2.5}$ concentration at the location i at time t, $VIS_{i,t}$, $AT_{i,t}$, and $WS_{i,t}$ denote the visibility (m), air temperature (°C), and surface wind speed (m/s), respectively, at location i at time t. $\beta_{0,i,t}$, $\beta_{1,i,t}$, $\beta_{2,i,t}$, and $\beta_{3,i,t}$ are corresponding regression coefficients at location i at time t.

A 10-fold validation analysis [45] was adopted to evaluate the modeling performance by comparing the estimated and measured $PM_{2.5}$ concentrations (details can be found in Supplementary Materials). With the iterative cross validations, the optimal coefficients in each time point were retrieved to interpolate the entire study areas with a spatial resolution of 30 arc-second (~1.2 km), and then were used to estimate gridded $PM_{2.5}$ concentrations.

2.6. Estimation of Real-Time Population Distribution by Integrating MPL and Census Data

The mobile phone locating-request (MPL) data can be served as an indicator to delineate the spatiotemporal pattern of population distribution, however, the MPL data do not represent the actual population sizes. In this study, we first aggregated the 5-min MPL data into 3-h MPL data, making its temporal resolution consistent with that of the estimated $PM_{2.5}$ concentrations, and calculated the pixel-based population density using the MPL data, and then applied the MPL-based population density map to downscale the census data. Consequently, we can obtain the 3-h pixel-based population approximations. Given the difference of physical environment and socio-economic development in various areas of China, downscaling the MPL data with population census at the national scale will undoubtedly result in the underestimation of population in under- and less-developed areas and overestimation of population in those developed areas. To solve this problem, we decided to estimate real-time population distribution by integrating MPL and census data at the city level. The 3-h MPL map was used to redistribute the census data for each city by Equations (2) and (3), under the assumption that the inter-city mobility will not dramatically influence the total population of a city within a short time window. Finally, we could obtain the 3-h pixel-based population approximation for each city, and then conducted the image mosaic to produce the 3-h national-scale population distribution map in China.

$$W_{ij} = \frac{p_{ij}}{\sum_{i=1}^{n} p_{ij}} \tag{2}$$

$$pop_{ij} = TR \times W_{ij} \tag{3}$$

where $p_{i,j}$ is the amount of locating-request times within the i-th pixel at the hour j, n is the total number of pixels within a city, $W_{i,j}$ is the weight for redistributing population and TR is the total population in the city from the census data. $Pop_{i,j}$ denotes the population approximation in the i-th pixel at the hour j.

2.7. Real-Time Estimation of Population Exposure to PM$_{2.5}$

Since the levels of PM$_{2.5}$ concentration and population distribution are spatially and temporally varied, here we adopted the population-weighted metric (Equation (4)) to estimate the real-time exposure risks to PM$_{2.5}$ concentrations, which was likely to be more representative of population exposure to PM$_{2.5}$ across different temporal scales [46]:

$$PWP = \sum_{i=1}^{N} (pop_i \cdot pm_i) / \sum_{i=1}^{N} pop_i \tag{4}$$

where pop_i and pm_i denote the population and PM$_{2.5}$ concentration level in the i-th pixel, N is the total number of pixels within the corresponding administrative unit. PWP is the population-weighted PM$_{2.5}$ concentration level for the targeted administrative unit.

With the PM$_{2.5}$ concentrations and population distribution estimated in previous sections, we could integrate them based on Equation (4) to provide the estimation of population exposure to PM$_{2.5}$ with a 3-h updating frequency, thereby being able to track the real-time dynamics of exposure risks by considering the spatiotemporal variation of PM$_{2.5}$ concentration and population distribution.

2.8. Estimation of Cumulative Inhaled PM$_{2.5}$

PM$_{2.5}$ concentration causes acute and chronic adverse effects on human health mainly by means of inhalation exposure. To our understanding, deriving the estimations of cumulative inhaled PM$_{2.5}$ masses will be one of the most important prerequisites to model the accurate relationship between PM$_{2.5}$ exposure and human health [47–49]. Thus, we proposed to incorporate human respiratory volume and the spatiotemporal variation of PM$_{2.5}$ concentration and population density to present a better estimation of cumulative inhaled PM$_{2.5}$:

$$InPM_{2.5} = \sum_{i=1}^{N} \sum_{t=1}^{T} p_i(t) \cdot h_i \cdot d_i(t) \cdot m(t) + p_i(t) \cdot h_i \cdot (1 - d_i(t)) \cdot m(t) \cdot \alpha \tag{5}$$

where p_i and h_i denote the population and the inhaled volume of air for the i-th age group, N is the total number of the age group. t denotes the time (hours in this study), $m(t)$ denotes the PM$_{2.5}$ concentration level at time t, T is the target temporal period, d_i is the percentage of outdoor population, α is the outdoor-indoor ratio of PM$_{2.5}$ concentration.

However, recent advances regarding the outdoor-indoor ratio of $PM_{2.5}$ concentrations are all limited to local scales for the purpose of experimental tests [50], as it is difficult to acquire such valid observations relating this ratio on a large scale. More importantly, the outdoor-indoor ratio is influenced by several factors such as geographic location, building structures, and living habits. In addition, the inhaled volume of air is also different, not only in terms of age differences but of physical activities, gender, and size, all of these factors would affect the inhaled value [51,52]. Thus, we have to simplify the ideal model in Equation (5) for being suitable to nationwide estimates of cumulative inhaled $PM_{2.5}$ masses by neglecting the difference between outdoor and indoor $PM_{2.5}$ concentration exposure and the inhaled volume of air among different age groups, gender, and other related factors. In this way, we can directly obtain the estimation of cumulative inhaled $PM_{2.5}$ masses using the following equation:

$$InPM'_{2.5} = \sum_{t=1}^{T} p_i(t) \cdot h \cdot m(t) \qquad (6)$$

where $InPM'_{2.5}$ denotes the cumulative inhaled $PM_{2.5}$ mass from the simplified model, and h denotes the empirical inhaled volume of air. A measurement conducted by Adams [51] based on 200 individuals showed that the hourly average volume of air breathed by adults when they are sitting or resting were ranging from 0.42 to 0.63 m^3 (i.e., 10.08 to 15.12 m^3/day), and the volumes for walking were from 1.20 to 1.44 m^3/h, and for running were from 3.10 to 3.48 m^3/h. Thus, the average inhaled volume of air for an individual is assumed to be 15 m^3/day in this study [52].

2.9. Comparison of Exposure Assessments from the MPL-Based and Census-Based Methods

In order to investigate whether the improvement of incorporating dynamic population distributions does make a difference in the exposure assessment, we intuitively compared the MPL-based and census-based calculations of cumulative inhaled $PM_{2.5}$ masses and population-weighted $PM_{2.5}$ exposure concentrations in China's 359 cities across different temporal scales (i.e., 3-h, 1-day, 1-week, and 1-month). For each city, the population from the census data was directly used in the census-based method, while the redistributed population dynamics was used in the MPL-based method.

3. Results

3.1. Different Facets of Population Exposure to PM2.5

The spatiotemporal integration of $PM_{2.5}$ concentration and population density was used to produce thematic information that document different facets of population exposure to $PM_{2.5}$. Figure 2 shows an extracted example from the time-series analysis of population exposure to $PM_{2.5}$ in China.

Figure 2a shows the real-time nationwide estimation of population distribution (11:00 a.m.) on 1 March 2016, which is derived by integrating MPL and census data at a city-level scale in Section 2.6. The intensity represents the specific population number in each gridded pixel with stretched colors from blue to red denoting varied population size. Figure 2b shows the real-time nationwide estimation of $PM_{2.5}$ concentrations (11:00 a.m.), which is derived from incorporating ground-station $PM_{2.5}$ measurements and meteorological variables based on GWR models in Section 2.5. Figure 2c shows the nationwide estimation of 24-h cumulative inhaled $PM_{2.5}$ masses. Figure 2d shows the estimation of 24-h cumulative inhaled $PM_{2.5}$ masses based on the census data. Figure 2e–h show insets from Figure 2a–d for part of the Northern China as a zoomed visualization in different facets of population exposure to $PM_{2.5}$ concentrations.

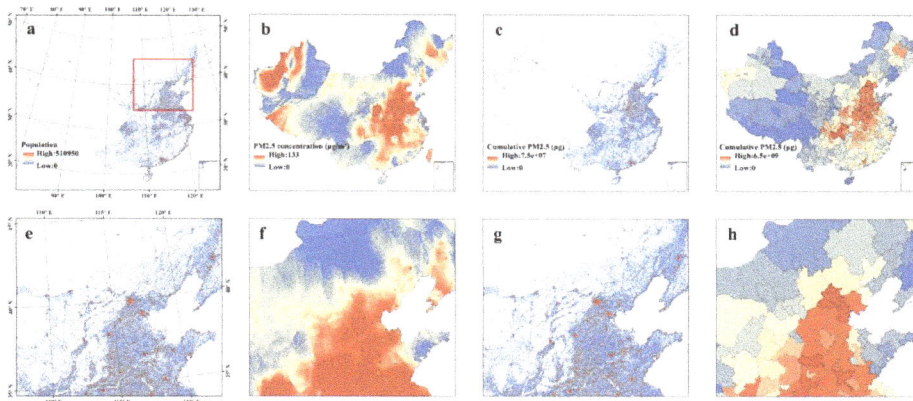

Figure 2. Different facets of population exposure to PM$_{2.5}$. (**a**) Map of population distribution in China on 1 March 2016 (11:00 a.m.). (**b**) Map of PM$_{2.5}$ concentration levels in China on 1 March 2016 (11:00 a.m.). (**c**) Map of cumulative inhaled PM$_{2.5}$ masses in China based on the MPL data on 1 March 2016. (**d**) Map of cumulative inhaled PM$_{2.5}$ in China based on the census data on 1 March 2016. (**e–h**) show the insets from (**a–d**) for part of the Northern China.

3.2. Temporal Dynamics of Population Exposure to PM$_{2.5}$

In the form of Figure 2a–c, we can also provide the temporal variation of population, PM$_{2.5}$ concentrations, and cumulative inhaled PM$_{2.5}$ masses with a 3-h temporal resolution from 1 March to 31 March 2016. In this way, the pixel-based dynamics of population exposure to PM$_{2.5}$ concentrations at the nationwide scale with a nearly real-time updating frequency (i.e., 3-h in this study) were retrieved. In order to better present the experimental results with an entire month in March 2016, we further aggregated the pixel-based estimations into 359 cities in this study. Results demonstrate that both the population-weighted PM$_{2.5}$ concentrations (Figure 3a) and cumulative inhaled PM$_{2.5}$ masses (Figure 3b) exist distinguished diurnal and daily variations, which also verify the necessity of considering the spatiotemporal variability of both air pollution and population distribution in air pollution exposure assessments.

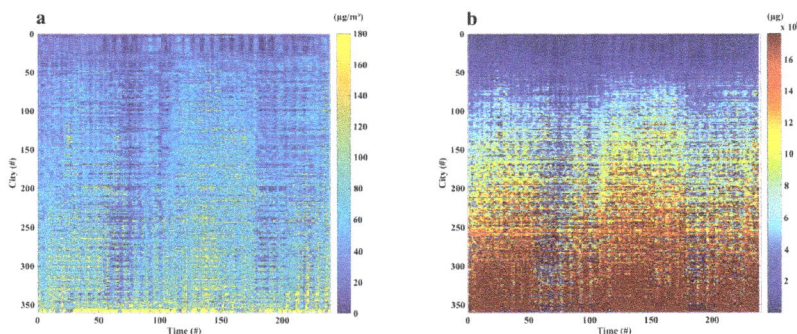

Figure 3. The estimated population-weighted PM$_{2.5}$ concentrations (**a**) and cumulative inhaled PM$_{2.5}$ masses (**b**) for 359 cities in China with every 3 h from 1 March to 31 March 2016. Note that the *x* axis represents the time from the first 3-h (2:00 a.m. 1 March 2016) to the last 3-h (23:00 p.m. 31 March 2016), and *y* axis represents the order of 359 cities.

3.3. Comparison of Exposure Assessment Methods

From the visual inspection from Figure 2c,d, it can be found out that the MPL-based method yields the gridded cumulative inhaled $PM_{2.5}$ masses, whereas the census-based assessments are only based on administrative units (cities in this study), which informs us that the MPL-based method improves the spatial resolution of basic cells from administrative units to gridded pixels in exposure assessments. In addition, by comparing the cumulative inhaled $PM_{2.5}$ masses and population-weighted $PM_{2.5}$ exposure concentrations in China's 359 cities across different temporal scales, results in Figure 4 show that without introducing the dynamics of population distribution into the exposure assessment, the maximum biases (over- or under- estimation) of cumulative inhaled $PM_{2.5}$ mass reach to over 100% across different temporal scales. Meanwhile, the maximum biases of population-weighted $PM_{2.5}$ concentrations will be approximately 30 $\mu g/m^3$. By aggregating the experimental tests in China's 359 cities from 1 March to 31 March 2016, the biased percentage between the MPL-based and the census-based estimations will be the level of 14.9% (3-h), 5.8% (1-day), 4.7% (1-week), and 3.9% (1-month) on average.

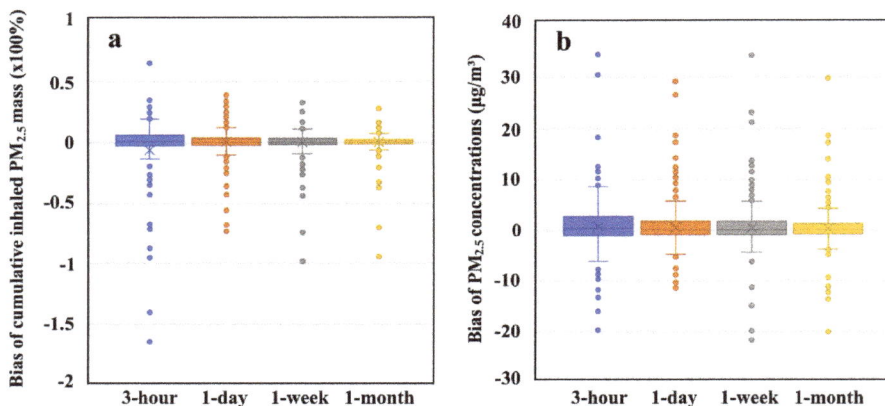

Figure 4. The biases of cumulative inhaled $PM_{2.5}$ mass (**a**) and the per capita $PM_{2.5}$ exposure concentration (**b**) between the MPL-based estimations and the census-based estimations in China's cities across different temporal scales.

4. Discussion

Compared with previous methods for air pollution exposure assessment, the proposed method in this study considered well the spatiotemporal variability of both population distribution and $PM_{2.5}$ concentration levels, thereby contributing to a better exposure assessment. The relative reasonability of our method may be due to the following strengths. First, the spatiotemporal variability of $PM_{2.5}$ concentrations and population distribution are incorporated in air pollution exposure assessments. Given that the level of $PM_{2.5}$ concentrations is continuously changing over space and time and human beings are also mobile across spatiotemporal scales [14], both of these dynamic characteristics and their interactions at finer spatiotemporal scales should be well considered to estimate population exposure risks. However, many previous studies always used the census data with the assumption that people are non-mobile or moving within regions of generally the same air quality throughout a day or other time periods, thus leading to considerable biases in actual air pollution exposure assessments. In reality, people in different areas experience different levels of $PM_{2.5}$ concentrations across different temporal scales. In order to characterize the interaction between population dynamics and $PM_{2.5}$ concentrations, here we used the mobile-phone locating-request (MPL) big data to quantify the dynamics of population distribution. By integrating the MPL and census data, we then derived real-time pixel-based population dynamics at the nationwide scale. Combing this nationwide population dynamic information and surface-based $PM_{2.5}$ concentrations simultaneously will be of great importance to assess the actual population exposure to $PM_{2.5}$ at different temporal scales. Second, the characterized dynamics of $PM_{2.5}$ concentrations and population dynamics in the proposed method keep a consistent spatiotemporal scale. The MPL data used in this study were initially retrieved at a 5-min updating temporal resolution from the Tencent big data platform. We further aggregated the 5-min updating MPL data into 3-h synthetic data, making it temporally comparable to the updating frequency of the nationwide surface-based $PM_{2.5}$ concentrations. Meanwhile, the spatial resolution of $PM_{2.5}$ concentrations is also set to be with a 30 arc-second (~1.2 km) spatial resolution, which is the same with that of MPL data. These efforts contribute much to achieving near real-time (3-h) estimates of national population exposure to $PM_{2.5}$ at the pixel-based level in China. Third, the presented model incorporated human respiratory volume and the spatiotemporal variation of $PM_{2.5}$ concentration and population density to estimate cumulative inhaled $PM_{2.5}$ masses. It will contribute to advancing the development of modelling the relationship between $PM_{2.5}$ exposures, health risks, and life expectancies quantitatively.

Besides $PM_{2.5}$, the ground monitoring stations are always coupled with sensors measuring other air pollutants such as PM_{10}, SO_2, NO_2, and O_3. With the similar framework by integrating mobile phone big data and air pollutant concentrations, the proposed method can also be customized to estimate population exposure risks to these ambient pollutants in China. Compared with the census-based method, the MPL-based method can yield near real-time estimations of population exposure to ambient pollutants. That is, we can achieve the estimation of air pollution exposure risks at any specific location and time on a large scale by combining the spatiotemporal variability of population distribution and air pollutant concentrations. By aggregating the short-term exposure assessments into longer temporal scales, we can also derive more robust and reliable estimations related to the chronic effects from air pollutants. Additionally, the proposed framework can be also applied to estimate the real-time number of people exposed to poor air quality as a result of updating the population distribution and air pollutant concentrations.

Meanwhile, some potential concerns regarding the implementation of the proposed method should be pointed out. First, in order to redistribute the census data to derive real-time population dynamics using the MPL data, we assume that the total population of each administrative unit (359 cities in this study) is constant since the inter-city mobility (the trade-off of inflow and outflow population) will not dramatically influence the total population of a city within a short time window. Thus, human movements and migrations across administrative units are neglected in this study. Second, volunteer-produced geospatial big data, such as MPL records in this study tend to leave out some population groups of the society because the children, the elderly, and the poor are less-frequent active users. Nevertheless, such data can still well quantify actual population distribution patterns [35,37,38] because of the massive volumes of data records. Here we take the MPL records in China on 1 March 2016 for example, the total number of locating-request records reaches 1.71 billion. By aggregating all MPL records from 1 March to 31 March 2016, the total number of locating-request records will be approximately 60 billion, thereby providing a robust measurement of population dynamics. Third, although the nationwide $PM_{2.5}$ concentrations used in this study are estimated by incorporating the meteorological variables and ground-based $PM_{2.5}$ measurements with the GWR models, the spatial interpolations are still the limits to affect the estimation accuracy in areas without sufficient inputs of station-based variables. As a result, even there is much greater spatial variations in the population data, there will be relatively less spatial variations in $PM_{2.5}$ concentrations, which may lead to no significant impacts on the exposure assessments. However, with·the comparison of exposure assessments between the MPL-based and the census-based methods, we can still figure out considerable differences. Thus, if we can further improve the estimation of $PM_{2.5}$ concentrations, such as developing spatial-temporal integrated method by combing satellite-based and station-based observations guided with the diurnal change pattern of $PM_{2.5}$ concentrations, land cover/use types, landscape topography, and related meteorological variables, the combination of the mobile phone big data and the improved air pollutant concentrations will contribute to a more reliable exposure assessment. Finally, the simplified model without considering outdoor-indoor ratio of $PM_{2.5}$ concentrations and the difference of inhaled volumes of air among different population groups may be biased to the assessment of actual cumulative inhaled $PM_{2.5}$ masses. As the Tencent-based MPL dataset was recorded by aggregating the real-time locations of active apps users within a mesh grid at a spatial resolution of 30 arc-second (~1.2 km) without differentiating individual's moving trajectories and population groups, it was impractical to apply empirical parameters into the exposure assessment at a nationwide scale since the outdoor-indoor ratio of $PM_{2.5}$ concentrations is influenced by several factors such as geographical locations, building materials, living habits, and so on. Similarly, the gridded MPL data without tracking individuals' trajectories also prevented us from considering the commuting patterns or choices of different transports. However, the MPL dataset represents the unique data source having the best spatial resolution with real-time updating population distribution we can access right now. Meanwhile, the estimates in the experimental test also represent the trade-off between over- and under-estimated cumulative inhaled $PM_{2.5}$ masses. On the one hand, these estimates are the highest estimates of cumulative inhaled $PM_{2.5}$ masses since we do not consider the situations that people are with indoor environments or commuting transportations. On the other hand, the cumulative inhaled $PM_{2.5}$ masses could be even higher because we use the constant value representing a low level of the inhaled air volume for an adult without considering factors such as physical activity, gender, and size [51]. Thus, these over and under estimates help balance each out in terms of cumulative inhaled $PM_{2.5}$ masses to provide the general assessment at large scales.

5. Conclusions

This study sought to combine mobile phone big data and station-based $PM_{2.5}$ measurements to achieve real-time estimations of population exposure to $PM_{2.5}$ concentrations in China. The results showed that the proposed method can well quantify dynamics of the real-time population distribution and yield the estimation of population exposure to $PM_{2.5}$ concentrations and cumulative inhaled $PM_{2.5}$ masses with a 3-h updating frequency. This study provides a novel framework for environmental exposure assessments by considering the spatiotemporal variability of both population distribution and $PM_{2.5}$ concentrations, which can also be customized to estimate other ambient pollutant exposure risks. These findings and methods may hold potential utilities in supporting the environmental exposure assessment and related policy-driven environmental actions.

Supplementary Materials: The following are available online at http://www.mdpi.com/1660-4601/15/4/573/s1, Table S1. Accuracy of the fitting and 10-fold cross-validation for eight periods. Figure S1: Scatterplots of the observed and predicted $PM_{2.5}$ for eight-time periods.

Acknowledgments: The authors thank Tencent Inc. for making the mobile phone location data publicly available. This work was supported by the Ministry of Science and Technology of China under the National Key Research and Development Program (2016YFA0600104) and was also supported by a project funded by the China Postdoctoral Science Foundation (2017M620739). The authors also thank three anonymous reviewers and editors for providing valuable suggestions and comments, which have greatly improved this manuscript.

Author Contributions: Bin Chen and Bing Xu conceived and designed the experiments; Bin Chen and Yimeng Song performed the experiments and wrote the paper; Tingting Jiang, Bo Huang, Ziyue Chen and Bing Xu contributed to the data analysis and manuscript revision.

Conflicts of Interest: The authors declare no conflict of interest.

References

1. Kampa, M.; Castanas, E. Human health effects of air pollution. *Environ. Pollut.* **2008**, *151*, 362–367. [CrossRef] [PubMed]
2. Pope, C.A., III; Dockery, D.W. Health effects of fine particulate air pollution: Lines that connect. *J. Air Waste Manag. Assoc.* **2006**, *56*, 709–742. [CrossRef] [PubMed]

3. Apte, J.S.; Marshall, J.D.; Cohen, A.J.; Brauer, M. Addressing global mortality from ambient *Environ. Sci. Technol.* **2015**, *49*, 8057–8066. [CrossRef] [PubMed]

4. Brook, R.D.; Rajagopalan, S.; Pope, C.A.; Brook, J.R.; Bhatnagar, A.; Diez-Roux, A.V.; Holguin, F.; Hong, Y.; Luepker, R.V.; Mittleman, M.A. Particulate matter air pollution and cardiovascular disease. *Circulation* **2010**, *121*, 2331–2378. [CrossRef] [PubMed]

5. Liu, C.; Yang, C.; Zhao, Y.; Ma, Z.; Bi, J.; Liu, Y.; Meng, X.; Wang, Y.; Cai, J.; Kan, H. Associations between long-term exposure to ambient particulate air pollution and type 2 diabetes prevalence, blood glucose and glycosylated hemoglobin levels in China. *Environ. Int.* **2016**, *92*, 416–421. [CrossRef] [PubMed]

6. Pope, C.A., III; Burnett, R.T.; Thun, M.J.; Calle, E.E.; Krewski, D.; Ito, K.; Thurston, G.D. Lung cancer, cardiopulmonary mortality, and long-term exposure to fine particulate air pollution. *JAMA* **2002**, *287*, 1132–1141. [CrossRef] [PubMed]

7. Pope, C.A., III; Ezzati, M.; Dockery, D.W. Fine-particulate air pollution and life expectancy in the United States. *N. Engl. J. Med.* **2009**, *2009*, 376–386. [CrossRef] [PubMed]

8. Xu, B.; Yang, J.; Zhang, Y.; Gong, P. Healthy cities in China: A lancet commission. *Lancet* **2016**, *388*, 1863–1864. [CrossRef]

9. Xu, P.; Chen, Y.; Ye, X. Haze, air pollution, and health in China. *Lancet* **2013**, *382*, 2067. [CrossRef]

10. Ministry of Environmental Protection of the People's Republic of China. *China's Environmental Bulletin in 2014*; Ministry of Environmental Protection: Beijing, China, 2014.

11. Babu, S.S.; Manoj, M.; Moorthy, K.K.; Gogoi, M.M.; Nair, V.S.; Kompalli, S.K.; Satheesh, S.; Niranjan, K.; Ramagopal, K.; Bhuyan, P. Trends in aerosol optical depth over Indian region: Potential causes and impact indicators. *J. Geophys. Res. Atmos.* **2013**, *118*. [CrossRef]

12. World Health Organization; UNAIDS. *Air Quality Guidelines: Global Update 2005*; World Health Organization: Geneva, Switzerland, 2006.

13. Zhang, Q.; Crooks, R. *Toward an Environmentally Sustainable Future: Country Environmental Analysis of the People's Republic of China*; Asian Development Bank: Mandaluyong, Philippines, 2012.

14. Park, Y.M.; Kwan, M.-P. Individual exposure estimates may be erroneous when spatiotemporal variability of air pollution and human mobility are ignored. *Health Place* **2017**, *43*, 85–94. [CrossRef] [PubMed]

15. Zhang, A.; Qi, Q.; Jiang, L.; Zhou, F.; Wang, J. Population exposure to $PM_{2.5}$ in the urban area of Beijing. *PLoS ONE* **2013**, *8*, e63486. [CrossRef] [PubMed]

16. Van Donkelaar, A.; Martin, R.V.; Brauer, M.; Kahn, R.; Levy, R.; Verduzco, C.; Villeneuve, P.J. Global estimates of ambient fine particulate matter concentrations from satellite-based aerosol optical depth: Development and application. *Environ. Health Perspect.* **2010**, *118*, 847–855. [CrossRef] [PubMed]

17. Van Donkelaar, A.; Martin, R.V.; Park, R.J. Estimating ground-level $PM_{2.5}$ using aerosol optical depth determined from satellite remote sensing. *J. Geophys. Res. Atmos.* **2006**, *111*. [CrossRef]

18. Wang, J.; Christopher, S.A. Intercomparison between satellite-derived aerosol optical thickness and $PM_{2.5}$ mass: Implications for air quality studies. *Geophys. Res. Lett.* **2003**, *30*. [CrossRef]

19. Liu, Y.; Park, R.J.; Jacob, D.J.; Li, Q.; Kilaru, V.; Sarnat, J.A. Mapping annual mean ground-level $PM_{2.5}$ concentrations using multiangle imaging spectroradiometer aerosol optical thickness over the contiguous united states. *J. Geophys. Res. Atmos.* **2004**, *109*. [CrossRef]

20. Lin, C.; Li, Y.; Yuan, Z.; Lau, A.K.; Li, C.; Fung, J.C. Using satellite remote sensing data to estimate the high-resolution distribution of ground-level $PM_{2.5}$. *Remote Sens. Environ.* **2015**, *156*, 117–128. [CrossRef]

21. Tian, J.; Chen, D. A semi-empirical model for predicting hourly ground-level fine particulate matter ($PM_{2.5}$) concentration in southern ontario from satellite remote sensing and ground-based meteorological measurements. *Remote Sens. Environ.* **2010**, *114*, 221–229. [CrossRef]

22. Chu, Y.; Liu, Y.; Li, X.; Liu, Z.; Lu, H.; Lu, Y.; Mao, Z.; Chen, X.; Li, N.; Ren, M. A review on predicting ground $PM_{2.5}$ concentration using satellite aerosol optical depth. *Atmosphere* **2016**, *7*, 129. [CrossRef]

23. Hu, Z. Spatial analysis of modis aerosol optical depth, $PM_{2.5}$, and chronic coronary heart disease. *Int. J. Health Geogr.* **2009**, *8*, 27. [CrossRef] [PubMed]

24. Kloog, I.; Koutrakis, P.; Coull, B.A.; Lee, H.J.; Schwartz, J. Assessing temporally and spatially resolved $PM_{2.5}$ exposures for epidemiological studies using satellite aerosol optical depth measurements. *Atmos. Environ.* **2011**, *45*, 6267–6275. [CrossRef]

25. Kloog, I.; Nordio, F.; Coull, B.A.; Schwartz, J. Incorporating local land use regression and satellite aerosol optical depth in a hybrid model of spatiotemporal $PM_{2.5}$ exposures in the mid-atlantic states. *Environ. Sci. Technol.* **2012**, *46*, 11913–11921. [CrossRef] [PubMed]

26. Lee, H.; Liu, Y.; Coull, B.; Schwartz, J.; Koutrakis, P. A novel calibration approach of modis aod data to predict $PM_{2.5}$ concentrations. *Atmos. Chem. Phys.* **2011**, *11*, 7991. [CrossRef]

27. Ma, Z.; Hu, X.; Huang, L.; Bi, J.; Liu, Y. Estimating ground-level $PM_{2.5}$ in China using satellite remote sensing. *Environ. Sci. Technol.* **2014**, *48*, 7436–7444. [CrossRef] [PubMed]

28. Hu, X.; Waller, L.; Lyapustin, A.; Wang, Y.; Liu, Y. 10-year spatial and temporal trends of $PM_{2.5}$ concentrations in the southeastern us estimated using high-resolution satellite data. *Atmos. Chem. Phys.* **2014**, *14*, 6301–6314. [CrossRef] [PubMed]

29. Dewulf, B.; Neutens, T.; Lefebvre, W.; Seynaeve, G.; Vanpoucke, C.; Beckx, C.; Van de Weghe, N. Dynamic assessment of exposure to air pollution using mobile phone data. *Int. J. Health Geogr.* **2016**, *15*, 14. [CrossRef] [PubMed]

30. Gariazzo, C.; Pelliccioni, A.; Bolignano, A. A dynamic urban air pollution population exposure assessment study using model and population density data derived by mobile phone traffic. *Atmos. Environ.* **2016**, *131*, 289–300. [CrossRef]

31. Dewulf, B.; Neutens, T.; Van Dyck, D.; De Bourdeaudhuij, I.; Panis, L.I.; Beckx, C.; Van de Weghe, N. Dynamic assessment of inhaled air pollution using gps and accelerometer data. *J. Transp. Health* **2016**, *3*, 114–123. [CrossRef]

32. Lu, Y.; Fang, B.T. Examining personal air pollution exposure, intake, and health danger zone using time geography and 3D geovisualization. *ISPRS Int. J. Geo-Inf.* **2015**, *4*, 32–46. [CrossRef]

33. Erlander, S.; Stewart, N.F. *The Gravity Model in Transportation Analysis: Theory and Extensions*; VSP: Rancho Cordova, CA, USA, 1990; Volume 3.

34. Simini, F.; González, M.C.; Maritan, A.; Barabási, A.-L. A universal model for mobility and migration patterns. *Nature* **2012**, *484*, 96–100. [CrossRef] [PubMed]

35. Lee, R.; Sumiya, K. Measuring Geographical Regularities of Crowd Behaviors for Twitter-Based Geo-Social Event Detection. In Proceedings of the 2nd ACM SIGSPATIAL International Workshop on Location Based Social Networks, San Jose, CA, USA, 2 November 2010; ACM: New York, NY, USA, 2010; pp. 1–10.

36. Stefanidis, A.; Crooks, A.; Radzikowski, J. Harvesting ambient geospatial information from social media feeds. *GeoJournal* **2013**, *78*, 319–338. [CrossRef]

37. Cheng, Z.; Caverlee, J.; Lee, K.; Sui, D.Z. Exploring millions of footprints in location sharing services. *ICWSM* **2011**, *2011*, 81–88.

38. Frias-Martinez, V.; Soto, V.; Hohwald, H.; Frias-Martinez, E. Characterizing Urban Landscapes Using Geolocated Tweets. In Proceedings of the Privacy, Security, Risk and Trust (PASSAT), 2012 International Conference on and 2012 International Confernece on Social Computing (SocialCom), Amsterdam, The Netherlands, 3–5 September 2012; pp. 239–248.

39. Preoţiuc-Pietro, D.; Cohn, T. Mining User Behaviours: A Study of Check-in Patterns in Location Based Social Networks. In Proceedings of the 5th Annual ACM Web Science Conference, Paris, France, 2–4 May 2013; ACM: New York, NY, USA, 2013; pp. 306–315.

40. Yu, H.; Russell, A.; Mulholland, J.; Huang, Z. Using cell phone location to assess misclassification errors in air pollution exposure estimation. *Environ. Pollut.* **2018**, *233*, 261–266. [CrossRef] [PubMed]

41. Kwan, M.-P. How GIS can help address the uncertain geographic context problem in social science research. *Ann. GIS* **2012**, *18*, 245–255. [CrossRef]

42. Tencent. *Annual Report*; Tencent: Shenzhen, China, 2016.

43. Wackernagel, H. *Multivariate Geostatistics: An Introduction with Applications*; Springer Science & Business Media: Berlin, Germany, 2013.

44. Brunsdon, C.; Fotheringham, A.S.; Charlton, M.E. Geographically weighted regression: A method for exploring spatial nonstationarity. *Geogr. Anal.* **1996**, *28*, 281–298. [CrossRef]

45. Rodriguez, J.D.; Perez, A.; Lozano, J.A. Sensitivity analysis of k-fold cross validation in prediction error estimation. *IEEE Trans. Pattern Anal. Mach. Intell.* **2010**, *32*, 569–575. [CrossRef] [PubMed]

46. Chafe, Z.A.; Brauer, M.; Klimont, Z.; Van Dingenen, R.; Mehta, S.; Rao, S.; Riahi, K.; Dentener, F.; Smith, K.R. Household cooking with solid fuels contributes to ambient $PM_{2.5}$ air pollution and the burden of disease. *Environ. Health Perspect.* **2014**, *122*, 1314–1320. [CrossRef] [PubMed]

47. Gamble, J.F. $PM_{2.5}$ and mortality in long-term prospective cohort studies: Cause-effect or statistical associations? *Environ. Health Perspect.* **1998**, *106*, 535–549. [CrossRef] [PubMed]
48. Gavett, S.H.; Koren, H.S. The role of particulate matter in exacerbation of atopic asthma. *Int. Archiv. Allergy Immunol.* **2001**, *124*, 109–112. [CrossRef] [PubMed]
49. Wong, J.Y.; De Vivo, I.; Lin, X.; Christiani, D.C. Cumulative $PM_{2.5}$ exposure and telomere length in workers exposed to welding fumes. *J. Toxicol. Environ. Health Part A* **2014**, *77*, 441–455. [CrossRef] [PubMed]
50. Zhang, L.; Wang, F.; Ji, Y.; Jiao, J.; Zou, D.; Liu, L.; Shan, C.; Bai, Z.; Sun, Z. Phthalate esters (paes) in indoor PM_{10}/$PM_{2.5}$ and human exposure to paes via inhalation of indoor air in Tianjin, China. *Atmos. Environ.* **2014**, *85*, 139–146. [CrossRef]
51. Adams, W.C. *Measurement of Breathing Rate and Volume in Routinely Performed Daily Activities: Final Report*; Contract NO. A033-205; University of California: Davis, CA, USA, 1993.
52. Marty, M.A.; Blaisdell, R.J.; Broadwin, R.; Hill, M.; Shimer, D.; Jenkins, M. Distribution of daily breathing rates for use in California's air toxics hot spots program risk assessments. *Hum. Ecol. Risk Assess.* **2002**, *8*, 1723–1737. [CrossRef]

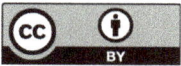

International Journal of
Environmental Research and Public Health

MDPI

Article

An Innovative Context-Based Crystal-Growth Activity Space Method for Environmental Exposure Assessment: A Study Using GIS and GPS Trajectory Data Collected in Chicago

Jue Wang [1], Mei-Po Kwan [1] and Yanwei Chai [2,*]

[1]   Department of Geography and Geographic Information Science, Natural History Building,
      1301 W Green Street University of Illinois at Urbana-Champaign, Urbana, IL 61801, USA;
      kingjue.w@gmail.com (J.W.); mpk654@gmail.com (M.-P.K.)
[2]   Department of Urban and Economic Geography, College of Urban and Environmental Sciences,
      Peking University, Beijing 100871, China
*   Correspondence: chyw@pku.edu.cn

Received: 9 March 2018; Accepted: 3 April 2018; Published: 9 April 2018

Abstract: Scholars in the fields of health geography, urban planning, and transportation studies have long attempted to understand the relationships among human movement, environmental context, and accessibility. One fundamental question for this research area is how to measure individual activity space, which is an indicator of where and how people have contact with their social and physical environments. Conventionally, standard deviational ellipses, road network buffers, minimum convex polygons, and kernel density surfaces have been used to represent people's activity space, but they all have shortcomings. Inconsistent findings of the effects of environmental exposures on health behaviors/outcomes suggest that the reliability of existing studies may be affected by the uncertain geographic context problem (UGCoP). This paper proposes the context-based crystal-growth activity space as an innovative method for generating individual activity space based on both GPS trajectories and the environmental context. This method not only considers people's actual daily activity patterns based on GPS tracks but also takes into account the environmental context which either constrains or encourages people's daily activity. Using GPS trajectory data collected in Chicago, the results indicate that the proposed new method generates more reasonable activity space when compared to other existing methods. This can help mitigate the UGCoP in environmental health studies.

Keywords: GIS; GPS; activity space; environmental exposure; the uncertain geographic context problem

---

1. Introduction

In the fields of epidemiology and health geography, understanding environmental exposure is a nontrivial issue involving the investigation of environmental effects on human health. Researchers have examined the relationships among human movement, environmental context, and health outcomes over the past decades. Abundant research has shown that physical activity, tobacco use, obesity, mental health and many other health behaviors or issues are related to environmental exposure [1–4]. For instance, it has been found that the built environment influences physical activity and health [5,6]—e.g., obesity is more prevalent in areas that lack physical activity facilities [7] or are unfriendly to walking [8,9]. One of the fundamental questions in this research area is how to measure environmental exposure.

Despite the existence of many methods, the residential neighborhood is predominantly utilized as the contextual unit for environmental exposure measurement. It is often represented by administration areas, such as census tracts and postal units, because of the availability and easy access to routine administrative data. The readily available spatial delineations of administrative areas and the lack of detailed mobility data are other reasons for the popularity of administrative areas in environmental health research. With the help of advanced geospatial technologies (e.g., geographic information systems [GIS] and global positioning system [GPS]), there has been a methodological shift in health research, moving from using fixed administrative areas as contextual units to ego-centered definitions [10–12]. An ego-centered neighborhood is usually represented by a buffer area centered on an individual's home with a given threshold of specific distance or travel time [13], which may reflect more accurately the exposure area rather than administrative units. Due to the ongoing debate as to the best way to define geographic context [14–17] and the availability of activity diary and GPS tracking data, many researchers have now adopted the idea that the residential neighborhood can only partially capture people's exposure to environmental context, and daily activities that take place at other locations also contribute to their environmental exposures [10,18,19]. The shift from a static measuring approach to a dynamic one has inspired researchers to explore and develop exposure assessment methods using individual GPS tracking data [20–22].

Although there are many ways to measure environmental exposure, activity space based on GPS tracking data (movement data) appears to be a promising way to assess the environment utilized by individuals, and to which they are exposed [23,24]. Activity space is defined as "the local areas within which people move or travel in the course of their daily activities" [25]. Because activity space indicates where and how people have contact with their social and physical environments [26], it can be used as a measure of "people's degree of mobility" [27]. The activity space of an individual can thus be used to explore the interaction between human activity and environmental context [28,29]. Conventionally, standard deviational ellipses, GPS trajectory buffers, minimum convex polygons, and kernel density surfaces have been used to represent human activity space [13,28,30]. Notwithstanding the improvements in the theory and methodology to assess environmental exposure and in the investigation of the contextual effects on health outcomes with activity space, substantial challenges remain.

Even with advanced activity space methods to assess individual environmental exposure, inconsistent findings of the environmental effects on health behaviors/outcomes have been observed in recent studies [31–33]. This suggests that the reliability of existing studies may be affected by the misspecification of the geographic context [34], which was recently articulated as the uncertain geographic context problem (UGCoP) by Kwan [14]. The UGCoP refers to the problem that findings of the effects of area-based environmental variables (e.g., land-use mix) on health outcomes or behavior (e.g., physical activity) can be affected by how contextual units are geographically delineated. The problem "arises because of the spatial uncertainty in the actual areas that exert contextual influences on the individuals being studied and the temporal uncertainty in the timing and duration in which individuals experienced these contextual influences" [35]. Existing activity space methods have limitations that may compromise their ability to mitigate the UGCoP both spatially and temporally. From the perspective of spatial uncertainty, conventional methods ignore the accessibility of different locations in the study area and thus may include locations that may not be accessible to people. Moreover, arbitrary cut-off distances are often used for delineating activity space. Temporally, the duration of environmental exposure is treated merely as the multiplier of exposure while individuals' interactions with space during particular periods of time (the more time spent at the location, the more familiar with the sounding area) is not considered.

This paper proposes the context-based crystal-growth (CCG) activity space as an innovative method for generating individual activity space based on both GPS tracking and environmental context. To mitigate the UGCoP, portable GPS devices are utilized to trace human movement accurately, and advanced GIS methods are used to relate these data to high-resolution data of relevant environmental contexts [14,36]. The integration of GPS and GIS provides a powerful means for examining the relationships between environmental contexts and health outcomes [22,37].

In contrast to other existing methods, and in order to address spatial uncertainty, activity space is generated considering not only people's actual daily activity patterns based on GPS tracks but also the environmental contexts that either constrain or encourage people's daily activity. Instead of using arbitrary cut-off distance, activity space is delineated based on the features of individual movement patterns. To mitigate temporal uncertainty, the duration of the environmental context in which individuals experienced and with which individuals interact are taken into account by abstracting the core areas of their daily activities. The size of activity space is based on the accumulated time an individual spent at the location (the more time a person spent there, the larger the activity space). To the best of our knowledge, this is the first study to introduce the context-based crystal-growth method and consider both people's daily activity patterns and environmental context in activity space and environmental health research. The results indicate that the proposed new method generates more reasonable activity space and more accurate exposure assessment when compared to other existing methods. It can help mitigate the UGCoP spatially and temporally in environmental exposure measures. The accurate assessment of environmental exposures sheds light on the investigation of environmental effects in the field of epidemiology and health geography. The method is a new tool for activity space delineation and can be used for exploring the relationships among human movement patterns, environmental context, and health outcomes.

2. Methodology

This research proposes an innovative method for delineating individual activity space based on GPS tracking data, accessibility-related contextual data, and a crystal-growth algorithm. Due to the capability of incorporating GPS tracking and contextual data, as well as the flexibility to adaptively adjust the activity space based on the context of accessibility, this method is suitable for generating activity space while mitigating the UGCoP. In this method, accessibility-related contexts are incorporated into weighted planes, in which space is tiled into fine regular-grid cells (e.g., hexagonal cells). The weighted planes use hexagon grids to achieve higher accuracy in representing the spatial features of the land surface and minimize orientation bias and sampling bias from edge effects. The method is also capable of handling different transportation modes (e.g., walking, driving, taking the bus or train) while generating the activity space. Two accessibility-weighted planes are generated for public transport users and private transport users, respectively, considering the different effects of context for various groups of residents. Based on the weighted planes, space is delineated by the growth of cells from one or more seed points to neighbor cells through a sequence of growth cycles. The crystal-growth method is suitable for this study because the growth speed of each cell can be dynamically adjusted according to the accessibility-weighted planes, and the growth extent can be feasibly defined based on travel time. Figure 1 illustrates the workflow of the proposed context-based crystal-growth method. As people's frequently visited locations are essential for understanding their daily activity, these places are considered as the core areas of their activity space, as identified by the kernel density analysis of an individual's 7-day GPS trajectories. Thus, the activity space is grown from the core areas, and they will grow to their neighbor cells cycle by cycle. The crystal-growth process is either constrained or encouraged based on the accessibility-weighted planes. The merging of the crystal-growth space of all core areas generates the activity space.

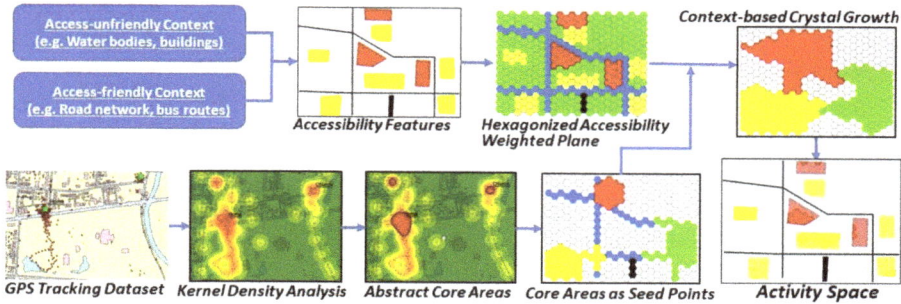

Figure 1. Workflow of the context-based crystal-growth activity space method.

2.1. GPS Tracking and Context Data

The individual GPS tracking dataset used in this research was collected as part of a larger study that examines the relationship among the exposure to environmental stressors, neighborhood quality, and individual health in Chicago. The larger study seeks to understand how the neighborhoods people live in and visit in their daily life affect their health and wellbeing. It focuses on the noise and air quality that people are exposed to in their daily life—not just at their residence, but also while they undertake their daily activities at other locations (e.g., travel to work, shopping, or running errands). The data were collected from October to December 2017 in the Chicago metropolitan area using surveys, GPS-equipped mobile phones, and portable noise and air pollutant sensors. The GPS tracking dataset is not recorded in even temporal duration but somewhat random over time depending on participants' movement for prolonging battery life. To be specific, if a subject moves more than 1 m from the previous record within 3 s, a tracking point will be recorded by the tracking device. If the subject does not move more than 1 m from the last record in 3 s, a new tracking point is still recorded. In the GPS tracking dataset, each subject was tracked with GPS-equipped mobile phones for seven days. Because most people have highly routinized daily activities [38], 7-day continuous activity tracking, which covers both weekdays and weekends, can capture most of the participants' weekly routine activities and is typically used for activity space research [38–44]. Consistent with previous studies, GPS tracks for 7 consecutive days were used to generate individual activity space in this study.

To compare the activity space generated by different methods, as some of them are sensitive to participants' movement patterns, four representative participants are selected from the dataset, as their movement trajectories have very different patterns (the spatial arrangement of the GPS points). The movement trajectories of Person A show a compact clustered pattern, those of Person B exhibit a modest clustered pattern, those of Person C display a one-directional pattern, and those of Person D present a multi-directional pattern. Note that due to the Institutional Review Board's (IRB) requirements for protecting data confidentiality and participants' privacy, we can describe the patterns but cannot include these maps in this paper.

Further, the activity spaces are used to assess environmental exposure with the whole dataset. The exposure to physical-activity-friendly contexts is used as a proxy for the comparison of activity space methods. Physical activity has been intensively studied in environmental health research [45–47] because it is highly related to many chronic diseases, such as type-II diabetes, obesity and cardiovascular diseases [8,48–51]. Although the results are inconsistent, most previous studies have observed a positive association between physical-activity-friendly environments and the level of physical activity [1,44,52–57]; the effectiveness of activity space for environmental exposure assessment can be evaluated by examining whether the association between exposure to the context and physical activity is captured. Physical-activity-friendly contexts include green spaces, blue spaces and other leisure facilities such as urban parks, playgrounds, swimming pools, and sports centers. The level of physical activity, which was reported by participants in the questionnaire before the GPS tracking, is measured by the number of days over a typical week in which a participant is physically active for a total of at least 30 min. There are 31 participants whose GPS tracking data in the dataset are used for such evaluation. The sociodemographic characteristics of these participants are shown in Table 1. The physical-activity-friendly contexts are just an example used to illustrate the usefulness of the proposed activity space method for environmental exposure assessment, which can also be applied to examine the effects of other environmental influences on other kinds of health behaviors or outcomes. For example, to explore the environmental influences on people's body weight, we can include the availability of different types of food outlets or shops (e.g., fast-food outlets that sell unhealthy foods and supermarkets that provide more selections of healthy foods. To examine people's exposure to air pollution, we can include traffic-related sources (e.g., highways) and various point sources (e.g., industrial plants; oil refineries) as environmental influences.

Table 1. Sociodemographic characteristics of the participants in this study.

Sociodemographic Variables		Percentage
Gender	Male	61.3%
	Female	38.7%
Age	18–30	17.2%
	31–40	17.2%
	41–50	24.1%
	51–65	41.4%
Race	White	9.7%
	African American	41.9%
	Latino/Hispanic	41.9%
	Other	6.5%
Education	Elementary School	6.5%
	High School	58.1%
	College/University	32.3%
	Graduate School	3.2%
Marital Status	Married	17.9%
	Divorced	14.3%
	Single	67.9%
Annual Income	Less than $10,000	58.1%
	$10,000–$24,999	19.4%
	$25,000–$50,000	9.7%
	$50,000–$99,000	9.7%
	$100,000 or more	3.2%

To generate a consistent and consecutive time series for the GPS trajectories, data cleaning and interpolation of GPS points was conducted so that there is one GPS tracking point each second for every participant for the 7-day tracking period. A Python program is developed to test every consecutive pair of GPS records and calculate the time difference. If the time difference between two consecutive GPS records is N seconds, which is longer than 1 s and shorter than 1800 s (half hour), linear interpolation in both spatial and temporal dimension is performed between the GPS records so that N-1 more records are inserted. After the interpolation process, each participant has one GPS tracking point for every second for the entire tracking period.

The environmental context data for this study were derived from a comprehensive digital geographic database of Chicago from the Chicago Data Portal as well as the volunteered geographic information website of OpenStreetMap. This includes the geographic location and footprint of buildings, water bodies, woods, restricted area (e.g., airport), and ground railways, which can be considered as barrier factors for accessibility; while the various levels of road networks, walkable areas, public transport routes are considered as the access friendly context that encourages accessibility. These contextual data are used to generate the two context-based hexagonal accessibility-weighted planes.

2.2. Core Areas of Daily Activities

People's frequently-visited locations are crucial for understanding their daily activity and the delineation of their activity space. Therefore, these locations (core areas) are first abstracted from the GPS trajectories using kernel density analysis. The results of the kernel density analysis of the GPS trajectories are not distributed normally and skewed to the low-density values, so the geometric interval classification is a suitable method for classifying the density values by minimizing the sum of squares of the number of elements in each class. The algorithm creates geometric intervals to ensure that each class range has approximately the same number of values while keeping the change between intervals consistent [58]. The core areas are abstracted from the results of the kernel density analysis as the collection of cells with density value larger than the 3/4 cut point of the geometric interval classification of all non-zero values. These core areas will be used as the seed points in the following crystal-growth delineation. Further, the number of the growth cycle of each core area is weighted based on the accumulated time the individual spent at these locations. The more time a person spent there, the more cycles the activity space grows. The crystal-growth cycle of each core area is calculated based on the normalized sojourn time (NST) at each core area. For instance, one individual spent 600 min daily at home on average, so the normalized sojourn time at home (NST_h) is 600. The growth extent (GE) is dependent on the NST. We assume the growth extent from home location is GE_h, so the GE_i of other core areas can be calculated based on the following formula:

$$a = \sqrt[GE_h]{NST_h} \tag{1}$$

$$GE_i = \log_a NST_i \tag{2}$$

where GE_i is the growth extent of seed point i in minutes, NST_i is the normalized sojourn time at core area i, NST_h is the normalized sojourn time at home, GE_h is the growth extent from the home location.

As the only parameter for defining the growth extent of all the core areas, the GE_h can be fixed universally for all subjects, and it can also be determined based on personal mobility. For the purpose of illustration, this study uses 10-mins' travel as the universal value of GE_h. Although the GE_h could be different for people with different mobility, 10-mins' travel distance is a reasonable assumption that people are familiar with the environment and activity opportunities of the areas around the home, and it is highly possible that people choose to undertake the daily activity and are exposed to the context in this area.

2.3. Context-Based Hexagonal Accessibility-Weighted Planes

The accessibility-weighted plane, as a representation of the accessibility-friendliness of the environmental context, considers the effect of many kinds of environmental contexts (e.g., rivers as barriers, roads as thoroughfares) on the accessibility of the study area. The context of buildings, water bodies, woods, restricted areas, ground railways, road networks, public transport routes (metro and bus) and walkable areas are critical factors for the accessibility-weighted plane. Further, considering the different effects of environmental contexts for various groups of people (e.g., the expressway is considered as a thoroughfare for car users, while it is a barrier for public transport users), two context-based hexagonal accessibility-weighted planes are generated respectively for private transport users and public transport users.

For private transport users, on the one hand, among all these contexts, buildings, water bodies, woods, restricted areas (e.g., airport, private land) and ground railways are considered as barrier factors that are normally hard to trespass by people. On the other hand, various levels of road networks and walkable areas are accessibility-friendly context since they increase the general approachability of various sites. Road networks are further classified into expressways, primary roads, secondary roads and tertiary roads with various travel speeds. On the accessibility-weighted plane, as illustrated in Table 2, seed point cells are assigned a value of 100. The barrier cells (e.g., restricted areas and water bodies) are designated a value from 10 to 14 with a growth speed of 0. The transport network cells are assigned a value of 21 to 24, and the growth speed varies with their average travel speed. For pedestrian trails and walkable areas, cell values of 30 and 31 are assigned, respectively, and the growth speed is 1 cell per cycle (3 miles/h).

In contrast to private transport users, for public transport users, expressways, buildings, water bodies, woods, restricted areas and ground railways are considered as barriers, while metro routes and bus routes are considered as thoroughfares with higher accessibility. On the weighted plane for public transport users, all kinds of local road (including primary roads, secondary roads, tertiary roads, and pedestrian trails) are considered as walkable area only, since they do not have cars to drive on them. As listed in Table 3, local roads and walkable areas are assigned a value of 30 and 31, with a growth speed of 1 cell per cycle. Bus routes have a growth speed of 3 cells per cycle with a cell value of 23, while metro routes have a growth speed of 6 cells per cycle with a cell value of 21. Metro stations are also marked in the weighted plane (cell value: 22; growth speed: 1), since citizens can only get on or get off the metro system at stations. On the contrary, bus stations are not considered, since buses stop frequently and the distance between bus stations are only about 100 to 200 m in Chicago.

Table 2. Cell attributes of the hexagonal accessibility-weighted plane for private transport users.

Context Type	Cell Value	Average Moving Velocity	Growth Speed (Cells/Cycle)
Out of Research Area	0	-	0
Restricted Area	10	-	0
Water Bodies	11	-	0
Woods	12	-	0
Buildings	13	-	0
Railway	14	-	0
Expressway	21	About 35 miles/h	12
Primary Road	22	About 25 miles/h	8
Secondary Road	23	About 15 miles/h	5
Tertiary Road	24	About 9 miles/h	3
Pedestrian Trail	30	About 3 miles/h	1
Walkable Area	31	About 3 miles/h	1
Seed Points	100	About 3 miles/h	1

Table 3. Cell attributes of the hexagonal accessibility-weighted plane for public transport users.

Context Type	Cell Value	Average Moving Velocity	Growth Speed (Cells/Cycle)
Out of Research Area	0	-	0
Restricted Area	10	-	0
Water Bodies	11	-	0
Woods	12	-	0
Buildings	13	-	0
Railway	14	-	0
Expressway	15	-	0
Metro Routes	21	About 18 miles/h	6
Metro Stations	22	About 3 miles/h	1
Bus Routes	23	About 9 miles/h	3
Local Roads	30	About 3 miles/h	1
Walkable Area	31	About 3 miles/h	1
Seed Points	100	About 3 miles/h	1

The geographical location and footprint of the environmental contexts are utilized to generate the hexagon-grid-based accessibility-weighted plane. The hexagonal grid, different from the raster grid, tiles the land surface with regularly sized hexagonal cells. They are the most compact regular polygons that can fill the land surface [59]. Hexagonal cells are closer in shape to circles [60,61], and they have only one kind of neighbor cells that share the same edge. Further, the distance to the centroid of a cell from the six neighboring cells is the same. The hexagon grid can achieve high accuracy in representing the spatial features of land surface from the perspective of spatial analysis [60], and it reduces the complexity in defining neighbor cells when compared to the raster grid. Thus, it is suitable for the crystal-growth algorithms used in this study. Figure 2 illustrates the environmental contexts of a neighborhood in Chicago, and the generated hexagonal accessibility-weighted plane for private transport users (see Figure 3) and public transport users (see Figure 4). The hexagonal cells in the weighted planes have a fine resolution of 10 × 10 m to ensure the accuracy of the calculation, and were generated using ArcMap. The context-based hexagonal accessibility-weighted planes of Chicago are shown in Figure 5; there are about 6 million hexagonal cells for each weighted plane that covers the city.

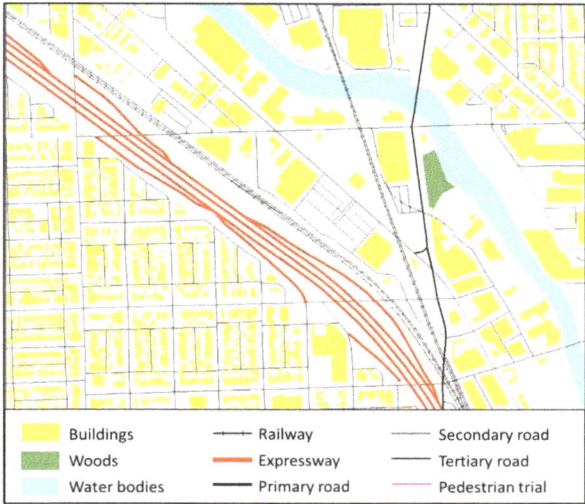

Buildings	Railway	Secondary road
Woods	Expressway	Tertiary road
Water bodies	Primary road	Pedestrian trial

Figure 2. Accessibility-related environmental contexts.

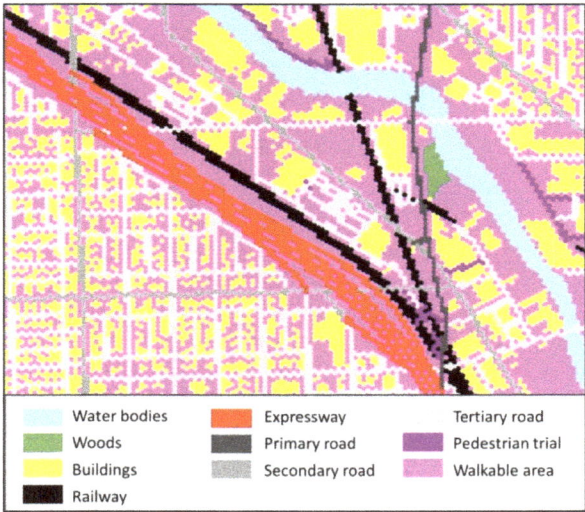

Water bodies	Expressway	Tertiary road
Woods	Primary road	Pedestrian trial
Buildings	Secondary road	Walkable area
Railway		

Figure 3. Hexagonal accessibility-weighted plane for private transport users.

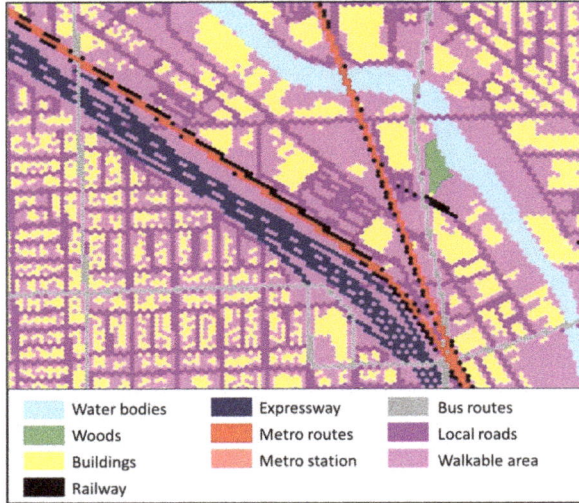

Figure 4. Hexagonal accessibility-weighted plane for public transport users.

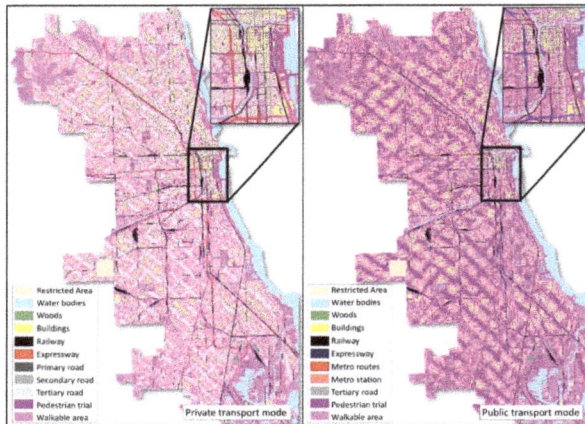

Figure 5. The context-based hexagonal accessibility-weighted plane of Chicago.

2.4. Hexagon-Grid Crystal-Growth Activity Space

The crystal-growth method is a tool for space partitioning and was used for Voronoi diagrams [62], spatial delineation [63], and spatial optimization [64]. The method is suitable for this study because the growth speed of each cell could be adjusted based on the context of accessibility. Since the context of accessibility is one of the critical factors for accurately generating activity space, which is rarely considered in previous research, this study utilizes the crystal-growth algorithm based on the hexagon-grid accessibility-weighted planes.

Figure 6 illustrates this crystal-growth algorithm. In the method, the activity space is grown from all seed point cells (the location of the core areas), the service area of each seed point cell will grow to their neighbor cells cycle by cycle. Because the weighted planes simulate the road network and other physical barriers (Figure 6a), the growth speed of each location can be adjusted in real time based on the attributes of the cells. For instance, roads speed up growth, while rivers or lakes block the growth. For illustration, the road network is rendered as blue cells, while black cells represent barriers in the figure. As illustrated, crystal-growth starts from the seed point cells to their six immediate neighbor cells, and the growth continues cycle by cycle (Figure 6a,b illustrates one crystal-growth cycle). In contrast to other cells, the growth speed of transport network cells is faster due to the higher accessibility they enable (Figure 6b,c). Growth is constrained by natural barrier cells because it is usually challenging to travel through barriers such as rivers and lakes (Figure 6c,d). The growth of each seed point will stop when its maximum growth extent reached. The merging of the crystal-growth area of all core areas generates the final activity space.

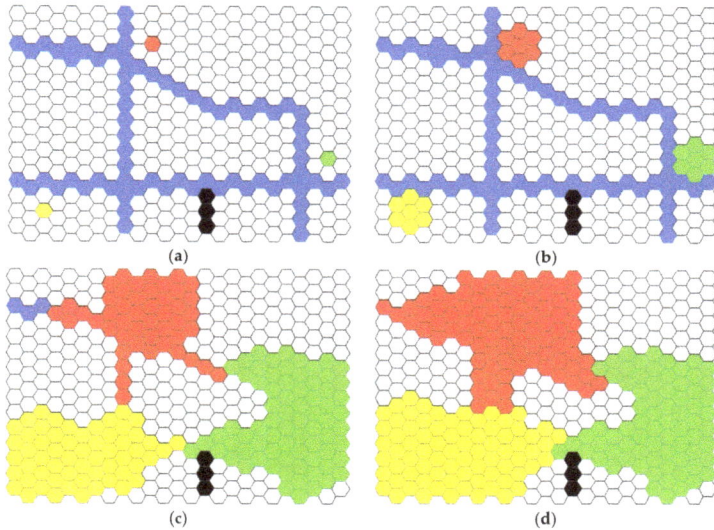

Figure 6. Illustration of the context-based crystal-growth activity space method. (**a**) The initial status with three seed cells; (**b**) crystal growth after one cycle; (**c**) crystal growth after several cycles; (**d**) the final result of crystal-growth. The red, yellow and green cells are three seed cells. Blue cells represent transport network, while black cells illustrate the physical barriers. The other white cells imply the walkable area.

According to the generation method of the context-based crystal-growth method discussed above, activity space is generated according to the following growth rules. (1) Based on participants' travel mode, choose the context-based hexagonal accessibility-weighted plane accordingly for either private transport users or public transport users. (2) The crystal-growth starts from all the seed points (core area cells) separately. Seed point cells are the hexagon cells that intersect with the locations of the centroids of core areas. (3) For each crystal-growth cycle, if a neighbor cell is a barrier cell or a cell that has already been labeled as a grown area, it will be skipped. Otherwise, the neighbor cell will be marked as the grown area. (4) The crystal-growth speed of each cell is determined by the cell value, which was defined on the accessibility-weighted planes. (5) The crystal-growth will finish if the growth of all the seed cells reached their maximum growth extent. (6) The final activity space is generated by merging all the crystal-growth areas.

2.5. Other Existing Activity Space Methods

To compare the proposed context-based crystal-growth (CCG) activity space method with other existing methods, four commonly used delineations of activity space are implemented with the same

GPS dataset, including GPS trajectory buffers (GTB), standard deviational ellipses (SDE), kernel density surfaces (KDS) and minimum convex polygons (MCP). GTB was created for each selected participant by covering the subject's GPS trajectories with a 200-m buffer area, which covers all the locations that a participant visited or passed by during the study period. SDE is a commonly used method for delineating individual activity space. The SDE captures the geographic distribution and directional trend of all activity locations. The ellipse was obtained based on one or two standard deviations of the distances between each point and the transformed mean center along the rotated major and minor axes of the point set. Since past studies have used either one standard deviation SDE (SDE1) or two standard deviations SDE (SDE2), we derived both in this study for comparative purposes. KDS is a density surface derived from the activity locations and an associated weight using a kernel function and a predetermined search radius. In this study, the KDS was generated based on the duration spent at each GPS point as the weight on a raster layer at the spatial resolution of 10×10 m and search radius of 1000 m. MCP for a subject is the smallest convex polygon that contains all of the person's GPS tracking points. It represents the smallest area that includes all activity destinations of a participant.

3. Results

3.1. Context-Based Crystal-Growth Activity Space

The CCG activity spaces delineated based on the four selected participants are illustrated in Figure 7. For person A, whose daily activity is highly concentrated around the home location, it shows a compact clustered pattern. Based on the collected demographic characteristics, this person is a retired female in her 60s, who spends most of her time at home and only visits the public library regularly. Only two core areas are detected, and they are close to each other. Thus, the CCG activity space is a grown area centered at these two locations within the travel distance of 10 min from home (one of the core areas) and the corresponding travel distance (calculated based on the normalized sojourn time) from the other core area (library). Because the growth is based on the accessibility-weighted plane, the activity space protrudes along major roads due to their higher accessibility than other contexts. There are several hollow areas in the activity space, which are barrier contexts, such as water bodies and private houses, that could not be easily trespassed. In contrast to the compact clustered pattern, person B presents a modest clustered pattern. Although the movement is also clustered around the home, this person has more activity locations and travels much further than person A to undertake daily activities. According to the participant's profile, this subject is an unemployed male in his 40s. He visits his mother's home frequently in the west of the city about half-hours' drive from home. He also visits the downtown area to visit doctors and friends. Not surprisingly, three core areas are identified, and his CCG activity space is composed of three separate grown areas centered at home, mother's house and downtown. The largest sub-area is the one centered at home (in the middle of the map) based on the fact that he spends the largest amount of time at home. He also spends much time at his mother's house, and the sub-area should be larger than the current form, which is truncated due to edge effects. His mother's home is close to the boundary of the study area, and thus only part of the sub-area is captured due to the lack of contextual information outside the border of the study area. Since the time he spends in the downtown area is much less when compared to the time spends in the other two core areas, this sub-area is much smaller. With a one-directional pattern, the CCG activity space of person C is exhibited in Figure 7. This person is a middle-aged male. He does grocery shopping and other personal activities around the home neighborhood. That is probably the reason why many core areas are identified around his residential neighborhood. What's more, with his close relatives living in the southeastern part of the city, he needs to drive there and visit them regularly, and that is why we find another core area there. Thus, his activity space has a significant part centered at home and another small portion in the southeastern part of the city. Finally, person D is a female adult, who has a full-time job at downtown. With considerable mobility and travel around the city for daily activities, this participant's movement shows a multi-directional pattern. As shown in the figure, the two largest portions of her activity space are the ones around home and workplace, since a significant amount of time is spent at these two locations. Other small parts of her activity space are scattered around the city for different daily activities. As a married woman, she needs to take care of the family, which includes grocery shopping and other household-related activities. It is noted that even though she traveled to the further north of the city, no activity space is identified, because she only spends limited time there, and it is not recognized as a core area. It is reasonable to exclude this kind of location from the activity space if the subject only visits the place with limited time on a nonregular basis.

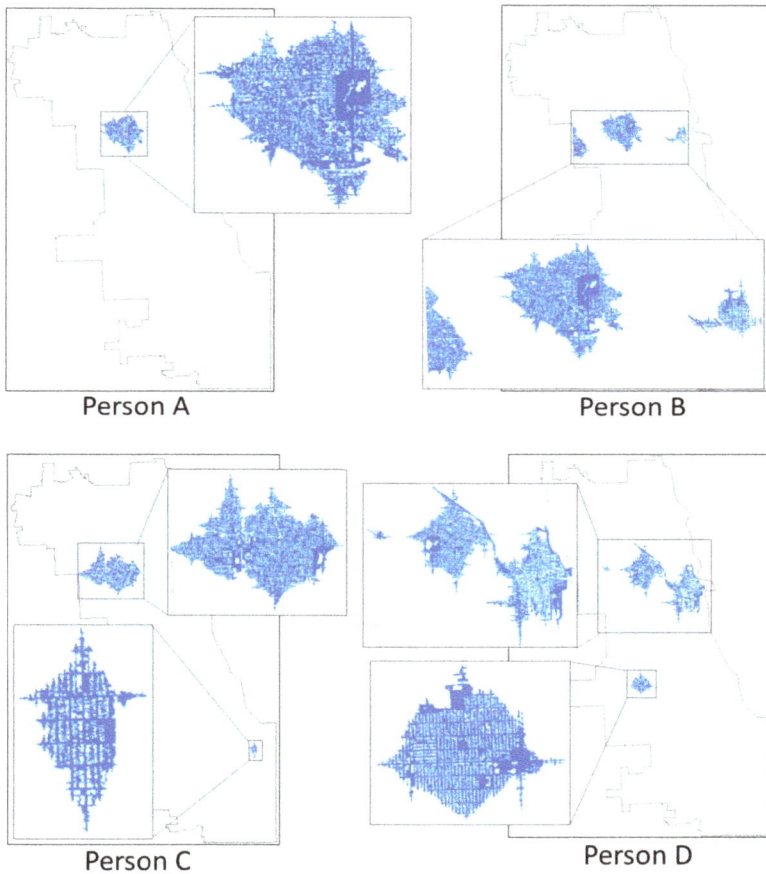

Figure 7. The context-based crystal-growth activity spaces of the four representative participants.

To compare and illustrate the difference of CCG based on accessibility-weighted planes for private transport users and public transport users, respectively, as shown in Figure 8, both activity spaces are generated with the same core areas at the same locations. For private transport users, the activity space is grown and enlarged along primary and secondary roads. On the contrary, the public transport users relied heavily on the bus and metro systems, so the activity space extends along the bus and metro routes instead of the roads. It can be seen from the figure that the CCG activity space of public transport users is much smaller than that of private transport users.

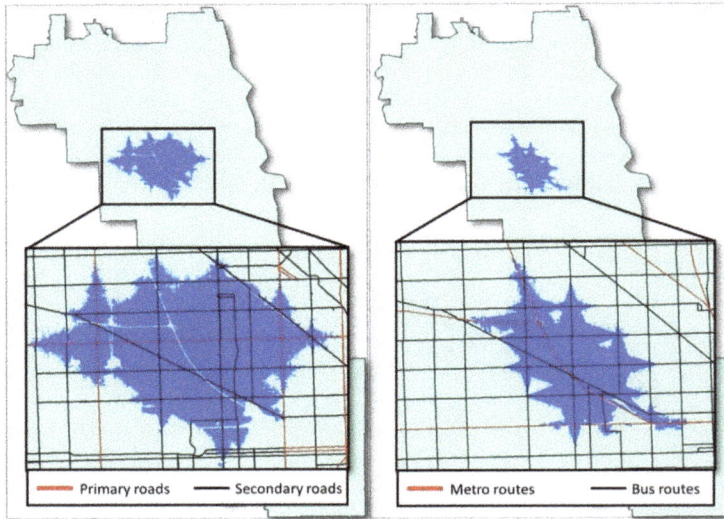

Figure 8. Crystal-growth activity space based on accessibility-weighted plane for private transport users (**left**) and public transport users (**right**).

3.2. Comparing the CCG Activity Spaces with Other Activity Spaces

3.2.1. Comparing the Activity Spaces

The commonly used methods for activity space delineations are implemented with the four representative participants' GPS tracking trajectory to compare with the proposed CCG method. The comparison is based on the geometric characteristics of the activity spaces, matching them with subjects' daily activity, and visual interpretation. The activity spaces of the four participants are illustrated in Figure 9, and the comparison results are listed in Table 4. Note that the resulting maps of GTB, due to the risk of re-identification for the subjects, are not included in Figure 9 in order to protect their privacy. The activity spaces of person A are similar among the different methods because of the simplicity of the daily movement. Since person A has low mobility, and the GPS trajectories have a compact clustered pattern, all five methods generate activity spaces that are nearly circular, while focusing on the home location of the subject. The area of activity spaces generated by CCG (8.21 km^2) and KDS (6.58 km^2) are significantly larger than the area of activity spaces generated by the other two methods, while they cover almost all of the total GPS tracking points. For more complicated movement patterns (persons B, C, and D), the CCG is capable of generating multiple areas to portray individual activity space, whereas all the other methods only create a single continuous region. The area of the activity space of person B is larger than the one of person A. KDS (66.66 km^2) and MCP (65.52 km^2) have the largest area, while CCG (11.74 km^2) has the smallest area. CCG activity spaces have the highest coverage of the total GPS tracking points except for the GTB, KDS, and MCP. For person C, the GTB, KDS, and MCP include not only the area for daily activity, but also the places along the travel trajectories between activity locations, leading to their larger areas. The directional pattern of the GPS trajectories makes the SDE highly compressed. Although the SDE does not include the places along the travel trajectory, it ignores the activity location in the southeastern part of the city and covers a lot of unrelated sites in the northwestern part. Still, the CCG activity spaces have the smallest size among all the activity spaces (18.76 km^2) for person D. The dispersed GPS trajectories around the city make the area of the activity spaces generated with KDS, MCP, and SDE extremely huge, which covers many irrelevant city spaces. On average, the CCG has the smallest area (12.65 km^2) among all the methods and the highest coverage (94.04%) of total GPS tracking points except for GTB, KDS, and MCP. Because of the nature of the techniques themselves, GTB, KDS, and MCP always cover all the GPS tracking points. On the contrary, CCG, and SDE include only the prominent parts of the points since they are more focused on the characteristics of the movement patterns instead of every single GPS point.

Table 4. Comparing the representative participants' activity spaces generated by different methods.

		CCG	GTB	KDS	MCP	SDE1	SDE2
Person A	Area (km²)	8.21	0.91	6.58	0.52	0.0373	0.15
	%GTPC	100%	100%	100%	100%	93.28%	93.45%
Person B	Area (km²)	11.74	31.14	66.66	65.52	12.704	50.82
	%GTPC	87.97%	100%	100%	100%	76.47%	85.71%
Person C	Area (km²)	11.89	19.14	81.20	105.10	7.71	30.83
	%GTPC	96.60%	100%	100%	100%	82.04%	93.72%
Person D	Area (km²)	18.76	28.92	101.28	109.16	39.12	156.48
	%GTPC	91.69%	100%	100%	100%	75.69%	90.83%
Average	Area (km²)	12.65	20.03	63.93	70.08	14.89	59.57
	%GTPC	94.04%	100%	100%	100%	81.87%	90.93%

Note: the area of KDS is measured as the total area with positive density, which is consistent with Schonfelder and Axhausen [65]; %GTPC: percent of total GPS tracking points covered.

For a more comprehensive comparative analysis, the activity spaces of the 31 participants in the dataset are also generated by CCG and the other five methods. Figure 10 illustrates the differences in the size of the activity spaces for private transport and public transport users. Considering the median size of the activity spaces, private transport users have larger activity spaces than those of public transport users for all the six methods; while the average size of the activity spaces of private transport users is still larger when compared to that of public transport users for all the methods except MCP. However, as shown in the boxplot in Figure 10, the difference is only significant for CCG.

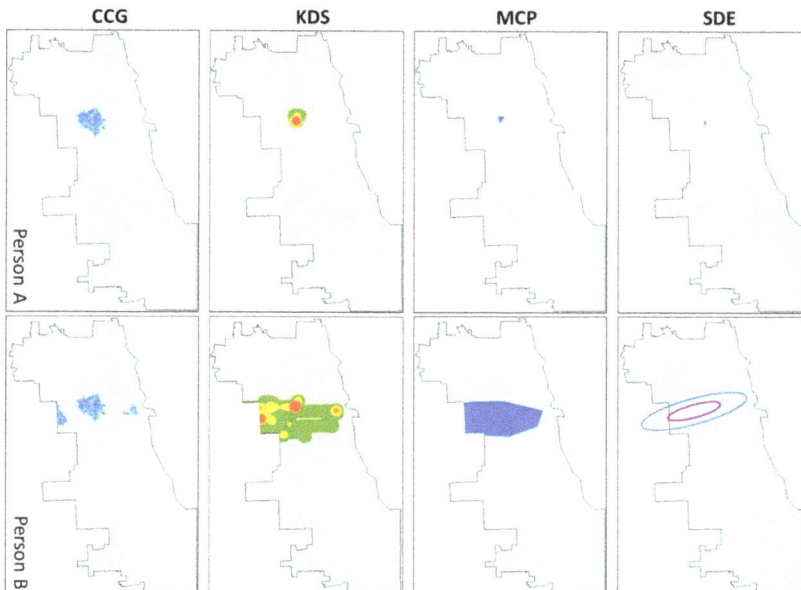

Figure 9. *Cont.*

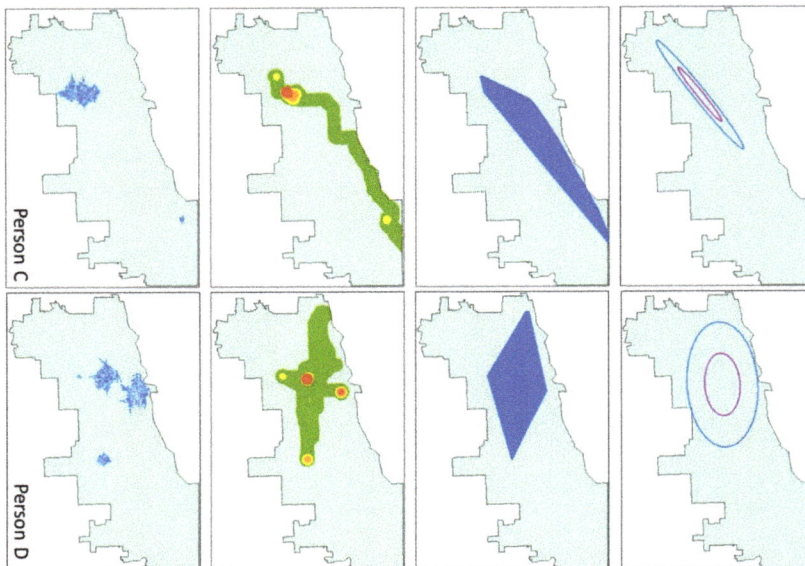

Figure 9. The four representative persons' activity spaces generated by different methods.

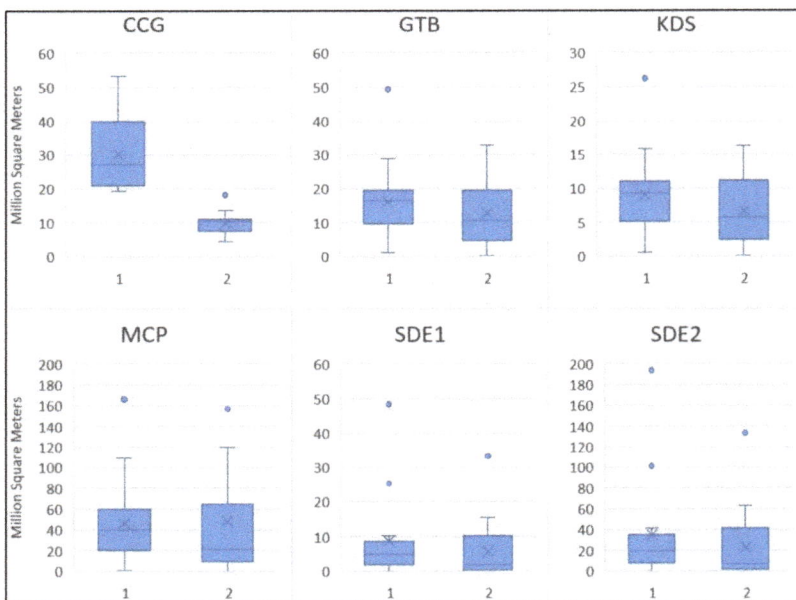

Figure 10. The differences in size of activity space for private transport (1) and public transport users (2).

3.2.2. Comparing Physical-Activity-Friendly Contextual Exposures Measured by Different Activity Spaces

Physical-activity-friendly contextual exposures are assessed for the 31 participants by CCG activity spaces, as well as the other five methods. The assessment is based on the intersection between activity space polygon features and the physical-activity-friendly context polygon features. Contextual exposures are evaluated as the ratio of the area of the intersection polygons to the area of the activity space. In other words, they are calculated by the percentage of a participant's activity space that is physical-activity-friendly. The higher the percentage value, the higher the assessed contextual exposure. The assessment results of the 31 participants are displayed in Figure 11. The top section illustrates the physical-activity-friendly contextual exposures assessed by the different activity space methods, while the bottom section depicts the number of days in which the participant is physically active for 30 min or more in a typical week. As indicated in the figure, CCG-assessed contextual exposures match the number of physically active days well. For instance, Participant 1 has a high physical activity level, while CCG is the only method that yielded high contextual exposure when compared to all other methods. For Participant 14, who has a medium level of physical activity, CCG estimated a reasonable level of contextual exposure, whereas SDE gave very high levels of exposure. Again, CCG is the only method that yielded moderate exposures, while all other methods gave extremely low values for Subject 25.

To further investigate the performance of the methods for discovering the relationship between physical-activity-friendly contextual exposures assessed by the different activity space methods and physical activity level is examined using a scatter plot with trend lines (Figure 12). As indicated in the figure, the contextual exposures measured by CCG and KDS show a positive correlation with physical activity level, while SDE1 and SDE2 reveal a negative association. For GTB and MCP, inconsistent relationships are observed. Although both CCG and KDS reveal the positive correlation between physical-activity-friendly contextual exposures and physical activity level, CCG has more robust results based on the trend lines and plot points in the figure.

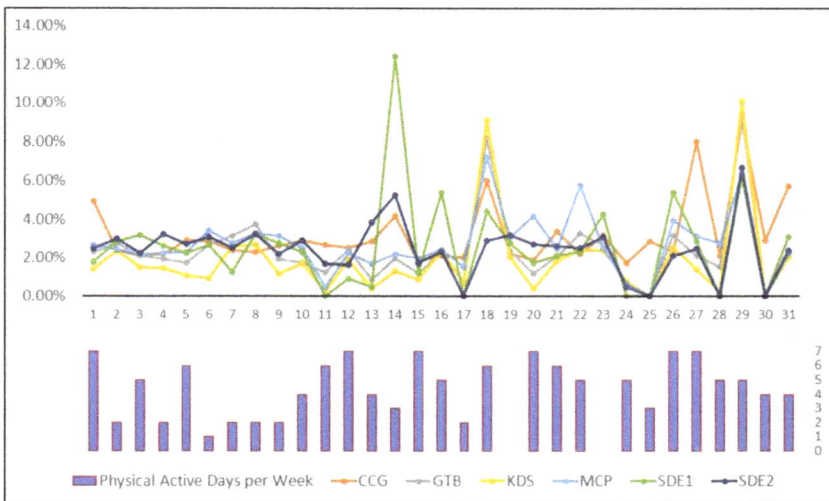

Figure 11. The physical-activity-friendly contextual exposures assessed by the different activity space methods and the physical active days per week for the 31 participants.

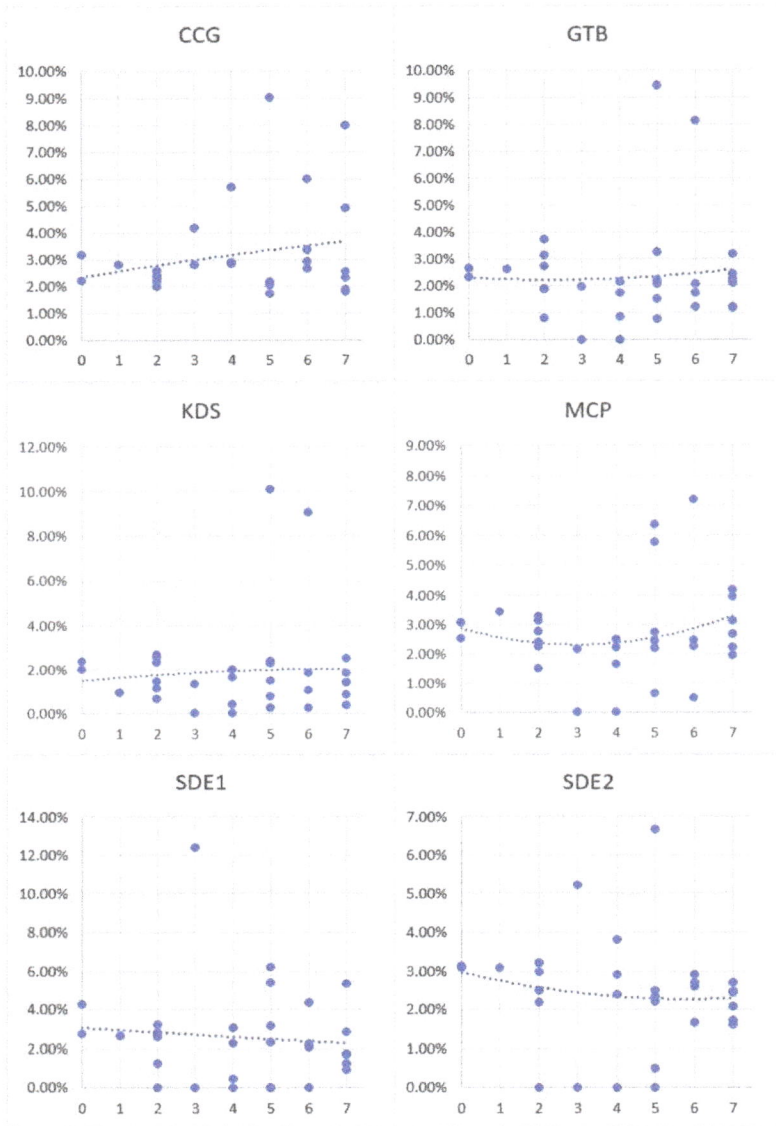

Figure 12. The correlation between physical-activity-friendly contextual exposures and physical activity level. (Vertical axis: the physical-activity-friendly contextual exposures level; horizontal axis: physical active days per week; trend lines are generated using the 2nd order polynomial fitting method.)

4. Discussion

This study proposed an innovative method for delineating activity space for environmental exposure assessment based on GIS and GPS tracks data. By implementing the method with a GPS tracking dataset collected in Chicago, the proposed method generates more reasonable and reliable results when compared with other methods.

The proposed method focuses on movement pattern mining and core-area abstraction using the entire GPS trajectory patterns instead of individual GPS points. As listed in Table 4, the activity spaces derived with GTB, KDS, MCP are large and cover all the GPS tracking points. In these methods, each GPS point is indifferently considered as part of the activity space. The consequence of this is that the result includes not only the critical activity locations but also areas that participants passed by when traveling between activity locations. In contrast to other approaches, and by abstracting core areas based on GPS tracking data, the proposed method generates activity spaces based on the core areas that cover only the prominent parts of the points. All frequently visited activity destinations and more than 90% of the total GPS tracking records are covered in the CCG activity spaces. Further, the CCG can generate multiple areas to portrait individual activity space instead of a single continuous region, so the places that participants only passed by can be excluded. All other activity space techniques generate one activity space that unavoidably includes a large area of irrelevant space. This error can be exacerbated, as shown in Figure 9, when dealing with highly mobile subjects whose movement pattern is dispersed or strongly directional.

While other methods ignore the potential activity opportunities and environmental exposure around a person's critical activity locations, which are also crucial factors for environmental exposure assessment, this study includes these potential areas to generate activity space by innovatively utilizing the crystal-growth algorithm. The idea is developed based on the fact that people are familiar with the environment and activity opportunities of the areas around their core activity locations (e.g., home, workplace). Even though they are not captured by their GPS trajectories during the tracking period, it is highly possible that people chose or will choose to undertake the daily activity and are or will be exposed to the contextual environments in these areas. For instance, in Figure 9, the CCG activity space of Person D contains a sub-area on the south of the city. According to the sojourn time spent in that area and the context of accessibility, an independent activity area is generated, which is centered at that core area and includes the potential activity opportunities. For other methods, GTB, KDS, and MCP activity spaces only include the actual GPS-tracked locations, while SDE doesn't even cover that area, since it is so isolated from other activity locations.

By incorporating the hexagon-grid-based accessibility-weighted plane, this is the first study that takes into account the context of accessibility for activity space delineation. Accessibility is a critical but disregarded factor in previous research. Inaccessible areas in a study area may include private houses, water bodies and restricted areas (e.g., airport). Since people can only access and undertake daily activities at accessible locations, including inaccessible areas in the activity space introduces error for delineating people's activity space as well as environmental exposure assessment. Further, the CCG method generates activity space from core areas based on specific travel time distance represented on the accessibility-weighted planes. Various levels of road networks and walkable areas are regarded as accessibility-friendly contexts with different travel speeds for private and public transport users, while people cannot trespass barrier contexts and need to bypass them, so more accurate results can be achieved by considering the context of accessibility. Additionally, the CCG method uses a hexagon grid for the weighted planes instead of the conventional raster grid to represent the context of accessibility more accurately.

The CCG method takes into account the ownership of automobiles, which is a critical factor that influences the size of people's activity space but was widely ignored in previous studies. Although living in the same neighborhood, the transportation network and facilities have different effects on the accessibility of different groups of residents. For private transport users, road networks are treated as a high-accessibility context. Thus, their activity spaces grow and are enlarged along road networks. Notice that there is a primary road passing through the area from east to west in Figure 8, so the activity space extends in an east-west direction. While public transport users rely heavily on the bus and metro system, their activity space extends along the bus and metro routes. Further, different from private transport users who could utilize all the road networks effectively by driving their own cars, the public transport users can only increase their travel speed by taking buses or the metro. Although the bus routes are densely distributed in the area, the average travel speed is much lower than that of private cars. Not surprisingly, the CCG activity space of public transport users is much smaller than the ones of private transport users. By considering the different environmental effects of accessibility on different residents, as indicated in Figure 10, the CCG activity spaces of private transport users are significantly larger than those of public transport users, which highlights the fact that residents with automobiles have high accessibility and thus a large activity space. Whereas none of the other activity space methods consider the effects of automobile ownership on activity space, which introduces error in both the delineation of activity space and the assessment of environmental exposures.

In this study, the exposure to physical-activity-friendly contexts is utilized as an example for comparing different activity space methods. Physical activity has been intensively investigated in past research, and it is highly related to obesity. The associations between physical-activity-friendly contexts and physical activity/obesity were found to be inconsistent and influenced by different delineations of activity space in environmental exposure assessment [66]. For instance, Zenk et al. [44] explored the environmental influences on dietary and physical activity through comparing the results generated by two different activity space methods (standard deviation ellipses and daily path areas), and inconsistent results were found. In Oliver et al.'s [67] study, the influence of land use on walking behaviors was examined by using 1-km circular and line-based road network buffers. The author found that the selection of activity space methods has considerable influences on the analytical results [67]. In addition, different kinds of activity space methods for built environment assessment were compared by analyzing their relationship with energy balance and obesity in other studies, e.g., [66,68]. These results indicate that activity space delineations have a significant influence on the observed associations between environmental exposures and health outcomes or behaviors [66,68]. Although the results are inconsistent, many past studies have observed the positive relationship between people's exposures to physical-activity-friendly contexts and their physical activity level [44,52–57]. CCG is the only activity space method that discovered such positive association in this study. The comparative results in Figures 11 and 12 support the idea that the proposed context-based crystal-growth activity space method performs better than other activity space methods in environmental exposure assessment. Although it is not feasible to use regression models to investigate the relationship between contextual exposures and participants' physical activity due to the small sample size and the lack of other independent variables, this study obtained results that reasonably justify the usefulness and effectiveness of the proposed CCG activity space method for exposure assessment and environmental health studies. Further, although this study only implements the new method for assessing environmental influences on physical activity, it can be easily applied in other environmental health studies.

In summary, the CCG activity space method achieves a balance between the actual activities captured by GPS trajectories and the context-based potential activity opportunities around core areas, which are both crucial factors for environmental exposure assessment. According to the results, the SDE and MCP are too sensitive to the pattern of the GPS trajectories; they always include much irrelevant space that makes the activity space too large. Remote activity sites that are far from the other activity locations tend to be ignored by SDE. GTB is more focused on travel behavior and therefore ignores the important activity locations. With respect to KDS, similar to all other conventional methods, it disregards the context of accessibility.

As discussed above, the existing activity space methods fail to mitigate the UGCoP. Spatially, the context of accessibility is ignored, and thus the activity spaces derived indifferently include many areas that may not be accessible. Furthermore, the effects of automobile ownership on activity space are ignored, therefore introducing uncertainty in the delineation of activity space. Moreover, arbitrary cut-off distance is used for the delineation of activity space, which adds error in the assessment of environmental exposures. Temporally, the duration in which individuals experienced environmental context is treated merely as a multiplier of exposure, while the interactions with space during the time (the more time spent at the location, the more familiar with the surrounding area) is overlooked.

The CCG activity space method addresses these issues and delineates individual activity space more reasonably. It thus helps mitigate the UGCoP when assessing environmental exposure by people's activity space.

Finally, this research has several limitations that need to be explored or addressed in future studies. First, this study implements the proposed activity space method based on the 7-day GPS trajectories of a small sample of participants and compares the results with other existing methods from the aspects of the geometric characteristics of the activity space, its correspondence with subjects' daily activity, and visual interpretation. However, a larger dataset with the GPS trajectories of more subjects and further utilizing of the proposed technique for environmental exposure assessment are needed in future research to further evaluate and justify the method. Second, although the CCG is compared with other existing approaches based on GPS tracking data, there are also methods that don't rely on GPS or GIS. For instance, studies that used map-based electronic questionnaires [38,69], mobility surveys [70] and activity space questionnaires [71] also yielded useful results. Although these qualitative methods based on self-reported information may include recall bias and not be geographically accurate, they can capture more background information about participants' activities [38], such as the transportation modes and social interactions [72]. Thus, further study is needed to compare these qualitative methods or integrate them with CCG to generate more accurate activity space. Third, the final activity space is hexagon-grid based, so distance decay functions can be applied optionally to the results to generate a weighted activity space, in which the core areas have a weigh according to their NST values. The weights of other cells can be calculated with specific distance decay functions based on travel distance from the core areas. Fourth, as the only parameter when calculating the growth extent of all core areas, for the purpose of illustration, GE_h is set to 10-mins' travel distance for all subjects in this study. However, it can also be determined based on personal mobility (such as age and health condition) to increase accuracy. Fifth, the method is based on the assumption that people are familiar with the environment and activity opportunities of the areas around the core areas, and it is highly possible that people choose to undertake the daily activity and expose to the context in these areas. However, even if only rarely, it is possible that one person may spend a lot of time at one location but is still not familiar with the surrounding area. This problem could be addressed by cross-validation with an activity diary data in future studies.

5. Conclusions

This study proposed an innovative method for delineating activity space using individual GPS trajectories and a crystal-growth algorithm based on hexagon-grid accessibility-weighted planes. It generates a more reasonable activity space and captures people's environmental exposures more accurately when compared to other methods. It is a new tool for activity space delineation that can be used for exploring the relationships between human movement patterns and environmental context as well as accessibility. It has considerable potential for making a groundbreaking contribution to the advancement of methods by introducing and developing a new analytical framework that allows the examination of activity space and individual environmental exposures while mitigating the UGCoP.

Acknowledgments: This research was supported by the National Natural Science Foundation of China (41529101). In addition, Mei-Po Kwan was supported by a John Simon Guggenheim Memorial Foundation Fellowship. The Chicago project was conducted with the help of Lirong Kou, Xue Zhang, Rebecca Shakespeare, Kangjae Lee, Ruoxin Li, and Yoo Min Park. Rachael Wilson of the Latin United Community Housing Association (LUCHA) in Chicago provided essential assistance in the entire data collection process.

Author Contributions: M.-P.K. and Y.C. conceived, designed and implemented the larger Chicago study that collected the data used in the paper. J.W. also contributed to the methodology design and implementation of data collection for the project. In addition, J.W. designed the method and performed the analyses presented in this paper. J.W. wrote the paper with M.-P.K., who also contributed to refining and revising the paper.

Conflicts of Interest: The authors declare no conflicts of interest.

References

1. Koohsari, M.J.; Mavoa, S.; Villianueva, K.; Sugiyama, T.; Badland, H.; Kaczynski, A.T.; Owen, N.; Giles-Corti, B. Public open space, physical activity, urban design and public health: Concepts, methods and research agenda. *Health Place* **2015**, *33*, 75–82. [CrossRef] [PubMed]
2. Millstein, R.A.; Yeh, H.-C.; Brancati, F.L.; Batts-Turner, M.; Gary, T.L. Food availability, neighborhood socioeconomic status, and dietary patterns among blacks with type 2 diabetes mellitus. *Medscape J. Med.* **2009**, *11*, 15. [PubMed]
3. Epstein, D.H.; Tyburski, M.; Craig, I.M.; Phillips, K.A.; Jobes, M.L.; Vahabzadeh, M.; Mezghanni, M.; Lin, J.L.; Furr-Holden, C.D.M.; Preston, K.L. Real-time tracking of neighborhood surroundings and mood in urban drug misusers: Application of a new method to study behavior in its geographical context. *Drug Alcohol Depend.* **2014**, *134*, 22–29. [CrossRef] [PubMed]
4. Shareck, M.; Kestens, Y.; Vallée, J.; Datta, G.; Frohlich, K.L.; Vallee, J.; Datta, G.; Frohlich, K.L. The added value of accounting for activity space when examining the association between tobacco retailer availability and smoking among young adults. *Tob. Control* **2015**, *25*, 1–7. [CrossRef] [PubMed]
5. Lee, C.; Moudon, A.V. Correlates of walking for transportation or recreation purposes. *J. Phys. Act. Health* **2006**, *3*, S77–S98. [CrossRef] [PubMed]
6. Saelens, B.E.; Sallis, J.F.; Frank, L.D. Environmental correlates of walking and cycling: Findings from the transportation, urban design, and planning literatures. *Ann. Behav. Med.* **2003**, *25*, 80–91. [CrossRef] [PubMed]
7. Giles-Corti, B.; Broomhall, M.H.; Knuiman, M.; Collins, C.; Douglas, K.; Ng, K.; Lange, A.; Donovan, R.J. Increasing walking: How important is distance to, attractiveness, and size of public open space? *Am. J. Prev. Med.* **2005**, *28*, 169–176. [CrossRef] [PubMed]
8. Ewing, R.; Schmid, T.; Killingsworth, R.; Zlot, A.; Raudenbush, S. Relationship between urban sprawl and physical activity, obesity, and morbidity. *Am. J. Health Promot.* **2003**, *18*, 47–57. [CrossRef] [PubMed]
9. Frank, L.D.; Andresen, M.A.; Schmid, T.L. Obesity relationships with community design, physical activity, and time spent in cars. *Am. J. Prev. Med.* **2004**, *27*, 87–96. [CrossRef] [PubMed]
10. Chaix, B.; Merlo, J.; Evans, D.; Leal, C.; Havard, S. Neighbourhoods in eco-epidemiologic research: Delimiting personal exposure areas. A response to Riva, Gauvin, Apparicio and Brodeur. *Soc. Sci. Med.* **2009**, *69*, 1306–1310. [CrossRef] [PubMed]
11. Lee, B.A.; Reardon, S.F.; Firebaugh, G.; Farrell, C.R.; Matthews, S.A.; O'Sullivan, D. Beyond the Census Tract: Patterns and Determinants of Racial Segregation at Multiple Geographic Scales. *Am. Sociol. Rev.* **2008**, *73*, 766–791. [CrossRef] [PubMed]
12. Miller, H. Place-Based versus People-Based Geographic Information Science. *Geogr. Compass* **2007**, *3*, 503–535. [CrossRef]
13. Perchoux, C.; Chaix, B.; Cummins, S.; Kestens, Y. Conceptualization and measurement of environmental exposure in epidemiology: Accounting for activity space related to daily mobility. *Health Place* **2013**, *21*, 86–93. [CrossRef] [PubMed]
14. Kwan, M. The Uncertain Geographic Context Problem. *Ann. Assoc. Am. Geogr.* **2012**, *102*, 958–968. [CrossRef]
15. Weber, J.; Kwan, M.-P. Evaluating the Effects of Geographic Contexts on Individual Accessibility: A Multilevel Approach 1. *Urban Geogr.* **2003**, *24*, 647–671. [CrossRef]
16. Inagami, S.; Cohen, D.A.; Finch, B.K. Non-residential neighborhood exposures suppress neighborhood effects on self-rated health. *Soc. Sci. Med.* **2007**, *65*, 1779–1791. [CrossRef] [PubMed]
17. Saarloos, D.; Kim, J.-E.; Timmermans, H. The built environment and health: Introducing individual space-time behavior. *Int. J. Environ. Res. Public Health* **2009**, *6*, 1724–1743. [CrossRef] [PubMed]
18. Houston, D. Implications of the modifiable areal unit problem for assessing built environment correlates of moderate and vigorous physical activity. *Appl. Geogr.* **2014**, *50*, 40–47. [CrossRef]
19. Rainham, D.; McDowell, I.; Krewski, D.; Sawada, M. Conceptualizing the healthscape: Contributions of time geography, location technologies and spatial ecology to place and health research. *Soc. Sci. Med.* **2010**, *70*, 668–676. [CrossRef] [PubMed]
20. Chaix, B.; Méline, J.; Duncan, S.; Jardinier, L.; Perchoux, C.; Vallée, J.; Merrien, C.; Karusisi, N.; Lewin, A.; Brondeel, R.; et al. Neighborhood environments, mobility, and health: Towards a new generation of studies in environmental health research. *Rev. Epidemiol. Sante Publique* **2013**, *61*, 139–145. [CrossRef] [PubMed]

21. Duncan, M.J.; Badland, H.M.; Mummery, W.K. Applying GPS to enhance understanding of transport-related physical activity. *J. Sci. Med. Sport* **2009**, *12*, 549–556. [CrossRef] [PubMed]
22. Maddison, R.; Ni Mhurchu, C. Global positioning system: A new opportunity in physical activity measurement. *Int. J. Behav. Nutr. Phys. Act.* **2009**, *6*, 73. [CrossRef] [PubMed]
23. Krause, C. An Activity Space Based Approach for Capturing Long Distance Travel Using Longitudinal GPS Survey Data. In Proceedings of the Transportation Research Board 92nd Annual Meeting, Washington, DC, USA, 13–17 January 2012; pp. 1–23.
24. Shen, Y.; Chai, Y.W. Daily activity space of suburban mega-community residents in Beijing based on GPS data. *Acta Geogr. Sin.* **2013**, *68*, 506–516.
25. Albert, D.P.; Gesler, W.M. How spatial analysis can be used in medical geography. In *Spatial Analysis, GIS and Remote Sensing*; CRC Press: Boca Raton, FL, USA, 2003; pp. 19–46.
26. Golledge, R.G. *Spatial Behavior: A Geographic Perspective*; Guilford Press: New York, NY, USA, 1997; ISBN 1572300507.
27. Gesler, W.M.; Meade, M.S. Locational and population factors in health care-seeking behavior in Savannah, Georgia. *Health Serv. Res.* **1988**, *23*, 443–462. [PubMed]
28. Sharp, G.; Denney, J.T.; Kimbro, R.T. Multiple contexts of exposure: Activity spaces, residential neighborhoods, and self-rated health. *Soc. Sci. Med.* **2015**, *146*, 204–213. [CrossRef] [PubMed]
29. Tamura, K.; Elbel, B.; Chaix, B.; Regan, S.D.; Al-Ajlouni, Y.A.; Athens, J.K.; Meline, J.; Duncan, D.T. Residential and GPS-Defined Activity Space Neighborhood Noise Complaints, Body Mass Index and Blood Pressure Among Low-Income Housing Residents in New York City. *J. Commun. Health* **2017**, *42*, 974–982. [CrossRef] [PubMed]
30. Cummins, S. Commentary: Investigating neighbourhood effects on health—Avoiding the "local trap". *Int. J. Epidemiol.* **2007**, *36*, 355–357. [CrossRef] [PubMed]
31. Adams, B.; Kapan, D.D. Man bites mosquito: Understanding the contribution of human movement to vector-borne disease dynamics. *PLoS ONE* **2009**, *4*, e6763. [CrossRef] [PubMed]
32. Diez Roux, A.V. Investigating Neighbourhood and Area Effects on Health. *Am. J. Public Health* **2001**, *91*, 1783–1789. [CrossRef] [PubMed]
33. Oakes, J.M.; Forsyth, A.; Schmitz, K.H. The effects of neighborhood density and street connectivity on walking behavior: The Twin Cities walking study. *Epidemiol. Perspect. Innov.* **2007**, *4*, 16. [CrossRef] [PubMed]
34. Spielman, S.; Yoo, E. The spatial dimensions of neighborhood effects. *Soc. Sci. Med.* **2009**, *68*, 1098–1105. [CrossRef] [PubMed]
35. Kwan, M. How GIS can help address the uncertain geographic context problem in social science research. *Ann. GIS* **2012**, *18*, 245–255. [CrossRef]
36. Almanza, E.; Jerrett, M.; Dunton, G.; Seto, E.; Ann Pentz, M. A study of community design, greenness, and physical activity in children using satellite, GPS and accelerometer data. *Health Place* **2012**, *18*, 46–54. [CrossRef] [PubMed]
37. Wiehe, S.E.; Hoch, S.C.; Liu, G.C.; Carroll, A.E.; Wilson, J.S.; Fortenberry, J.D. Adolescent Travel Patterns: Pilot Data Indicating Distance from Home Varies by Time of Day and Day of Week. *J. Adolesc. Health* **2008**, *42*, 418–420. [CrossRef] [PubMed]
38. Kestens, Y.; Thierry, B.; Shareck, M.; Steinmetz-Wood, M.; Chaix, B. Integrating activity spaces in health research: Comparing the VERITAS activity space questionnaire with 7-day GPS tracking and prompted recall. *Spat. Spatiotemporal. Epidemiol.* **2018**, *25*, 1–9. [CrossRef]
39. Kestens, Y.; Thierry, B.; Chaix, B. Re-creating daily mobility histories for health research from raw GPS tracks: Validation of a kernel-based algorithm using real-life data. *Health Place* **2016**, *40*, 29–33. [CrossRef] [PubMed]
40. Ta, N.; Chai, Y.; Kwan, M.P. Suburbanization, daily lifestyle and space-behavior interaction: A study of suburban residents in Beijing, China. *Acta Geogr. Sin.* **2015**, *70*, 1271–1280.
41. Shen, Y.; Chai, Y.; Kwan, M.P. Space-time fixity and flexibility of daily activities and the built environment: A case study of different types of communities in Beijing suburbs. *J. Transp. Geogr.* **2015**, *47*, 90–99. [CrossRef]
42. Tana; Kwan, M.P.; Chai, Y. Urban form, car ownership and activity space in inner suburbs: A comparison between Beijing (China) and Chicago (United States). *Urban Stud.* **2016**, *53*, 1784–1802. [CrossRef]
43. Shen, Y.; Kwan, M.P.; Chai, Y. Investigating commuting flexibility with GPS data and 3D geovisualization: A case study of Beijing, China. *J. Transp. Geogr.* **2013**, *32*, 1–11. [CrossRef]

44. Zenk, S.N.; Schulz, A.J.; Matthews, S.A.; Odoms-Young, A.; Wilbur, J.E.; Wegrzyn, L.; Gibbs, K.; Braunschweig, C.; Stokes, C. Activity space environment and dietary and physical activity behaviors: A pilot study. *Health Place* **2011**, *17*, 1150–1161. [CrossRef] [PubMed]

45. Rodriguez, D.A.; Brown, A.L.; Troped, P.J. Portable global positioning units to complement accelerometry-based physical activity monitors. *Med. Sci. Sports Exerc.* **2005**, *37*, S572–S581. [CrossRef] [PubMed]

46. Rodríguez, D.A.; Cho, G.-H.; Evenson, K.R.; Conway, T.L.; Cohen, D.; Ghosh-Dastidar, B.; Pickrel, J.L.; Veblen-Mortenson, S.; Lytle, L.A. Out and about: Association of the built environment with physical activity behaviors of adolescent females. *Health Place* **2012**, *18*, 55–62. [CrossRef] [PubMed]

47. Wheeler, B.W.; Cooper, A.R.; Page, A.S.; Jago, R. Greenspace and children's physical activity: A GPS/GIS analysis of the PEACH project. *Prev. Med. (Baltim)* **2010**, *51*, 148–152. [CrossRef] [PubMed]

48. Arem, H.; Moore, S.C.; Patel, A.; Hartge, P.; Berrington De Gonzalez, A.; Visvanathan, K.; Campbell, P.T.; Freedman, M.; Weiderpass, E.; Adami, H.O.; et al. Leisure time physical activity and mortality: A detailed pooled analysis of the dose-response relationship. *JAMA Intern. Med.* **2015**, *175*, 959–967. [CrossRef] [PubMed]

49. O'Donovan, G.; Lee, I.M.; Hamer, M.; Stamatakis, E. Association of "weekend warrior" and other leisure time physical activity patterns with risks for all-cause, cardiovascular disease, and cancer mortality. *JAMA Intern. Med.* **2017**, *177*, 335–342. [CrossRef] [PubMed]

50. Lahti, J.; Holstila, A.; Lahelma, E.; Rahkonen, O. Leisure-time physical activity and all-cause mortality. *PLoS ONE* **2014**, *9*, e101548. [CrossRef] [PubMed]

51. Moore, S.C.; Lee, I.M.; Weiderpass, E.; Campbell, P.T.; Sampson, J.N.; Kitahara, C.M.; Keadle, S.K.; Arem, H.; De Gonzalez, A.B.; Hartge, P.; et al. Association of leisure-time physical activity with risk of 26 types of cancer in 1.44 million adults. *JAMA Intern. Med.* **2016**, *176*, 816–825. [CrossRef] [PubMed]

52. Roberts, H.V. Using Twitter data in urban green space research: A case study and critical evaluation. *Appl. Geogr.* **2017**, *81*, 13–20. [CrossRef]

53. Maroko, A.R.; Maantay, J.A.; Sohler, N.L.; Grady, K.L.; Arno, P.S. The complexities of measuring access to parks and physical activity sites in New York City: A quantitative and qualitative approach. *Int. J. Health Geogr.* **2009**, *8*, 34. [CrossRef] [PubMed]

54. Mota, J.; Almeida, M.; Santos, P.; Ribeiro, J.C. Perceived neighborhood environments and physical activity in adolescents. *Prev. Med. (Baltim)* **2005**, *41*, 834–836. [CrossRef] [PubMed]

55. Santos, M.P.; Page, A.S.; Cooper, A.R.; Ribeiro, J.C.; Mota, J. Perceptions of the built environment in relation to physical activity in Portuguese adolescents. *Health Place* **2009**, *15*, 548–552. [CrossRef] [PubMed]

56. Handy, S.L.; Boarnet, M.G.; Ewing, R.; Killingsworth, R.E. How the built environment affects physical activity: Views from urban planning. *Am. J. Prev. Med.* **2002**, *23*, 64–73. [CrossRef]

57. Berke, E.M.; Koepsell, T.D.; Moudon, A.V.; Hoskins, R.E.; Larson, E.B. Association of the built environment with physical activity and obesity in older persons. *Am. J. Public Health* **2007**, *97*, 486–492. [CrossRef] [PubMed]

58. ESRI Data Classification Methods. Available online: http://pro.arcgis.com/en/pro-app/help/mapping/layer-properties/data-classification-methods.htm (accessed on 31 January 2017).

59. Birch, C.P.D.; Oom, S.P.; Beecham, J.A. Rectangular and hexagonal grids used for observation, experiment and simulation in ecology. *Ecol. Modell.* **2007**, *206*, 347–359. [CrossRef]

60. Zook, M. Small Stories in Big Data: Gaining Insights From Large Spatial Point Pattern Datasets. *Cityscape A J. Policy Dev. Res.* **2015**, *17*, 151–160.

61. Feick, R.; Robertson, C. A multi-scale approach to exploring urban places in geotagged photographs. *Comput. Environ. Urban Syst.* **2015**, *53*, 96–109. [CrossRef]

62. Schaudt, B.F.; Drysdale, R.L.S. Multiplicatively weighted crystal growth Voronoi diagrams (extended abstract). In Proceedings of the Seventh Annual Symposium on Computational Geometry—SCG '91; North Conway, NH, USA, 10–12 June 1991; ACM Press: New York, NY, USA, 1991; pp. 214–223.

63. Wang, J.; Kwan, M.-P.; Ma, L. Delimiting service area using adaptive crystal-growth Voronoi diagrams based on weighted planes: A case study in Haizhu District of Guangzhou in China. *Appl. Geogr.* **2014**, *50*, 108–119. [CrossRef]

64. Lin, C.; Huang, I. A Crystal Growth Approach for Topographical Global Optimization. *J. Glob. Optim.* **1998**, *13*, 255–267. [CrossRef]

65. Schönfelder, S.; Axhausen, K.W. Activity spaces: Measures of social exclusion? *Transp. Policy* **2003**, *10*, 273–286. [CrossRef]

66. James, P.; Berrigan, D.; Hart, J.E.; Aaron Hipp, J.; Hoehner, C.M.; Kerr, J.; Major, J.M.; Oka, M.; Laden, F. Effects of buffer size and shape on associations between the built environment and energy balance. *Health Place* **2014**, *27*, 162–170. [CrossRef] [PubMed]

67. Oliver, L.N.; Schuurman, N.; Hall, A.W. Comparing circular and network buffers to examine the influence of land use on walking for leisure and errands. *Int. J. Health Geogr.* **2007**, *6*, 41. [CrossRef] [PubMed]

68. Zhao, P.; Kwan, M.P.; Zhou, S. The uncertain geographic context problem in the analysis of the relationships between obesity and the built environment in Guangzhou. *Int. J. Environ. Res. Public Health* **2018**, *15*, 308. [CrossRef] [PubMed]

69. Chaix, B.; Kestens, Y.; Perchoux, C.; Karusisi, N.; Merlo, J.; Labadi, K. An Interactive Mapping Tool to Assess Individual Mobility Patterns in Neighborhood Studies. *Am. J. Prev. Med.* **2012**, *43*, 440–450. [CrossRef] [PubMed]

70. Kestens, Y.; Lebel, A.; Chaix, B.; Clary, C.; Daniel, M.; Pampalon, R.; Theriault, M.; p Subramanian, S.V. Association between activity space exposure to food establishments and individual risk of overweight. *PLoS ONE* **2012**, *7*, e41418. [CrossRef] [PubMed]

71. Shareck, M.; Kestens, Y.; Frohlich, K.L. Moving beyond the residential neighborhood to explore social inequalities in exposure to area-level disadvantage: Results from the Interdisciplinary Study on Inequalities in Smoking. *Soc. Sci. Med.* **2014**, *108*, 106–114. [CrossRef] [PubMed]

72. Kestens, Y.; Wasfi, R.; Naud, A.; Chaix, B. "Contextualizing Context": Reconciling Environmental Exposures, Social Networks, and Location Preferences in Health Research. *Curr. Environ. Health Rep.* **2017**, *4*, 51–60. [CrossRef] [PubMed]

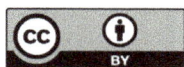

International Journal of
*Environmental Research
and Public Health*

MDPI

Article

A Multilevel Analysis of Perceived Noise Pollution, Geographic Contexts and Mental Health in Beijing

Jing Ma [1], Chunjiang Li [2], Mei-Po Kwan [3,4] and Yanwei Chai [2,*]

[1]   Beijing Key Laboratory for Remote Sensing of Environment and Digital Cities, Faculty of Geographical
     Science, Beijing Normal University, Beijing 100875, China; jing.ma@bnu.edu.cn
[2]   College of Urban and Environmental Sciences, Peking University, Beijing 100871, China; lcjiang@pku.edu.cn
[3]   Department of Geography and Geographic Information Science, University of Illinois at Urbana-Champaign,
     Natural History Building, MC-150, 1301 W Green Street, Urbana, IL 61801, USA; mpk654@gmail.com
[4]   Department of Human Geography and Spatial Planning, Faculty of Geosciences, Utrecht University,
     P.O. Box 80125, 3508 TC Utrecht, The Netherlands
*   Correspondence: chyw@pku.edu.cn

Received: 15 June 2018; Accepted: 8 July 2018; Published: 13 July 2018

Abstract: With rapid urbanization and increase in car ownership, ambient noise pollution resulting from diversified sources (e.g., road traffic, railway, commercial services) has become a severe environmental problem in the populated areas in China. However, research on the spatial variation of noise pollution and its potential effects on urban residents' mental health has to date been quite scarce in developing countries like China. Using a health survey conducted in Beijing in 2017, we for the first time investigated the spatial distributions of multiple noise pollution perceived by residents in Beijing, including road traffic noise, railway (or subway) noise, commercial noise, and housing renovation (or construction) noise. Our results indicate that there is geographic variability in noise pollution at the neighborhood scale, and road traffic and housing renovation/construction are the principal sources of noise pollution in Beijing. We then employed Bayesian multilevel logistic models to examine the associations between diversified noise pollution and urban residents' mental health symptoms, including anxiety, stress, fatigue, headache, and sleep disturbance, while controlling for a wide range of confounding factors such as socio-demographics, objective built environment characteristics, social environment and geographic context. The results show that perceived higher noise-pollution exposure is significantly associated with worse mental health, while physical environment variables seem to contribute little to variations in self-reported mental disorders, except for proximity to the main road. Social factors or socio-demographic attributes, such as age and income, are significant covariates of urban residents' mental health, while the social environment (i.e., community attachment) and housing satisfaction are significantly correlated with anxiety and stress. This study provides empirical evidence on the noise-health relationships in the Chinese context and sheds light on the policy implications for environmental pollution mitigation and healthy city development in China.

Keywords: noise pollution; mental disorders; built environment; multilevel model; China

1. Introduction

Noise pollution in cities is an important environmental risk that is detrimental to people's health and well-being [1]. The World Health Organization (WHO) reported in 2011 that about 1.0–1.6 million disability-adjusted life-years (DALYs) were lost every year in Europe due to noise pollution [2]. More than 30% of the population in Europe was exposed to road traffic noise louder than 55 dB during the night, which would cause severe sleep disturbance and adverse health effects [3]. In China, noise pollution resulting from the rapid urbanization, industrialization and increase in car ownership has become a serious environmental problem, and there is increasing concern over it among the general public and policymakers.

In China, some prior studies found that the L_{eq24h} values (Leq—equivalent 24-h noise level) were higher than 70 dB in Beijing and the majority of urban residents were influenced by excessive noise [4]. Construction noise has become the second most serious acoustic pollution in many Chinese cities, which could cause significant DALYs loss, health damage and social costs [5]. In particular, the road traffic noise in Beijing far exceeded the standard value of noise level and spread outwards with urban sprawls as well as the construction of ring roads [6,7]. The 2016 Reports on the State of the Environment in China showed that approximately 50% of functional zones where highways, railways or urban roads crossing were exposed to high noise pollution during night-time [8]. It suggested that community noise and nocturnal traffic noise were important environmental risk factors to public health. However, research on the noise-health relationship in a rapidly urbanizing context like China has been quite scarce to date [9–11].

Much literature on noise pollution exists predominantly in developed countries, particularly in Europe. It provides empirical evidence on the adverse effects of noise pollution on public health in residential areas [12]. Noise has been identified as one of the main environmental stressors that have adverse psychological and physiological effects on human health, including annoyance, cardiovascular and metabolic diseases, sleep disturbance, hearing loss and tinnitus, birth outcomes, and cognitive impairments [13–19]. However, compared to the physical health or physiological effects which have received considerable attention in academia, the relationship between noise-pollution exposure and population's mental health or mental disorders has only received modest attention, and the results are inconclusive [20–23].

Mental disorders are a major health risk for urban populations [24]. It was estimated that one in every four persons worldwide would be affected by mental disorders during their lifetime [25]. In China, mental and behavioral disorders were responsible for a large proportion of all years lived with disability (YLDs) in 2010, while major depression was the second leading cause of YLDs [26]. Regarded as a part of the indirect pathway from noise to health, examining the noise effects on mental health or psychological disorders can also be helpful for a better understanding of the influences of noise on physical health, e.g., cardiovascular disease [27].

Aircraft noise, the focus in early research, was found to cause some mental disorders among different populations, such as annoyance, depression, anxiety, nervousness, as well as sleep disturbance [28–30]. Recent studies have attempted to extend the noise sources to include traffic noise from roads and railways as well [31–35]. In particular, much research has investigated road traffic noise in different contexts and its correlation with population's health and wellbeing [36,37]. Studies have shown that higher exposure to road traffic noise could significantly increase annoyance and have harmful effects on people's sleep quality, wellbeing and other health outcomes [38–40].

Objective measures of noise pollution have been used in some studies to quantify the health effects of traffic noise in different contexts using various statistical methods [13–15]. Prior comparative studies showed that annoyance was associated with objectively measured noise level in noisy streets, but not in quiet streets [41,42]. Meta-analyses of noise and health suggested that night-time road traffic noise was positively associated with sleep disturbance, as well as aircraft noise and railway noise [15,43]. Recent years have also seen a growing number of empirical studies on the health effects of subjectively reported community or neighborhood noise [13–18]. Perceived neighborhood noise was found to be associated with poor self-rated health and some mental health symptoms (e.g., depression) in Delhi, India [44,45].

However, although some studies provide relatively consistent evidence on the effects of noise on more serious health outcomes (e.g., ischemic heart disease, hypertension), the evidence concerning various mental health symptoms (e.g., depression) or general health outcomes has been inconclusive [46–48]. While some studies have shown a significant relationship between annoyance from a few noise sources and anxiety and depression [28,49], other cohort research reported weak associations between traffic noise exposure and mental health assessed by SF-36 [50] and no significant association or linear trend for psychiatric disorders [51]. Concerning children's mental health, the results have also been equivocal. Traffic noise exposure and increased noise annoyance were linked to deteriorations of children's mental health as well as behavioral and emotional symptoms in some cross-sectional analyses [52–54], while a longitudinal study reported no significant associations between aircraft noise level and psychological health [55].

In addition to objective or subjective measures of noise-pollution exposure, characteristics of the physical built environment, such as housing quality, proximity to green space, land-use mix, and accessibility to public transit, have also been found to be covariates of mental health symptoms or mental disorders, such as stress and depression [56–59]. Moreover, social environment like social contact or community attachment can influence population's mental health as well [60,61]. Nonetheless, such variables of the physical built environment and social environment have rarely been taken into account simultaneously in prior research on noise pollution and mental health, particularly in developing countries like China [62].

To conclude, the results on the associations between mental disorders and noise pollution from multiple sources (e.g., road traffic, railways, industries, neighbors, and aircraft) have been inconsistent to date [21,59,63,64]. This is possibly because these studies used different concepts of mental health and different measures (e.g., objective versus subjective) of noise-pollution exposure, and most of them are ecological or cross-sectional studies with poor adjustments in the statistical models and no mediator/moderator variables in the analysis. Relatively few empirical attempts have been made so far to consider multiple noise pollution sources simultaneously and explore their relationships with a wide range of mental health outcomes, while controlling for various confounding factors such as socio-demographics, physical environment, and social environment.

In this study, we aim to extend the literature by exploring the socio-spatial variations of diversified noise pollution in Beijing and developing a comprehensive conceptual framework to examine the relationships between noise pollution and self-reported symptoms of mental health, taking into account a wide range of objective and subjective measures [47,65]. As shown in Figure 1, we consider the mental health correlations with socio-demographics, social environment, objective measures of the physical built environment, and perceived pollution exposure to multiple noise sources, including road traffic, railways (or subways), commercial services (e.g., restaurants, shops), and housing renovation and construction work, which have rarely been examined together in the Chinese context. Moreover, we measure a wide range of self-reported symptoms of mental health in the analysis, including anxiety, stress, fatigue, headache, and sleep disturbance, to understand the connections between noise pollution and urban residents' mental disorders in Beijing, China.

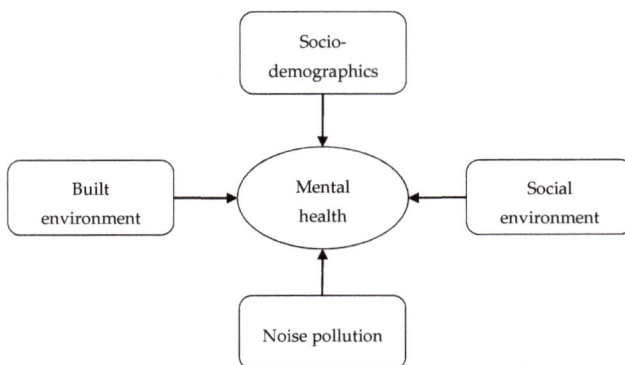

Figure 1. Conceptual framework.

Drawing upon a health survey conducted in 26 communities of Beijing in 2017, we for the first time demonstrated the spatial distributions of noise pollution from multiple sources at the community level in Beijing. Then we employed rigorous Bayesian multilevel logistic models to investigate the associations between self-reported mental disorders and a wide range of objective and subjective measures, including socio-demographics, social environment, objective physical built environment, perceived noise-pollution exposure, as well as geographic context (or unobserved community effect). We aim to present an empirical noise-health study using rigorous statistical analysis based on a comprehensive conceptual framework and make a timely contribution to a better understanding of the mental health–noise relationships in urban China.

2. Data and Variables

2.1. Data Sources

Beijing has experienced rapid urbanization, industrialization and increase in car ownership in recent decades, subjecting people to a wide range of environmental hazards and health risks [66]. In this study, we adopted a health survey conducted in Beijing in 2017 to investigate residents' evaluation of various types of noise pollution in their surrounding environment and their associations with self-reported symptoms of mental health. The survey was implemented by research teams at Peking University and Tsinghua University from March to May in 2017, using a spatial stratified random sampling strategy. First, 26 communities were selected based on their spatial location, housing condition, community type and built environment. These selected communities are representative of the diversified urban neighborhoods in Beijing, including work-unit compounds, commodity housing neighborhoods, affordable housing and mixed neighborhoods.

Then, in each neighborhood, approximately 50 household members aged between 18 and 65 years old were randomly selected to answer the questionnaire, which contains much information on the household and individual socio-demographics, social networks, evaluations on housing and community environment, noise pollution, and physical and mental health status. In total, surveys of 1280 individuals from 26 communities were collected with valid answers. Here, our analysis comprised 1125 respondents with valid and complete information on socio-demographics, housing conditions and evaluations on noise pollution and mental health. Table 1 presents the distribution of key socio-demographic attributes and variables on housing satisfaction and community attachment in the survey. The majority of participants were married, employed, local residents, house owners, and satisfied with their housing conditions. About 75% of the residents rated the traffic congestion near the community as serious or very serious, while about 63% reported they had feelings of community attachment or belongings.

Table 1. Key socio-demographics and community environment evaluation in the survey.

Variables	Description	Proportion (%)
Gender	Female as the base category	50.0
Age	<30	11.5
	30–39	26.9
	40–49	18.5
	50–59	20.9
	60+	22.3
Monthly income (RMB)	<3000	7.9
	3000–6000	18.8
	6000–10,000	35.7
	10,000–15,000	14.8
	15,000+	22.7

Table 1. *Cont.*

Variables	Description	Proportion (%)
Education	Primary	16.9
	Secondary	29.9
	Tertiary	53.2
Marital status	Married	84.6
Residence status	Migrants	28.2
Housing tenure	Owners	74.3
Employment	Employed	61.0
Housing satisfaction	Satisfied or very satisfied with housing	72.7
Community traffic congestion	Perceived serious or very serious traffic congestion around the community	74.7
Community attachment	Have feelings of community attachment	63.4

Note: RMB = renminbi, the official Chinese currency.

In addition to the health survey, point of interest (POI) data in Beijing and GIS-based spatial analysis have also been employed to derive multi-dimensional measures of objective built environment characteristics for each surveyed neighborhood (Table 2). Four aspects of the built environment are considered at the neighborhood scale: public transit accessibility (measured by the distance from each surveyed neighborhood to the nearest subway station), road connection (calculated by the distance to the nearest main road), accessibility to facilities (measured by the distance to the nearest restaurant) and proximity to park. As shown in Table 2, the surveyed communities are characterized by different configurations of these four characteristics. Moreover, these variables are also considered as proxies of objective measures of pollution exposure to various noise sources, such as railways, road traffic, and commercial services. As these objective measures of built environment characteristics might have influences on residents' mental health, they are included in the statistical analysis and transformed to a standard Normal distribution to reduce the potential problem of heteroscedasticity.

2.2. Measuring Noise Pollution

While the objective data on noise pollution is usually not available at the fine spatial resolution in Beijing in particular and in China more generally, we derived individuals' subjective evaluations of multiple noise sources in their surrounding environment from the surveys. Perceived noise pollution considered in this study focuses on four dimensions: road traffic noise, railway or subway noise, commercial noise (from restaurants, shops, and other commercial establishments) and housing renovation/construction noise. Therefore, perceived pollution exposures to various types of noise are assessed by the following questions: How would you evaluate the levels of noise pollution (from road traffic, railways or subways, commercial facilities, and housing renovation or construction, respectively) in your neighborhood? Answers are given on a 5-point Likert scale ranging from 1 (very low noise level) to 5 (very high noise level).

Figure 2 presents the proportions of each category in various types of noise-pollution exposures perceived by survey respondents. A noticeable variation exists between the proportions of each category for the four types of noise pollution. The percentages of urban residents rating the levels of housing renovation noise pollution and road traffic noise pollution in their neighborhoods as high or very high are 30% and 37% respectively. In contrast, there are only 12% and 16% of residents reporting serious commercial and railway noise pollution in their surrounding environment. This suggests that road traffic and housing renovation are the principal sources of noise pollution in Beijing, possibly due to high usage of private cars and the prosperous second-hand housing market in China's capital city.

Table 2. Built environment characteristics of 26 surveyed communities.

Surveyed Communities	Distance to the Nearest Point of Interest (m)			
	Main Road	Park	Subway Station	Restaurant
Jin Yu Chi (JYC)	86.8	306.2	479.9	104.9
Xi Yuan Zi (XYZ)	120.8	378.5	462.6	77.3
Liang Jia Yuan (LJY)	167.4	1546.3	367.1	169.9
Xiang Lu Ying (XLY)	189.7	1623.0	325.7	152.7
Sheng Gu Zhuang (SGZ)	221.4	485.4	416.6	165.2
Ping Le Yuan (PLY)	374.2	86.7	708.4	93.1
Bai Zi Wan (BZW)	728.2	2185.3	936.1	7.5
Guan Dong Dian (GDD)	72.5	425.4	199.2	57.0
Gan Lu Yuan (GLY)	50.4	306.1	735.4	21.4
Jia Ming Yuan (JMY)	461.2	499.2	157.7	94.3
Mei He Yuan (MHY)	83.8	303.1	259.3	168.6
Zhu Fang (ZF)	257.4	665.8	819.1	18.0
Hua Yuan Lou (HYL)	441.9	769.3	1710.4	236.4
Xue Fu Shu (XFS)	63.7	605.2	951.2	146.4
Pu Hui Nan (PHN)	234.5	179.5	555.9	45.0
Pu Hui Si (PHS)	317.7	296.4	596.7	52.2
Jing Xi Bin Guan (JXBG)	86.9	614.7	499.9	98.2
Yun Yun Guo Ji (YYGJ)	348.1	770.9	1161.8	108.9
Xiao Yue Yuan (XYY)	796.8	1319.3	1237.8	297.4
Fei Cheng (FC)	220.0	502.1	1430.5	221.0
Sen Lin Da Di (SLDD)	151.0	1255.4	2320.3	267.4
Du Shi Fang Yuan (DSFY)	1918.4	1625.1	1847.8	416.6
Lv Zhou Jia Yuan (LZJY)	1885.5	771.9	1781.1	49.5
Hong Xing Lou (HXL)	69.5	853.7	2766.0	29.6
Qing Xin Yuan (QXY)	163.0	529.4	1749.7	58.9
Run Xing Jia Yuan (RXJY)	1216.6	297.2	1790.1	291.6

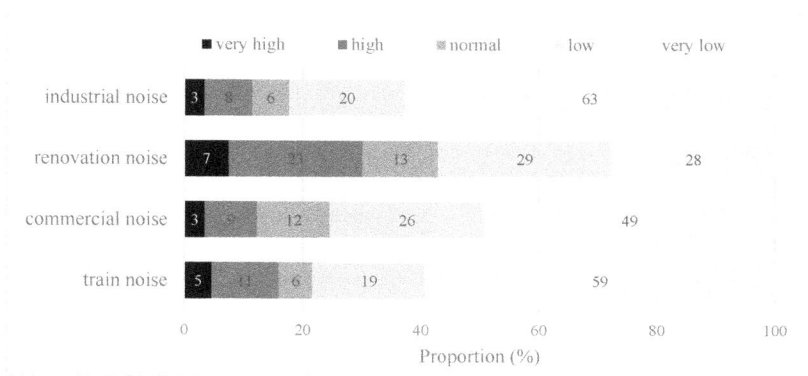

Figure 2. Population (%) in perceived noise-pollution levels of different categories.

Moreover, we further recoded the original noise-pollution variables into three categories: 1 for no or very low noise pollution, 2 for moderate noise pollution (including low and normal), and 3 for high noise pollution (including high and very high). Figure 3 shows, by quantile, the spatial distributions of the respondents (%) reporting high pollution exposure to noise (including road traffic, railways, commercial services and housing renovation) at the community level in Beijing. The non-uniform patterns of exposure to various types of noise pollution are evident. For instance, Figure 3A illustrates the proportion of residents reporting the road noise level in their surrounding environment as high or very high for each surveyed community. It suggests the cluster of communities with a high proportion (ranging from 45% to 70%) of high road traffic noise pollution is mainly located in the inner city and areas in the north, where car ownership has been higher than other areas and people make greater use of private vehicles [67]. Figure 3B–D present geographic variability of respondents' pollution exposures to railway noise, commercial noise and housing renovation noise in Beijing, respectively.

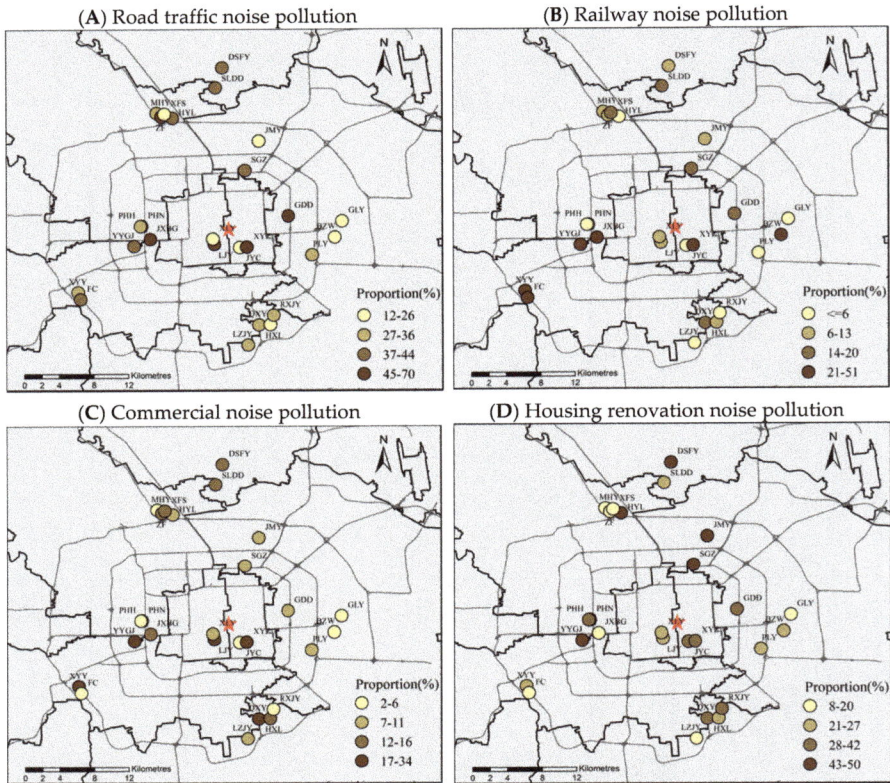

Figure 3. Spatial distribution of the population (%) reporting high or very high noise pollution at the community level in Beijing.

2.3. Measuring the Outcome Variables of Mental Health

In this study, we measured the self-reported symptoms of mental health or mental disorders with five dimensions: anxiety, stress, fatigue, headache, and sleep disturbance. These variables were measured by the frequency of being bothered by such feelings over the past four weeks through asking the questions: In general, how frequently have you suffered from the following mental health problems, such as anxiety, stress, fatigue, headache, and sleep disturbance, respectively. The responses are quantified on a 4-point scale: 1 = never, 2 = rarely, 3 = sometimes, and 4 = often. Figure 4 illustrates the proportion of the respondents in each category for different mental disorder variables. The majority (>70%) of respondents reported no feelings of headache in a recent month, while about half of the respondents reported they had suffered from the mental disorders of anxiety, stress and sleep disturbance. These results suggest that people more frequently suffer from the mental health problems of stress and sleep disturbance than headache in Beijing. To have better comparability with prior research in this area and facilitate the multilevel model implementation, the outcome variables of five mental health measures have been recoded into binary variables, respectively: 1 refers to having suffered from mental disorders (including rarely, sometimes and often) and 0 represents no such mental health symptoms (i.e., never).

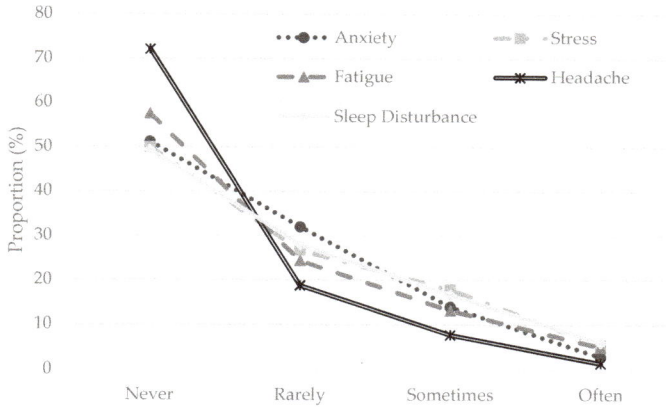

Figure 4. Population (%) in mental health categories.

2.4. Statistical Model

In our analysis, due to the two-level structure of our survey data (e.g., individual-level socio-demographics and community-level built environment characteristics) and the binary outcome variables of mental health, we employed a Bayesian multilevel logistic model to investigate the relationships between noise pollution and mental health. The five measures of mental health are modeled as binomial distributions with a logit link function, respectively. Let p_{jk} represent the mental health status of individual j living in community k, and the Bayesian multilevel logistic model is expressed as [66,68]:

$$Y_{j,k} \sim \text{Binomial} (1, p_{jk}); \text{ for } j = 1, \dots, J; k = 1, \dots, K, \tag{1}$$

$$\text{Log} \left\{ p_{jk}/(1 - p_{jk}) \right\} = \eta_{jk} = \alpha + P'_{jk}\beta + S'_{jk}\gamma + E'_{jk}\delta + C'_k\phi + u_k,$$
$$u_k \sim N(0, \sigma^2), \{\alpha, \beta, \gamma, \delta, \phi\} \sim N(0, b); \sigma^2 \sim \text{Inverse Gamma} (e, f),$$

The log odds are related to a linear predictor (η_{jk}), which depends on a set of additive covariate effects. P represents perceived exposure to various types of noise pollution (road traffic, railways, commercial services and housing renovation), S refers to a set of socio-demographic attributes (e.g., age, gender, income, education, employment, marital status, residential status or migrants, housing tenure), E represents residents' subjective evaluations of housing conditions (e.g., housing satisfaction) and community environment (traffic congestion and community attachment), and C includes the objective measures of the built environment at the community level (distances to the nearest subway station, main road, restaurant and park).

Vectors of $\{\alpha, \beta, \gamma, \delta, \phi\}$ are fixed regression coefficients to be estimated, which quantify the effects of corresponding covariates on mental health on the logistic scale. Relatively diffuse priors are usually specified for fixed regression coefficients; for instance, a normal distribution with mean zero and very large variance (i.e., $b = 10,000$). The unobserved effect from community k on residents' mental health is indicated by u_k, which follows a normal distribution with mean zero and variance σ^2 [69]. The prior distribution for the variance parameter σ^2 is an Inverse Gamma distribution with scale and shape parameters being e and f, following [69]. We note that given the above model specification, the regression coefficients are interpreted as cluster- or group-specific associations between independent variables and an outcome variable (i.e., the effect on the log-odds that Y equals to one from a one unit change in a predictor variable for a given community) [70,71].

The Bayesian multilevel logistic model was implemented using the R-INLA package (http://www.r-inla.org/), which is an interface of the C package INLA with R [72]. Five Bayesian multilevel logistic models were estimated for the five measures of self-reported mental health symptoms (anxiety, stress, fatigue, headache, and sleep disturbance), respectively.

3. Results

3.1. Mental Disorders and Socio-Demographics

The estimates of odds ratios (OR) with corresponding 95% credible intervals (95% CI) from the five Bayesian multilevel logistic models are provided in Table 3. As shown in the table, most of the socio-demographic attributes are significantly associated with self-reported mental health symptoms or mental disorders in Beijing. Distinctness in odds of reporting various mental disorders is found between different age cohorts: middle-aged respondents (aged 40–49 years old) have significantly higher odds of reporting a wide range of mental health problems, including anxiety, stress, fatigue, headache, as well as sleep disturbance, than the young respondents (aged 18–30). Moreover, older respondents (aged 50 years old and above) tend to be more likely to suffer from sleep disturbance, fatigue and headache than the young respondents.

A significant link between mental health and people with different levels of monthly income has been identified. Compared to respondents with medium-level income (between 6000 RMB and 10,000 RMB), the odds of reporting mental health problems for respondents with the highest income level increase by 45.6 %, 66.8% and 74.0% for anxiety, sleep disruption and fatigue, respectively, all else being equal. However, respondents with low income are not significantly distinguishable from medium-income respondents, which indicates a threshold effect of income on mental health. This suggests that the correlation between income and health is likely to be nonlinear.

Gender, marital and migrant status are not significant covariates with various mental health symptoms, whereas employed residents are more likely to report the feelings of stress than their counterparts. Housing tenure is found to be significantly associated with some mental disorders, such as anxiety and sleep disturbance, while residents' subjective evaluation of their housing conditions does not seem to make a significant difference to mental disorders, except for stress. The odds of reporting stress for residents with housing satisfaction significantly decrease by 30.1% compared to people who are not satisfied with their housing conditions. While many people cannot afford to purchase a commodity house with large floor space and good housing quality due to its very high price in Beijing, overall evaluation on housing satisfaction seems to be a significant predictor of stress or a main stressor for urban residents in Chinese megacities.

Moreover, with respect to the social environment, community attachment is found to be significantly associated with good mental health, as people with feelings of community attachment or social cohesion are less likely to report various mental health problems, particularly for anxiety and fatigue. This demonstrates that detachment from one's community may be detrimental to mental well-being in Beijing.

3.2. Mental Disorders and Noise Pollution

Regarding the community-level objective built environment characteristics, proximity to the main road is a significant covariate of urban residents' mental disorders in Beijing. Respondents residing in neighborhoods far from the main road have lower odds of reporting various mental health problems, such as anxiety, fatigue, and sleep disturbance, than residents living close to the main road. In contrast, accessibility to green space or parks is not significantly correlated with people's mental health, although the correlations are positive. Other built environment variables, such as close proximity to public transit or commercial facilities like restaurants, which can be regarded as objective measures of exposure to railway noise or commercial noise, seem to be insignificant correlates of mental health in Beijing.

Table 3. Multilevel modeling results for five types of mental disorders.

Variables	Anxiety		Stress		Fatigue		Headache		Sleep Disturbance	
	OR	95% CI	OR	95% CI	OR	95% CI	OR	95% CI	OR	95% CI
Gender										
Female	1.000	reference	1.000	reference	1.000	reference	1.000	reference	1.000	reference
Male	0.919	0.706–1.196	0.993	0.761–1.295	0.840	0.648–1.090	0.888	0.667–1.181	0.839	0.649–1.084
Age										
<30	1.000	reference	1.000	reference	1.000	reference	1.000	reference	1.000	reference
30–39	1.208	0.715–2.045	1.028	0.605–1.739	1.433	0.848–2.443	1.303	0.704–2.471	**1.804**	**1.077–3.053**
40–49	**2.320**	**1.307–4.138**	**1.796**	**1.008–3.203**	**2.512**	**1.424–4.481**	**2.689**	**1.422–5.231**	**2.843**	**1.628–5.019**
50–59	1.376	0.745–2.546	1.069	0.577–1.980	**2.505**	**1.362–4.656**	**2.248**	**1.134–4.558**	**3.585**	**1.964–6.625**
60+	1.170	0.604–2.266	0.806	0.413–1.568	**2.759**	**1.427–5.394**	**3.266**	**1.573–6.951**	**3.127**	**1.631–6.061**
Income (RMB)										
<3000	1.069	0.632–1.803	1.350	0.795–2.293	0.837	0.492–1.410	1.557	0.908–2.646	1.221	0.734–2.040
3000–6000	0.836	0.573–1.217	0.875	0.598–1.276	0.912	0.626–1.322	1.391	0.935–2.064	0.949	0.660–1.360
6000–10,000	1.000	reference	1.000	reference	1.000	reference	1.000	reference	1.000	reference
10,000–15,000	**1.772**	**1.181–2.669**	**1.885**	**1.252–2.853**	1.469	0.986–2.188	1.092	0.686–1.716	1.351	0.912–2.004
15,000+	**1.456**	**1.011–2.101**	1.388	0.962–2.006	**1.740**	**1.214–2.499**	1.332	0.889–1.989	**1.668**	**1.171–2.382**
Education										
Primary	1.000	reference	1.000	reference	1.000	reference	1.000	reference	1.000	reference
Secondary	0.683	0.452–1.030	**0.506**	**0.331–0.768**	0.865	0.578–1.296	0.808	0.531–1.231	0.746	0.500–1.109
Tertiary	1.051	0.669–1.652	0.957	0.606–1.507	0.981	0.629–1.533	0.870	0.544–1.393	0.790	0.510–1.223
Employment status										
Unemployed	1.000	reference	1.000	reference	1.000	reference	1.000	reference	1.000	reference
Employed	1.003	0.671–1.497	**1.724**	**1.157–2.573**	1.279	0.862–1.907	1.053	0.687–1.620	1.028	0.696–1.521
Marital status										
Unmarried	1.000	reference	1.000	reference	1.000	reference	1.000	reference	1.000	reference
Married	0.778	0.499–1.208	0.788	0.503–1.231	0.818	0.528–1.266	0.915	0.569–1.486	0.715	0.463–1.098
Residence status										
Migrants	1.000	reference	1.000	reference	1.000	reference	1.000	reference	1.000	reference
Local residents	0.970	0.682–1.378	0.819	0.574–1.164	1.086	0.770–1.531	0.914	0.628–1.331	0.733	0.519–1.028
Housing tenure										
Renters	1.000	reference	1.000	reference	1.000	reference	1.000	reference	1.000	reference
Housing owners	**1.454**	**1.011–2.101**	1.294	0.898–1.873	1.215	0.853–1.740	1.249	0.848–1.867	**1.737**	**1.231–2.471**

Table 3. *Cont.*

Variables	Anxiety OR	95% CI	Stress OR	95% CI	Fatigue OR	95% CI	Headache OR	95% CI	Sleep Disturbance OR	95% CI
Perceived community traffic congestion										
Not serious	1.000	reference	1.000	reference	1.000	reference	1.000	reference	1.000	reference
Serious	0.953	0.715–1.269	0.818	0.612–1.091	0.843	0.634–1.120	0.765	0.558–1.046	1.038	0.790–1.362
Housing satisfaction										
Unsatisfied	1.000	reference	1.000	reference	1.000	reference	1.000	reference	1.000	reference
Satisfied	0.947	0.687–1.308	**0.699**	**0.505–0.966**	0.872	0.640–1.190	0.778	0.563–1.080	0.937	0.693–1.270
Community attachment										
No such feelings	1.000	reference	1.000	reference	1.000	reference	1.000	reference	1.000	reference
Have such feelings	**0.736**	**0.549–0.984**	0.913	0.681–1.224	**0.677**	**0.507–0.901**	0.872	0.638–1.193	0.878	0.662–1.164
Standardized distance to the main road	**0.780**	**0.605–0.995**	0.789	0.614–1.003	**0.796**	**0.634–0.989**	0.828	0.666–1.024	**0.791**	**0.660–0.942**
Standardized distance to the nearest park	1.091	0.864–1.382	1.117	0.887–1.411	1.001	0.812–1.236	1.021	0.835–1.254	1.049	0.889–1.238
Standardized distance to the nearest subway station	1.123	0.881–1.436	1.044	0.821–1.327	1.157	0.932–1.441	1.069	0.866–1.317	1.005	0.846–1.193
Standardized distance to the nearest restaurant	0.897	0.710–1.126	1.010	0.805–1.266	0.932	0.758–1.145	1.001	0.820–1.226	1.012	0.859–1.192
Perceived noise pollution										
Very low road noise	1.000	reference	1.000	reference	1.000	reference	1.000	reference	1.000	reference
Moderate road noise	0.899	0.617–1.311	0.886	0.605–1.296	1.378	0.943–2.023	1.165	0.760–1.801	0.970	0.674–1.394
High road noise	0.667	0.435–1.021	1.045	0.683–1.599	**1.627**	**1.067–2.492**	1.534	0.962–2.467	0.771	0.513–1.157
Very low train noise	1.000	reference	1.000	reference	1.000	reference	1.000	reference	1.000	reference
Moderate train noise	1.257	0.888–1.781	1.193	0.839–1.699	1.100	0.779–1.554	1.016	0.694–1.482	1.034	0.737–1.452
High train noise	**2.659**	**1.639–4.354**	**2.272**	**1.390–3.758**	1.404	0.886–2.230	1.447	0.894–2.347	**1.854**	**1.178–2.955**
Very low commercial noise	1.000	reference	1.000	reference	1.000	reference	1.000	reference	1.000	reference
Moderate commercial noise	**1.793**	**1.296–2.485**	**1.549**	**1.116–2.151**	1.307	0.947–1.805	**1.513**	**1.060–2.164**	**1.558**	**1.139–2.133**
High commercial noise	0.951	0.560–1.607	0.943	0.548–1.614	1.018	0.610–1.693	1.555	0.905–2.655	1.330	0.797–2.214
Very low renovation noise	1.000	reference	1.000	reference	1.000	reference	1.000	reference	1.000	reference
Moderate renovation noise	**2.572**	**1.805–3.689**	**2.053**	**1.444–2.931**	**1.792**	**1.264–2.552**	1.301	0.884–1.924	**1.632**	**1.167–2.289**
High renovation noise	**2.625**	**1.756–3.951**	**2.263**	**1.517–3.394**	**2.057**	**1.390–3.058**	1.401	0.908–2.166	**1.494**	**1.023–2.184**
Community-level variance	0.194		0.185		0.136		0.100		0.050	
Median Odds Ratio (MOR)	52.0%		50.5%		42.0%		35.1%		23.7%	

Note: Bold font reflects statistically significant results at $p < 0.05$. OR represents odds ratios (median) and 95% CI refers to the 95% credible interval in the Bayesian inference paradigm.

With respect to the subjective measures of perceived noise pollution, most of them are found to be significantly associated with self-reported mental health symptoms or mental disorders (Table 3). For instance, the odds of reporting fatigue for respondents with perceived high pollution exposure to road traffic noise increase by 62.7%, compared to people who rated the road noise pollution in their neighborhoods as very low. Residents who perceived higher exposure to railway or commercial noise tend to be more likely to suffer from mental disorders, such as anxiety, stress and sleep disturbance. These results demonstrate that perceived pollution exposure to multiple noise sources is negatively associated with self-reported mental health symptoms in Beijing, China.

Moreover, housing renovation noise pollution, which has rarely been investigated to date in the Chinese context, shows significant correlations with various types of mental health symptoms in Beijing. Respondents who perceived both moderate and high exposure to housing renovation noise tend to have significantly worse mental health, or more likely suffer from various mental disorders than those who reported very low housing renovation noise levels in their surrounding environment. Since the second-hand housing market is prosperous in urban Beijing, housing renovation is popular and widespread for urban residents. As a result, housing renovation noise has become a serious environmental problem in many Chinese cities, which has potential adverse effects on the population's mental health.

3.3. Mental Disorders and Geographic Context

Geographic context effects, as measured by the distribution of community-level residuals, quantify how individuals' mental health outcomes would vary across places net of their socio-demographic and economic characteristics. The geographic context effects on mental health are quantified by the median odds ratio (MOR), which transforms the community-level variance on the logit scale to a more interpretable odds ratio scale, thus offering an intuitive quantification of the magnitude of geographic context effects [73]. MOR is interpreted as the increased risks that would occur when moving residents from a low-risk area to a high-risk area. Here, it means an elevated odds of reporting mental health problems if an individual is relocated from a community with a small residual (i.e., low proportion of reporting mental disorders net of included covariate effects) to a community with a large residual. As shown in Table 3, the MOR values indicate that, on average, there is an increase of 52.0% (anxiety), 50.5% (stress), 42.0% (fatigue), 35.1% (headache), and 23.7% (sleep disturbance) in the odds of reporting mental health problems for the urban residents if they are relocated from a community (or a geographic context) that enhances mental health to one with undesirable environment. These results suggest a significant geographic context effect on mental well-being in Beijing, China.

4. Discussion

In prior studies, only the evidence on the associations between road traffic noise and sleep disturbance, annoyance, and cognitive performance was sufficient [13,15,18]. There has been little research concerning the linkage of noise pollution from housing renovation/construction and commercial services with a wide range of mental disorders, such as anxiety, stress, fatigue and headache. Even fewer studies have examined the spatial distribution of multiple noise pollution at fine geographic resolution and their associations with various mental health symptoms, especially in developing countries like China [5,9].

This study contributes to the literature in several dimensions. First, it presents the geographic variations in people's subjective evaluations of noise pollution from diverse sources, including road traffic, railways, housing renovation, and commercial services at the community level in Beijing. It shows that road traffic noise and housing renovation noise are the principal noise stressors in the capital city of China, and there is geographic variability in pollution exposure to multiple noise sources. Second, this paper develops a broad conceptual framework to investigate the relationships between mental health and various objective and subjective measures, including socio-demographics, social environment, the objective physical built environment characteristics, and perceived noise-pollution evaluations [66,67]. It also examines the associations between these variables and multiple self-reported symptoms of mental health, such as anxiety, stress, fatigue, headache, as well as sleep disturbance. Finally, as mental health is associated with various factors at both the individual and community scales, Bayesian multilevel logistic models were employed to capture the hierarchical structure of our survey data and the unobserved effects of geographic context on the survey respondents [74].

Our results show that some social factors or socio-demographic attributes, such as age and income, are significant covariates of mental disorders for urban residents in Beijing. People with the highest income level have significantly increased odds of reporting mental health problems, such as anxiety, fatigue, and sleep disturbance. This seems to be in contrast with the findings from some prior studies, which found that people with high levels of income tend to have good health, although the correlation is likely to be nonlinear [66,75]. This result might be due to the potential bias of subjectively reported data on mental disorders and occupational stress for people with higher income levels [76]. Moreover, people with higher income levels have been found to suffer from more personal exposure to traffic-related air pollution, which might worsen their subjective health evaluations [77].

Housing tenure and satisfaction evaluation with housing conditions are significantly correlated with some mental health symptoms, such as anxiety, stress, as well as sleep disturbance. Social environment or community attachment is also a significant correlate of mental health, which is in agreement with previous findings [33]. Objective built environment variables seem to contribute little to the variation of self-reported mental disorders, except for proximity to the main road. People residing in neighborhoods close to the main road have significantly higher odds of reporting various mental health problems, such as anxiety, fatigue, and sleep disturbance.

Regarding the subjective measure of perceived noise exposure, it might produce a potential bias for different subpopulations. Therefore, before reporting the estimation results in Table 3, we ran a series of regression models to examine the associations between perceived noise pollution and some key socio-demographics, such as age, education and income, and found no systematic bias in our measurement of noise perception assessment. The Bayesian multilevel logistic modeling results show that residents' perceived high exposures to road traffic noise tend to significantly increase their odds of reporting fatigue, while residents who perceived high exposure to railway noise are more likely to suffer from mental disorders such as anxiety, stress and sleep disturbance. Housing renovation and construction noise, which has rarely been investigated before, is a significant covariate of a wide range of mental health symptoms. As China is experiencing a rapid urbanization process, there are numerous ongoing construction projects that have led to an increase in environmental complaints, and construction noise has become a serious problem in many Chinese cities [5]. This type of noise pollution is a feature that reflects rapid urbanization in China and is different from the noise problems in Europe and North America, and thus needs more investigation in the Chinese context. Furthermore, the multilevel modeling results also suggest a significant geographic context effect on mental well-being in Beijing.

This study has some limitations. Since objective data on noise pollution at a fine geographic resolution is usually not available in China, it poses an important constraint on noise-health interaction research in the Chinese context. Although characteristics of the objective physical built environment may be regarded as proxies of people's objective exposure to various noise sources, the inaccurate measure of objective noise exposure might weaken the mental health effects of the noise pollution in statistical models [47]. Moreover, due to the unavailability of some health-relevant confounders in the survey data, such as body mass index, smoking and drug use, these variables are missing in the analysis. However, the effects of such variables might be included in the residuals of the statistical models. Future research will need to collect both objective and subjective data on noise pollution at a fine spatiotemporal resolution to explore their combined effects on mental health, while controlling for a wide range of confounding variables.

5. Conclusions

China's rapid urbanization and increase in car ownership have given rise to a wide range of environmental hazards, such as air and noise pollution, which pose significant health risks to the population. While the health effects of environmental pollution, particularly ambient air pollution, have received considerable attention in past research, the detrimental effects of noise pollution on people's mental health need more investigation. This study attempts to shed light on the relationships between exposures to multiple sources of noise pollution and mental disorders in a Chinese megacity. Overall, road traffic and housing renovation are found to be the principal noise polluting sources influencing the urban living environment in Beijing. Higher noise-pollution exposures are significantly associated with the worse mental health of urban residents in general. The results also have some policy implications for the construction of transportation infrastructure, noise abatement interventions, and public health promotion. We argue that, while pursuing GDP growth and economic development in China, it is also important for the government to develop sustainable healthy environments and cities for promoting public health and well-being in the future.

Author Contributions: J.M., M.-P.K. and Y.C. conceived and designed the experiments; J.M. and C.L. performed the experiments, analyzed the data and wrote the paper. J.M. and M.-P.K. contributed to revising the paper.

Funding: This work was funded by the National Natural Science Foundation of China (Grants No. 41601148, 41529101 and 41571153). In addition, Mei-Po Kwan was supported by a John Simon Guggenheim Memorial Foundation Fellowship.

Acknowledgments: The authors would like to thank Dr. Zhilin Liu from Tsinghua University for providing the survey data used in this research.

Statement: There is no human subject protection or ethics requirements in China concerning this research, so a project identification code is not available. The data were collected from the participants with their consent.

Conflicts of Interest: The authors declare no conflicts of interest.

References

1. Giles-Corti, B.; Vernez-Moudon, A.; Reis, R.; Turrell, G.; Dannenberg, A.L.; Badland, H.; Foster, S.; Lowe, M.; Sallis, J.F.; Stevenson, M.; et al. City planning and population health: A global challenge. *Lancet* **2016**, *388*, 2912–2924. [CrossRef]

2. Organization, W.H. Burden of disease from environmental noise: Quantification of healthy life years lost in Europe. In *Burden of Disease from Environmental Noise: Quantification of Healthy Life Years Lost in Europe*; World Health Organization: Geneva, Switzerland, 2011; p. 126.

3. Pirrera, S.; De Valck, E.; Cluydts, R. Nocturnal road traffic noise: A review on its assessment and consequences on sleep and health. *Environ. Int.* **2010**, *36*, 492–498. [CrossRef] [PubMed]

4. Zheng, D.; Cai, X.; Song, H.; Chen, T. Study on personal noise exposure in China. *Appl. Acoust.* **1996**, *48*, 59–70. [CrossRef]

5. Xiao, J.; Li, X.; Zhang, Z. Daly-based health risk assessment of construction noise in Beijing, China. *Int. J. Environ. Res. Public Health* **2016**, *13*, 1045. [CrossRef] [PubMed]

6. Li, B.; Tao, S.; Dawson, R. Evaluation and analysis of traffic noise from the main urban roads in Beijing. *Appl. Acoust.* **2002**, *63*, 1137–1142. [CrossRef]

7. Li, B.; Tao, S. Influence of expanding ring roads on traffic noise in Beijing city. *Appl. Acoust.* **2004**, *65*, 243–249. [CrossRef]

8. Ministry of Environment Protection of China. 2016 Report on the State of the Environment in China. Available online: http://english.sepa.gov.cn/Resources/Reports/soe/ReportSOE/201709/P020170929573904364594.pdf (accessed on 10 June 2018).

9. Guoqing, D.; Xiaoyi, L.; Xiang, S.; Zhengguang, L.; Qili, L. Investigation of the relationship between aircraft noise and community annoyance in China. *Noise Health* **2012**, *14*, 52. [CrossRef] [PubMed]

10. Di, G.; Liu, X.; Lin, Q.; Zheng, Y.; He, L. The relationship between urban combined traffic noise and annoyance: An investigation in Dalian, north of China. *Sci. Total Environ.* **2012**, *432*, 189–194. [CrossRef] [PubMed]

11. Li, H.-J.; Yu, W.-B.; Lu, J.-Q.; Zeng, L.; Li, N.; Zhao, Y.-M. Investigation of road-traffic noise and annoyance in Beijing: A cross-sectional study of 4th ring road. *Arch. Environ. Occup. Health* **2008**, *63*, 27–33. [CrossRef] [PubMed]

12. Basner, M.; Babisch, W.; Davis, A.; Brink, M.; Clark, C.; Janssen, S.; Stansfeld, S. Auditory and non-auditory effects of noise on health. *Lancet* **2014**, *383*, 1325–1332. [CrossRef]

13. Guski, R.; Schreckenberg, D.; Schuemer, R. Who environmental noise guidelines for the European region: A systematic review on environmental noise and annoyance. *Int. J. Environ. Res. Public Health* **2017**, *14*, 1539. [CrossRef] [PubMed]

14. Kempen, E.V.; Casas, M.; Pershagen, G.; Foraster, M. Who environmental noise guidelines for the European region: A systematic review on environmental noise and cardiovascular and metabolic effects: A summary. *Int. J. Environ. Res. Public Health* **2018**, *15*, 379. [CrossRef] [PubMed]

15. Basner, M.; McGuire, S. Who environmental noise guidelines for the European region: A systematic review on environmental noise and effects on sleep. *Int. J. Environ. Res. Public Health* **2018**, *15*, 519. [CrossRef] [PubMed]

16. Śliwińska-Kowalska, M.; Zaborowski, K. Who environmental noise guidelines for the European region: A systematic review on environmental noise and permanent hearing loss and tinnitus. *Int. J. Environ. Res. Public Health* **2017**, *14*, 1139. [CrossRef] [PubMed]

17. Nieuwenhuijsen, M.J.; Ristovska, G.; Dadvand, P. Who environmental noise guidelines for the European region: A systematic review on environmental noise and adverse birth outcomes. *Int. J. Environ. Res. Public Health* **2017**, *14*, 1252. [CrossRef] [PubMed]

18. Clark, C.; Paunovic, K. Who environmental noise guidelines for the European region: A systematic review on environmental noise and cognition. *Int. J. Environ. Res. Public Health* **2018**, *15*, 285. [CrossRef] [PubMed]

19. Davies, H.; Van Kamp, I. Noise and cardiovascular disease: A review of the literature 2008–2011. *Noise Health* **2012**, *14*, 287. [CrossRef] [PubMed]

20. McLean, E.; Tarnopolsky, A. Noise, discomfort and mental health: A review of the socio-medical implications of disturbance by noise. *Psychol. Med.* **1977**, *7*, 19–62. [CrossRef] [PubMed]

21. Stansfeld, S.; Haines, M.; Burr, M.; Berry, B.; Lercher, P. A review of environmental noise and mental health. *Noise Health* **2000**, *2*, 1. [PubMed]

22. Clark, C.; Myron, R.; Stansfeld, S.; Candy, B. A systematic review of the evidence on the effect of the built and physical environment on mental health. *J. Public Ment. Health* **2007**, *6*, 14–27. [CrossRef]

23. Van Kamp, I.; Davies, H. Environmental noise and mental health: Five year review and future directions. In Proceedings of the 9th International Congress on Noise as a Public Health Problem, Mashantucket, CT, USA, 21–25 July 2008.

24. Gu, L.; Xie, J.; Long, J.; Chen, Q.; Chen, Q.; Pan, R.; Yan, Y.; Wu, G.; Liang, B.; Tan, J. Epidemiology of major depressive disorder in mainland China: A systematic review. *PLoS ONE* **2013**, *8*, e65356. [CrossRef] [PubMed]

25. Organization, W.H. *The World Health Report 2001: Mental Health: New Understanding, New Hope*; World Health Organization: Geneva, Switzerland, 2001.

26. Yang, G.; Wang, Y.; Zeng, Y.; Gao, G.F.; Liang, X.; Zhou, M.; Wan, X.; Yu, S.; Jiang, Y.; Naghavi, M. Rapid health transition in China, 1990–2010: Findings from the global burden of disease study 2010. *Lancet* **2013**, *381*, 1987–2015. [CrossRef]

27. Münzel, T.; Gori, T.; Babisch, W.; Basner, M. Cardiovascular effects of environmental noise exposure. *Eur. Heart J.* **2014**, *35*, 829–836. [CrossRef] [PubMed]

28. Beutel, M.E.; Junger, C.; Klein, E.M.; Wild, P.; Lackner, K.; Blettner, M.; Binder, H.; Michal, M.; Wiltink, J.; Brahler, E.; et al. Noise annoyance is associated with depression and anxiety in the general population- the contribution of aircraft noise. *PLoS ONE* **2016**, *11*, e0155357. [CrossRef] [PubMed]

29. Schreckenberg, D.; Meis, M.; Kahl, C.; Peschel, C.; Eikmann, T. Aircraft noise and quality of life around Frankfurt airport. *Int. J. Environ. Res. Public Health* **2010**, *7*, 3382–3405. [CrossRef] [PubMed]

30. Schreckenberg, D.; Griefahn, B.; Meis, M. The associations between noise sensitivity, reported physical and mental health, perceived environmental quality, and noise annoyance. *Noise Health* **2010**, *12*, 7. [CrossRef] [PubMed]

31. Oiamo, T.H.; Luginaah, I.N.; Baxter, J. Cumulative effects of noise and odour annoyances on environmental and health related quality of life. *Soc. Sci. Med.* **2015**, *146*, 191–203. [CrossRef] [PubMed]

32. Sygna, K.; Aasvang, G.M.; Aamodt, G.; Oftedal, B.; Krog, N.H. Road traffic noise, sleep and mental health. *Environ. Res.* **2014**, *131*, 17–24. [CrossRef] [PubMed]

33. Dzhambov, A.; Tilov, B.; Markevych, I.; Dimitrova, D. Residential road traffic noise and general mental health in youth: The role of noise annoyance, neighborhood restorative quality, physical activity, and social cohesion as potential mediators. *Environ. Int.* **2017**, *109*, 1–9. [CrossRef] [PubMed]

34. Lercher, P.; Brink, M.; Rudisser, J.; Van Renterghem, T.; Botteldooren, D.; Baulac, M.; Defrance, J. The effects of railway noise on sleep medication intake: Results from the alpnap-study. *Noise Health* **2010**, *12*, 110. [CrossRef] [PubMed]

35. Sørensen, M.; Hvidberg, M.; Hoffmann, B.; Andersen, Z.J.; Nordsborg, R.B.; Lillelund, K.G.; Jakobsen, J.; Tjønneland, A.; Overvad, K.; Raaschou-Nielsen, O. Exposure to road traffic and railway noise and associations with blood pressure and self-reported hypertension: A cohort study. *Environ. Health* **2011**, *10*, 92. [CrossRef] [PubMed]

36. Bocquier, A.; Cortaredona, S.; Boutin, C.; David, A.; Bigot, A.; Sciortino, V.; Nauleau, S.; Gaudart, J.; Giorgi, R.; Verger, P. Is exposure to night-time traffic noise a risk factor for purchase of anxiolytic–hypnotic medication? A cohort study. *Eur. J. Public Health* **2013**, *24*, 298–303. [CrossRef] [PubMed]

37. Evandt, J.; Oftedal, B.; Krog, N.H.; Skurtveit, S.; Nafstad, P.; Schwarze, P.E.; Skovlund, E.; Houthuijs, D.; Aasvang, G.M. Road traffic noise and registry based use of sleep medication. *Environ. Health* **2017**, *16*, 110. [CrossRef] [PubMed]

38. Yoshida, T.; Osada, Y.; Kawaguchi, T.; Hoshiyama, Y.; Yoshida, K.; Yamamoto, K. Effects of road traffic noise on inhabitants of Tokyo. *J. Sound Vib.* **1997**, *205*, 517–522. [CrossRef]

39. Lercher, P.; Kofler, W. Behavioral and health responses associated with road traffic noise exposure along alpine through-traffic routes. *Sci. Total Environ.* **1996**, *189*, 85–89. [CrossRef]

40. Héritier, H.; Vienneau, D.; Frei, P.; Eze, I.C.; Brink, M.; Probst-Hensch, N.; Röösli, M. The association between road traffic noise exposure, annoyance and health-related quality of life (hrqol). *Int. J. Environ. Res. Public Health* **2014**, *11*, 12652–12667. [CrossRef] [PubMed]

41. Öhrström, E.; Skånberg, A.; Svensson, H.; Gidlöf-Gunnarsson, A. Effects of road traffic noise and the benefit of access to quietness. *J. Sound Vib.* **2006**, *295*, 40–59. [CrossRef]

42. Paunović, K.; Jakovljević, B.; Belojević, G. Predictors of noise annoyance in noisy and quiet urban streets. *Sci. Total Environ.* **2009**, *407*, 3707–3711. [CrossRef] [PubMed]

43. Miedema, H.M.; Vos, H. Associations between self-reported sleep disturbance and environmental noise based on re-analyses of pooled data from 24 studies. *Behav. Sleep Med.* **2007**, *5*, 1–20. [CrossRef] [PubMed]

44. Firdaus, G.; Ahmad, A. Temporal variation in risk factors and prevalence rate of depression in urban population: Does the urban environment play a significant role? *Int. J. Ment. Health Promot.* **2014**, *16*, 279–288. [CrossRef]

45. Firdaus, G. Built environment and health outcomes: Identification of contextual risk factors for mental well-being of older adults. *Ageing Int.* **2017**, *42*, 62–77. [CrossRef]

46. Welch, D.; Shepherd, D.; Dirks, K.N.; McBride, D.; Marsh, S. Road traffic noise and health-related quality of life: A cross-sectional study. *Noise Health* **2013**, *15*, 224. [CrossRef] [PubMed]

47. Brink, M. Parameters of well-being and subjective health and their relationship with residential traffic noise exposure—A representative evaluation in Switzerland. *Environ. Int.* **2011**, *37*, 723–733. [CrossRef] [PubMed]

48. Halonen, J.I.; Lanki, T.; Yli-Tuomi, T.; Turunen, A.W.; Peniti, J.; Kivimäki, M.; Vahtera, J. Associations of traffic noise with self-rated health and psychotropic medication use. *Scand. J. Work Environ. Health* **2014**, *40*, 235–243. [CrossRef] [PubMed]

49. Persson, R.; Björk, J.; Ardö, J.; Albin, M.; Jakobsson, K. Trait anxiety and modeled exposure as determinants of self-reported annoyance to sound, air pollution and other environmental factors in the home. *Int. Arch. Occup. Environ. Health* **2007**, *81*, 179–191. [CrossRef] [PubMed]

50. Roswall, N.; Høgh, V.; Envold-Bidstrup, P.; Raaschou-Nielsen, O.; Ketzel, M.; Overvad, K.; Olsen, A.; Sørensen, M. Residential exposure to traffic noise and health-related quality of life—A population-based study. *PLoS ONE* **2015**, *10*, e0120199. [CrossRef] [PubMed]

51. Stansfeld, S.; Gallacher, J.; Babisch, W.; Shipley, M. Road traffic noise and psychiatric disorder: Prospective findings from the caerphilly study. *BMJ* **1996**, *313*, 266–267. [CrossRef] [PubMed]

52. Lercher, P.; Evans, G.; Meis, M.; Kofler, W. Ambient neighbourhood noise and children's mental health. *Occup. Environ. Med.* **2002**, *59*, 380–386. [CrossRef] [PubMed]

53. Hjortebjerg, D.; Andersen, A.M.N.; Christensen, J.S.; Ketzel, M.; Raaschou-Nielsen, O.; Sunyer, J.; Julvez, J.; Forns, J.; Sørensen, M. Exposure to road traffic noise and behavioral problems in 7-year-old children: A cohort study. *Environ. Health Perspect.* **2016**, *124*, 228. [CrossRef] [PubMed]

54. Dreger, S.; Meyer, N.; Fromme, H.; Bolte, G. Environmental noise and incident mental health problems: A prospective cohort study among school children in Germany. *Environ. Res.* **2015**, *143*, 49–54. [CrossRef] [PubMed]

55. Clark, C.; Head, J.; Stansfeld, S.A. Longitudinal effects of aircraft noise exposure on children's health and cognition: A six-year follow-up of the UK ranch cohort. *J. Environ. Psychol.* **2013**, *35*, 1–9. [CrossRef]

56. Weich, S.; Blanchard, M.; Prince, M.; Burton, E.; Erens, B.; Sproston, K. Mental health and the built environment: Cross–sectional survey of individual and contextual risk factors for depression. *Br. J. Psychiatry* **2002**, *180*, 428–433. [CrossRef] [PubMed]

57. Galea, S.; Ahern, J.; Rudenstine, S.; Wallace, Z.; Vlahov, D. Urban built environment and depression: A multilevel analysis. *J. Epidemiol. Community Health* **2005**, *59*, 822–827. [CrossRef] [PubMed]

58. Melis, G.; Gelormino, E.; Marra, G.; Ferracin, E.; Costa, G. The effects of the urban built environment on mental health: A cohort study in a large northern Italian city. *Int. J. Environ. Res. Public Health* **2015**, *12*, 14898–14915. [CrossRef] [PubMed]

59. Evans, G.W. The built environment and mental health. *J. Urban Health* **2003**, *80*, 536–555. [CrossRef] [PubMed]

60. Araya, R.; Dunstan, F.; Playle, R.; Thomas, H.; Palmer, S.; Lewis, G. Perceptions of social capital and the built environment and mental health. *Soc. Sci. Med.* **2006**, *62*, 3072–3083. [CrossRef] [PubMed]

61. Xiao, Y.; Miao, S.; Sarkar, C.; Geng, H.; Lu, Y. Exploring the impacts of housing condition on migrants' mental health in nanxiang, shanghai: A structural equation modelling approach. *Int. J. Environ. Res. Public Health* **2018**, *15*, 225. [CrossRef] [PubMed]

62. Kamimura, A.; Armenta, B.; Nourian, M.; Assasnik, N.; Nourian, K.; Chernenko, A. Perceived environmental pollution and its impact on health in China, Japan, and South Korea. *J. Prev. Med. Public Health* **2017**, *50*, 188. [CrossRef] [PubMed]

63. Niemann, H.; Bonnefoy, X.; Braubach, M.; Hecht, K.; Maschke, C.; Rodrigues, C.; Robbel, N. Noise-induced annoyance and morbidity results from the pan-European lares study. *Noise Health* **2006**, *8*, 63. [CrossRef] [PubMed]

64. Stansfeld, S.; Clark, C. Mental health effects of noise. *Encycl. Environ. Health* **2011**, *20*, 683–689.

65. Mouratidis, K. Rethinking how built environments influence subjective well-being: A new conceptual framework. *J. Urban.* **2018**, *11*, 24–40. [CrossRef]

66. Ma, J.; Mitchell, G.; Dong, G.; Zhang, W. Inequality in Beijing: A spatial multilevel analysis of perceived environmental hazard and self-rated health. *Ann. Am. Assoc. Geogr.* **2017**, *107*, 109–129. [CrossRef]

67. Ma, J.; Heppenstall, A.; Harland, K.; Mitchell, G. Synthesising carbon emission for mega-cities: A static spatial microsimulation of transport CO_2 from urban travel in Beijing. *Comput. Environ. Urban Syst.* **2014**, *45*, 78–88. [CrossRef]

68. Congdon, P. *Applied Bayesian Modelling*; John Wiley & Sons: Hoboken, NJ, USA, 2014; Volume 595.

69. Gelman, A.; Carlin, J.B.; Stern, H.S.; Dunson, D.B.; Vehtari, A.; Rubin, D.B. *Bayesian Data Analysis*; CRC Press: Boca Raton, FL, USA, 2014; Volume 2.

70. Steele, F. Multilevel models for longitudinal data. *J. R. Stat. Soc. Ser. A Stat. Soc.* **2008**, *171*, 5–19. [CrossRef]

71. Goldstein, H. *Multilevel Statistical Models*; John Wiley & Sons: Hoboken, NJ, USA, 2011; Volume 922.

72. Rue, H.; Martino, S.; Lindgren, F.; Simpson, D.; Riebler, A.; Krainski, E. INLA: Functions Which Allow to Perform a Full Bayesian Analysis of Structured Additive Models Using Integrated Nested Laplace Approximation. 2014. Available online: http://www.r-inla.org/ (accessed on 10 June 2018).

73. Merlo, J.; Chaix, B.; Ohlsson, H.; Beckman, A.; Johnell, K.; Hjerpe, P.; Råstam, L.; Larsen, K. A brief conceptual tutorial of multilevel analysis in social epidemiology: Using measures of clustering in multilevel logistic regression to investigate contextual phenomena. *J. Epidemiol. Community Health* **2006**, *60*, 290–297. [CrossRef] [PubMed]

74. Zhao, P.; Kwan, M.-P.; Zhou, S. The uncertain geographic context problem in the analysis of the relationships between obesity and the built environment in Guangzhou. *Int. J. Environ. Res. Public Health* **2018**, *15*, 308. [CrossRef] [PubMed]

75. Subramanian, S.V.; Kawachi, I. Income inequality and health: What have we learned so far? *Epidemiol. Rev.* **2004**, *26*, 78–91. [CrossRef] [PubMed]

76. Cesaroni, G.; Badaloni, C.; Romano, V.; Donato, E.; Perucci, C.A.; Forastiere, F. Socioeconomic position and health status of people who live near busy roads: The Rome Longitudinal Study (RoLS). *Environ. Health* **2010**, *9*, 41. [CrossRef] [PubMed]

77. Tonne, C.; Milà, C.; Fecht, D.; Alvarez, M.; Gulliver, J.; Smith, J.; Beevers, S.; Anderson, H.R.; Kelly, F. Socioeconomic and ethnic inequalities in exposure to air and noise pollution in London. *Environ. Int.* **2018**, *115*, 170–179. [CrossRef] [PubMed]

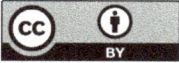

International Journal of
Environmental Research and Public Health

MDPI

Article

Understanding the Influence of Crop Residue Burning on PM$_{2.5}$ and PM$_{10}$ Concentrations in China from 2013 to 2017 Using MODIS Data

Yan Zhuang [1,2], Danlu Chen [1,2], Ruiyuan Li [1,2], Ziyue Chen [1,2,*], Jun Cai [3], Bin He [1,2], Bingbo Gao [4], Nianliang Cheng [5] and Yueni Huang [6]

[1] State Key Laboratory of Earth Surface Processes and Resource Ecology, College of Global Change and Earth System Science, Beijing Normal University, 19 Xinjiekouwai Street, Haidian, Beijing 100875, China; yzhuang@mail.bnu.edu.cn (Y.Z.); dlchen@mail.bnu.edu.cn (D.C.); leeruiyuan@bjfu.edu.cn (R.L.); hebin@bnu.edu.cn (B.H.)

[2] Joint Center for Global Change Studies, Beijing 100875, China

[3] Department of Earth System Science, Tsinghua University, Beijing 100084, China; cai-j12@mails.tsinghua.edu.cn

[4] National Engineering Research Center for Information Technology in Agriculture, 11 Shuguang Huayuan Middle Road, Beijing 100097, China; gaobb@nercita.org.cn

[5] College of Water Sciences, Beijing Normal University, 19 Xinjiekouwai Street, Haidian, Beijing 100875, China; 15001195306@163.com

[6] Department of Physics, Beijing Normal University, 19 Xinjiekouwai Street, Haidian, Beijing 100875, China; huangyueni@mail.bnu.edu.cn

* Correspondence: zychen@bnu.edu.cn

Received: 5 June 2018; Accepted: 14 July 2018; Published: 17 July 2018

Abstract: In recent years, particulate matter (PM) pollution has increasingly affected public life and health. Therefore, crop residue burning, as a significant source of PM pollution in China, should be effectively controlled. This study attempts to understand variations and characteristics of PM$_{10}$ and PM$_{2.5}$ concentrations and discuss correlations between the variation of PM concentrations and crop residue burning using ground observation and Moderate Resolution Imaging Spectroradiometer (MODIS) data. The results revealed that the overall PM concentration in China from 2013 to 2017 was in a downward tendency with regional variations. Correlation analysis demonstrated that the PM$_{10}$ concentration was more closely related to crop residue burning than the PM$_{2.5}$ concentration. From a spatial perspective, the strongest correlation between PM concentration and crop residue burning existed in Northeast China (NEC). From a temporal perspective, the strongest correlation usually appeared in autumn for most regions. The total amount of crop residue burning spots in autumn was relatively large, and NEC was the region with the most intense crop residue burning in China. We compared the correlation between PM concentrations and crop residue burning at inter-annual and seasonal scales, and during burning-concentrated periods. We found that correlations between PM concentrations and crop residue burning increased significantly with the narrowing temporal scales and was the strongest during burning-concentrated periods, indicating that intense crop residue burning leads to instant deterioration of PM concentrations. The methodology and findings from this study provide meaningful reference for better understanding the influence of crop residue burning on PM pollution across China.

Keywords: PM concentrations; crop residue burning; correlation analysis; interannual and seasonal variations; China

1. Introduction

Recently, particulate matter (PM) pollution has become a hot spot concerning people's life and health [1–3]. Both PM_{10} (coarse particles with aerodynamic diameter between 2.5 μm and 10 μm) and $PM_{2.5}$ (fine particles with aerodynamic diameter equal to or less than 2.5 μm) have been considered as major air pollutants in China [4]. A great deal of research [5–7] has proved that in addition to haze-induced low visibility, sustained exposure to high concentrations of PM_{10} and $PM_{2.5}$ is harmful for human's physical and mental health. On the other hand, short-term exposure or low-concentration exposure also adversely affects corporeity or even birth outcomes [8–10]. Furthermore, the morbidity of respiratory disease, cardiovascular disease, and lung cancer are strongly correlated with severe $PM_{2.5}$ pollution [11]. However, although the government has taken some effective emission-reduction measures to alleviate the air pollution, PM concentrations still significantly exceed the guideline value proposed by the World Health Organization (WHO) in many cities of China [12]. There are two major drivers for the PM pollution, anthropogenic activities, and unfavorable meteorological conditions [13–15]. With increasing anthropogenic emission, PM pollution is hard to ameliorate in a short time [16]. Specifically, biomass burning and secondary pollutant formation are two main sources for PM pollution in China [17].

Crop residue burning, as one type of biomass burning, is a convenient, yet less environmentally friendly way to dispose massive agricultural wastes. For China, agricultural production plays an important role in the national economy, which means a large number of crop residues, such as paddy straws, wheat straws, and corn stalks, are generated and piled up on bare croplands. Following this, substantial crop residues are burnt directly to fertilize the soil and prepare for next crop-planting season. However, the burning of crop residues has seriously influenced the local and regional air quality during harvest seasons, especially in Northeast China [18–20]. During the burning process, severe haze episodes are further aggravated because SO_2 and NO_X can be oxidized into secondary inorganic/organic aerosol (SIA/SOA), which are important sources for generating secondary $PM_{2.5}$ [17]. In addition, other aerosol emissions from crop residue burning result in the decline of local precipitation to a certain extent, leading to the further increase of $PM_{2.5}$ concentrations [21,22]. In other words, the change of meteorological conditions caused by crop residue burning may further exacerbate PM pollution. Therefore, in order to mitigate the current ambient air pollution, it is highly urgent to take effective and targeted measures to control crop residue burning in China.

Due to the vast territory of China, PM concentrations and the condition of crop residue burning demonstrate notable temporal and spatial difference across China. Given the potential risk PM exert on public health, it is essential to explore correlations between crop residue burning and PM concentrations. Yin et al. revealed the spatial distribution of crop residue burning and $PM_{2.5}$ concentrations in China at a seasonal pattern [23], and Chen et al. discussed the influence of crop residue burning on $PM_{2.5}$ concentration in Heilongjiang Province of China during a severe haze episode [24]. Zhuang et al. analyzed the trend of crop residue burning in different regions of China from 2003 to 2017 [18]. Meanwhile, some related studies have been conducted in other countries, such as India and Thailand. Awasthi et al. explored the effect of crop residue burning on pulmonary function tests of youth in North West India [25]. Although many scholars [26–28] have discussed the emissions from crop residue burning, limited studies have been conducted on understanding correlations between crop residue burning and PM concentrations. To fill this gap, we attempt to understand the spatio-temporal variation of PM concentrations across China and its correlation with crop residue burning. Firstly, from a regional perspective, we conducted spatio-temporal trend analyses of PM (including $PM_{2.5}$ and PM_{10}) concentrations in China during 2013 to 2017. Next, we analyzed interannual and seasonal variations of crop residue burning in different regions across China. Following this, we analyzed the correlation between PM concentrations and crop residue burning in different regions at different temporal scales.

2. Materials and Methods

2.1. Study Area

China has a vast territory area of about 9.6 million square kilometers with complicated terrain and climatic characteristics in different regions, which leads to different-periods of agricultural crops-planting and reaping. Considering the notable spatio-temporal patterns of crop residue burning in China, we divided the study area into seven regions (Figure 1) according to Chinese administrative divisions [29]. The seven regions are named as follows: Northeast China (NEC, including Heilongjiang Province, Jilin Province, Liaoning Province), North China (NC, including The Inner Mongolia Autonomous Region, Shanxi Province, Hebei Province, Beijing, Tianjin), Northwest China (NWC, including Shaanxi Province, Gansu Province, The Ningxia Hui Autonomous Region, Qinghai Province, The Xinjiang Uygur Autonomous Region), East China (EC, including Shandong Province, Jiangsu Province, Zhejiang Province, Fujian Province, Anhui Province, Jiangxi Province), Central China (CC, including Henan Province, Hubei Province, Hunan Province), South China (SC, including Guangdong Province, The Guangxi Zhuang Autonomous Region, Hainan Province), and Southwest China (SWC, including Sichuan Province, Guizhou Province, Yunnan Province, The Tibet Autonomous Region).

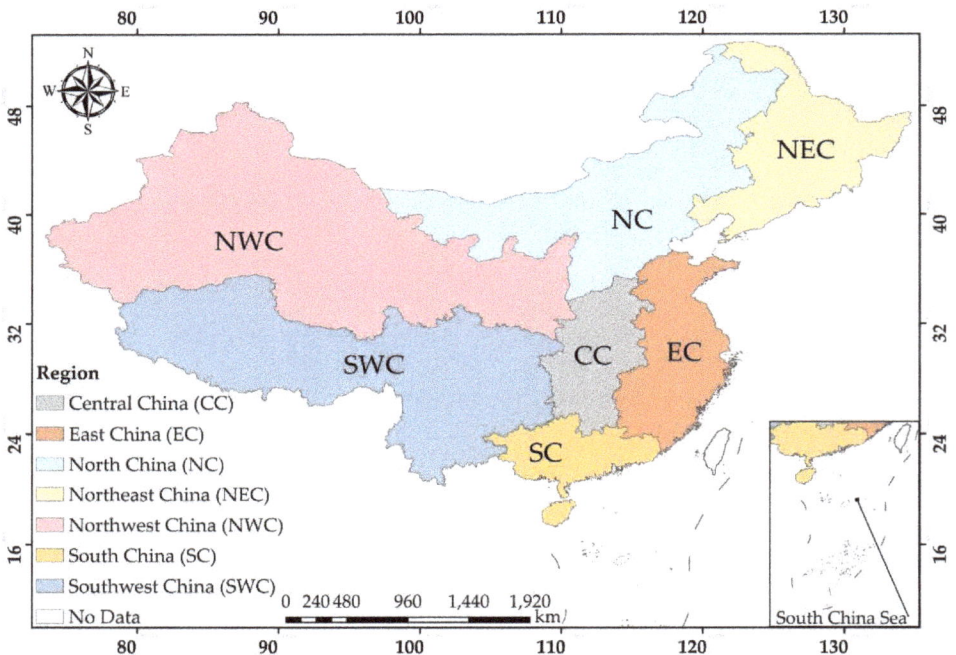

Figure 1. Geographical locations of seven regions in China.

2.2. Data Sources

2.2.1. Ground-Observed PM$_{2.5}$ and PM$_{10}$ Concentrations Data

The PM$_{2.5}$ and PM$_{10}$ concentrations data used for this study were obtained from website PM25.in (http://pm25.in/about), which collects official real-time air quality data provided by China National Environmental Monitoring Center (CNEMC). The real-time air quality data include hourly PM$_{2.5}$

concentration data (μg/m^3), hourly PM$_{10}$ concentration data (μg/m^3), Air Quality Index (AQI), and other airborne pollutants concentration data. Before 1 January 2015, the published PM data supplied by PM25.in (http://pm25.in/about), covered 190 monitoring cities in China, and this number has increased to 367 since 1 January 2015 [30]. The location of ground-monitoring air quality stations can be seen in Figure 2.

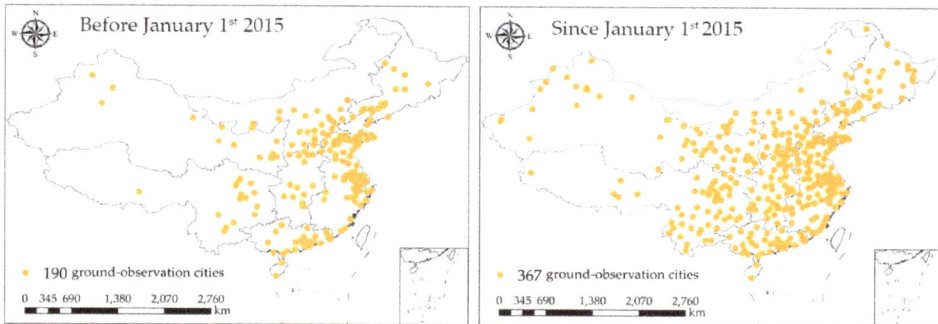

Figure 2. The location of ground-monitoring air quality stations.

By calling the specific API document on website PM25.in (http://pm25.in/about), we collected hourly PM$_{2.5}$ and PM$_{10}$ concentrations data for all monitoring cities in China from 18 January 2013 to 31 December 2017. The daily PM concentration data for each region were calculated by averaging all available hourly PM data from all monitoring cities.

2.2.2. MODIS Active Fire Data

The Moderate Resolution Imaging Spectroradiometer (MODIS) is an optical remote sensing instrument widely used in the fields of Geoscience, Environmental Science, and so on. Owing to its multi-spectral bands (36) and broad spectrum, ranging from 0.4 μm (visible band) to 14.4 μm (thermal infrared band), MODIS can provide a great deal of geographic and atmospheric information. Meanwhile, terra (AM) and aqua (PM) with MODIS transits China four times per day on 10:30, 22:30, 01:30, and 13:30, respectively [31]. Concerning the capability of fire detection, MODIS can monitor conflagration areas over 1000 m^2. If the weather is suitable (e.g., little/no smoke and relative homogeneous land surface) for observing, one tenth of burning fire spots would be detected. Light fires covering around 50 m^2 can be detected under the most favorable weather conditions [32].

We utilized MOD14A1/MYD14A1 daily Level 3 fire products (MODIS Thermal Anomalies/Fire products) with a spatial resolution of 1 km, which are available at NASA's LAADS DACC ftp server [33], to extract crop residue burning spots in China. In addition, a contextual algorithm was applied to detect fire spots according to the strong radiation from mid-infrared bands [34]. The products also classified the reliability of fire detection into three levels, including low-confidence fires, nominal-confidence fires, and high-confidence fires. MOD14A1/MYD14A1 were stored as a single file that consisted of eight days' data for convenience, representing eight-day continuous collection of fire data. To get daily fire spots map (Figure 3a), a maximum value composite method was employed for processing the data integration of MOD14A1/MYD14A1 products.

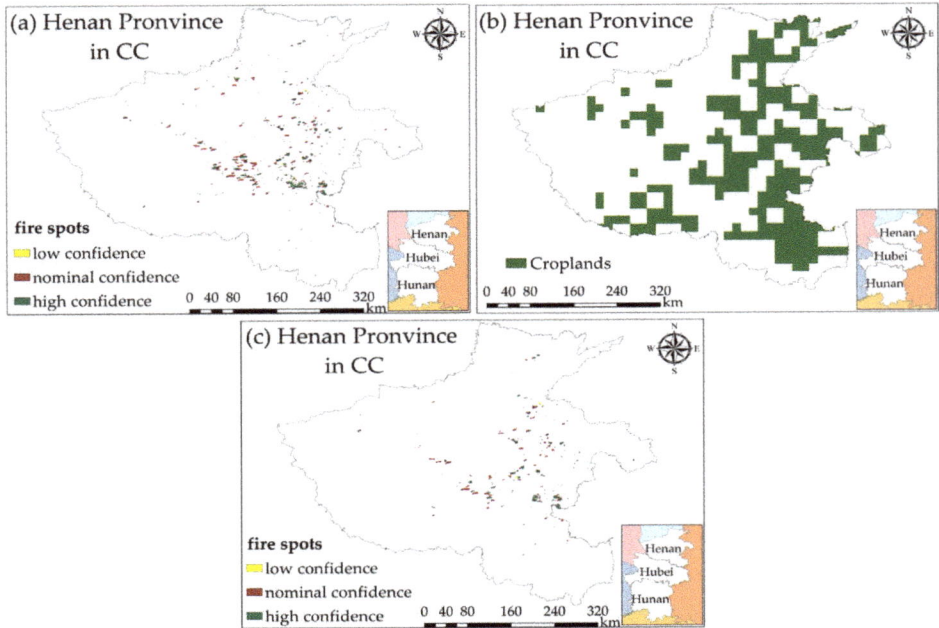

Figure 3. Extraction of crop residue burning spots in China. (**a**) Fire spots extracted from Moderate Resolution Imaging Spectroradiometer (MODIS) fire products; (**b**) Croplands extracted from Land-Use and Land-Cover Change (LUCC) dataset in 2015; (**c**) Crop residue burning spots extracted by combining MODIS fire products and LUCC dataset.

2.2.3. Land-Use and Land-Cover Data

Although fire spots could be extracted from MODIS fire products, it cannot be directly defined as the crop residue burning spots. Owing to the existence of such burning types as forest fire and urban solid waste incineration, the extraction of crop residue burning spots was further processed with a dataset of Land-Use and Land-Cover Change (LUCC) provided by Resources and Environmental Sciences Data Center, Chinese Academy of Sciences (RESDC) [35]. The dataset reflects changes of land-use and land-cover in China every five years with a high spatio-resolution of 1 km, which is similar to that of MODIS fire products'. This data set has six classes, including cropland, forest, grassland, waters, urban and rural & industrial and residential areas, and unused land. The classification precision of this dataset for each region varies from 73% to 89%, and the overall accuracy of whole nation is up to 81% [36]. In this study, for more reliable extraction of crop residue burning spots, we used the LUCC data in year 2010 and year 2015 (Figure 3b) to generate cropland-masks on study area. Here, the extracted fire spots in year 2013 and 2014 corresponded to cropland-mask in 2010, and fire spots in other years corresponded to cropland-mask in 2015 (Figure 3c).

2.3. Methods

Firstly, due to a tremendous amount of pixels comprised, we conducted mosaic processes to compose complete remote sensing images of China. Meanwhile, we extracted "fire-mask" from Science Dataset for obtaining fire spots maps of the study area. Given the long research period and the large quantity of data, we employed batch processing using a specific tool named MODIS Reprojection Tool (MRT) provided by the Land Processes Distributed Active Archive Center. Secondly, in order to summarize overall fire spots in one day, a maximum value composite strategy was proposed and developed to count the number of daily fire spots [18]. The principle of this strategy is to set corresponding attribute values (7 means low-confidence fire spots, 8 means nominal-confidence fire spots, and 9 means high-confidence fire spots) to each pixel based on the maximum value in the daily four observations. In the process of composite, if fire spots detected in the same pixel were recorded several times for a day, we only counted them as one spot to avoid repeat counting. Clouds and haze had significant influences on the detection of fire spots. Since the same area was rarely covered by clouds in the four observations per day, this strategy reduced the occlusion effects and guaranteed the accuracy of fire spots detection. Thirdly, we employed LUCC dataset for extracting crop residue burning spots from the preprocessed data. Cropland-masks were selected from the dataset and combined with corresponding fire spots maps, then daily fire pixels located in croplands (daily crop residue burning spots) were extracted. On the other hand, hourly $PM_{2.5}$ and PM_{10} concentration data were collated into a daily format and the city-level observation data were also recalculated into a regional scale. Finally, we employed statistical and Spearman's rank correlation analysis to examine the correlation between crop residue burning and PM pollution for each region at different temporal scales.

3. Results

To better understand the following study, the spatial distribution of crop residue burning and PM concentrations in the different regions of China was shown in Figure 4.

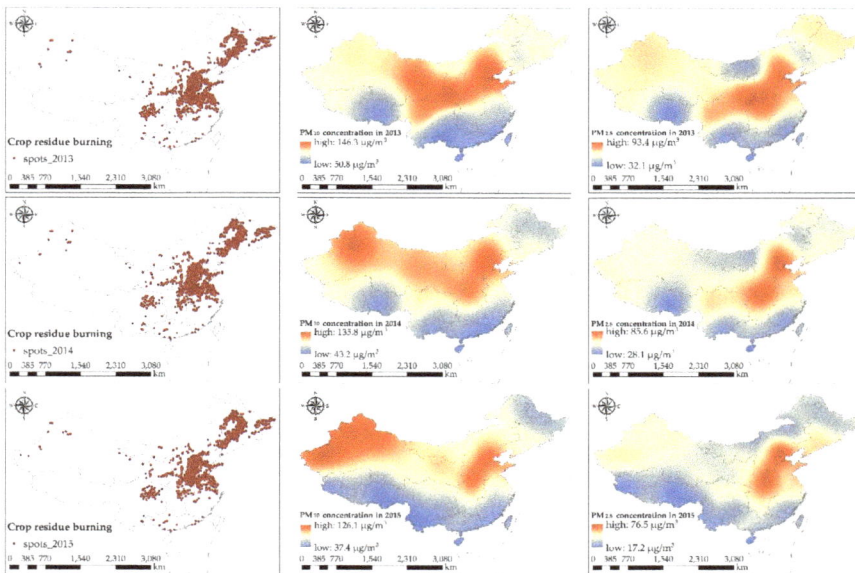

Figure 4. *Cont.*

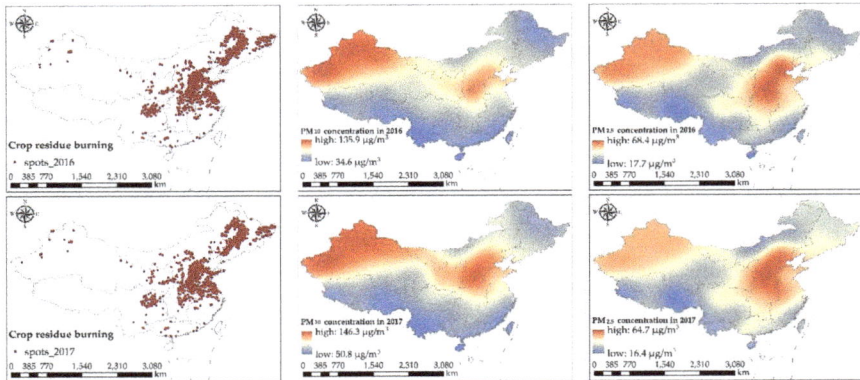

Figure 4. The spatial distribution of crop residue burning and particulate matter (PM) concentrations in the different regions of China. The left column shows the spatial distribution of crop residue burning spots in mainland China. The middle and right columns show the spatial distribution of PM_{10} concentration and $PM_{2.5}$ concentration, respectively, in China by interpolating.

3.1. The 5-Years' Variations and Characteristics of $PM_{2.5}$ and PM_{10} in China from a Regional Perspective

3.1.1. Interannual Variations and Characteristics

According to Figure 5, one can see a remarkable downtrend of PM concentrations in all of these seven regions from 2013 to 2017. Specially, during the first three years, PM concentrations in each region decreased dramatically. Afterwards, the decline rate decreased and such regions as SC even demonstrated a slight rise of PM concentrations in 2017. Different from variations of $PM_{2.5}$ concentrations, PM_{10} concentrations from 2016 to 2017 presented a slight upward trend in most regions. The peak value of $PM_{2.5}$ concentrations usually appears in CC and NC. The region with highest PM_{10} concentration is NWC. Similarly, a clear decline of $PM_{2.5}$ concentrations and PM_{10} concentrations was witnessed in CC and NWC, respectively. The decrease of PM concentrations in NEC was relatively higher than that of other regions. Furthermore, we analyzed the $PM_{2.5}/PM_{10}$ ratio, which could reveal different characteristics and origins of particle pollution [36]. A higher ratio usually indicated that PM pollution was caused by anthropogenic activities, while a lower ratio demonstrated that natural factors were the main contribution source of PM pollution [37]. According to Figure 6, the $PM_{2.5}/PM_{10}$ ratio in each region all dropped to a much lower level with small fluctuations that occasionally arose during 5-year period. Meanwhile, the most obvious decline of $PM_{2.5}/PM_{10}$ ratio was shown in CC (from 0.85 in 2013 to 0.63 in 2017) and the lowest ratio appeared in NWC (average value is about 0.47) for each year.

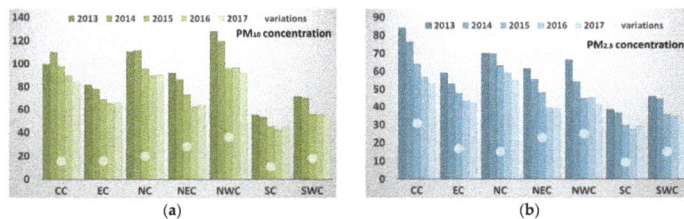

Figure 5. The overall variations of PM_{10} (a) and $PM_{2.5}$ (b) concentrations in different regions of China from 2013 to 2017. The histogram represents mean PM concentration ($\mu g/m^3$) and the circle refers to the difference between the annual mean PM concentration in 2017 and that in 2013.

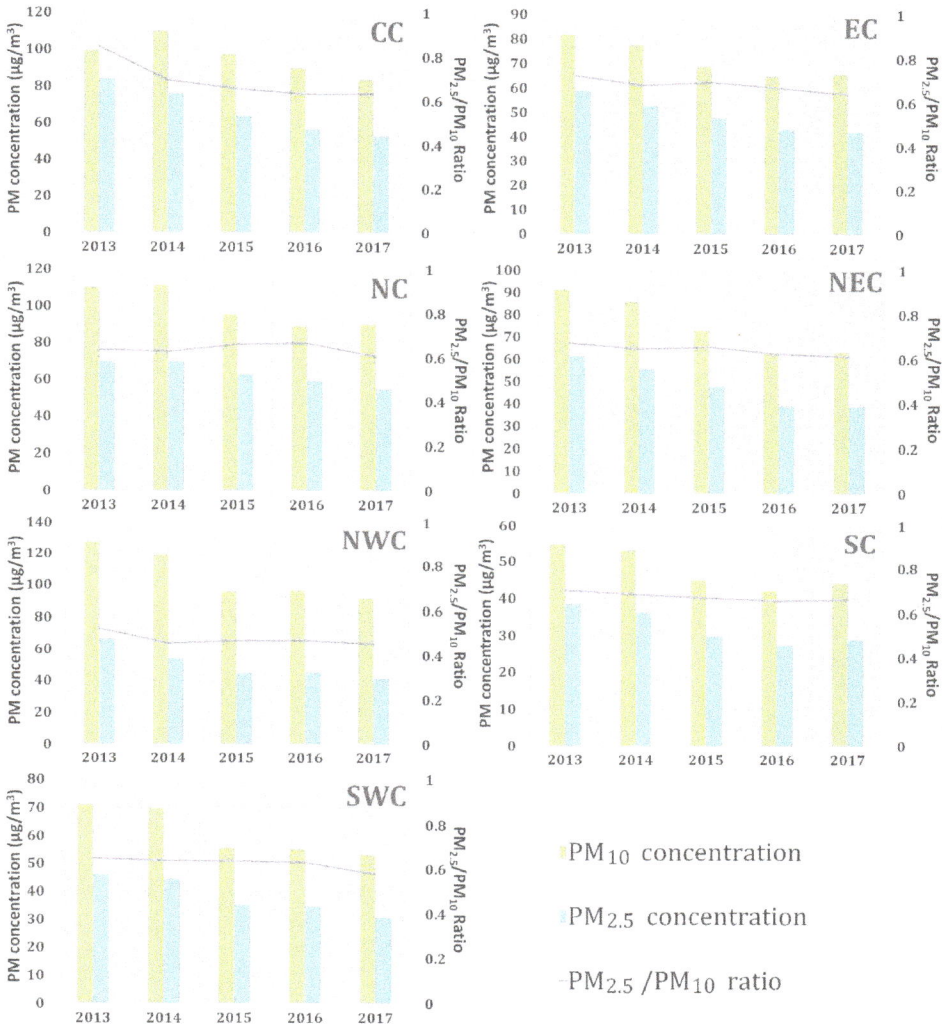

Figure 6. The 5-year variations of $PM_{2.5}/PM_{10}$ Ratio and Difference Value (PM_{10}–$PM_{2.5}$) in each region of study area.

3.1.2. Seasonal Variations and Characteristics

For better understanding seasonal variations and characteristics of $PM_{2.5}$ and PM_{10} concentrations, we divided twelve months into four seasons as follows: Spring (March, April, May), summer (June, July, August), autumn (September, October, November), and winter (December, January, February). As can be seen from Figure 7, the seasonal variation of PM_{10} concentrations in the same region is similar to that of $PM_{2.5}$ concentrations, whereas seasonal characteristics and variations of these two PM concentrations vary significantly across regions. Besides, concentrations of PM_{10} and $PM_{2.5}$ in each region both demonstrated a generally decreasing tendency in each season, despite some obvious concentration-growth in such years as 2014 and 2016.

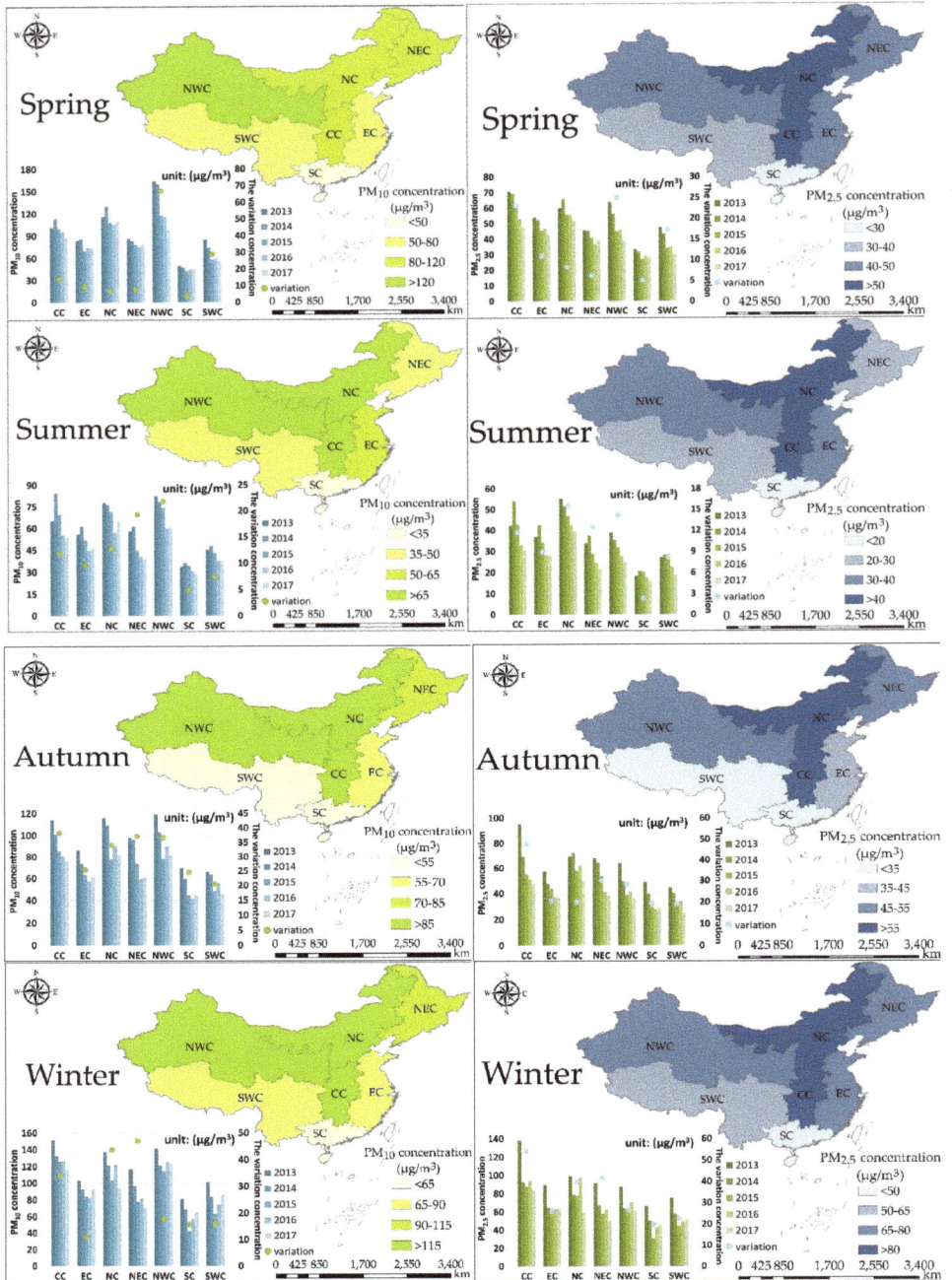

Figure 7. The characteristics and variations of PM$_{10}$ and PM$_{2.5}$ concentrations in different regions of China from seasonal and interannual perspectives.

Regarding characteristics of PM_{10} concentrations in different regions, the highest value always appeared in NWC and the lowest concentration of PM_{10} was usually observed in SC. In addition, throughout a whole year, the average PM_{10} concentration of NC always maintained a much higher level than that of other regions'. For CC and NEC, the PM_{10} pollution usually deteriorated in autumn and winter. Moreover, from a temporal perspective, the maxima of PM_{10} concentrations in each region appeared in winter, and the minima appeared in summer. In spring, PM_{10} concentrations evidently decreased in NWC and slightly decreased in other regions. For the decline of PM_{10} concentration in summer, the maximum change appeared in NWC, with NEC in the second place. In autumn, the declines from 2013 to 2015 were evident in all regions and increases appeared in northern and western China in 2016, when PM_{10} concentrations in CC, NEC, and NWC greatly reduced (40 $\mu g/m^3$ approximately) compared to the previous high concentration. For winter, the major decrease of PM_{10} concentrations was witnessed in NEC, NC, and CC.

Similar to PM_{10} concentrations, $PM_{2.5}$ concentrations in different regions were the lowest in summer and highest in winter. Spatially, the peak of $PM_{2.5}$ concentrations usually appeared in CC and NC, which was different from that of PM_{10} concentrations. Meanwhile, the lowest $PM_{2.5}$ concentration showed in SC, which was similar to that of PM_{10} concentrations. For other regions, the $PM_{2.5}$ concentration of NEC always kept at a much higher level in spring, autumn, and winter. Although the $PM_{2.5}$ concentration of NWC was not the highest in these seven regions, it remained at a relatively high level throughout the year. The higher $PM_{2.5}$ concentration was also observed in EC in spring, summer, and winter. $PM_{2.5}$ concentration in SWC was lower than other regions except for SC. For spring, the notable decline of $PM_{2.5}$ concentrations was witnessed in NWC and CC, whilst the decrease in other regions was much smaller. For summer, the decline of $PM_{2.5}$ concentrations was very small in each region and the largest decrease of 16 $\mu g/m^3$ appeared in NC. Different from slight variations in spring and summer, $PM_{2.5}$ concentrations in autumn and winter decreased significantly in each region. Particularly, maximum changes were observed in CC (reduced about 50 $\mu g/m^3$) and NEC (reduced about 35 $\mu g/m^3$). Besides, for NC, the decreased-concentration in winter was much higher than that in autumn. Other seasonal-interannual variations of PM concentrations could be found in Figure 7.

3.2. The 5-Year Variations of Crop Residue Burning in China from Regional Perspective

3.2.1. Interannual Variations

According to Figure 8, the most serious region of crop residue burning was NEC, with an annual average number of crop residue burning spots up to 30,569 during the five years period. Meanwhile, throughout China the number of crop residue burning spots progressively reduced from east to west. Specifically, the decline of burning spots in NWC and EC was the most obvious without large fluctuations. The number of crop residue burning spots in CC decreased significantly in the past five years, whereas during the first three years, the number actually increased gradually until 2016, when a significant decrease showed up. The number of crop residue burning spots in NEC increased significantly from 2014 to 2015. Although the number dropped to a relatively low level in 2016, it rose in 2017 to three times of the number in 2013. Similarly, the number of crop residue burning spots in NC also increased generally, except for the decrease in 2014. Compared with the north of China, the number of crop residue burning spots distributed in SC and SWC were small and interannual variations of burning spots in these two regions were very slight.

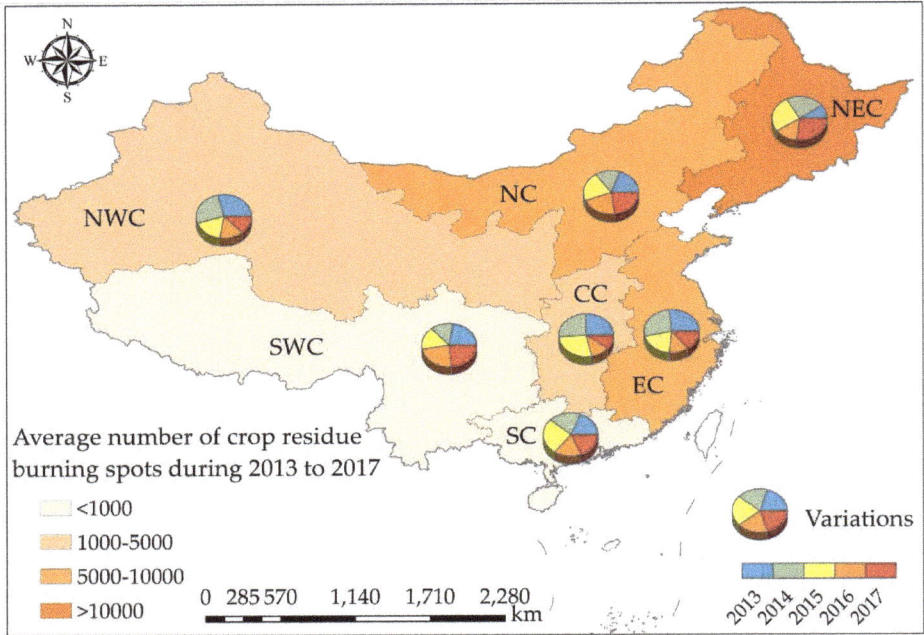

Figure 8. Interannual variations of crop residue burning spots in different regions of study area.

3.2.2. Seasonal Variations

According to Figure 9, we can see clear seasonal variations of crop residue burning spots for each region. Crop residue burning in CC usually took place in summer and autumn. During 2013 to 2017, the proportion of crop residue burning in spring increased gradually, and decreased notably in summer and autumn, whilst it demonstrated slight variations in winter. The variation of crop residue burning in EC were generally consistent with that in CC. For NC, crop residues were often burnt in summer and autumn. However, the proportion of crop residue burning spots in these two seasons decreased year by year, while the ratio in spring gradually increased to one third of the total amount. The number of crop residue burning spots were limitedly distributed in winter. As an agriculturally developed region, NEC experienced very intense crop residue burning, which mainly concentrated in spring and autumn. Meanwhile, the proportion of crop residue burning in autumn decreased from 67% in 2013 to 34% in 2017, and the proportion in spring increased from 27% in 2013 to 64% in 2017. For NWC, crop residue burning mainly took place in spring and autumn. A sudden increase appeared in the spring of 2014, whilst the proportion in autumn plummeted to 20%. Following this, crop residue burning in spring and autumn decreased dramatically, and gradually concentrated in summer. During this period, the proportion of crop residue burning in autumn decreased whilst the proportion in spring stabilized between 30% and 40%. Finally, crop residue burning spots in NWC presented similar proportion in spring, summer and winter in 2017. Unlike the northern part of China, crop residue burning in SC was usually observed in winter. Whereas, in recent years, proportions of crop residue burning in other seasons increased without clear pattern. Furthermore, crop residue burning of SWC usually concentrated in spring and summer. During this period, the proportion of crop residue burning increased in summer and decreased in spring.

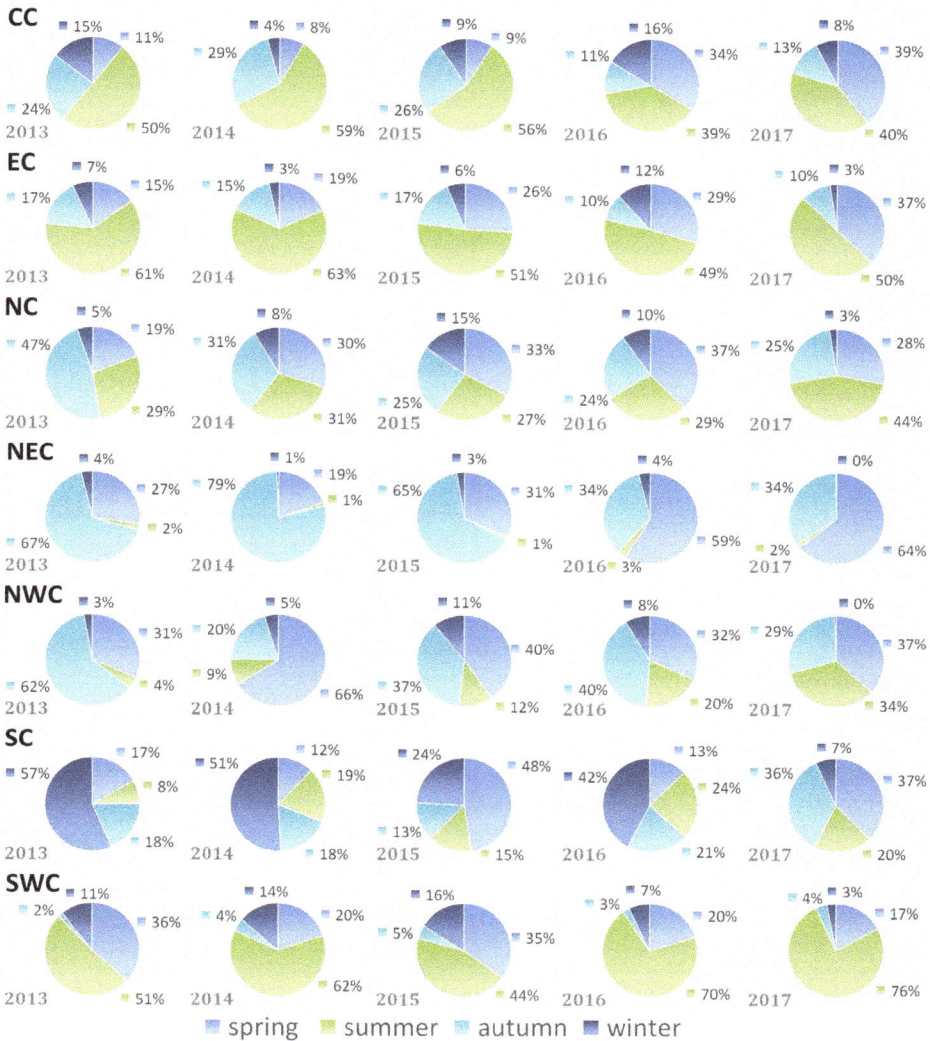

Figure 9. Seasonal variations of crop residue burning spots in different regions of study area.

3.3. The Correlation between PM Concentration and Crop Residue Burning at Different Temporal Scales

3.3.1. The Correlation between PM Concentrations and Crop Residue Burning at an Annual Scale

We employed Spearman's rank correlation for establishing the correlation between daily PM data and daily crop residue burning spots data. The result (Table 1) showed that the correlation between PM concentration and crop residue burning in NEC and SC were much stronger than that in other regions. According to Figure 10, variations were different in these two regions. In NEC, correlations between PM_{10} concentration and crop residue burning were generally upward with fluctuations, except for a notable decrease in 2015. The overall trend of the correlation between crop residue burning and $PM_{2.5}$ concentrations was similar, yet the significance of this correlation was much weaker. In SC, correlation coefficients between PM concentrations and crop residue burning generally decreased, except for a slight increase in 2015. In addition, a significant phenomenon was that the correlation between PM_{10} concentrations and crop residue burning was stronger than that between $PM_{2.5}$ concentrations and crop residue burning.

Table 1. The correlation between particulate matter (PM) concentrations and crop residue burning occurred in different regions of China during 2013 to 2017.

		CC	EC	NC	NEC	NWC	SC	SWC
Spearman	PM10	0.095 **	0.110 **	−0.011	0.218 **	−0.027	0.260 **	−0.019
	PM2.5	−0.015	0.002	−0.106 **	0.124 **	−0.134 **	0.228 **	−0.068 **

Note: ** $p < 0.01$.

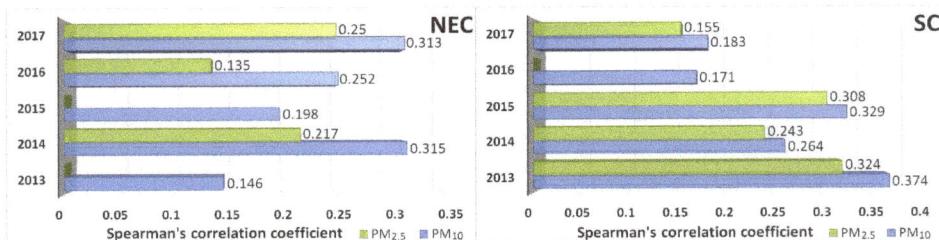

Figure 10. Interannual variations of correlation coefficient between PM concentrations and crop residue burning in Northeast China (NEC) and South China (SC).

3.3.2. The Correlation between PM Concentrations and Crop Residue Burning at a Seasonal Scale

We analyzed correlations between PM concentrations and crop residue burning for each region from a seasonal perspective. The results (in Figure 11 and Table 2) showed that correlations in autumn were significantly stronger for the north part of China, including CC, EC, and NEC. For SC, correlations were stronger throughout four seasons and the largest correlation coefficient appeared in winter. Correlations in SWC were relatively poor and only significant in spring and summer. The correlation coefficient in NEC was the strongest among seven regions and the strongest correlation usually appeared in spring and autumn, when crop residues were intensely burnt in NEC. For EC, the correlation between PM concentrations and crop residue burning was significant in four seasons and were much stronger in autumn and winter. Similar to annual analysis, PM_{10} concentrations were more strongly correlated with crop residue burning than $PM_{2.5}$ concentrations.

Table 2. The seasonal variation of correlation coefficients in different regions from 2013 to 2017.

		Spring	Summer	Autumn	Winter
CC	PM_{10}	0.063	0.214 **	0.426 **	0.148 **
	$PM_{2.5}$	−0.056	0.124 **	0.321 **	0.003
EC	PM_{10}	0.199 **	0.193 **	0.397 **	0.363 **
	$PM_{2.5}$	0.125 **	0.153 **	0.255 **	0.283 **
NC	PM_{10}	0.019	0.088	0.186 **	−0.159 **
	$PM_{2.5}$	0.035	−0.009	0.040	−0.239 **
NEC	PM_{10}	0.398 **	0.032	0.486 **	−0.132 **
	$PM_{2.5}$	0.435 **	−0.060	0.464 **	−0.158 **

Table 2. *Cont.*

		Spring	Summer	Autumn	Winter
NWC	PM_{10}	−0.106 *	−0.013	0.139 **	0.186 **
	$PM_{2.5}$	−0.151 **	−0.114 *	0.087	0.007
SC	PM_{10}	0.236 **	0.187 **	0.214 **	0.418 **
	$PM_{2.5}$	0.177 **	0.180 **	0.194 **	0.391 **
SWC	PM_{10}	0.179 **	0.130 **	0.068	0.042
	$PM_{2.5}$	0.119 *	0.023	0.063	0.091

Note: * $p < 0.05$; ** $p < 0.01$.

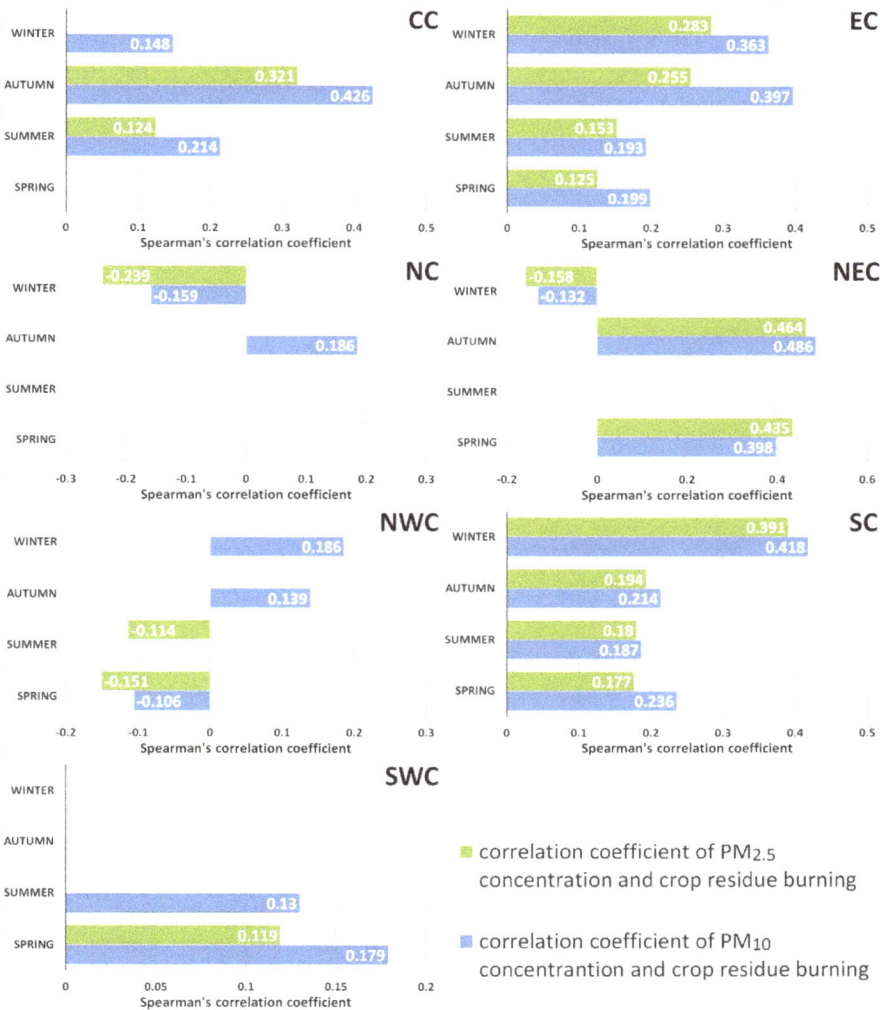

Figure 11. Seasonal variations of correlation coefficient between PM concentrations and crop residue burning among seven regions of China.

3.3.3. The Correlation between PM Concentrations and Crop Residue Burning in Burning-Concentrated Periods

With different time of crop ripening in each region, periods of crop residue burning are different accordingly. Therefore, in order to better analyze the change of PM concentrations when crop residues were intensely combusted, for each year, we selected a burning-concentrated period for each region during 2013–2017. The principle of selection was based on the appearance of peak months of crop residue burning spots and prior knowledge of agricultural production. In total, we acquired five periods for each region and analyzed the correlation between the number of crop residue burning spots during the burning-concentrated period and corresponding $PM_{2.5}$ concentrations. The results are shown in Table 3. Except for NC, correlations between PM concentrations and crop residue burning were significant in all regions. Generally, correlations in NC and SWC were the weakest, and correlations in NEC were the strongest. Meanwhile, the correlation between PM_{10} concentrations and crop residue burning was significantly stronger than that of $PM_{2.5}$ concentrations. This result indicated that the variation of PM_{10} concentrations was more sensitive to crop residue burning than that of $PM_{2.5}$ concentrations during the process of crop residue burning. Correlation between PM concentrations and crop residue burning increased significantly with the narrowing temporal scales and was the strongest during burning-concentrated periods, indicating that intense crop residue burning exerts a much stronger influence on the short-term than long-term variation of PM concentrations.

Table 3. The correlation between PM concentrations and crop residue burning occurred in different regions of China during burning-concentrated periods.

		CC	EC	NC	NEC	NWC	SC	SWC
Spearman	PM_{10}	0.362 **	0.444 **	0.236 **	0.491 **	0.347 **	0.436 **	0.234 **
	$PM_{2.5}$	0.335 **	0.404 **	0.044	0.446 **	0.407 **	0.400 **	0.169 *

Note: * $p < 0.05$; ** $p < 0.01$.

4. Discussion

4.1. The Attribution of Variations of PM_{10} and $PM_{2.5}$ Concentrations during 5-Year Period

In this study, we analyzed variations and characteristics of PM concentrations from interannual and seasonal perspectives. Meanwhile, we selected some crop residue burning-concentrated periods to explore variations of PM concentrations during the burning processes. Generally, concentrations of PM_{10} and $PM_{2.5}$ have decreased notably since 2013. Besides, $PM_{2.5}/PM_{10}$ ratios also declined during the 5-year period which indicates that the composition of PM_{10} occupied by $PM_{2.5}$ is decreasing. Meanwhile, some studies have shown that the high $PM_{2.5}/PM_{10}$ ratio can be attributed to human activities, while the lower ratio is related to natural factors [37,38]. In other words, $PM_{2.5}$ pollution has been mitigated significantly, due to a series of emission-reduction measures. Firstly, in autumn and winter, the variation of PM concentrations in northern China can be attributed to the control of crop residue burning, traffic exhaust, and coal combustion for large-scale central heating [39]. Secondly, with the implementation of Red and Orange alert measures for reducing PM pollution, $PM_{2.5}$ concentrations have decreased remarkably [40]. Thirdly, as a result of traffic control, the exhaust-emission of vehicles has been cut down dramatically and leads to the reduction of PM concentrations [41]. Fourthly, some environmental-meteorological projects have been implemented to address PM pollution issues [42]. In burning-concentrated periods, the variation trend of PM concentrations is consistent with that of crop residue burning in all regions, indicating intensive crop residue burning leads to instant deterioration of PM concentrations. Hence, more strict and effective policies should be proposed and implemented to encourage more efficient utility of crop residues and reduce large scale and intensive crop residue burning.

4.2. The Attribution of Correlations between PM Concentration and Crop Residue Burning

The correlation between PM concentrations and crop residue burning was discussed in this paper. Firstly, it is found that the correlation between PM concentrations and crop residue burning is significant and strong, especially in burning-concentrated periods, which is consistent with findings from previous studies [43]. Awasthi et al. (2010) found PM_{10}, $PM_{2.5}$, $PM_{10-2.5}$ concentrations increased significantly during crop residue burning in India. Strong correlation between crop residue burning and PM concentrations was observed. Different from this research, Awasthi et al. (2010) found that the $PM_{2.5}$ concentration was more sensitive to crop residue burning than PM_{10} concentrations. This difference may result from pollution level and meteorological diffusion conditions in India. However, our finding about the very strong correlation between crop residue burning and PM concentrations during the intensive crop residue burning period in all regions across China proved that, despite other influencing factors such as emission sources and meteorological factors, intensive and large-scale crop residue burning could be a dominant emission sources for PM pollution across China. Secondly, correlations between different particulate matters and crop residue burning are distinct. PM_{10} concentrations are much strongly correlated with crop residue burning than $PM_{2.5}$ concentrations, indicating crop residue burning in China may produce more PM_{10} than $PM_{2.5}$. From a temporal perspective, crop residue burning in autumn usually presents a higher correlation with PM concentration, which is consistent with the findings from Yin et al. Whereas, different from this research, Yin et al.'s research [23] mainly introduced the temporal variation of both crop residue burning and $PM_{2.5}$ concentrations in China and did not discuss the correlation from different temporal scales. From a spatial perspective, the correlation in NEC is the strongest among the seven regions, especially in spring and autumn, suggesting that the PM concentration is closely related to crop residue burning in the burning-concentrated periods. This phenomenon was consistent with findings from previous studies suggesting that crop residue burning is related to $PM_{2.5}$ concentration [23,24]. The main reason for the poor correlation in NC is that the source of PM is high exhaust-emission of vehicles and industrial production, instead of crop residue burning [41]. For NWC, petroleum exploitation is also an important contributor to PM pollution [44], which may be the reason why PM_{10} demonstrates a weaker correlation with crop residue burning than $PM_{2.5}$. To sum up, the burning of crop residues has a great contribution to PM pollution, though the relative contribution of crop residue burning to PM concentrations, compared with other emission sources, including industry and traffic exhaust, should be further investigated.

4.3. Limitations and Prospect

Although the paper comprehensively examined correlations between PM concentration and crop residue burning, some limitations remain. Firstly, due to the fact that crop residue burning usually lasts for a short period, the correlation analysis should be more reliable if it is conducted based on a finer temporal resolution, such as hourly. Thus, considering the finer temporal resolution of Himawari-8, it is a better choice to extract fire spots on the hourly scale. Secondly, due to the limited spatial resolution of MODIS data, some actual burning spots may be lost in the process of fire spots extraction and statistics. That means remote sensing data with higher temporal resolution are required for extracting fine-scale crop reside burning spots. Furthermore, due to complicated interactions between PM and meteorological factors, commonly used correlation analysis may be biased significantly. To reduce the influence from other factors and better investigate the influence of crop residue burning on PM concentrations, advanced causality methods, such as cross convergent mapping (CCM) [45] and chemical transport models (CTM), such as WRF-CAMx [46], should be employed in future studies. Whereas, the difficulty for examining the causality of crop residue burning on PM concentration without other influencing factors, using above models lies in the short time series of the concentrated crop residue burning periods. Meanwhile, the MODIS data extracted crop residue burning spots are mainly based on a daily scale and thus the time series of intensive crop residue burning is limited to less than 30 numbers, not sufficient for a robust CCM or CTM analysis.

Therefore, to implement CCM or CTM analysis, fire spots should be extracted using remote sensing data with a much higher temporal resolution, such as Himawari 8 with 10-min temporal resolution. In the future, with growing availability and accuracy of Himawari data sources, it is possible to conduct robust causality analysis based on CCM or CTM using long time series data of crop residue burning and PM pollution. In this case, the influence of crop residue burning on PM concentrations can be better extracted by filtering the biases of other influencing factors.

5. Conclusions

This paper analyzed interannual and seasonal variations of PM_{10} and $PM_{2.5}$ concentrations and simultaneous variations of crop residue burning in several regions across China. The results showed that the PM concentration was in a downward trend from interannual and seasonal perspectives and $PM_{2.5}/PM_{10}$ ratios in different regions decreased gradually. The peak value of PM_{10} concentrations usually appeared in NWC and winter whilst the peak value of $PM_{2.5}$ concentrations appeared in NC and CC. Temporal variations of $PM_{2.5}$ are similar to that of PM_{10} concentrations. For the number of crop residue burning spots in China, it remained a downward tendency during the 5-year period in most regions, except for an evident increase in NEC in 2017. Furthermore, we analyzed correlations between PM concentration and crop residue burning and explored at different temporal scales. The variation of PM_{10} concentration was more sensitive to crop residue burning than that of $PM_{2.5}$ concentrations and the strongest correlation between PM concentrations and crop residue burning appears in NEC. Correlation between PM concentrations and crop residue burning increased significantly with the narrowing temporal scales and was the strongest during burning-concentrated periods, indicating that intense crop residue burning exert a much stronger influence on the short-term than long-term variation of PM concentrations. The methodology and conclusions from this study provide useful reference for better understanding the influence of crop residue burning on PM concentrations at different scales and suggest that intensive crop residue burning leads to instant increases of PM concentrations. Given the major contribution of crop residue burning to PM pollution, more strict and effective policies should be proposed and implemented to encourage more efficient utility of crop residues and reduce large scale and intensive crop residue burning.

Author Contributions: Conceptualization, Z.C.; Data curation, J.C.; Formal analysis, Y.Z.; Methodology, R.L. and J.C.; Visualization, Y.Z., D.C. and R.L.; Writing—original draft, Y.Z.; Writing—review & editing, Z.C., B.H., B.G., N.C. and Y.H.

Funding: This research was funded by the National Natural Science Foundation of China (grant No. 210100066), State Key Laboratory of Earth Surface Processes and Resource Ecology (2017-KF-22), the Fundamental Research Funds for the Central Universities, Ministry of Environmental Protection (201409005), and the Beijing Training Support Project for Excellent Scholars (2015000020124G059).

Acknowledgments: This research is supported by the National Natural Science Foundation of China (grant No. 210100066), State Key Laboratory of Earth Surface Processes and Resource Ecology (2017-KF-22), the Fundamental Research Funds for the Central Universities, Ministry of Environmental Protection (201409005), and the Beijing Training Support Project for Excellent Scholars (2015000020124G059).

Conflicts of Interest: The authors declare no conflicts of interest.

References

1. Song, C.B.; He, J.J.; Wu, L.; Jin, T.S.; Chen, X.; Li, R.P.; Ren, P.P.; Zhang, L.; Mao, H.J. Health burden attributable to ambient $PM_{2.5}$ in China. *Environ. Pollut.* **2017**, *223*, 575–586. [CrossRef] [PubMed]
2. Zheng, S.; Pozzer, A.; Cao, C.X.; Lelieveld, J. Long-term (2001–2012) concentrations of fine particulate matter (PM2.5) and the impact on human health in Beijing, China. *Atmos. Chem. Phys.* **2015**, *15*, 5715–5725. [CrossRef]
3. Xing, Y.F.; Xu, Y.H.; Shi, M.H.; Lian, Y.X. The impact of PM2.5 on the human respiratory system. *J. Thorac. Dis.* **2016**, *8*, E69–E74. [CrossRef] [PubMed]
4. Wang, Y.G.; Ying, Q.; Hu, J.L.; Zhang, H.L. Spatial and temporal variations of six criteria air pollutants in 31 provincial capital cities in China during 2013–2014. *Environ. Int.* **2014**, *73*, 413–422. [CrossRef] [PubMed]

5. Zhao, H.J.; Che, H.Z.; Ma, Y.J.; Wang, Y.F.; Yang, H.B.; Liu, Y.C.; Wang, Y.Q.; Wang, H.; Zhang, X.Y. The Relationship of PM Variation with Visibility and Mixing-Layer Height under Hazy/Foggy Conditions in the Multi-Cities of Northeast China. *Int. J. Environ. Res. Public Health* **2017**, *14*, 471. [CrossRef] [PubMed]

6. An, Z.; Jin, Y.F.; Li, J.; Li, W.; Wu, W.D. Impact of Particulate Air Pollution on Cardiovascular Health. *Curr. Allergy Asthma Rep.* **2018**, *18*, 15–22. [CrossRef] [PubMed]

7. Pun, V.C.; Manjourides, J.; Suh, H. Association of Ambient Air Pollution with Depressive and Anxiety Symptoms in Older Adults: Results from the NSHAP Study. *Environ. Health Perspect.* **2017**, *125*, 342–348. [CrossRef] [PubMed]

8. Mariania, J.; Faveroa, C.; Spinazzèc, A.; Cavalloc, D.M.; Carugnoa, M.; Mottaa, V.; Bonzinia, M.; Cattaneoc, A.; Pesatoria, A.C.; Bollati, V. Short-term particulate matter exposure influences nasal microbiota in a population of healthy subjects. *Environ. Res.* **2018**, *162*, 119–126. [CrossRef] [PubMed]

9. Chen, G.B.; Guo, Y.M.; Abramson, M.J.; Williams, G.; Li, S.S. Exposure to low concentrations of air pollutants and adverse birth outcomes in Brisbane, Australia, 2003–2013. *Sci. Total Environ.* **2018**, *622*, 721–726. [CrossRef] [PubMed]

10. Shang, Y.; Sun, Z.W.; Cao, J.J.; Wang, X.M.; Zhong, L.J.; Bi, X.H.; Li, H.; Liu, W.X.; Zhu, T.; Huang, W. Systematic review of Chinese studies of short-term exposure to air pollution and daily mortality. *Environ. Int.* **2013**, *54*, 100–111. [CrossRef] [PubMed]

11. Huang, F.F.; Pan, B.; Wu, J.; Chen, E.G.; Chen, L.Y. Relationship between exposure to PM2.5 and lung cancer incidence and mortality: A meta-analysis. *Oncotarget* **2017**, *8*, 43322–43331. [CrossRef] [PubMed]

12. Cao, S.S.; Zhao, W.J.; Guan, H.L.; Hu, D.Y.; Mo, Y.; Zhao, W.H.; Li, S.S. Comparison of remotely sensed PM2.5 concentrations between developed and developing countries: Results from the US, Europe, China, and India. *J. Clean. Prod.* **2018**, *182*, 672–681. [CrossRef]

13. Tian, G.J.; Qiao, Z.; Xu, X.L. Characteristics of particulate matter (PM10) and its relationship with meteorological factors during 2001–2012 in Beijing. *Environ. Pollut.* **2014**, *192*, 266–274. [CrossRef] [PubMed]

14. Chen, Z.; Xie, X.M.; Cai, J.; Chen, D.L.; Gao, B.B.; He, B.; Cheng, N.L.; Xu, B. Understanding meteorological influences on PM2.5 concentrations across China: A temporal and spatial perspective. *Atmos. Chem. Phys.* **2018**, *18*, 5343–5358. [CrossRef]

15. Lee, J.; Kim, K.Y. Analysis of source regions and meteorological factors for the variability of spring PM10 concentrations in Seoul, Korea. *Atmos. Environ.* **2018**, *175*, 199–209. [CrossRef]

16. Zhao, Y.B.; Gao, P.P.; Yang, W.D.; Ni, H.G. Vehicle exhaust: An overstated cause of haze in China. *Sci. Total Environ.* **2018**, *612*, 490–491. [CrossRef] [PubMed]

17. Chen, J.M.; Li, C.L.; Ristovski, Z.; Milic, A.; Gu, Y.; Islam, M.S.; Wang, S.; Hao, J.; Zhang, H.; He, C.; et al. A review of biomass burning: Emissions and impacts on air quality, health and climate in China. *Sci. Total Environ.* **2017**, *579*, 1000–1034. [CrossRef] [PubMed]

18. Zhuang, Y.; Li, R.Y.; Yang, H.; Chen, D.L.; Chen, Z.Y.; Gao, B.B.; He, B. Understanding Temporal and Spatial Distribution of Crop Residue Burning in China from 2003 to 2017 Using MODIS Data. *Remote Sens.* **2018**, *10*, 390. [CrossRef]

19. Department of Environmental Protection of Heilongjiang Province. Heavy Straw. Available online: http://www.hljdep.gov.cn/xwzx/hjyw/2016/04/12292.html (accessed on 1 April 2016).

20. Chen, W.W.; Tong, D.Q.; Zhang, S.C.; Zhang, X.L.; Zhao, H.M. Local PM10 and PM2.5 emission inventories from agricultural tillage and harvest in northeastern China. *J. Environ. Sci.* **2017**, *57*, 15–23. [CrossRef] [PubMed]

21. Hodnebrog, Ø.; Myhre1, G.; Forster, P.M.; Sillmann, J.; Samset, B.H. Local biomass burning is a dominant cause of the observed precipitation reduction in southern Africa. *Nat. Commun.* **2016**, *7*, 11236. [CrossRef] [PubMed]

22. Zhang, B.E.; Jiao, L.M.; Xu, G.; Zhao, S.L.; Tang, X.; Zhou, Y.; Gong, C. Influences of wind and precipitation on different-sized particulate matter concentrations (PM2.5, PM10, PM2.5–10). *Meteorol. Atmos. Phys.* **2018**, *130*, 383–392. [CrossRef]

23. Yin, S.; Wang, X.F.; Xiao, Y.; Tani, H.; Zhong, G.S.; Sun, Z.Y. Study on spatial distribution of crop residue burning and PM$_{2.5}$ change in China. *Environ. Pollut.* **2017**, *220*, 204–221. [CrossRef] [PubMed]

24. Chen, Z.Y.; Chen, D.L.; Zhuang, Y.; Cai, J.; Zhao, N.; He, B.; Gao, B.B.; Xu, B. Examining the Influence of Crop Residue Burning on Local PM$_{2.5}$ Concentrations in Heilongjiang Province Using Ground Observation and Remote Sensing Data. *Remote Sens.* **2017**, *9*, 971. [CrossRef]

25. Awasthi, A.; Singh, N.; Mittal, S.; Gupta, P.K.; Agarwal, R. Effects of agriculture crop residue burning on children and young on PFTs in North West India. *Sci. Total Environ.* **2010**, *408*, 4440–4445. [CrossRef] [PubMed]

26. Huang, X.; Li, M.M.; Li, J.F.; Song, Y. A high-resolution emission inventory of crop burning in fields in China based on MODIS Thermal Anomalies/Fire products. *Atmos. Environ.* **2012**, *50*, 9–15. [CrossRef]

27. Zhang, H.F.; Hu, J.; Qi, Y.X.; Li, C.L.; Chen, J.M.; Wang, X.M.; He, J.W.; Wang, S.X.; Hao, J.M.; Zhang, L.L.; et al. Emission characterization, environmental impact, and control measure of $PM_{2.5}$ emitted from agricultural crop residue burning in China. *J. Clean. Prod.* **2017**, *149*, 629–635. [CrossRef]

28. Yang, S.J.; He, H.P.; Lu, S.L.; Chen, D.; Zhu, J.X. Quantification of crop residue burning in the field and its influence on ambient air quality in Suqian, China. *Atmos. Environ.* **2008**, *42*, 1961–1969. [CrossRef]

29. Qiu, X.H.; Duan, L.; Chai, F.; Wang, S.X.; Yu, Q.; Wang, S.L. Deriving High-Resolution Emission Inventory of Open Biomass Burning in China based on Satellite Observations. *Environ. Sci. Technol.* **2016**, *50*, 11779–11786. [CrossRef] [PubMed]

30. PM25.in. Available online: http://pm25.in/about (accessed on 20 May 2018).

31. Justice, C.; Giglio, L.; Boschetti, L.; Roy, D.; Csiszar, I.; Morisette, J.; Kaufman, Y. Algorithm Technical Background Document MODIS FIRE PRODUCTS. MODIS Science Team: Washington, DC, USA. Available online: ftp://ladsweb.nascom.nasa.gov (accessed on 10 October 2017).

32. Giglio, L. *MODIS Collection 6 Active Fire Product User's Guide*; Revision, A., Ed.; Department of Geographical Sciences, University of Maryland: College Park, MD, USA, 2015.

33. LAADS DACC ftp Server. Available online: ftp://ladsweb.nascom.nasa.gov (accessed on 10 October 2017).

34. Dozier, J. A Method for Satellite Identification of Surface Temperature Fields of Subpixel Resolution. *Remote Sens. Environ.* **1981**, *11*, 221–229. [CrossRef]

35. Resources and Environmental Sciences, Chinese Academy of Sciences. Data Center. Land-Use and Land-Cover Change. Available online: http://www.resdc.cn (accessed on 10 October 2017).

36. Liu, J.Y.; Liu, M.L.; Deng, X.Z.; Zhuang, D.F.; Zhang, Z.X.; Luo, D. The land use and land cover change database and its relative studies in China. *J. Geogr. Sci.* **2002**, *12*, 275–282. [CrossRef]

37. Xu, G.; Jiao, L.M.; Zhang, B.E.; Zhao, S.L.; Yuan, M.; Gu, Y.Y.; Liu, J.F.; Tang, X. Spatial and Temporal Variability of the $PM_{2.5}/PM_{10}$ Ratio in Wuhan, Central China. *Aerosol. Air Qual. Res.* **2017**, *17*, 741–751. [CrossRef]

38. Sugimoto, N.; Shimizu, A.; Matsui, I.; Nishikawa, M. A method for estimating the fraction of mineral dust in particulate matter using $PM_{2.5}$-to-PM_{10} ratios. *Particuology* **2016**, *28*, 114–120. [CrossRef]

39. Zheng, M.; Yan, C.Q.; Wang, S.X.; He, K.B.; Zhang, Y.H. Understanding $PM_{2.5}$ sources in China: Challenges and perspectives. *Natl. Sci. Rev.* **2017**, *4*, 801–803. [CrossRef]

40. Cheng, N.L.; Zhang, D.W.; Li, Y.T.; Xie, X.M.; Chen, Z.Y.; Meng, F.; Gao, B.B.; He, B. Spatio-temporal variations of $PM_{2.5}$ concentrations and the evaluation of emission reduction measures during two red air pollution alerts in Beijing. *Sci. Rep.* **2017**, *7*, 8220–8232. [CrossRef] [PubMed]

41. Wu, Y.; Zhang, S.J.; Hao, J.M.; Liu, H.; Wu, X.M.; Hu, J.N.; Walsh, M.P.; Wallington, T.J.; Zhang, K.M.; Stevanovic, S. On-road vehicle emissions and their control in China: A review and outlook. *Sci. Total Environ.* **2017**, *574*, 332–349. [CrossRef] [PubMed]

42. Beijing Plans Ventilation Corridors to Blow Away Smog. Available online: http://en.people.cn/n3/2016/0221/c90882-9019126.html (accessed on 21 February 2016).

43. Awasthi, A.; Agarwal, R.; Mittal, S.K.; Singh, N.; Singh, K.; Guptab, P.K. Study of size and mass distribution of particulate matter due to crop residue burning with seasonal variation in rural area of Punjab, India. *J. Environ. Monit.* **2011**, *13*, 1073–1081. [CrossRef] [PubMed]

44. Zhou, X.; Zhang, T.J.; Li, Z.Q.; Tao, Y.; Wang, F.T.; Zhang, X.; Xu, C.H.; Ma, S.; Huang, J. Particulate and gaseous pollutants in a petrochemical industrialized valley city, Western China during 2013–2016. *Environ. Sci. Pollut. Res.* **2018**, *25*, 15174–15190. [CrossRef] [PubMed]

45. Chen, Z.Y.; Cai, J.; Gao, B.B.; Xu, B.; Dai, S.; He, B.; Xie, X.M. Detecting the causality influence of individual meteorological factors on local PM2.5 concentration in the Jing-Jin-Ji region. *Sci. Rep.* **2017**, *7*, 40735–40746. [CrossRef] [PubMed]

46. Xu, J.M.; Chang, L.Y.; Qu, Y.H.; Yan, F.X.; Wang, F.Y.; Fu, Q.Y. The meteorological modulation on PM2.5 interannual oscillation during 2013 to 2015 in Shanghai, China. *Sci. Total Environ.* **2016**, *572*, 1138–1149. [CrossRef] [PubMed]

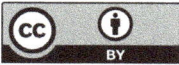

International Journal of
Environmental Research and Public Health

MDPI

Communication

The Neighborhood Effect Averaging Problem (NEAP): An Elusive Confounder of the Neighborhood Effect

Mei-Po Kwan

Department of Geography and Geographic Information Science, Natural History Building, 1301 W Green Street, University of Illinois at Urbana-Champaign, Urbana, IL 61801, USA; mpk654@gmail.com

Received: 30 July 2018; Accepted: 23 August 2018; Published: 27 August 2018

Abstract: Ignoring people's daily mobility and exposures to nonresidential contexts may lead to erroneous results in epidemiological studies of people's exposures to and the health impact of environmental factors. This paper identifies and describes a phenomenon called neighborhood effect averaging, which may significantly confound the neighborhood effect as a result of such neglect when examining the health impact of mobility-dependent exposures (e.g., air pollution). Several recent studies that provide strong evidence for the neighborhood effect averaging problem (NEAP) are discussed. The paper concludes that, due to the observed attenuation of the neighborhood effect associated with people's daily mobility, increasing the mobility of those who live in disadvantaged neighborhoods may be helpful for improving their health outcomes.

Keywords: the neighborhood effect averaging problem (NEAP); human mobility; environmental exposure; the uncertain geographic context problem; UGCoP

The neighborhood effect is a central analytic notion in epidemiological studies for assessing people's exposures to and the health impact of environmental factors. Past studies have largely used the residential neighborhood, often operationalized as static administrative areas such as the home census tract, as the contextual area to examine people's environmental exposures. For health behaviors or outcomes that are heavily influenced by environmental factors in a person's residential neighborhood or the areas nearby (e.g., social capital and collective efficacy at the neighborhood level), this approach may be adequate. However, using this residence-based approach may lead to erroneous results for health outcomes that are also influenced by exposures to environmental factors in neighborhoods other than the residential neighborhood (e.g., air pollution) because most people move around to undertake their daily activities and come under the influence of many different neighborhood contexts outside their home neighborhoods [1–4].

As recent studies have shown, ignoring people's daily mobility and exposures to nonresidential contexts may lead to erroneous results. For instance, Park and Kwan [5] compared individual air pollution exposures in Los Angeles (CA, USA) using four combinations of spatial and temporal attributes: residence-based hourly levels, residence-based daily levels, mobility-based hourly levels, and mobility-based daily levels (where an hourly exposure level was estimated using cokriging for each of the 24 h of a day while the daily level was the average of these 24 hourly exposure levels for the day). The results indicated that these four exposure estimates are significantly different, suggesting that individual exposures may be under- or over-estimated if human mobility and the spatiotemporal variability of air pollution levels are not taken into account. The study argued that ignoring human mobility may lead to misleading results in air pollution studies. Another study in Israel by Shafran-Nathan et al. [6] observed that differences between home-based and work-based exposures to nitrogen oxides are considerable for over 50% of the subjects, and it is equally likely that a subject's residence-based exposure is either higher or lower than the mobility-based exposure (which takes into account a subject's work/school location). The study concluded that estimating air pollution exposures at subjects' home location may under- or overestimate exposures when compared to exposure estimates that take their daily mobility into account.

Several recent studies not only provide evidence on how ignoring daily human mobility may lead to misleading results in exposure and health impact assessments but also highlight a specific reason that contributes to estimation errors [6–8]. This phenomenon may be called neighborhood effect averaging, which operates as follows.

Given that most people move around to undertake their daily activities (e.g., shop, attend school, or go to work), they are exposed to the environmental contexts of many different areas outside their residential neighborhoods in the course of a day. As a person travels to areas outside of his or her residential neighborhood, the person may experience similar or different levels of exposure when compared to that of his or her residential neighborhood. Because of the diversity in the intensity of the environmental factor in question (e.g., air pollution) over space in any study area, a person's exposure level in nonresidential neighborhoods may be higher, lower, or similar when compared to the exposure level experienced in his or her residential neighborhood. As indicated by recent studies, the probability distribution of individual residence-based exposure approximates a bell-shaped distribution, which means that many people have exposure levels around the mean value for the population of the study area, while fewer people have very high or low exposure levels [6–8]. Therefore, a person who lives in a neighborhood with a high level of an environmental factor (and thus exposure) will visit areas that are more likely to have lower levels of such environmental factor as a result of his or her daily mobility, while a person who lives in a neighborhood with a low level of the environmental factor will visit areas that are more likely to have higher levels of such environmental factor. For those who have residence-based exposure levels around the mean value, their exposure levels in nonresidential neighborhoods tend to be similar to those of their residential neighborhoods because they will visit areas that are less likely to have significantly different levels of such environmental factor in their daily life.

As a result, the neighborhood effect assessed with a traditional residence-based approach for individuals whose residence-based exposures are much higher than the mean exposure will be overestimated because these individuals tend to experience lower levels of exposure outside their residential neighborhoods, which attenuates their high exposures in their residential neighborhoods [7,8]. On the other hand, the neighborhood effect for individuals whose residence-based exposures are much lower than the mean exposure will be underestimated because these individuals tend to experience higher levels of exposure outside their residential neighborhoods, which moderates their low exposures in their residential neighborhoods [7,8].

Taking people's daily mobility into account (which will generate more accurate assessments for mobility-dependent exposures) will therefore lead to an overall tendency toward the mean exposure because exposure levels for people whose residence-based exposures are lower or higher than the mean exposure will tend toward the mean exposure, thus moderating the influence of the environmental factor in their residential neighborhoods on their health behaviors or outcomes. This is neighborhood effect averaging. It means that for health outcomes that are also affected by exposures to environmental factors in people's nonresidential neighborhoods as they move around in their daily life (mobility-dependent exposures), using residence-based neighborhoods to estimate individual exposures to and the health impact of environmental factors will tend to overestimate the statistical significance and effect size of the neighborhood effect because it ignores the confounding effect of neighborhood effect averaging that arises from human daily mobility. This is a fundamental methodological issue when examining the health effects of mobility-dependent exposures and may be called the neighborhood effect averaging problem (NEAP).

Two recent studies have observed the phenomenon of neighborhood effect averaging. A study in Belgium found that exposures to NO_2 for mobile phone users with low residence-based NO_2 exposures are 54.5% higher when their daily mobility is taken into account, while exposures to NO_2 for mobile phone users with high residence-based NO_2 exposures are 33.1% lower when their daily mobility is taken into account [7]. Another study in China found that residence-based estimates of individual exposures to six air pollutants (carbon monoxide, nitrogen dioxide, sulfur dioxide, ozone, particulate matter with aerodynamic diameter less than 2.5 μm [$PM_{2.5}$], and elemental carbon) tend to overestimate exposures for people with high residence-based exposures and underestimate exposures for people with low residence-based exposures [8]. The study also observed that the range between the maximum and minimum as well as the 5th and 95th percentile exposure estimates is smaller for the mobility-based approach than for the residence-based approach, indicating that individual exposures are less variable when people's mobility is taken into account. These two studies thus provide strong evidence for the neighborhood effect averaging problem (NEAP) when assessing individual-based mobility-dependent exposures.

However, given that these studies are both on air pollution and cover only two study areas, further evidence is needed for assessing whether the NEAP also holds true for mobility-dependent exposures other than air pollution and in other study areas. It is also important to note that while the probability distribution of individual residence-based exposure approximates a bell-shaped distribution [7,8], it may be a normal or non-normal (i.e., skewed) distribution. For instance, the distribution of individual residence-based exposures across a city may be skewed and non-normal as a result of the particular geographic distribution of its population and specific environmental factors. However, even when the probability distribution of individual residence-based exposures is a non-normal bell-shaped distribution, many people would still have exposure levels close to the mean value for the population, and fewer people would have very high or low exposure levels as far as such distribution is slightly to moderately skewed. As a result, it is likely that neighborhood effect averaging would hold for slightly to moderately skewed distributions of individual residence-based exposures across a study area; but again, further evidence is needed to evaluate the extent to which this is true.

Further, neighborhood effect averaging may operate over different time scales: exposures to different neighborhood contexts via a person's daily mobility may reduce the influence of the residential context, while the effect of exposure to a person's current residential neighborhood may be mitigated by exposures to the residential contexts experienced earlier in life (e.g., childhood or previous residences). Considering the effects of daily human mobility and mobility over the life course (residential mobility and migration) is thus essential in certain epidemiological studies, especially when examining environmental contexts that are highly mobility-dependent (e.g., air pollution, noise pollution, healthy food outlets, green spaces, and cancer risk) [3,4,9].

The implications of neighborhood effect averaging for public health policies is that increasing the mobility of those who live in disadvantaged neighborhoods through better, safer, and more reliable public transit, in addition to improving neighborhood quality *in situ*, may be helpful for improving their health outcomes. Recent studies on the activity spaces and segregation experiences of disadvantaged social groups found that people who live in highly segregated neighborhoods tend to work or conduct many of their daily activities in relatively integrated urban areas (when compared to their residential neighborhoods) [10,11]. This observation supports the view that increasing the daily mobility of marginalized social groups or racial minorities to diverse parts of an urban area may mitigate the social disadvantages they experience, including disproportionate exposures to health risks [10,11]. However, as Wang et al. [12] recently found, even when residents of disadvantaged neighborhoods regularly travel to advantaged neighborhoods, their relative isolation and segregation may persist. Thus, concerted policies of social integration that mitigate racial discrimination and reduce segregation are ultimately critical, and more research on the positive and negative implications of neighborhood effect averaging is sorely needed.

Acknowledgments: The author would like to thank the four anonymous reviewers for their helpful comments. This work was supported by a John Simon Guggenheim Memorial Foundation Fellowship.

Conflicts of Interest: The author declares no conflicts of interest.

References

1. Cummins, S.; Curtis, S.; Diez-Roux, A.V.; Macintyre, S. Understanding and representing 'place' in health research: A relational approach. *Soc. Sci. Med.* **2007**, *65*, 1825–1838. [CrossRef] [PubMed]
2. Matthews, S.A. The salience of neighborhood: Some lessons from sociology. *Am. J. Prev. Med.* **2008**, *34*, 257–259. [CrossRef] [PubMed]
3. Kwan, M.-P. The uncertain geographic context problem. *Ann. Am. Assoc. Geogr.* **2012**, *102*, 958–968. [CrossRef]
4. Kwan, M.-P. Beyond space (as we knew it): Toward temporally integrated geographies of segregation, health, and accessibility. *Ann. Am. Assoc. Geogr.* **2013**, *103*, 1078–1086. [CrossRef]
5. Park, Y.M.; Kwan, M.-P. Individual exposure estimates may be erroneous when spatiotemporal variability of air pollution and human mobility are ignored. *Health Place* **2017**, *43*, 85–94. [CrossRef] [PubMed]
6. Shafran-Nathan, R.; Levy, I.; Broday, D.M. Exposure estimation errors to nitrogen oxides on a population scale due to daytime activity away from home. *Sci. Total Environ.* **2017**, *580*, 1401–1409. [CrossRef] [PubMed]
7. Dewulf, B.; Neutens, T.; Lefebvre, W.; Seynaeve, G.; Vanpoucke, C.; Beckx, C.; Van de Weghe, N. Dynamic assessment of exposure to air pollution using mobile phone data. *Int. J. Health Geogr.* **2016**, *15*, 14. [CrossRef] [PubMed]
8. Yu, H.; Russell, A.; Mulholland, J.; Huang, Z. Using cell phone location to assess misclassification errors in air pollution exposure estimation. *Environ. Pollut.* **2018**, *233*, 261–266. [CrossRef] [PubMed]
9. Kwan, M.-P. The limits of the neighborhood effect: Contextual uncertainties in geographic, environmental health, and social science research. *Ann. Am. Assoc. Geogr.* **2018**, *108*. [CrossRef]
10. Jones, M.; Pebley, A.R. Redefining neighborhoods using common destinations: Social characteristics of activity spaces and home census tracts compared. *Demography* **2014**, *51*, 727. [CrossRef] [PubMed]
11. Park, Y.M.; Kwan, M.-P. Beyond residential segregation: A spatiotemporal approach to examining multi-contextual segregation. *Comput. Environ. Urban Syst.* **2018**, *71*, 98–108. [CrossRef]
12. Wang, Q.; Phillips, N.E.; Small, M.L.; Sampson, R.J. Urban mobility and neighborhood isolation in America's 50 largest cities. *Proc. Natl. Acad. Sci. USA* 2018. [CrossRef] [PubMed]

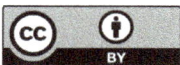

International Journal of
Environmental Research and Public Health

MDPI

Article

Exploring the Influence of Built Environment on Car Ownership and Use with a Spatial Multilevel Model: A Case Study of Changchun, China

Xiaoquan Wang [1], Chunfu Shao [2,*], Chaoying Yin [1,*] and Chengxiang Zhuge [3]

1   MOE Key Laboratory for Urban Transportation Complex Systems Theory and Technology, Beijing Jiaotong University, Beijing 100044, China; 15120886@bjtu.edu.cn
2   Key Laboratory of Transport Industry of Big Data Application Technologies for Comprehensive Transport, Beijing Jiaotong University, Beijing 100044, China
3   Department of Geography, University of Cambridge, Downing Place, Cambridge CB2 3EN, UK; zgcx615@126.com
*   Correspondence: cfshao@bjtu.edu.cn (C.S.); 15114226@bjtu.edu.cn (C.Y.)

Received: 22 July 2018; Accepted: 27 August 2018; Published: 29 August 2018

Abstract: Although the impacts of built environment on car ownership and use have been extensively studied, limited evidence has been offered for the role of spatial effects in influencing the interaction between built environment and travel behavior. Ignoring the spatial effects may lead to misunderstanding the role of the built environment and providing inconsistent transportation policies. In response to this, we try to employ a two-step modeling approach to investigate the impacts of built environment on car ownership and use by combining multilevel Bayesian model and conditional autocorrelation (CAR) model to control for spatial autocorrelation. In the two-step model, the predicting car ownership status in the first-step model is used as a mediating variable in the second-step car use model. Taking Changchun as a case study, this paper identifies the presence of spatial effects in influencing the effects of built environment on car ownership and use. Meanwhile, the direct and cascading effects of built environment on car ownership and use are revealed. The results show that the spatial autocorrelation exists in influencing the interaction between built environment and car dependency. The results suggest that it is necessary for urban planners to pay attention to the spatial effects and make targeted policy according to local land use characteristics.

Keywords: car ownership; car use; built environment; spatial autocorrelation; multilevel Bayesian model

1. Introduction

Car dependency is one of the most influential contributing factors to air pollution, traffic congestion, and energy consumption [1]. Additionally, it is widely believed that car use can increase the risk of health problem due to more sedentary behavior than other travel modes [2]. A growing body of literature has focused on the link between built environment and travel behavior in order to reduce car dependency through promoting sustainable urban planning strategies in developed countries [3–5]. It is also viewed as a long-term effective solution to the negative effect of car dependency on the environment to promote high-density and compact urban development strategies due to the likelihood to engage in active travel. Especially in developing country like China, many cities are experiencing urban sprawl with urbanization process, thus increasing more motorized travel demand and transport-related environmental issues. Reducing car ownership and use has recently become the emerging national concern [6]. On the other hand, it is a good opportunity for policy makers and urban planners to shape the interaction between the built environment and car dependency in developing countries due to the changes in built environment along with rapid urbanization [7].

However, to the best of our knowledge, few studies have been conducted in developing countries although many studies have investigated the link between built environment and travel behavior [8,9]. China is the largest developing country and experiencing an explosive increase in motorized travel demand with rapid urbanization in recent years. These dramatic transformations lead to a different situation where empirical studies in Western cities could provide few evidences [10]. Second, a very limited number of empirical studies have paid attention to the influence of spatial effects on the link between built environment and car dependency [11–13]. Although some existing studies have paid increasing attention to spatial context and attempted to capture the spatial heterogeneity by applying multilevel models, it is still a challenge to address spatial autocorrelation, which is important for capturing the potential correlation of observations located in nearby locations in the geographic data context. The study contributes to the literature by addressing the spatial effects when investigating the influence of built environment on car ownership and use in Changchun, China. To achieve this, we employed a two-step model based on Changchun Household Travel Survey, in which the multilevel Bayesian model combined with conditional autocorrelation (CAR) model is used to address spatial autocorrelation.

The remainder of the paper is organized as follows. In Section 2, we review related studies on the effects of built environment and the spatial effects. Then, we describe the data in Section 3, while Section 4 presents the methodology used for this study. Section 5 presents the model results, followed by policy implications and future work in Section 6.

2. Literature Review

2.1. Built Environment, Other Factors, and Car Dependency

Over the past few decades, important conclusions have been reached on the interaction between the built environment and travel behavior [14–18]. In the existing studies, it is acknowledged that the built environment mainly consists of physical and social elements that make up the structure of a community and it can influence travel behavior. Additionally, the built environment has been summarized as "D variables", developing from "three Ds" defined by Cervero [19] to "six Ds" in recent studies including diversity, density, design, destination accessibility, distance to transit, and demand management [20,21]. Numerous existing studies have also confirmed that the built environment plays a remarkable role in car ownership and use decision [1,3,4,22–26]. Although some debatable conclusions are reached in existing studies, some built environment characteristics show significant influences, directly or indirectly, on a range of outcomes including car ownership, mode choice, vehicle miles traveled (VMT), vehicle hours traveled (VHT), car trip frequencies et al. Especially in the context of Chinese cities, the influence of built environment on car dependency is attracting more and more attention due to the concerns about environmental and health issues brought by the rapid growth of car ownership and use. For instance, Jiang et al. [26] employed the multinomial logistic model and double-hurdle model to investigate the effect of the land use and street characteristics on car ownership and use in Jinan respectively and found that along with the proximity to regional transport infrastructures, most land use characteristics could influence the car dependency. Additionally, Li et al. [1] found that higher land use mix and accessibility of living facilities could help reduce the car dependency for people living near metro stations in Beijing.

Apart from built environment, a body of other factors has been found to be significantly associated with car ownership and use, including individual factors, household factors, travel-related factors and self-selection factors. Moreover, some of these factors may be more influential than the built environment factors. Many previous studies have explored the influence of socio-economic characteristics on car ownership and use, in which household income is found to be one of the most key factors [27–29]. The influence of household structure is also well studied from different aspects, consisting of household size [30], household workers [31], household children [25], and household composition [32]. Hukou is a special system conducted in China to ensure the reasonable migration, which is a term that attracts the attention of scholars due to its relation with urbanization [33]. Hukou is a population policy to control the movement of the rural population into the city. It is also a direct factor on the distribution of the state's welfare. In some Chinese cities, it can determine purchase qualification of house and car.

Additionally, travel-related factors have a significantly association with car dependency, which is also confirmed by some existing studies [7,18,34]. Moreover, the self-selection effect, which is characterized by the phenomenon that residents would choose their residence location according to their preferences for travel mode and land use patterns, can influence car dependency further [35,36]. For example, Hong et al. examined the relationship between built environment and travel behavior, in which self-selection was found to have significant influence on household VMT [37]. Additionally, Cao et al. [38] used Guangzhou as a case and found that built environment and self-selection effects influenced car ownership and commuting distance, further producing influence on emissions.

2.2. Spatial Effects

Spatial autocorrelation is an explanation for the phenomenon that observations at nearby locations tend to have similar characteristics, which is documented in the literature [37,39–41]. The observations are not independent when spatial autocorrelation occurs. Therefore, statistical methods ignoring spatial effects may lead to inefficient or even biased estimated results due to their assumption that the observations are independent. For instance, Bhat [11] employed a multilevel cross-classified model to analyze commuting model choice considering spatial clustering of observations. The results indicate that spatial clustering exists and should be taken into account to avoid inferior data fit. To address the challenge and incorporate the spatial context, researchers have developed several methods to resolve the problem of spatial autocorrelation in spatial data [42–44]. For instance, Wu et al. [13] conducted two rounds of surveys to identify the effect of public transit improvement on car dependency and found that spatial dependency existed between adjacent neighborhoods. In another example, Wang et al. [40] employed a Poisson log-normal conditional autoregressive model to investigate the determinants of safety impacts of roadway network and found that spatial autocorrelation existed in crashes on highways. In addition, the spatial autocorrelation has also been studied in land use and emission analysis. For instance, Hong et al. [41] examined the relationship between residential density and transportation emissions and utilized a multilevel Bayesian model with spatial random effects to address the spatial autocorrelation. The results suggest that spatial autocorrelation can influence the effect of residential density on emission. Eboli et al. employed the geographically weighted regression model to evaluate transit service quality considering spatial variation of passengers' responses across the study area and it could provide more appropriate results compared with ordinary least square model [45]. Additionally, Eboli et al. found the existing clusters of similar values in the distribution of the service quality attributes based on passenger satisfaction survey data from Milan [46].

However, there are few efforts having been made to handle the spatial autocorrelation existing in influencing the role of the built environment to play in car ownership and use decision. In response to this, this study will contribute to current literature in two aspects. First, statistic models have their own disadvantages in capturing spatial effects, which may lead to a biased estimation. To address the spatial autocorrelation, we employ a two-step Bayesian multilevel model with spatial random term to explore the determinants of car ownership and use in this study. Second, there are many differences between China and Western countries, including the level of economic development, urbanization, hukou system, and the culture context. Although there is a growing body of literature investigating the influence of built environment on car dependency in developed countries, studies about the impacts in China are away from reaching the consensus. What's more, rapid urbanization in Chinese cities provides a good chance to explore the link between built environment and car dependency.

Based on our literature review, we identified a number of research gaps which are detailed below: (1) from the influential variable side, previous studies are mainly conducted in developed countries and not much attention has been paid to the influential variables about China-specific issues like hukou [47]; (2) From the methodology side, previous studies use discrete choice model [6,17,31,48], structural equation model (SEM) [4,25], and regression model [1,26,49,50] to investigate the relationship between land use and transport characteristics. SEM can take into the mediating effects of car ownership when investigating the influencing factors, but have a limitation of recognizing the spatial effects. Additionally, although discrete choice methods and regressions methods can model the spatial effects, they cannot take into account mediating effects. In this study, a two-step modeling approach with spatial random effects is proposed to investigate the determinants of car ownership and use and address the spatial effects in the unified analytical framework.

3. Data and Variable

3.1. Study Region

The study region in this study is Changchun city as shown in Figure 1, which is a mid-sized city in Northeast China. It covers approximately 20,565 km^2 and has more than 7 million people [51]. As the capital of Jilin province, Changchun continues to exhibit economic growth and urban sprawl which are relative to the rapid urbanization process in China. Additionally, motorized travel demand has explosively grown over the past decade due to the rapid economic growth and urban expansion in Changchun. Changchun has been chosen as a member of "Transit Metropolis" program and invested huge amounts of capital in public transit construction in order to reduce car dependency. However, similar to many Chinese cities, the growth in car ownership and use still leads to notorious traffic congestion and air pollution. Therefore, Changchun is chosen as the study region to provide references for similar cities in China.

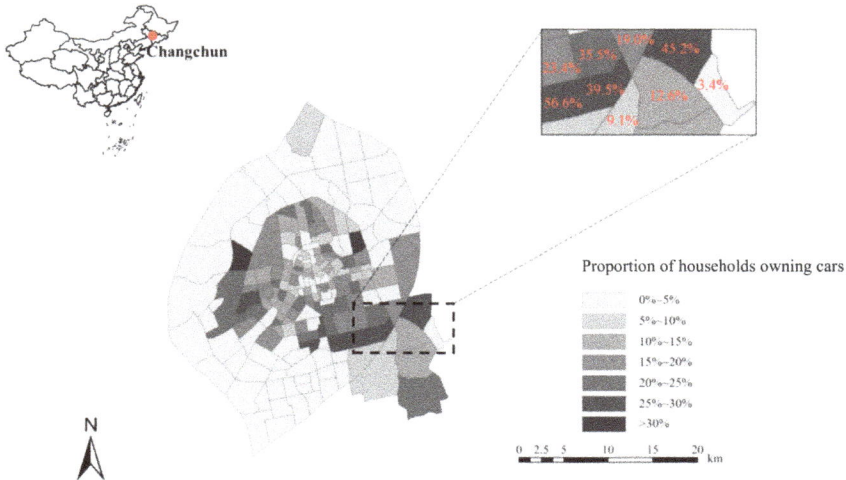

Figure 1. Study region and traffic analysis zones.

3.2. Data and Descriptive Statistics

The primary data used for the empirical explosion is extracted from the 2012 Changchun household travel survey conducted by Beijing Transport Institute. The survey is part of a comprehensive traffic model report undertaken by Beijing Transport Institute and Changchun

Institute of Urban Planning and Design to monitor comprehensive traffic network, travel demand, and travel behavior. The survey is conducted from 1 May 2012 to 13 May 2012. The survey provided socio-economic characteristics consisting of household income, household size, hukou type. Additionally, completed travel information of all members in the respondent's household was collected on the assigned day, including travel modes, trip purposes, departure time, arrival time, and origin and destination of a trip. In the dataset, travel information of 20,000 households is available. About 18.2% of the total sample owned one or more cars. As shown in Figure 1, the proportion of households that own at least one car in the traffic analysis zones is presented. After error-checking and clearing the raw data, a total of 100,058 complete trip records of 16,732 households are used in this study. Socio-economic characteristics are described in Table 1.

Table 1. Descriptive statistics of socio-economic and travel-related characteristics.

Variable Name	Variable Description	Min	Max	Mean
Car ownership	1, if one or more cars are available; 0, otherwise	0	1	0.18
Hukou	1, local hukou; 0, otherwise	0	1	0.95
Household income 1	1, household income yearly is less than 20,000 (RMB); 0, otherwise (around US$3 thousand)	0	1	0.25
Household income 2	1, household income yearly is between 20,000–100,000 (RMB); 0, otherwise (around US$3–15 thousand)	0	1	0.73
Household income 3	1, household income yearly is less than 100,000 (RMB); 0, otherwise (around US$15 thousand)	0	1	0.02
Household size	Number of household members	1	9	2.71
Household student	Number of household students	0	4	0.33

Built environment measurements are collected from two major sources: AMAP.com and Changchun traffic map. As shown in Figure 1, there are 237 traffic analysis zones (TAZs) in the study region and the average area of each TAZ is 2.46 km^2. The data reflects five dimensions of built environment characteristics, including population density, intersection density, transit station density, distance to central business district (CBD), and land use mix at the TAZ level. Intersection density is obtained based on Changchun traffic map using the ArcGIS platform (Environmental Systems Research Institute, Redlands, CA, USA) and only four-way intersections are used in this analysis. Transit station density is measured by the ratio of the number of bus stops and metro stations within the TAZ. Distance to CBD represents the location of residence, which is measured based on the Euclidean distance between the household's TAZ centroid and CBD. Due to the limitations of data acquisition, the entropy index was used based on the point of interest (POI) to measure land use mix, following Cao et al. [38]. The POIs were extracted from AMAP includes residential buildings, hotels, restaurants, supermarkets, parks, squares, malls, schools, hospitals, banks, and government departments. The index is a measurement of the distribution evenness of different land use types in a given TAZ.

$$\text{Land use mix} = -\sum_{i=1}^{N} p_i \ln p_i / \ln N \tag{1}$$

where i corresponds to POI types and p_i is the proportion of a specific POI type from the total area of a given TAZ. N is the total number of possible POI types. The index value ranges from 0 to 1 and a higher value means a more balanced land use pattern in the TAZ.

The descriptive statistics of built environment measurements are described in Table 2.

Table 2. Descriptive statistics of built environment characteristics.

Variable Name	Variable Description	Mean	Standard Deviation
Population density	Population density per square kilometer at the TAZ level	0.34	0.22
Intersection density	Intersection density per square kilometer at the TAZ level	0.59	0.17
Transit station density	Transit station density per square kilometer at the TAZ level	10.50	5.91
Distance to CBD	Euclidean distance from residence to CBD (unit: km)	4.8	2.91
Land use mix	A measure of the composition of residential buildings, hotels, restaurants, supermarkets, parks, squares, malls, schools, hospitals, banks, and government departments	33.38	17.83

Note: CBD: central business district.

4. Methodology

The analysis was twofold. First, we used household characteristics and built environment characteristics to predict the household car ownership status using a Bayesian multilevel discrete choice model. In the first-step model, car ownership was used as a binary variable and treated as the dependent variable. Then we analyzed the determinants of household VMT, in which the predicted car ownership derived from the first model was used as a mediating variable instead of the observed car ownership status. The built environment and socio-economic characteristics were treated as independent variables. The two-step model can address the potential endogeneity bias and selection bias [52,53]. The endogeneity bias results from the endogeneity between car ownership and use due to the influence of unobserved factors on both car ownership and use. The second bias can be due to the fact that car use only happens when the household owns cars. Additionally, the two-step modeling approach can explicitly distinguish the direct effects of exogenous variables and indirect effects via car ownership on car use simultaneously [26,31]. Moreover, the proposed models assume that observations at nearby locations tend to have similar characteristics and TAZs vary as a function of built environment variables measured at the TAZ level [30]. The CAR model is used to specify the spatial autocorrelation. The detail models are described as follows.

In the first-step model, we performed a Bayesian multilevel discrete choice model on household car ownership by incorporating CAR model to address the spatial effects. In the model, we treated the household car ownership status as a binary variable and used relevant socio-economic and built environment characteristics as the independent variables. The socio-economic and built environment characteristics are treated as household and TAZ level variables respectively because households living in the same TAZ share a common environment. The car ownership model takes the Bayesian multilevel discrete choice model form, and the utility function is as below.

$$
\begin{aligned}
U_{ih} &= \alpha_{i|h} + \beta_{SD}^T X_{ih}^{SD} + s_{i|h} + \varepsilon_{ih} \\
\alpha_h &= \varphi + \gamma_{BE}^T X_h^{BE} + \sigma_h \\
s_h &= N(\overline{s_h}, \frac{\sigma_s^2}{n_h}) \\
\overline{s_h} &= \sum_{k \in \text{neighborhood}} \overline{w_{h,k}} s_k / n_h
\end{aligned}
\tag{2}
$$

where U_{ih} is the utility function of household i residing in TAZ j owning one or more cars. X_{ih}^{SD} and X_h^{BE} are the socio-economic and built environment characteristics, respectively. $\alpha_{i|h}$ is the varying intercept. β_{SD}^T and γ_{BE}^T are the vectors of parameters to be calibrated. The spatial autocorrelation term is represented by $s_{i|h}$, which means residents at nearby locations behave similarly due to their similar unobserved characteristics. s_h is assumed to follow a normal distribution in this study. ε_{ih} is the error term and assumed to follow a Gumbel distribution. $\overline{w_{h,k}}s_k$ is an element in the spatial adjacent matrix, representing the adjacent relation between TAZ h and k. n_h is the number of TAZs sharing common boundaries with TAZ h.

In this study, the household car ownership is treated as a binary variable according to whether the household owns cars or not. The household car ownership decision can be described as follows.

$$y_{ih} = \begin{cases} 1, \text{ if } U_{ih} > U_{jh}, \forall j \in A \\ 0, \text{ otherwise} \end{cases} \tag{3}$$

where y_{ih} is the choice indicator. If the household owns cars, y_{ih} takes the value of one, and zero otherwise.

Then, the probability of household i owning one or more cars can be obtained as follows.

$$p_{ih}\left(y_{ih} = 1 | X_{ni}^{SE}, X_{ni}^{BE}, X_{ni}^{PA}, CAR_{ni}, TD_{ni}, s_h, \varepsilon_{ni}, \sigma_h\right) = \frac{\exp(\varphi + \gamma_{BE}^T X_h^{BE} + \beta_{SD}^T X_{ih}^{SD} + \sigma_h + s_{i|h})}{\sum \exp(\varphi + \gamma_{BE}^T X_h^{BE} + \beta_{SD}^T X_{ih}^{SD} + \sigma_h + s_{i|h})} \tag{4}$$

In this study, common boundary matrix is used to measure the adjacent relation between two TAZs as below.

$$w_{h,k} = \begin{cases} \text{the length of common boundary, if TAZ } h \text{ is adjacent to TAZ } k \\ 0, \text{otherwise} \end{cases} \tag{5}$$

The spatial adjacent matrix can be obtained through standardizing the elements in common boundary matrix according to min-max normalization scheme.

Therefore, the predicted car ownership status can be calibrated as below.

$$X_{ih}^{CAR} = \begin{cases} 1, \text{ if } p_{ih} > 1 - p_{ih} \\ 0, \text{ otherwise} \end{cases} \tag{6}$$

where X_{ih}^{CAR} is the predicted car ownership status of household i living in TAZ h.

In the second-step model, a normal regression model with spatial random effects was employed to explore the determinants of car use. In the model, the dependent variable was derived based on all car-based trips conducted by the household members on the assigned day. According to the origin and destination of the trip in the dataset, vehicle kilometers traveled (VKT) was calibrated based on the shortest path on the road network. It is worth mentioning that log VKT was chosen as the dependent variable in this study because the VKT was found to be positively skewed to the right. In addition, the predicted car ownership status was used as an exogenous variable in the car use model. The model can address the potential influences of the exogenous variables, including the socio-economic and built environment characteristics, thus the indirect influence of socio-economic and built environment characteristics via car ownership can be revealed simultaneously. Therefore, the final car use model is as follows.

$$\begin{aligned} y_i &\sim N(\omega_{i|h} + \beta_{SD}^T X_{ih}^{SD} + \beta_{CAR}^T X_{ih}^{CAR} + v_{i|h}, \sigma_y^2) \\ \omega_h &\sim N(\varphi + \gamma_{BE}^T X_h^{BE}, \sigma_h^2) \\ v_h &= N(\overline{v_h}, \frac{\sigma_v^2}{n_h}) \\ \overline{v_h} &= \sum_{k \in \text{neighborhood}} \overline{w_{h,k}} v_k / n_h \end{aligned} \tag{7}$$

where X_{ih}^{CAR} is the predicted car ownership status for household i living in in TAZ h.

To estimate the car ownership model and car use model, multilevel Bayesian procedure based on the Markov Chain Monte Carlo (MCMC) method was conducted, which could overcome the deficiency resulting from the maximum likelihood estimation method [42,54]. The estimation method is based on Bayes' Theorem as follows.

$$\pi(\theta|y) = \frac{L(y|\theta)\pi(\theta)}{\int L(y|\theta)\pi(\theta)d\theta} \tag{8}$$

where y is a vector of observed variables. θ is the parameter vector of likelihood function. $\pi(\theta|y)$ is the posterior distribution under given y. $L(y|\theta)$ is the likelihood function. $\int L(y|\theta)\pi(\theta)d\theta$ is the edge probability distribution of the observed variables. $\pi(\theta)$ is the prior distribution. Based on the posterior distribution of parameters, MCMC method can generate a chain to make point and interval estimations through successive sampling [54,55]. Different from p value estimation based on the mean and the variance, MCMC method provides a more direct way through the posterior distributions of parameters. Moreover, the uncertainty can be obtained based on the MCMC method because it can provide a specific CI (Confidence Interval) for the estimated parameters. In this analysis, the mean of estimated parameters and 95% CI is presented instead of p value. It presents the 95% CI by providing the lower bound of 2.5% and upper bound of 97.5%. If the 95% CI does not include zero, it means that the influence of the corresponding independent variable on dependent variable is significant.

5. Result and Discussion

5.1. Car Ownership Model

The estimation result for car ownership model is presented in Table 3. With regard to spatial autocorrelation term, the parameter σ_s is found to be significant at the 95% significance level, which demonstrates that spatial autocorrelation exists in car ownership decision. The result confirms that households living in nearby areas tend to have similar decision on purchasing cars, which indicates that unobserved autocorrelation could moderate the influence of built environment on households' car ownership behavior.

Table 3. Multilevel Bayesian Logistic regression of household car ownership.

Variable	Mean	95% CI	
		2.5%	97.5%
Socio-demographics at household level			
Hukou	0.91	0.79	1.04
Household income 1 (reference: Household income 2)	−0.17	−0.25	−0.09
Household income 3 (reference: Household income 2)	0.43	0.30	0.56
Household size	0.03	−0.05	0.11
Household student	0.08	0.04	0.12
Built environment at TAZ level			
Residential density	−0.51	−0.31	−0.71
Land use mix	−0.23	−0.37	−0.10
Distance to CBD	0.09	−0.03	0.23
Transit station density	−0.09	−0.14	−0.04
Intersection density	−0.08	−0.14	−0.02
σ_h	0.09	0.07	0.11
σ_s	1.23	0.76	1.71

Note: CI: confidence interval. TAZ: traffic analysis zone.

According to Table 3, most coefficients of socio-economic characteristics show significant influences on household car ownership. For instance, it is found that the influence of hukou on car ownership is significantly positive, indicating that households with local hukou have a higher probability of owning cars. This may be explained by that hukou system ensure that households with local hukou enjoy better social welfares in China. Additionally, the results reveal that higher household income increases the likelihood of owning cars, which is consistent with existing studies [1,56,57]. Because many Chinese families still cannot afford to purchase a car [26], household income still serves as one of the primary determinants of household car ownership. Household size is found to have no significant influence on household car ownership. Although existing studies suggest that household size can increase the likelihood of owning cars [31], bigger household size means an increasing net income, thus decreasing the travel budget. Finally, household student has a positive influence on household car ownership at the significance level of 95%, indicating that the number of household students increases the likelihood of owning cars. This may be explained by that most parents tend to show concerns about the safety of children on the way to school and would like to drive them to school in China.

Turning to the built environment characteristics, residential density shows a significantly negative influence on car ownership. This means that households living in lower residential density areas are more likely to own cars because communities with higher residential density generally mean better living facilities in neighborhoods, thus reducing the motorized travel demand. Land use mix is found to be negatively associated with car ownership. It means that, when a household lives in a TAZ with compact land use, the probability of owning cars decreases. Distance to CBD shows no significant influence on car ownership, which is different from the existing study [34]. However, the existing studies also produce mixed results about the influence [31,34,57]. On one hand, living farther from CBD means a longer commuting distance due to the fact that most employments concentrate around CBD. Therefore, people living in these areas have to choose motorized mode because of the longer distance between origin and destination, thus increasing the likelihood of owning cars. On the other hand, commuting is only a factor that could influence car ownership. The other factors, including economical factor, should also be considered. Transit station density is found to have a significantly negative influence on car ownership. Also, higher intersection density reduces the likelihood of owning cars because higher intersection density generally provides a friendlier environment for active travel mode.

5.2. Car Use Model

The estimation result of car use model is presented in Table 4. The influence of σ_v at the 95% significance level suggests that spatial autocorrelation exists. The result indicates that households living in nearby areas have similar car use behavior.

The predicted household car ownership status, which is derived from the first-step model according to Equation (6) and estimated parameters, shows a strongly positive influence on the household total VKT. The result suggests household car ownership can affect household car use. Also, it is also found that hukou has significantly positive influence on household VKT. It is possible for the reason that households with local hukou generally tend to enjoy better welfares and have higher requirement for travel convenience and effectiveness. Similar with previous studies, the result shows that household income is positively associated with household car use. Compared with the influence of household size on car ownership, the result suggests that although household size shows no significant influence on car ownership, the households with bigger household size generate more car use. This may be explained by that bigger household size could generate more motorized travel demand such as education and social interaction purpose, but meanwhile bigger household size means more other household expenses and a limited budget for travel, thus constraining car-purchasing decision. Finally, household student on car use is not related with household VKT at the significance level of 95%, which is different from that in car ownership model. This indicates that the number of household students merely affects car use via the influence on car ownership.

After controlling for socio-economic factors, several built environment characteristics also show significant influence on car use. For instance, living in areas with higher residential density tends to be associated with a lower likelihood of car use. This may be due to the fact that areas with higher residential density generally have better living facilities to meet the demand of daily life and thus reduce the travel demand further. Similar with household student, land use mix and intersection density are both not associated with car use at the 95% significant level, yet they are associated with car ownership at the 95% significant level. In addition, distance to CBD has a positive influence on household car use at the 95% significant level, which suggests that multi-center compact development strategy may be an effective way to reduce VKT. Finally, it is found that as living in areas with higher transit station density is significantly associated with a lower likelihood of car use. This result suggests that investing on public transit may help reduce car use.

Table 4. Multilevel Bayesian Normal regression of household VKT (vehicle kilometers traveled).

Variable	Mean	95% CI	
		2.5%	97.5%
Socio-demographics at household level			
Predicted car ownership status	2.19	1.85	2.53
Hukou	0.07	0.04	0.11
Household income 1 (reference: Household income 2)	−0.19	−0.28	−0.11
Household income 3 (reference: Household income 2)	0.39	0.18	0.61
Household size	0.05	0.01	0.12
Household student	0.42	−0.09	0.93
Built environment at TAZ level			
Residential density	−0.10	−0.17	−0.03
Land use mix	−0.07	−0.15	0.01
Distance to CBD	0.05	0.01	0.09
Transit station density	−0.12	−0.17	−0.08
Intersection density	−0.11	−0.32	0.10
σ_h	0.29	0.09	0.49
σ_v	0.18	0.12	0.23

5.3. Combined Effects of Built Environment

To investigate the combined effects of built environment on household car use, including direct and indirect effects via car ownership, we estimated the cascading influences via simulation. Measuring elasticities of household car use with respect to the built environment characteristics are presented in Table 5, which are calibrated by combining the two models (the detailed calculation method can be seen in notes of Table 5).

Table 5. Elasticities of household VKT with built environment variables.

Variable	Elasticity of VKT via Car Ownership	Combined Elasticity of VKT
Residential density	−0.01	−0.02
Land use mix	−0.01	−0.01
Distance to CBD	−	0.12
Transit station density	−0.03	−0.08
Intersection density	−0.04	−0.04

Note: Adapted from [31], we used the $VKT_{baseline}$ and VKT_{new} represent the baseline total VKT generated and new VKT estimated after applying 10% increase for the variable of interest. The $VKT_{baseline}$ is obtained using the coefficient estimates from the regression model (Table 4), in which the predicted car ownership status is used. Then a 10% increase of the target variable and we update the new status of the predicted car ownership status according to the discrete choice model. VKT_{new} is generated by using the regression coefficients and the predicted number of car ownership. The elasticity can be calibrated by $((VKT_{new} − VKT_{baseline})/VKT_{baseline})/(0.10)$.

The estimated elasticities of VKT show that distance to CBD is the most influential contributing factor to VKT with a combined elasticity of 0.12. This means that households living farther from

CBD tend to generate more VKT and the influence is much greater than the other built environment characteristics. Therefore, it is necessary to promote tailor-made urban planning strategies according to the locations. Additionally, compared with the rest characteristics, transit station density could present relatively larger elasticities, indicating that transit station density is an important determinant of car use. Specifically, if we double the transit station density, it would reduce 8 percent of household VKT. Additionally, other built environment characteristics all may play a remarkable role in influencing car use. Therefore, the results suggest that promoting sustainable land use strategies can reduce car use effectively in urban areas.

6. Conclusions

This study aims to examine the direct and cascading effects of the built environment on car ownership and use based on a two-step model, in which CAR model is combined to the Bayesian multilevel model to address the spatial effects. Based on data from Changchun, the study can provide insightful results for the literature from two aspects: methodology implementations and policy implications.

First, a two-step model can provide an insight into the link between the built environment and travel behavior by revealing the direct and cascading effects of built environment on car ownership and use. Meanwhile, Bayesian multilevel model combined with CAR model provides evidence for the role of spatial effects play in influencing the impacts of built environment on car dependency. The results suggest that it is important to accommodate spatial autocorrelation that can moderate the influence of built environment on individual decision-making.

Second, as for policy implications, this paper provides concrete evidence on the interaction between built environment and car ownership and use for urban planners. The results indicate that promoting dense land use and transit-oriented development can reduce car ownership and use. In addition, communities nearer from CBD and with higher accessibility decline the car dependency for residents. However, it should be noted that one-size-fits-all design should not be the solution to reduce car dependency due to the fact that car ownership and use can vary over space. Therefore, urban planners should acknowledge the spatial effects and find the most suitable built environment sets according to the local land use characteristics.

The study also has some limitations. First, due to data limitation, self-selection effect is not addressed in the study. We control for the socio-demographics and spatial effects, but more attitude data is needed in future to address the self-selection effects. Second, it would be helpful to compare empirical results for spatial effects across cities because the spatial effects may vary with different cities.

Author Contributions: For this paper, X.W., C.S. and C.Y. proposed the method. X.W. wrote the paper. C.Y. provided data and revised advice for the paper. C.Z. provided revised advice for improving the paper.

Funding: This work was supported by the Hebei Natural Science Foundation under Grant E2016513016 and the National Natural Science Foundation of China under Grant 71621001.

Conflicts of Interest: The authors declare no conflict of interest.

References

1. Li, S.; Zhao, P. Exploring car ownership and car use in neighborhoods near metro stations in Beijing: Does the neighborhood built environment matter? *Transp. Res. Part D Transp. Environ.* **2017**, *56*, 1–17. [CrossRef]
2. Frederick, C.; Riggs, W.; Gilderbloom, J.H. Commute mode diversity and public health: A multivariate analysis of 148 US cities. *Int. J. Sustain. Transp.* **2018**, *12*, 1–12. [CrossRef]
3. Ewing, R.; Cervero, R. Travel and the built environment: A meta-analysis. *J. Am. Plan. Assoc.* **2010**, *76*, 265–294. [CrossRef]
4. Acker, V.V.; Witlox, F. Car ownership as a mediating variable in car travel behaviour research using a structural equation modelling approach to identify its dual relationship. *J. Transp. Geogr.* **2010**, *18*, 65–74. [CrossRef]

5. Pinjari, A.R.; Pendyala, R.M.; Bhat, C.R.; Waddell, P.A. Modeling residential sorting effects to understand the impact of the built environment on commute mode choice. *Transportation* **2007**, *34*, 557–573. [CrossRef]
6. Ding, C.; Chen, Y.; Duan, J.; Lu, Y.; Cui, J. Exploring the Influence of Attitudes to Walking and Cycling on Commute Mode Choice Using a Hybrid Choice Model. *J. Adv. Transp.* **2017**, *2017*, 1–8. [CrossRef]
7. Zhao, P. The impact of the built environment on individual workers' commuting behavior in Beijing. *Int. J. Sustain. Transp.* **2013**, *7*, 389–415. [CrossRef]
8. Liu, Q.; Wang, J.; Chen, P.; Xiao, Z. How does parking interplay with the built environment and affect automobile commuting in high-density cities? A case study in China. *Urban Stud.* **2016**, *54*, 1–19. [CrossRef]
9. Xiao, Z.; Liu, Q.; Wang, J. How do the effects of local built environment on household vehicle kilometers traveled vary across urban structural zones? *Int. J. Sustain. Transp.* **2018**, *12*, 1–11. [CrossRef]
10. Lu, Y.; Sun, G.; Sarkar, C.; Gou, Z.; Xiao, Y. Commuting Mode Choice in a High-Density City: Do Land-Use Density and Diversity Matter in Hong Kong? *Int. J. Environ. Public Health* **2018**, *15*, 920. [CrossRef] [PubMed]
11. Bhat, C.R. A multi-level cross-classified model for discrete response variables. *Transp. Res. Part B Method* **2000**, *34*, 567–582. [CrossRef]
12. Ding, C.; Wang, Y.; Yang, J.; Liu, C.; Lin, Y. Spatial heterogeneous impact of built environment on household auto ownership levels: Evidence from analysis at traffic analysis zone scales. *Transp. Lett.* **2016**, *8*, 26–34. [CrossRef]
13. Wu, W.; Hong, J. Does public transit improvement affect commuting behavior in Beijing, China? A spatial multilevel approach. *Transp. Res. Part D Transp. Environ.* **2017**, *52*, 471–479. [CrossRef]
14. Cervero, R. The built environment and travel: Evidence from the United States. *Eur. J. Transp. Infrastruct. Res.* **2003**, *3*, 119–137.
15. Cervero, R. Built environments and mode choice: Toward a normative framework. *Transp. Res. Part D Transp. Environ.* **2002**, *7*, 265–284. [CrossRef]
16. Cervero, R.; Lsarmiento, O.; Jacoby, E.; Gomez, L.F.; Nei-Man, A.; Xue, G. Influences of built environments on walking and cycling: Lessons from Bogotá. *Int. J. Sustain. Transp.* **2009**, *3*, 203–226. [CrossRef]
17. Cao, X.; Mokhtarian, P.L.; Handy, S.L. The relationship between the built environment and nonwork travel: A case study of Northern California. *Transp. Res. Part A Policy Pract.* **2009**, *43*, 548–559. [CrossRef]
18. Ding, C.; Lin, Y.; Liu, C. Exploring the influence of built environment on tour-based commuter mode choice: A cross-classified multilevel modeling approach. *Transp. Res. Part D Transp. Environ.* **2014**, *32*, 230–238. [CrossRef]
19. Cervero, R.; Kockelman, K. Travel demand and the 3ds: Density, diversity, and design. *Transp. Res. Part D Transp. Environ.* **1997**, *2*, 199–219. [CrossRef]
20. Sun, B.; Ermagun, A.; Dan, B. Built environmental impacts on commuting mode choice and distance: Evidence from Shanghai. *Transp. Res. Part D Transp. Environ.* **2017**, *52*, 441–453. [CrossRef]
21. Shay, E.; Khattak, A. Automobiles, trips, and neighborhood type: Comparing environmental measures. *Transp. Res. Rec. J. Transp. Res. Board* **2007**, *2010*, 73–82. [CrossRef]
22. Boarnet, M.G.; Sarmiento, S. Can Land-use Policy Really Affect Travel Behaviour? A Study of the Link between Non-work Travel and Land-use Characteristics. *Urban Stud.* **1998**, *35*, 1155–1169. [CrossRef]
23. Crane, R. Cars and Drivers in the New Suburbs: Linking Access to Travel in Neotraditional Planning. *J. Am. Plan. Assoc.* **1996**, *62*, 51–65. [CrossRef]
24. Potoglou, D.; Kanaroglou, P.S. Modelling car ownership in urban areas: A case study of Hamilton, Canada. *J. Transp. Geogr.* **2008**, *16*, 42–54. [CrossRef]
25. Ding, C.; Wang, D.; Liu, C.; Zhang, Y.; Yang, J. Exploring the influence of built environment on travel mode choice considering the mediating effects of car ownership and travel distance. *Transp. Res. Part A Policy Pract.* **2017**, *100*, 65–80. [CrossRef]
26. Jiang, Y.; Gu, P.; Chen, Y.; He, D.; Mao, Q. Influence of land use and street characteristics on car ownership and use: Evidence from Jinan, China. *Transp. Res. Part D Transp. Environ.* **2017**, *52*, 518–534. [CrossRef]
27. Dargay, J.; Gately, D. Income's effect on car and vehicle ownership, worldwide: 1960–2015. *Transp. Res. Part A Policy Pract.* **1999**, *33*, 101–138. [CrossRef]
28. Paulley, N.; Balcombe, R.; Mackett, R.; Titheridge, H.; Preston, J.; Wardman, M.; Shires, J.; White, P. The demand for public transport: The effects of fares, quality of service, income and car ownership. *Transp. Policy* **2006**, *13*, 295–306. [CrossRef]
29. Raphael, S.; Rice, L. Car ownership, employment, and earnings. *J. Urban Econ.* **2000**, *52*, 109–130. [CrossRef]

30. Wang, X.; Shao, C.; Yin, C.; Zhuge, C.; Li, W. Application of Bayesian Multilevel Models Using Small and Medium Size City in China: The Case of Changchun. *Sustainability* **2018**, *10*, 484. [CrossRef]

31. Zegras, C. The built environment and motor vehicle ownership and use: Evidence from Santiago de Chile. *Urban Stud.* **2010**, *47*, 1793–1817. [CrossRef]

32. Oakil, A.T.M.; Manting, D.; Nijland, H. Determinants of car ownership among young households in the Netherlands: The role of urbanisation and demographic and economic characteristics. *J. Transp. Geogr.* **2016**, *51*, 229–235. [CrossRef]

33. Jiang, Y.; Zhang, J.; Jin, X.; Ando, R.; Chen, L.; Shen, Z.; Ying, J.; Fang, Q.; Sun, Z. Rural migrant workers' intentions to permanently reside in cities and future energy consumption preference in the changing context of urban China. *Transp. Res. Part D Transp. Environ.* **2017**, *52*. [CrossRef]

34. Ding, C.; Wang, Y.; Tang, T.; Mishra, S.; Liu, C. Joint analysis of the spatial impacts of built environment on car ownership and travel mode choice. *Transp. Res. Part D Transp. Environ.* **2016**. [CrossRef]

35. Cao, X.J.; Mokhtarian, P.L.; Handy, S.L. Examining the impacts of residential self-selection on travel behaviour: A focus on empirical findings. *Transp. Rev.* **2009**, *29*, 359–395. [CrossRef]

36. Cao, X.J. Examining the impacts of neighborhood design and residential self-selection on active travel: A methodological assessment. *Urban Geogr.* **2015**, *36*, 236–255. [CrossRef]

37. Hong, J.; Shen, Q.; Zhang, L. How do built-environment factors affect travel behavior? A spatial analysis at different geographic scales. *Transportation* **2014**, *41*, 419–440. [CrossRef]

38. Cao, X.; Yang, W. Examining the effects of the built environment and residential self-selection on commuting trips and the related CO_2 emissions: An empirical study in Guangzhou, China. *Transp. Res. Part D Transp. Environ.* **2017**, *52*, 480–494. [CrossRef]

39. Xu, T.; Zhang, M.; Aditjandra, P.T. The impact of urban rail transit on commercial property value: New evidence from Wuhan, China. *Transp. Res. Part A Policy Pract.* **2016**, *91*, 223–235. [CrossRef]

40. Wang, X.; Yuan, J. Safety Impacts Study of Roadway Network Features on Suburban Highways. *China J. Highw. Transp.* **2017**, *30*, 106–114.

41. Hong, J.; Shen, Q. Residential density and transportation emissions: Examining the connection by addressing spatial autocorrelation and self-selection. *Transp. Res. Part D Transp. Environ.* **2013**, *22*, 75–79. [CrossRef]

42. Arcaya, M.; Brewster, M.; Zigler, C.M.; Subramanian, S.V. Area variations in health: A spatial multilevel modeling approach. *Health Place* **2012**, *18*, 824–831. [CrossRef] [PubMed]

43. Chaix, B.; Merlo, J.; Chauvin, P. Comparison of a spatial approach with the multilevel approach for investigating place effects on health: The example of healthcare utilisation in France. *J. Epidemiol. Commun. Health* **2005**, *59*, 517–526. [CrossRef] [PubMed]

44. Hong, J.; Goodchild, A. Land use policies and transport emissions: Modeling the impact of trip speed, vehicle characteristics and residential location. *Transp. Res. Part D Transp. Environ.* **2014**, *26*, 47–51. [CrossRef]

45. Eboli, L.; Forciniti, C.; Mazzulla, G. Spatial variation of the perceived transit service quality at rail stations. *Transp. Res. Part A Policy Pract.* **2018**, *114*, 67–83. [CrossRef]

46. Eboli, L.; Forciniti, C.; Mazzulla, G. Evaluating spatial association in passengers' perception of rail service quality at stations. *Ingeg. Ferr.* **2018**, *73*, 125–142.

47. Wang, D.; Zhou, M. The built environment and travel behavior in urban China: A literature review. *Transp. Res. Part D Transp. Environ.* **2017**, *52*, 574–585. [CrossRef]

48. Eboli, L.; Forciniti, C.; Mazzulla, G.; Calvo, F. Exploring the Factors That Impact on Transit Use through an Ordered Probit Model: The Case of Metro of Madrid. *Transp. Res. Procedia* **2016**, *18*, 35–43. [CrossRef]

49. Mazzulla, G.; Forciniti, C. Spatial association techniques for analysing trip distribution in an urban area. *Eur. Transp. Res. Rev.* **2012**, *4*, 217–233. [CrossRef]

50. Eboli, L.; Mazzulla, G.; Forciniti, C. Exploring the Relationship among Urban System Characteristics and Trips Generation through a GWR. *Int. J. Innov. Inf. Technol.* **2013**, *1*, 51–61.

51. National Bureau of Statistics. *China Statistic Yearbook 2014*; China Statistics Press: Beijing, China, 2014.

52. Chen, F.; Wu, J.; Chen, X.; Zegras, P.C.; Wang, J. Vehicle kilometers traveled reduction impacts of Transit-Oriented Development: Evidence from Shanghai City. *Transp. Res. Part D Transp. Environ.* **2017**, *55*, 227–245. [CrossRef]

53. Houston, D.; Ferguson, G.; Spears, S. Can compact rail transit corridors transform the automobile city? Planning for more sustainable travel in Los Angeles. *Urban Stud.* **2015**, *52*, 938–959. [CrossRef]

54. Wu, L.L.; Zhang, J.Y.; Chikaraishi, M. Representing the influence of multiple social interactions on monthly tourism participation behavior. *Tour. Manag.* **2013**, *36*, 480–489. [CrossRef]
55. Train, K.E. *Discrete Choice Methods with Simulation: GEV*; Cambridge University Press: Cambridge, UK, 2003; p. 54.
56. Shen, Q.; Chen, P.; Pan, H. Factors affecting car ownership and mode choice in rail transit-supported suburbs of a large Chinese city. *Transp. Res. Part A Policy Pract.* **2016**, *94*, 31–44. [CrossRef]
57. Yin, C.; Shao, C.; Wang, X. Built Environment and Parking Availability: Impacts on Car Ownership and Use. *Sustainability* **2018**, *10*, 2285. [CrossRef]

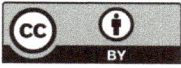

International Journal of
*Environmental Research
and Public Health*

MDPI

Article

Geographical Accessibility of Community Health Assist Scheme General Practitioners for the Elderly Population in Singapore: A Case Study on the Elderly Living in Housing Development Board Flats

Ong Ming Lee Deborah [1], Marcus Yu Lung Chiu [2,*] and Kai Cao [1,*]

[1]   Department of Geography, National University of Singapore, Singapore, Singapore
[2]   Department of Social and Behavioural Sciences, City University of Hong Kong, Hong Kong, China
*   Correspondence: mylchiu@cityu.edu.hk (M.Y.L.C.); geock@nus.edu.sg (K.C.)

Received: 9 August 2018; Accepted: 4 September 2018; Published: 12 September 2018

Abstract: Accessible primary healthcare is important to national healthcare in general and for older persons in particular, in societies where the population is ageing rapidly, as in Singapore. However, although much policy and research efforts have been put into this area, we hardly find any spatial perspective to assess the accessibility of these primary healthcare services. This paper analyzes the geographical accessibility of one major healthcare service in Singapore, namely, General Practitioners (GPs) services under the Community Health Assist Scheme (CHAS) for older persons. A Python script was developed to filter the website data of the Housing Development Board (HDB) of Singapore. The data derived was comprehensively analyzed by an Enhanced 2-Step Floating Catchment Area (E2SFCA) method based on a Gaussian distance-decay function and the GIS technique. This enabled the identification of areas with relatively weak geographical accessibility of CHAS-GPs. The findings are discussed along with suggestions for health practitioners, service planners and policy makers. Despite its initial nature, this study has demonstrated the value of innovative approaches in data collection and processing for the elderly-related studies, and contributed to the field of healthcare services optimization and possibly to other human services.

Keywords: geographical accessibility; Healthcare services; GIS; E2SFCA; CHAS; Singapore

1. Introduction

It is widely recognized that primary healthcare services are critical to national healthcare and play a vital role in support of elderly population [1–3]. Accessibility to healthcare services is variable across space and time, so it is affected by where health professionals are located (supply) and where people reside (demand) [4]. Besides, the value of healthcare professionals is dependent on the geographical accessibility of healthcare services [5], which depends on the impact of spatial gap between the supply and the demand sides of healthcare resource. In this regard, Geographical Information Systems (GIS) as well as spatial analysis technologies are particularly useful in addressing these kind of issues [6].

Rapid ageing is a key demographic challenge impacting Singapore. The ratio of seniors aged over 65 years, changed from 3.2% in 1970, to 13.0% in 2017, and will reach 24.1% in 2030 and 28.2% (over 900,000) in 2050 [7]. In addition to the challenge arising from the dramatic fall in Old-Age Support Ratio, demand for social and healthcare services is also rapidly increasing [8,9]. When home-based support and family caregiving are preferred to institutional care, policies of various types have been developed to enable seniors to age in place. In the case of Singapore, government seeks to maintain good health among older persons through health and exercise campaigns, building senior-friendly housing and towns, creating senior-friendly communities, and making quality and affordable healthcare services available.

Availability and accessibility of healthcare services is one of the major objectives of Singapore's national health plans and strategies in Singapore. Singapore's government is planning to add around 11,000 community hospitals and nursing home beds by 2020. In addition, the government is planning to expand home and community care with nursing homes as back up. One may assume that these additional resources will be accessible to meet the increasing need of the ageing population. However, this assumption may not be valid as revealed in other studies. Cheng [10] found that the distribution of the elderly population and residential care resources is geographically uneven across the districts in Beijing, so the supply of resources does not match with the needs. Similar studies have also been carried out in Hong Kong [11] and metro Atlanta [12]. It should therefore be beneficial to conduct a study on primary healthcare services in Singapore and examine how far the new provisions are meeting the changing spatial and temporal demand [13].

One common approach for assessing physical accessibility is to consider potential spatial accessibility. This approach has been used frequently while analyzing primary healthcare facilities in relation to the population of a catchment area on the basis of a variable of distance [14] that takes the availability as a supply-demand ratio within a region. However, it has been criticized for ignoring spatial variations within administrative boundaries as it assumes that people within the region do not seek healthcare services outside the boundaries [4,15]. Being an extension of accessibility-based approach, the regional accessibility approach considers the contribution and interactions of supply and demand between different regions [16,17]. By contrast, the gravity model integrates both the regional availability and regional accessibility as a unified measure of healthcare services accessibility. This measure has been widely employed in a variety of related studies [18,19].

In spite of the above mentioned advances in spatial analysis, most of the existing studies of the elderly in Singapore have focused on health and socio-economic correlates or determinants [20–26]. There have been some related studies, e.g., Wong, Heng [27], who used GIS to identify service gaps and suggest optimal sites for future polyclinics in Singapore. Koh, Leow [28] have also studied the mobility of the elderly in densely populated neighbourhoods in Singapore through a survey. Their study reflects more the perception of elderly subjects rather than objective effort to investigate the geographical accessibility of healthcare services for the elderly in Singapore.

In view of this dearth of spatial analysis for Singapore, this paper aims to assess the state of geographical accessibility of primary healthcare services for the elderly living in HDB flats in Singapore. This study is methodologically apt to the city-state of Singapore that is geographically confined with about 3 million resident populations.

2. Methodological Considerations

The early versions of a floating catchment area method have been used to measure geographical accessibility to calculate job accessibility. This is done by using the concept of a kernel density model estimation where the events within the kernel were used to represent the density at the center [29,30]. This has been considered a superior method for measuring geographical accessibility because it takes into consideration the cross-boundary demand and the distance decay effect [5,31].

Another popular method is the two-step floating catchment area (2SFCA) method, which is a gravity based model that takes into account both the accessibility and availability of population and service providers [4,32]. This method is intuitive while retaining the advantages of a gravity based model [18]. The 2SFCA method has been utilized in a variety of recent studies to measure healthcare services accessibility, e.g., measuring the accessibility of healthcare centers for villagers living in the Indian Alwar district of Rajasthan, the spatial accessibility of primary care physicians and mammography centers for women with breast cancer in the American Appalachian region, and the spatial accessibility of primary healthcare services for Australians [33–35]. However, caution is needed while using the method since it makes the unrealistic assumption of equal accessibility for all population living within each catchment area [4].

A distance decay function has been proposed in many studies to model continuous gradual decay within a threshold distance. The distance decay effect is dependent on the phenomena being studied and should be examined separately for each study to account for the different effect distance has on different groups of people for different types of services. Researchers have identified several common forms of the continuous distance decay function: linear decay, Butterworth filter, Gaussian function, inverse-power function, and negative exponential function [36,37]. The enhanced two-step floating catchment area (E2SFCA) method combines a chosen distance decay function with the 2SFCA method [21]. Researchers have used a kernel density function, a Gaussian function, a downward log-logistic function, amongst others, to model the distance decay function [5,38–41]. However, adjustments still need to be made to the final method to ensure a satisfactory real-world behaviour such as possibly adjusting the radius of a service area or even varying the catchment sizes [40,42,43].

The three-step floating catchment area (3SFCA) method attempts to overcome the possible overestimation of potential population demand in an area with access to multiple service facilities in view of lack of information about potential competition between service facilities by incorporating an extra step to calculate the selection weight in these situations [20]. However, Delamater [38] found that the 3SFCA method produced outcomes that do not necessarily match logic-based outcomes and overestimates the role of competition resulting in both and over- and under- estimation of spatial accessibility for the study area.

Therefore, considering the pros and cons of different approaches as well as the characteristics of our research context, we chose the E2SFCA method as adapted by incorporating a Gaussian distance decay function Equation (4) to estimate geographical accessibility.

The 2SFCA method is essentially a gravity-based accessibility measure of the spatial accessibility to healthcare resources [4,44]. In the first step, all population locations (k) that fall within a defined catchment area of a threshold travel time or distance (d_0) around physician location j are used to calculate the physician-to-population ratio (R_j) Equation (1):

$$R_j = \frac{S_j}{\sum_{j \in \{d_{kj} \leq d_0\}} P_k}$$

(1)

In the second step, for each population cluster (i), all physician-to-population ratios of facility locations (j) within the catchment area of a threshold travel time or distance (d_0) are summed to arrive at the spatial accessibility index of population cluster (A_i) Equation (2):

$$A_i = \sum_{j \in \{d_{ij} \leq d_0\}} R_j = \sum_{j \in \{d_{ij} \leq d_0\}} \frac{S_j}{\sum_{j \in \{d_{kj} \leq d_0\}} P_k}$$

(2)

Many studies have proposed a distance decay function (i.e., W_{kj}) to model the continuous gradual decay within a threshold distance, with no effect beyond the threshold distance. A possible model could use a continuous Gaussian distance-decay function. In Equation (3), $\beta = d_0/2$ and d_{kj} is the shortest network distance between population location k and physician location j:

$$W_{kj} = e^{\frac{-d_{kj}^2}{\beta^2}}$$

(3)

The distance decay function is then added into the 2SFCA method Equation (4):

$$A_i = \sum_{j \in \{d_{ij} \leq d_0\}} \frac{S_j}{\sum_{j \in \{d_{kj} \leq d_0\}} P_k W_{kj}}$$

(4)

Our study adopts an E2SFCA method based on the modified 2SFCA method proposed by Langford, Fry [37] and incorporates a Gaussian distance decay function Equation (4) to calculate geographical accessibility. These parameters will be introduced in the case study below.

3. Case Study

3.1. Background Information

The Singapore government has implemented several policies in light of city-state's ageing population, including increased healthcare support through an SGD$8 billion Pioneer Generation Fund [8,45]. All Singapore citizens born on or before the 31st of December 1949 and received their citizenship by 31 December 1986 are eligible for the benefits under the Pioneer Generation Scheme, which covers about 87% of the elderly in Singapore in 2017 [46,47]. With regard to healthcare, pioneers under this scheme can receive an additional 50% off on subsidized services at polyclinics, and special subsidies at private GPs participating in the CHAS.

In Singapore, there are two forms of primary healthcare services: private GP clinics and public polyclinics. Private GP clinics are dispersed in different neighbourhoods across the entire Singapore region. Normally, the patients can see the same doctor continuously, whereas public polyclinics provide subsidized services with less choices and convenience, and the patients are randomly allocated to a duty doctor [48–51]. It is necessary to note here that the elderly would benefit especially from the continuity of care [52] provided by GP clinics rather than public polyclinics.

Singapore's Ministry of Health acknowledges that only 20% of primary healthcare services is provided by government polyclinics while the remaining 80% is provided by private practitioners [48]. Although the elderly can already receive 50% off on subsidized services at polyclinics, there are only 18 polyclinics that they can choose from [50,51]. In addition, all Singaporeans and Permanent Residents receive subsidies at polyclinics to a very large extent, making polyclinics an attractive primary healthcare option for most Singaporean residents and increasing competition for medical attention [53]. On the other hand, only pioneers (predefined the elderly) and low-income individuals are eligible for subsidies at Private GP clinics participating in CHAS (henceforth referred to as "CHAS GPs"), with pioneers receiving the most subsidies [54]. Presently, there are 20 polyclinics, 1100 CHAS clinics, and 500 GP clinics [48].

Over the past decade, Singapore has seen an increasing doctor to population ratio, with an all-time high ratio of 1:430 in 2016 [55]. However, in a national survey commissioned by the Ministry of Social and Family Development in 2013, Singaporean elderly said that financial constraint and the lack of clinic or polyclinic near their homes were some of the major reasons for not seeking treatment [56]. While the subsidies under CHAS would ease the financial burden of seeing a doctor, the issue of the proximity to a clinic is still unclear despite the claim that there is a good geographical spread among CHAS GPs and more than 97% of pioneers have "more than one CHAS clinic within 1 km of their homes, or about 15 minutes by public transport" [57]. However, there are some elements that still worry the elderly, such as the difficulty in getting to a bus stop or MRT station, boarding or alighting, and maintaining their balance or obtaining a seat [58,59]. Singapore's elderly are mobile, with nearly 96% ambulant and physically independent, and 98% ambulant with the help of a walking aid [56]. Thus, if GP services are within walking distance, elderly in Singapore would be more willing to visit a doctor.

Furthermore, the Singapore's elderly living in HDB flats–Singapore's public housing–account for 80.6% of Singapore residents aged 65 or above, meaning that this group constitutes the majority of elderly population in Singapore [58]. Given that the average monthly income for HDB flats is less than half of the other dwelling types such as condominiums or landed properties, it stands to reason that elderly individuals living in HDB flats would face more financial constraints while seeking healthcare and would benefit two-fold from the CHAS subsidies, in terms of increased spatial accessibility, and more healthcare service options being made available to them [60].

3.2. Data Sources

The datasets used in this case study were provided by various Singapore government agencies—Housing Development Board (HDB), Singapore Land Authority (SLA), and Department of Statistics (SingStat). The unit of analysis used in this study is one HDB block.

3.2.1. Address Points

A shapefile containing all buildings in Singapore linking the address and postal code of the building to its geo-coded location was obtained from Singapore Land Authority (SLA).

3.2.2. HDB Address Points with Flat Type Information

HDB flats with flat type information cannot be collected directly nor purchased, but we managed to crawl the data by developing and using a Python script on the HDB website, which provides a map service where users can look at all the HDB flats in Singapore and obtain information about individual flats, such as the postal code and the number of each type of unit (Figure 1). This data is stored in XML files accessible through a URL that can be found in the Network tab under Developer Tools, and is available to anyone who accesses the website.

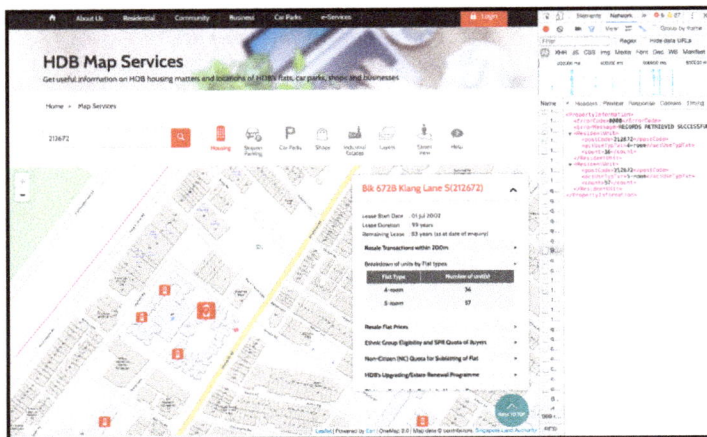

Figure 1. HDB's map service that shows detailed information about each flat. In the screenshot, a HDB flat with postal code "212672" was selected and the popup showing its information is displayed. The corresponding XML file was located in the Network tab of Developer Tools (Source: https://services2.hdb.gov.sg/web/fi10/emap.html last accessed on 12 November 2017).

A Python script was designed to run the URL for all postal codes in Singapore (obtained from the SLA Address Point dataset), read the XML file, and write the information into a csv file. If the building did not exist, then it was excluded from the output csv file. The script had to be run for over 24 h on three computers using PyCharm Community Edition 2017.2.4. Eventually, a csv containing the postal code and the number of each type of unit was produced.

3.2.3. Masterplan 2014 Planning Area

A shapefile containing Singapore's 2014 masterplan planning areas was obtained from data.gov.sg, a portal launched by the Singapore government to release publicly available datasets from various public agencies.

3.3. *Data Pre-Processing for Calculating Spatial Accessibility*

3.3.1. Location of HDBs in Singapore

A shapefile containing the location of HDBs in Singapore was produced by joining (1) SLA Address Point shapefile, (2) HDB postal codes with flat type information from the HDB website, and (3) URA's Masterplan 2014 Planning Areas. The map of all the HDBs can be seen from Figure 2.

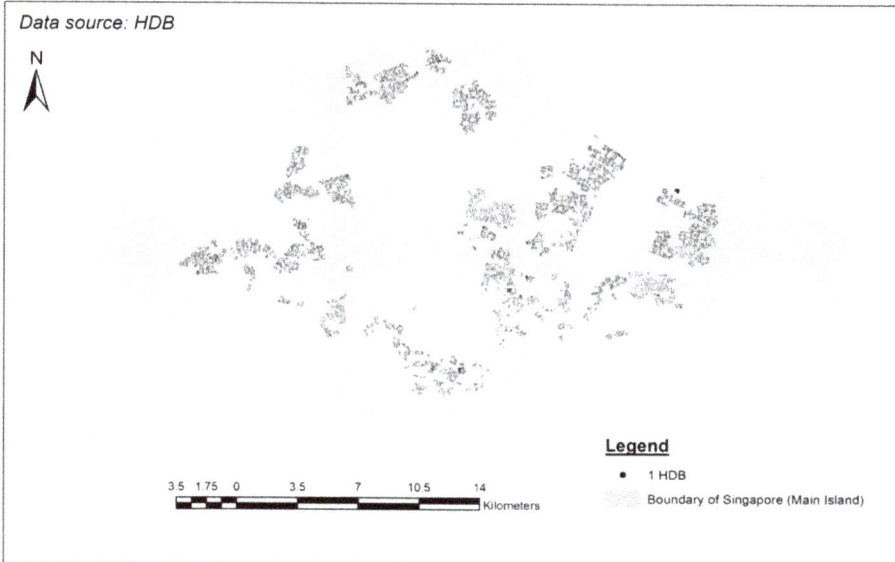

Figure 2. Map of HDBs in Singapore.

3.3.2. Population Density of Singapore Elderly Living in HDBs

A shapefile containing the population density of Singaporeans aged 65 and over per HDB block was produced using (1) a SingStat dataset categorizing the Singapore resident population by planning area, age group and type of dwelling in June 2017 and (2) URA's Masterplan 2014 Planning Areas. The map of the distribution of the elderly living in HDB flats can be seen from Figure 3.

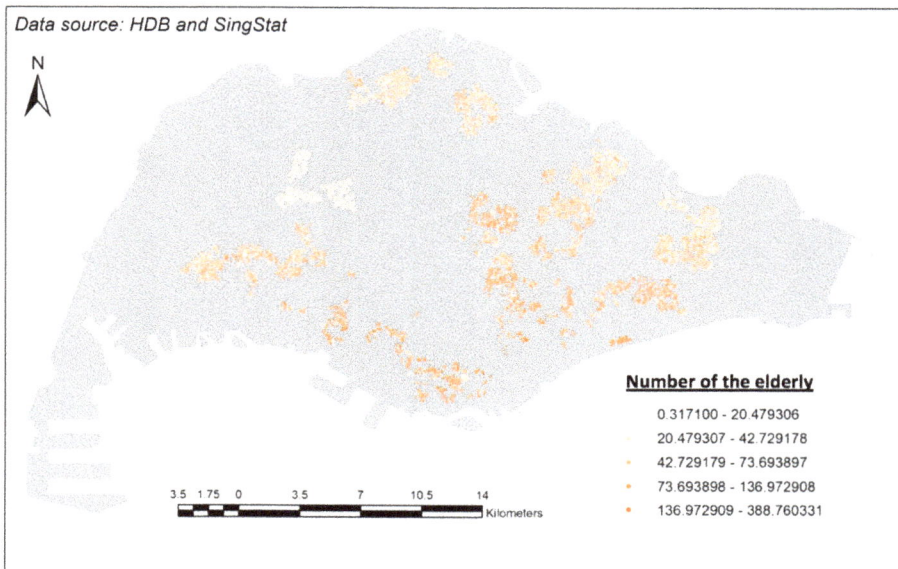

Figure 3. Density map of elderly living in HDB flats in Singapore.

3.3.3. Parameter Setting

In this study, A_i is the spatial accessibility index for a HDB at location i. P_k is the number of the elderly in a HDB flat at location k. S_j is assumed to be a constant value of 1 for all CHAS GPs because it is the minimum number of doctors that can possibly be available at each CHAS GP, ensuring there will not be an over-calculation of the physician-to-population ratio. d_{kj} is the distance between a CHAS GP at location j and a HDB flat at location k.

The threshold distance (d_0) was set at 400 m because the elderly prefer to live within 1 km of a healthcare center, and the distance covered by healthy Singaporeans up to age 85 in an assessment of their functional exercise capacity was 560–105 m, independent of age. The lower end of this range is 455 m. However, since no network dataset was used and it can be assumed that the route the elderly take to reach their chosen CHAS GP will not always be a straight line, 455 m was rounded down to 400 m. A distance threshold rather than a travel-time threshold was chosen because the elderly walk at a varied pace but, if healthy and willing, they are able to cover a certain distance in a given time [61–65].

3.4. Results

The A_i values ranged between 0.000027 and 0.351234. Figure 4 is a thematic map showing the A_i values; a darker shade of color represents a higher A_i value, and a lighter shade of color represents a lower A_i value.

A hot spot analysis was then performed on the A_i values. The Getis-Ord Gi* statistic for each HDB flat was calculated to find statistically significant hot spots of high or low value spatial clusters based on z-scores and p-values.

The result from hot spot analysis is shown in Figure 5, where the blue areas represent statistically significant clusters of cold spots, and the orange/red areas represent statistically significant clusters of hot spots. Within the clusters of cold spots, the lightest blue indicates a confidence level of 90%, while the darkest blue a confidence level of 99%, and so on. The yellow points represent areas where no statistically significant clusters are found.

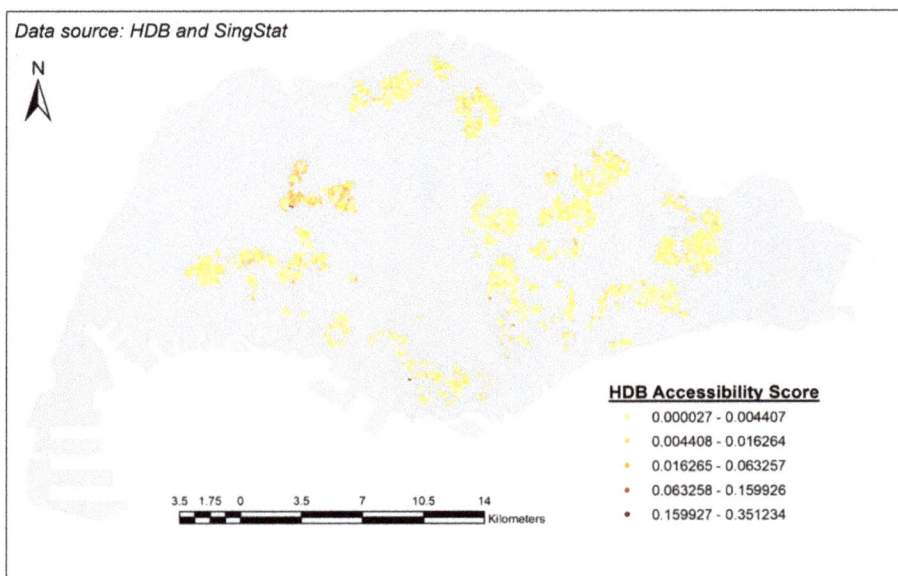

Figure 4. The A_i values of each HDB flat.

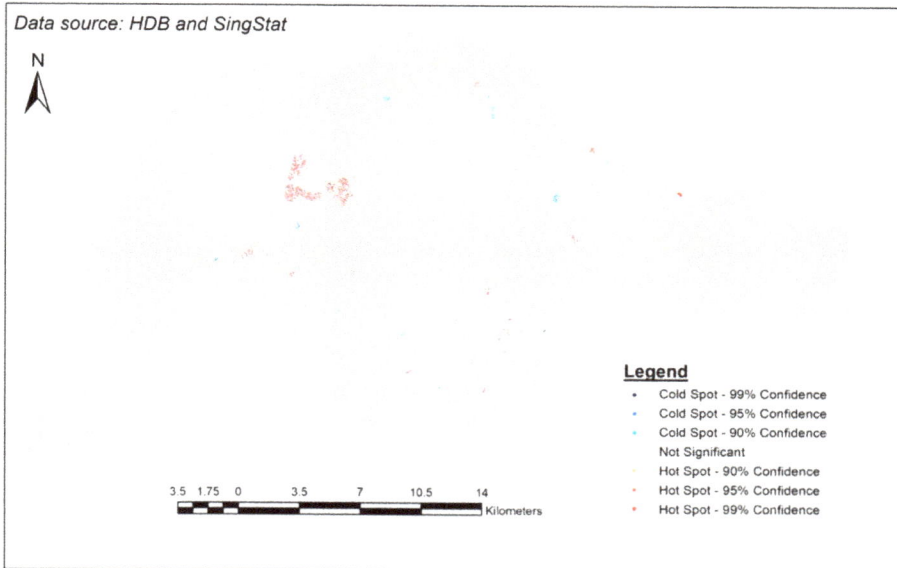

Figure 5. Results of the hot spot analysis.

4. Discussion

For further analysis and discussion, we produced a map demarcating the planning boundaries and displaying only the clusters of hot and cold spots (Figure 6).

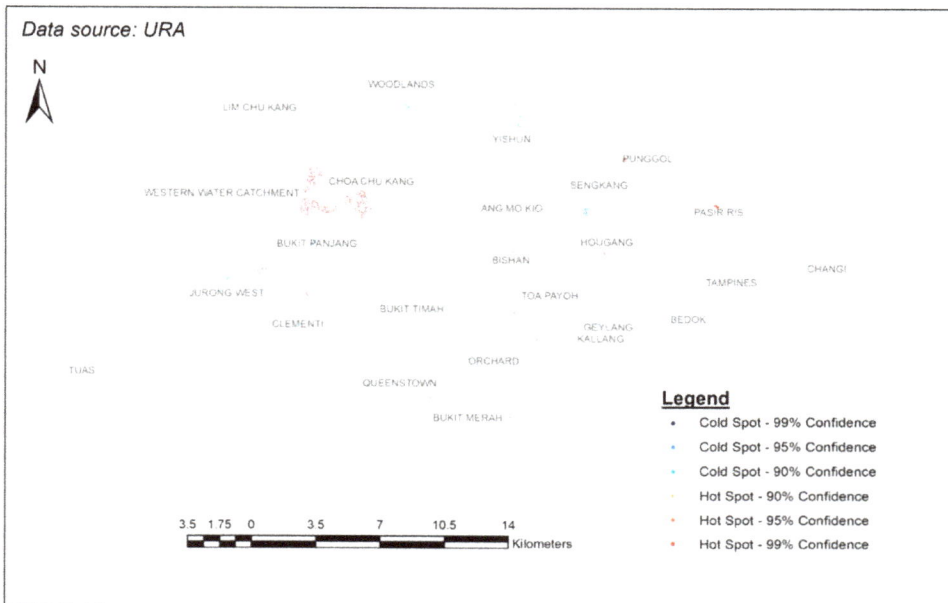

Figure 6. Results of hot spot analysis against the planning boundaries of Singapore.

4.1. Explanations on the Hot Spots

The hot spots could be a result of the maturity of the HDB Town. These spots are usually located in or near to towns and estates that were developed before the 1980s, In fact these towns are regarded as Mature Towns/Estates [66]. The Mature category includes areas such as Queenstown, Toa Payoh, Clementi, Kallang, and the Middle-Aged category includes areas such as Jurong West, Bukit Panjang, Choa Chu Kang, Hougang and Bukit Timah. In the map, these areas do have a cluster of hot spots, possibly due to the organic growth of businesses in the area over the years. Understandably it also includes GPs, and has a higher possibility of GPs in the area joining CHAS due to the larger number (competition per se) of GPs. Interestingly, some of these hot spots are very close to where the first HDB towns were built in the area. For example, the hot spot between Queenstown and Bukit Merah is located near Forfar Heights, which stands in the place of Forfar House, the very first high-rise apartment block built in 1956 [67,68]. Another example would be the hot spot in the north of Yishun, which is located very close to the Chong Pang area, where the first HDB flats were built in the 1980s [67].

Another reason for the hot spots could be the government's setting up of rejuvenation projects in the area. The Singapore government announced the Remaking Our Heartland (ROH) initiative in 2007 to help mature HDB towns keep up with modern designs [46]. This initiative tailors renewal plans based on the needs of the community and ensures that the areas remain relevant and sustainable while still maintaining their unique characteristics [69]. Areas like Punggol and Yishun were part of the first batch of the chosen towns in 2007, and Hougang was part of the second batch in 2011. An outcome of this initiative is that more GPs moved to these areas attracted by new facilities such as community plazas and the enhancement of community and connectivity. This would cause an increase in the number of people who would potentially visit the community plaza, thereby providing the GPs with a larger potential consumer market [70]. Such an increased number of GPs would once again result in more GPs in the area joining CHAS. With the ongoing and future projects under the ROH initiative, this could attract more GPs to new areas and provide more primary healthcare services.

4.2. Explanations on the Cold Spots

As for the cold spots, one very compelling reason could be the locations of polyclinics. The spread of polyclinics does seem to match the spread of cold spots (Figure 7). As mentioned earlier, it would be cheaper for elderly individuals to visit a polyclinic (further 50% subsidy on the already subsidized services). Thus, it makes sense that GPs would try to avoid being close to them. On the other hand, GPs may not have sufficient number of patients to join CHAS. This would then result in fewer GPs in the area participating in CHAS (cold spots). It is quite likely that additional incentives are needed if the government wants to encourage more GPs in the area to participate in CHAS.

Another reason for cold spots could relate to the government's city planning. For example, Punggol is considered a "young" area because it was one of the few areas that had build-to-order (BTO) HDB flats in around 2011. Since eligibility to purchase requires at least a nuclear family, the demographics of the area tend to be young families and their children. This is actually echoed in the figure where more than 11% of Punggol's residents are aged 4 and below [47,71]. Consequently, the infrastructure of the neighbourhood is featured with 52 childcare centers and two mega childcare centers with 1000 places in each [71]. This concentration of efforts for a certain demographic group may also mean overlooking the other, namely the elderly. A more balanced and comprehensive town planning may be required while planning future new towns.

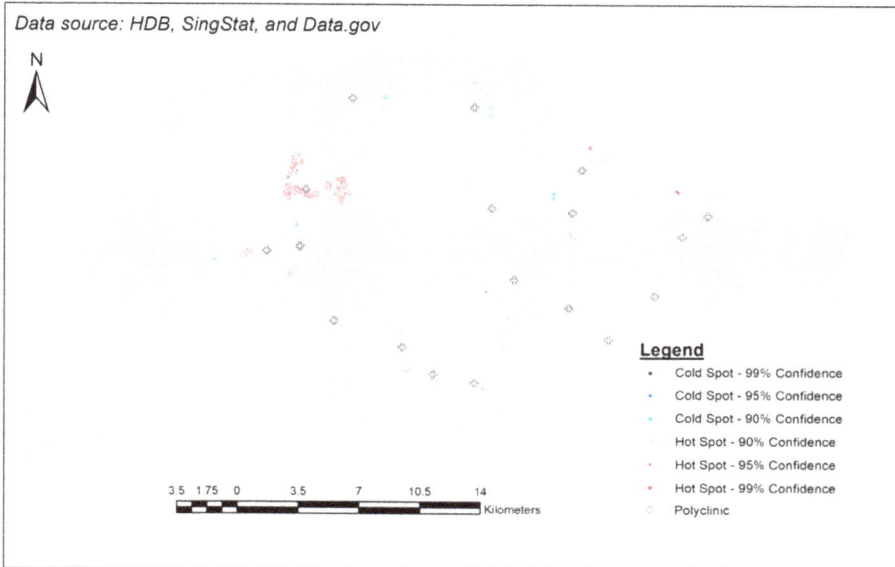

Figure 7. Results of hot spot analysis against locations of polyclinics.

4.3. More Implications

In this study, GIS concept and methods have been utilized to measure geographical accessibility of one major type of primary healthcare services, i.e., CHAS GPs, to a scale of HDB flats, i.e., the elderly living in HDB flats. This has worked better than in most other studies using the centroid of a census population tract to indicate the demand for all individuals within the same catchment area [4,18,43,44,72]. This advantage is a direct outcome of the finer scale this research has reached. Therefore, the results are considered more reliable for policy makers in the relevant fields. In the short term, more efforts could be put into convincing and incentivizing GPs located near areas with clusters of low accessibility scores to participate in CHAS so as to improve the elderly's geographical accessibility to a GP at a subsidized cost. In addition, it should be noted that even within the areas that do not have statistically significant clusters of high or low values, there are still individual places that may have low accessibility scores. These findings can also contribute the decision making process in terms of directing the current and future efforts in CHAS.

On the other hand, geographically (according to the map) more specific efforts should be put into increasing the number of CHAS GPs in certain areas. It is worth noting that cold-spot areas such as Woodlands, Hougang/Sengkang/Punggol, Geylang, and Bishan/Ang Mo Kio are quite far away from any hot spots, making it quite impossible to draw on the resources in the hot-spot areas. It is important to note that in a small city-state like Singapore, although planning boundaries were used to direct attention to specific hot or cold spots, people may not view area boundary as the administratively determined boundary. This could contribute to the existence of both hot and cold spots within one planning boundary. There is a need for greater flexibility with the administrative arrangement so that elderly citizens may draw on a nearby yet different administrative area.

In the long term, based on the hot spot analysis or accessibility scores, follow-up research efforts should be put into the optimization study to find out the best locations to set up GPs who are considering setting up new service centers. Carrying out a hot spot analysis on a regular basis, such as once per year, has the potential to inform/update the status of gaps between the demand from the elderly and the supply from existing CHAS GPs.

4.4. Limitations

One major limitation of the study relates to the distance decay function used, which reflects the willingness to access a medical service and its determinant should be a function of a variety of factors that is unique to the population under study. Ideally, the distance decay function should be generated following an empirical investigation possibly applying regression methods on the data collected. However, such a dataset was not available for this study, so a mathematical model had to be used in this study as in many other studies [18,33,73–78]. Secondly, this study is cross-sectional rather than a longitudinal study. There certainly are some dynamic factors that may bring about very different results over time. Among them are targeted healthcare policy, increased health hazards caused by global warming, and change in economy that may affect the contribution of income and savings to elderly parents. These are all beyond the scope and control of this study.

5. Conclusions

Rapid ageing is a major regional if not global demographic challenge; it is not just faced by Singapore, but many other countries. Primary healthcare services are critical to the elderly, and it is important not only to have the concerned services available, but also has to be geographically accessible. This study has examined the geographical accessibility of one representative healthcare service, i.e., CHAS GPs, for the elderly living in HDBs at the block level in Singapore by employing an enhanced 2-step floating catchment area method and a Gaussian distance-decay function in combination with the GIS technology. This research has succeeded in reflecting the current status of the geographical accessibility of CHAS GPs for elderly individuals living in HDBs across the entire Singapore. Areas with relatively weak geographical accessibility of CHAS GPs have been spotted, explained and discussed. Suggestions have been put forward for policy makers, and the value of using innovative technology and approaches has been demonstrated, along with recommendation for future studies. In the long run, the spatial analysis should also be repeated on a regular basis for better understanding the change in geographical accessibility of CHAS GPs alongside the change of the elderly demographics in Singapore. Similar geographical accessibility studies could be conducted with respect to a variety of healthcare resources such as general hospitals, polyclinics, post-acute care, with support from GIS, for meeting the needs of the elderly and other specific groups.

Author Contributions: O.M.L.D., M.Y.L.C. and K.C. conceived the research ideas and wrote the paper; O.M.L.D. and K.C. conceived and designed the experiments; O.M.L.D. performed the experiments and analyzed the data; M.Y.L.C. and K.C. contributed to subsequent manuscript revisions.

Acknowledgments: This work was supported by the research grant (R-101-000-054-720) from the Next Age Institute (NAI) at the National University of Singapore.

Conflicts of Interest: The authors declare no conflicts of interest.

References and Note

1. Bynum, J.; Chang, C.; Austin, A.; Carmichael, D.; Meara, E. Outcomes in Older Adults with Multimorbidity Associated with Predominant Provider of Care Specialty. *J. Am. Geriatr. Soc.* **2017**, *65*, 1916–1923. [CrossRef] [PubMed]
2. Edwards, S.; Landon, B. Seeking Value in Healthcare: The Importance of Generalists as Primary Care Physicians. *J. Am. Geriatr. Soc.* **2017**, *65*, 1900–1901. [CrossRef] [PubMed]
3. Deraas, T.; Berntsen, G.; Jones, A.; Førde, O.; Sund, E. Associations between primary healthcare and unplanned medical admissions in Norway: A multilevel analysis of the entire elderly population. *BMJ Open* **2014**, *4*, e004293. [CrossRef] [PubMed]
4. Luo, W.; Wang, F. Measure of spatial accessibility to healthcare in a GIS environment: Synthesis and a case study in the Chicago region. *Environ. Plan. B* **2003**, *30*, 865–884. [CrossRef]
5. Guagliardo, M. Spatial accessibility of primary care: Concept, methods and challenges. *Int. J. Health Geogr.* **2004**, *3*. [CrossRef] [PubMed]

6. Joseph, A.E.; Phillips, D.R. *Accessibility and Utilization: Geographical Perspectives on Health Care Delivery*; Sage: Newcastle upon Tyne, UK, 1984.

7. DOS. Population Trends. 2017. Available online: https://www.singstat.gov.sg/statistics/visualising-data/storyboards/population-trends (accessed on 12 November 2017).

8. NPTD. Ageing. 2017. Available online: https://www.population.sg/ageing (accessed on 12 November 2017).

9. MOH. Speech by Mr Gan Kim Yong, Minister for Health, at the SG50 Scientific Conference on Ageing, on 19 March 2015, 'Ageing in Singapore in the Next 50 Years'.

10. Cheng, Y. *Residential Care for Elderly People in Beijing*; A Study of the Relationship between Health and Place: Beijing, China, 2010.

11. Loo, B.P.; Lam, W.W.Y. Geographic accessibility around health care facilities for elderly residents in Hong Kong: A microscale walkability assessment. *Environ. Plan. B Plan. Des.* **2012**, *39*, 629–646.

12. Wei, Z. A Study of Accessibility to Health Facilities for Elderly People in Metro Atlanta Using a Categorical Multi-Step Floating Catchment Area Method. Master's Thesis, University of Georgia, Athens, GA, USA, 2013.

13. MOH. Life Expectancy in Singapore. 2016. Available online: http://www.singstat.gov.sg/docs/default-source/default-document-library/publications/publications_and_papers/births_and_deaths/lifetable15-16.pdf (accessed on 12 November 2017).

14. Khan, A. An integrated approach to measuring potential spatial access to health care services. *Soc.-Econ. Plan. Sci.* **1992**, *26*, 275–287. [CrossRef]

15. Wing, P.; Reynolds, C. The availability of physician services: A geographic analysis. *Health Serv. Res.* **1988**, *23*, 649–667. [PubMed]

16. Huff, D.L. A probabilistic analysis of shopping center trade areas. *Land Econ.* **1963**, *39*, 81–90. [CrossRef]

17. Huff, D.L. Defining and estimating a trading area. *J. Mark.* **1964**, *28*, 34–38. [CrossRef]

18. Luo, W.; Qi, Y. An enhanced two-step floating catchment area (E2SFCA) method for measuring spatial accessibility to primary care physicians. *Health Place* **2009**, *15*, 110–1107. [CrossRef] [PubMed]

19. Joseph, A.E.; Bantock, P.R. Measuring potential physical accessibility to general practitioners in rural areas: A method and case study. *Soc. Sci. Med.* **1982**, *16*, 85–90. [CrossRef]

20. Seow, L.S.E.; Subramaniam, M.; Abdin, E.; Vaingankar, J.A.; Chong, S.A. Hypertension and its associated risks among Singapore elderly residential population. *J. Clin. Gerontol. Geriatr.* **2015**, *6*, 125–132. [CrossRef]

21. Lim, W.S.; Ding, Y.Y. Evidence-balance Medicine: "Real" Evidence-based Medicine in the Elderly. *Ann. Acad. Med.* **2015**, *44*, 1–5.

22. Tan, N.E.; Sagayadevan, V.; Abdin, E.; Picco, L.; Vaingankar, J.; Chong, S.A.; Subramaniam, M. Employment status among the Singapore elderly and its correlates. *Psychogeriatrics* **2017**, *17*, 155–163. [CrossRef] [PubMed]

23. Kua, E.H. *Colours of Ageing: 30 Years of Research on the Mental Health of the Singapore Elderly*; Write Editions: Singapore, 2017. Available online: http://www.nlb.gov.sg/biblio/202747162 (accessed on 12 November 2017).

24. Chen, A.J.; Cheung PP, L. *The Elderly in Singapore*; ASEAN Population Co-ordinating Unit: Singapore, 1988.

25. Wee, L.E.; Yong, Y.Z.; Chng, M.W.X.; Chew, S.H.; Cheng, L.; Chua, Q.H.A.; Yek, J.J.L.; Lau, L.J.F.; Anand, P.; Hoe, J.T.M.; et al. Individual and area-level socioeconomic status and their association with depression amongst community-dwelling elderly in Singapore. *Aging Ment. Health* **2014**, *18*, 628–641. [CrossRef] [PubMed]

26. Yap, M.T. *State of the Elderly in Singapore 2008–2009*; Ministry of Community Development, Youth and Sports: Singapore, 2010.

27. Wong, L.Y.; Heng, B.H.; Cheah, J.T.S.; Tan, C.B. Using spatial accessibility to identify polyclinic service gaps and volume of under-served population in Singapore using Geographic Information System. *Int. J. Health Plan. Manag.* **2012**, *27*. [CrossRef] [PubMed]

28. Koh, P.; Leow, B.; Wong, Y. Mobility of the elderly in densely populated neighbourhoods in Singapore. *Sustain. Cities Soc.* **2015**, *14*, 126–132. [CrossRef]

29. Peng, Z. The job-housing balance and urban commuting. *Urban Stud.* **1997**, *34*, 1215–1235. [CrossRef]

30. Wang, F. Modeling commuting patterns in Chicago in a GIS environment: A job accessibility perspective. *Prof. Geogr.* **2000**, *52*, 120–133. [CrossRef]

31. Silverman, B.W. *Density Estimation for Statistics and Data Analysis*; Chapman and Hall: London, UK, 1986.

32. Luo, W.; Qi, Y. Using a GIS-based floating catchment method to assess areas with shortage of physicians. *Health Place* **2004**, *10*, 1–11. [CrossRef]
33. Kanuganti, S.; Sarkar, A.; Singh, A. Evaluation of access to health care in rural areas using enhanced two-step floating catchment area (E2SFCA) method. *J. Transp. Geogr.* **2016**, *56*, 45–52. [CrossRef]
34. Donohoe, J.; Marshall, V.; Tan, X.; Camacho, F.; Anderson, R.; Balkrishnan, R. Predicting Late-stage Breast Cancer Diagnosis and Receipt of Adjuvant Therapy: Applying Current Spatial Access to Care Methods in Appalachia. *Med. Care* **2015**, *53*, 980–988. [CrossRef] [PubMed]
35. McGrail, M.R.; Humphreys, J.S. Measuring spatial accessibility to primary healthcare services: Utilising dynamic catchment sizes. *Appl. Geogr.* **2014**, *54*, 182–188. [CrossRef]
36. Kwan, M.P. Space-time and integral measures of individual accessibility: A comparative analysis using a point-based framework. *Geogr. Anal.* **1998**, *30*, 191–216. [CrossRef]
37. Langford, M.; Fry, R.; Higgs, G. Measuring transit system accessibility using a modified two-step floating catchment technique. *Int. J. Geogr. Inf. Sci.* **2012**, *26*, 193–214. [CrossRef]
38. Delamater, P.L. Spatial accessibility in suboptimally configured health care systems: A modified two-step floating catchment area (M2SFCA) metric. *Health Place* **2013**, *24*, 30–43. [CrossRef] [PubMed]
39. Dai, D. Black residential segregation, disparities in spatial access to health care facilities, and late-stage breast cancer diagnosis in metropolitan Detroit. *Health Place* **2010**, *16*, 1038–1052. [CrossRef] [PubMed]
40. Wang, F. Measurement, optimization, and impact of health care accessibility: A methodological review. *Ann. Assoc. Am. Geogr.* **2012**, *102*, 1104–1112. [CrossRef] [PubMed]
41. Dai, D.; Wang, F. Geographic disparities in accessibility to food stores in southwest Mississippi. *Environ. Plan. B Plan. Des.* **2011**, *38*, 659–677. [CrossRef]
42. Yang, D.H.; Goerge, R.; Mullner, R. Comparing GIS-based methods of 187 measuring spatial accessibility to health services. *J. Med. Syst.* **2006**, *30*, 23–32. [CrossRef] [PubMed]
43. Luo, W.; Whippo, T. Variable catchment sizes for the two-step floating catchment area (2SFCA) method. *Health Place* **2012**, *18*, 789–795. [CrossRef] [PubMed]
44. Schuurman, N.; Bérubé, M.; Crooks, V. Measuring potential spatial access to primary health care physicians using a modified gravity model. *Can. Geogr. Géogr. Can.* **2010**, *54*, 29–45. [CrossRef]
45. MOF. Pioneer Generation Package is Adequately Funded and will be Transparent. 2014. Available online: http://www.mof.gov.sg/news-reader/articleid/1446/parentId/59/year/undefined?wmode=transparent (accessed on 12 November 2017).
46. Singapore_Government. Pioneer Generation Package Overview. 2017. Available online: https://www.pioneers.sg/en-sg/Pages/Overview.aspx (accessed on 12 November 2017).
47. DOS. *Resident Population by Planning Area, Age Group and Type of Dwelling Jun 2017*; DOS: Singapore, 2017.
48. MOH. Healthcare Institution Statistics. 2017. Available online: https://www.moh.gov.sg/content/moh_web/home/statistics/healthcare_institutionstatistics.html (accessed on 12 November 2017).
49. MOH. Polyclinics. 2011. Available online: https://www.moh.gov.sg/content/moh_web/home/pressRoom/Parliamentary_QA/2011/polyclinics.html (accessed on 12 November 2017).
50. NHGP. Our Clinics. 2017. Available online: https://www.nhgp.com.sg/Find_A_Polyclinic_Near_You/ (accessed on 12 November 2017).
51. SingHealth. About Us. 2014. Available online: https://polyclinic.singhealth.com.sg/aboutus/ourpolyclinics/Pages/home.aspx (accessed on 12 November 2017).
52. Saultz, J.; Lochner, J. Interpersonal Continuity of Care and Care Outcomes: A Critical Review. *Ann. Fam. Med.* **2005**, *3*, 159–166. [CrossRef] [PubMed]
53. MOH. Primary Care Subsidies. 2017. Available online: https://www.moh.gov.sg/content/moh_web/home/pressRoom/Current_Issues/2014/s-3ms-resources/primary-care-subsidies.html (accessed on 12 November 2017).
54. CHAS. About CHAS. 2017. Available online: http://www.chas.sg/content.aspx?id=636 (accessed on 12 November 2017).
55. MOH. Health Manpower. 2017. Available online: https://www.moh.gov.sg/content/moh_web/home/statistics/Health_Facts_Singapore/Health_Manpower.html (accessed on 12 November 2017).

56. Kang, S.; Tan, E.; Yap, M. National Survey of Senior Citizens 2011. 2013. Available online: Duke-nus.edu.sg: https://www.duke-nus.edu.sg/care/wp-content/uploads/National-Survey-of-Senior-Citizens-2011.pdf (accessed on 12 November 2017).

57. MOH. Bulk of Clinics Are in CHAS Scheme. 2017. Available online: https://www.moh.gov.sg/content/moh_web/home/pressRoom/Media_Forums/2017/bulk-of-clinics-are-in-chas-scheme.html (accessed on 12 November 2017).

58. LTA. Enhancing Physical Accessibility for All. Making Travel Easier For You; Public Transport; 2017. Available online: https://www.lta.gov.sg/content/ltaweb/en/public-transport/system-design/enhancing-physical-accessibility-for-all.html (accessed on 12 November 2017).

59. Krishnasamy, C.; Unsworth, C.; Howie, L. Exploring the mobility preferences and perceived difficulties in using transport and driving with a sample of healthy and outpatient older adults in Singapore. *Aust. Occup. Ther. J.* **2013**, *60*, 129–137. [CrossRef] [PubMed]

60. DOS. Table 11A. Average Monthly Household Income from Work (Including Employer CPF Contributions) Among Resident Employed Households by Type of Dwelling, 2000–2016. 2017. Available online: http://www.tablebuilder.singstat.gov.sg/publicfacing/createSpecialTable.action?refId=12315 (accessed on 12 November 2017).

61. Bollard, E.; Fleming, H. A study to investigate the walking speed of elderly adults with relation to pedestrian crossings. *Physiother. Theory Pract.* **2013**, *29*, 142–149. [CrossRef] [PubMed]

62. Fiser, W.; Hays, N.; Rogers, S.; Kajkenova, O.; Williams, A.; Evans, C.; Evans, W. Energetics of Walking in Elderly People: Factors Related to Gait Speed. *J. Gerontol. Ser. A Biol. Sci. Med. Sci.* **2010**, *65*, 1332–1337. [CrossRef] [PubMed]

63. Harwood, R.; Conroy, S. Slow walking speed in elderly people. *BMJ* **2009**, *339*, b4236. [CrossRef] [PubMed]

64. Lindemann, U.; Najafi, B.; Zijlstra, W.; Hauer, K.; Muche, R.; Becker, C.; Aminian, K. Distance to achieve steady state walking speed in frail elderly persons. *Gait Posture* **2008**, *27*, 91–96. [CrossRef] [PubMed]

65. Yeo, S.; He, Y. Commuter characteristics in mass rapid transit stations in Singapore. *Fire Saf. J.* **2009**, *44*, 183–191. [CrossRef]

66. HDB. *Public Housing in Singapore: Residents' Profile, Housing Satisfaction and Preferences*; HDB: Singapore, 2014.

67. HDB. History. 2017. Available online: http://www.hdb.gov.sg/cs/infoweb/about-us/history (accessed on 12 November 2017).

68. Remember_Singapore. From Villages to Flats (Part 2)—Public Housing in Singapore. 2012. Available online: https://remembersingapore.org/2012/05/11/from-villages-to-flats-part-2/ (accessed on 12 November 2017).

69. HDB. Remaking Our Heartland. 2017. Available online: http://www20.hdb.gov.sg/fi10/fi10349p.nsf/hdbroh/index.html (accessed on 12 November 2017).

70. Karthigayan, R. Remarking Our Heartland—Rejuvenating Singapore. 2017. Available online: https://www.gov.sg/news/content/remaking-our-heartlands-rejuvenating-singapore (accessed on 12 November 2017).

71. Abdullah, Z. *Punggol*: Singapore's Baby Town. *The Straits Times*. 8 June 2017. Available online: http://www.straitstimes.com/singapore/singapores-baby-town (accessed on 12 November 2017).

72. Kuai, X.; Zhao, Q. Examining healthy food accessibility and disparity in Baton Rouge, Louisiana. *Ann. GIS* **2017**, *23*, 103–116. [CrossRef]

73. Yu, J.C. GIS-Based Approach to the Characterisation of Spatial Accessibility to Primary Health Care Facilities in the Melbourne Metropolitan Area. Master's Thesis, RMIT University, RMIT University Research Repository, Melbourne, Australia, 2014.

74. Dai, D. Racial/ethnic and socioeconomic disparities in urban green space accessibility: Where to intervene. *Landsc. Urban Plan.* **2011**, *102*, 234–244. [CrossRef]

75. Ni, J.; Wang, J.; Rui, Y.; Qian, T.; Wang, J. An Enhanced Variable Two-Step Floating Catchment Area Method for Measuring Spatial Accessibility to Residential Care Facilities in Nanjing. *Int. J. Environ. Res. Public Health* **2015**, *12*, 14490–14504. [CrossRef] [PubMed]

76. Polo, G.; Acosta, C.M.; Ferreira, F.; Dias, R.A. Location-Allocation and Accessibility Models for Improving Spatial Planning of Public Health Services. *PLoS ONE* **2015**, *10*, e0119190. [CrossRef] [PubMed]

77. Zhan, Q.; Wang, X.; Sliuzas, R. A GIS-based method to assess the shortage areas of community health service. In Proceedings of the 2011 International Conference On Remote Sensing, Environment and Transportation Engineering, Nanjing, China, 24–26 June 2011; pp. 5654–5657. [CrossRef]
78. Polo, G.; Acosta, C.M.; Dias, R.A. Spatial accessibility to vaccination sites in a campaign against rabies in São Paulo city, Brazil. *Prev. Vet. Med.* **2013**, *111*, 10–16. [CrossRef] [PubMed]

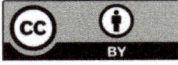

Article

International Journal of
*Environmental Research
and Public Health*

MDPI

An Analytical Framework for Integrating the Spatiotemporal Dynamics of Environmental Context and Individual Mobility in Exposure Assessment: A Study on the Relationship between Food Environment Exposures and Body Weight

Jue Wang * and Mei-Po Kwan

Department of Geography and Geographic Information Science, Natural History Building,
1301 W Green Street University of Illinois at Urbana-Champaign, Urbana, IL 61801, USA; mpk654@gmail.com
* Correspondence: kingjue.w@gmail.com

Received: 31 August 2018; Accepted: 13 September 2018; Published: 15 September 2018

Abstract: In past studies, individual environmental exposures were largely measured in a static manner. In this study, we develop and implement an analytical framework that dynamically represents environmental context (the environmental context cube) and effectively integrates individual daily movement (individual space-time tunnel) for accurately deriving individual environmental exposures (the environmental context exposure index). The framework is applied to examine the relationship between food environment exposures and the overweight status of 46 participants using data collected with global positioning systems (GPS) in Columbus, Ohio, and binary logistic regression models. The results indicate that the proposed framework generates more reliable measurements of individual food environment exposures when compared to other widely used methods. Taking into account the complex spatial and temporal dynamics of individual environmental exposures, the proposed framework also helps to mitigate the uncertain geographic context problem (UGCoP). It can be used in other environmental health studies concerning environmental influences on a wide range of health behaviors and outcomes.

Keywords: environmental health; food environment; environmental context cube; environmental context exposure index; the uncertain geographic context problem (UGCoP); GPS; GIS

---

1. Instruction

Environment-related chronic diseases are one of the biggest threats to public health. According to the World Health Organization (WHO), 22% of the global burden of disease is caused by environmental risks [1]. Because environmental exposure is a significant factor that influences health behaviors and outcomes, researchers in public health and health geography have put considerable effort into assessing environmental impacts on health [2–4]. Evidence shows that exposures to different environmental factors, such as air and noise pollution [5–7], the built environment [2,4,8,9] and the food environment [10–14], have significant associations with various health behaviors, including physical activity [2,15,16], tobacco and drug use [17–20], and health outcomes, which includes obesity and obesity-related disease [21–25] and mental health disorders [26–29].

The food environment, among different environmental factors, is one of the critical factors that could lead to obesity [30] and other obesity-related chronic diseases such as type II diabetes [31] and cardiovascular diseases [32], whose prevalence has increased rapidly in recent decades [33]. Increasing public concerns have prompted a growing number of studies on the effects of food environment exposures on obesity. Previous studies found that living in food desserts [34] and exposures to unhealthy food outlets [35] may encourage unhealthy food intake behavior that is associated with a higher likelihood of obesity. Furthermore, the association between food environment exposures and obesity has been utilized in developing intervention strategies to improve public health by numerous institutions worldwide [36–38].

However, the findings of the effects of food environment exposures on obesity are inconsistent [13,39,40]. Although a higher likelihood of obesity has been found to be significantly associated with exposures to unhealthy food (e.g., fast food restaurants) in many studies [12,41], it was not observed in other research [42–44]. For example, exposures to fast food restaurants were found to be positively associated with the prevalence of obesity in some studies [35,45,46], while no correlation [47,48] or even negative association [49] was observed in other studies. The inconsistent findings regarding the effects of the food environment on obesity bring enormous challenges on implementing effective policy to improve public health.

Many potential issues could cause these inconsistent findings (e.g., the modifiable areal unit problem [50], the uncertain geographic context problem [50], and spatial non-stationarity [51]). To examine whether the food environment has significant influences on obesity, an important task is to accurately measure individual exposure to relevant environmental factors [52]. Past studies that examine the effects of environmental exposures on health outcomes have predominantly used residential neighborhoods as contextual units [53]. In these studies, residential neighborhoods were defined either by the administration units (e.g., census tracts) in which people's homes are located or by buffer areas with a specific radius around people's home location [54–56]. However, residential neighborhoods only partially represent the environmental context that affects people's health, since people move around in their daily life [57–59]. Identifying environmental context based solely on the residential neighborhood may thus lead to inaccurate contextual exposure assessment and erroneous results concerning the relationships between environmental contexts and health outcomes [60,61]. This methodological issue may contribute to the inconsistent findings of past studies and has been articulated as the uncertain geographic context problem (UGCoP) by Kwan [62].

The UGCoP refers to the problem that findings about the effects of environmental factors (e.g., exposure to fast food restaurants) on individual health outcomes (e.g., obesity) could be affected by how contextual units are geographically delineated and the "temporal uncertainty in the timing and duration in which individuals experienced these contextual influences" [63]. In light of the dynamic nature of people's daily activity, people's movement in space and time should be taken into account while measuring their food environment exposures and its effects on obesity [60]. To mitigate the UGCoP, portable GPS devices can be utilized to accurately trace human movement in space and time, and advanced GIS methods can be used to relate activity locations to relevant environmental risk factors [63,64]. Further, GPS trajectories can be used to derive human activity space, which is more representative of people's daily context than the residential neighborhood [65]. The integration of GPS and GIS provides a powerful means for investigating the relationships between environmental contexts and health outcomes [58,66].

Individual GPS trajectories capture people's movement in space and time and thus help mitigate the UGCoP through more accurately delineating contextual units. A growing number of studies have started to adopt GPS-based activity space methods to investigate environmental effects on health outcomes [30,67,68]. However, environmental contexts can vary over time in a highly complex manner and are thus temporally uncertain [50]. Some contextual variables change over the 24-h period of a day (e.g., air pollution and the food environment), and some change over the seasons [7,69]. The temporal uncertainty of the environmental context is mostly ignored and not taken into account in environmental exposure assessment in previous studies. With regard to the food environment, food outlets open and close according to their daily schedules. Furthermore, many food outlets have different opening hours for weekdays and weekends. Given the complexity and spatiotemporal uncertainties of the food environment, it is highly challenging to accurately delineate the environmental context and assess individual exposures to the food environment. The UGCoP may introduce considerable errors to the results if the spatial and temporal variability of the food environment and people's daily movement in relation to such environment are not appropriately considered, but most previous research has paid little attention to them.

To address the challenges of the UGCoP, this paper proposes an analytical framework that utilizes GIS, time geography and GPS trajectory data to assess individual food environmental exposures for environmental health studies. In the framework, an environmental context cube (ECC) integrates variations in the food environment over space and time into a 3-D cube. By buffering individual GPS trajectories in 3-D to generate the individual space-time tunnel (ISTT) and projecting it into the ECC, environmental exposures can be derived and assessed by identifying the 3-D intersection of the ISTT and ECC. Based on the intersection, we calculate the environmental context exposure index (ECEI) as a standardized measure of individual exposure to the food environment. Considering both the spatiotemporal variations in the food environment and the dynamics of people's daily movement, the ECEI may provide a more accurate and reliable measurement of individual exposure to the food environment. The ECEI is utilized in this study to explore the relationship between individual food environment exposures and the overweight status for 46 participants using data collected with GPS in Columbus, Ohio, and binary logistic regression models. The results indicate that the proposed framework is effective for assessing individual exposures and investigating their health effects when compared with other widely used food environment exposures assessment methods. Addressing the spatiotemporal variations of contextual influences, the framework may help mitigate the spatial and temporal uncertainties in the food environment in public health studies. Further, the methodology is also useful in a wide range of environmental health research.

2. The Proposed Analytical Framework

This study proposes an analytical framework for assessing the effects of environmental exposures on individual health outcomes using food environment as an example. The framework seeks to more accurately measure individual food environment exposures so that more robust research findings can be obtained. Figure 1 illustrates the framework that integrates GIS, time geography, and GPS tracking. For this study, the food environment (BMI-unhealthy food outlets) is selected to generate 3-D environmental context cubes (ECC) for weekdays, Saturdays, and Sundays, which represent the spatial and temporal dynamics of the environmental contexts. By buffering individual GPS trajectories in 3-D, an individual space-time tunnel (ISTT) is generated to represent individual exposure space. By projecting the 3-D ISTT into the corresponding 3-D ECC and identifying their intersection, the individual environmental context exposure index (ECEI) can be derived as a standardized exposure measure. Based on the ECEI, the effect of the food environment on overweight is explored with statistical models, and the results are compared with other methods. Details of the dataset, the ECC, the ISTT and the ECEI are discussed in the following sections.

2.1. Study Area and Data

The study area for this research is Franklin County (Ohio, U.S.), which is part of the Columbus metropolitan area and where the city of Columbus is located. It is the second-most-populated county in Ohio where the percentage of obese or overweight adults is 63.9% [70]. The county includes urban, suburban, and some rural areas. This characteristic is helpful for a study that seeks to consider the influences of various land uses on people's health outcomes. In addition, Franklin County has a diverse racial composition, and also has both wealthy and impoverished communities. Further, there are 3727 food outlets in the county that include many kinds of food retailers (e.g., fast food restaurants, full-service restaurants, and supermarkets) that provide different types of foods. These features of Franklin County facilitate the identification of the spatial heterogeneity of the food environment and the differences in the levels of exposure among the county's population with various socio-economic statuses.

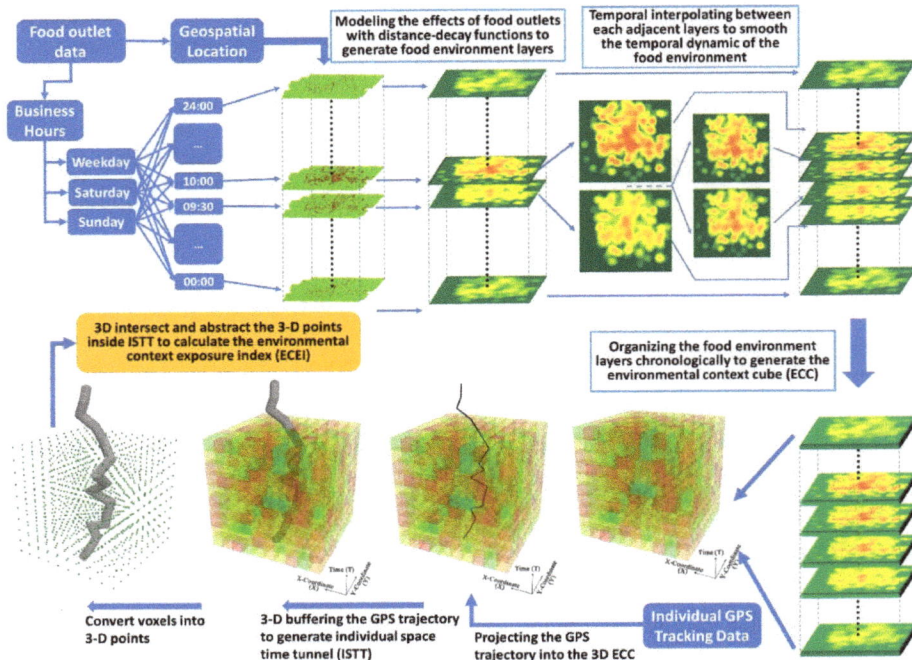

Figure 1. The proposed analytical framework.

The GPS trajectory dataset used in this research was collected as part of a larger study that examines the influence of parks on people's physical activity in four U.S. cities: Albuquerque (NM), Chapel Hill and Durham (NC), Columbus (OH), and Philadelphia (PA). In each of these cities, participants were recruited in person in selected public parks and neighborhoods surrounding these parks following household interviews. For each selected park and its surrounding neighborhoods, about 300 persons from different socio-economic backgrounds were randomly solicited to participate in the study. In the end, 238 subjects participated in the study and 51 of them were from the Columbus study site. Participants in the study were asked to wear a GPS and an accelerometer for three consecutive weeks. The data were collected from August 2009 to October 2010 in three selected seasons (spring, summer, and fall) to avoid the winter months in which people may undertake fewer outdoor physical activities (since the purpose of the larger project was to assess the influence of parks on people's physical activity). Geographic location was recorded by the GPS devices with a time interval of one minute. In addition, data about subjects' demographic, anthropometric and socio-economic statuses were also collected. Subjects' overweight status in the dataset was assessed by the Body Mass Index (BMI), which was calculated by dividing the subject's weight (kg) with his or her height in meters squared (m^2).

The environmental context data for this study were derived from a comprehensive digital geographic database of Franklin County maintained by the Franklin County Auditor's Office. It includes the attributes and physical boundaries of relevant environmental contexts. Food outlets data were derived from the food license data of Franklin County, and their business hours were collected and confirmed using Google Map and phone calls. These data include each food outlet's business name, geographic location, business hours and business category according to standard industrial classifications.

2.2. Data Pre-Processing

GPS signals may be absent in locations near tall buildings or under dense tree canopies, and this may lead to gaps in GPS tracking data. Data pre-processing is thus necessary to improve the reliability and usefulness of GPS data. Consistent with the procedures used by Wiehe et al. [71], missing GPS records in the Columbus GPS dataset were inserted at the location of the earlier point if the distance between two temporally adjacent records bounding a period of missing data was less than 30 m. If this distance was longer than 30 m and the gap between two recorded GPS points was less than 1 h, interim 1-min time points were imputed. Missing GPS points for time periods longer than an hour were considered missing and not imputed. Further, only survey days with eight or more hours of valid GPS records for each subject were included in the analysis.

Although the original dataset had 51 participants, only subjects with valid GPS records for at least five weekdays and two weekend days were included in the analysis. This ensured that there were sufficient data for the selected subjects for at least seven days that covered their daily activities in both weekdays and weekend days. As a result, 46 participants were finally selected as valid subjects for further analysis. Although the sample size is not large, the subjects cover a range of socio-economic attributes (e.g., age and education level) and are thus useful for this exploratory study of the proposed analytical framework for food environment exposure measurement.

Table 1 shows the demographic and socio-economic characteristics of the 46 participants in the sample used in the study. These participants are predominately female (60.87%) and younger people. All of them are adults, and only 2.18% are seniors older than 65. With respect to the education level, 56.52% of the subjects have a college degree or higher, while 43.58% of them have a high school degree or lower. The overweight status among the 46 participants is balanced in that half of them are overweight and the other half are not overweight.

Table 1. The socio-demographic characteristics of the participants in this study.

Socio-Demographic Variables		Percentage
Gender	Male	39.13%
	Female	60.87%
Age (years old)	18–30	56.52%
	31–65	41.30%
	65+	2.18%
Education	With College Degree or Higher (≥College Degree)	56.52%
	With High School Degree or Lower (<College Degree)	43.48%
OverweightStatus	Overweight	50%
	Non-overweight	50%

2.3. Representing Dynamic Environmental Contexts Using the Environmental Context Cube

Any attempt to measure exposures to the food environment needs to begin with representing the food environment, which in turn requires researchers to consider the location and distribution of food outlets as well as the kinds of food those outlets provide. The geographic range of influence from food outlets can be assessed by creating homogeneous buffer areas covering food outlet locations with a specific distance (such as 100 m or 1 km). Importantly, however, representation of food outlets' effects on health behavior should take into account the effect of distance decay rather than using arbitrary distance cutoffs: Environmental effects change as a function of distance, with locations farther from a food outlet less influenced by that outlet than nearer locations are. A few researchers have included distance-decay functions [30,72–77] as part of their food environment studies with a view to accounting for the effect of distance, but even these studies have treated the food environment statically and have failed to consider the dynamic features of the food environment (e.g., food outlets' opening and closing at different times of the day).

As some researchers have noted [39,62], environmental contexts undergo continuous change. For example, air pollution levels differ throughout the day. For this reason, exposure assessment may produce erroneous results if the variability of the environmental context is ignored [7]. Furthermore, the contextual influences of the food environment may also differ with time of day. Previous studies have largely ignored temporal variations in the food environment, although most food outlets operate on specific schedules and offer their services only during certain hours. Some even feature different schedules for weekdays and weekends. Accordingly, Chen and Clark [78], arguing that conventional space-only methods of exposure assessment overlook the dynamic features of the food environment, proposed a spatiotemporal method that takes into account food outlets' business hours when measuring access to food retailers. Although portrayal of the food environment spatiotemporally in Chen and Clark's [78] study is an important step forward for the study of environmental health, the study measures food access using census tracts as its contextual units and thus may still be susceptible to the UGCoP. As a result, further development is need to more accurately assess individual exposures to the food environment and to mitigate the UGCoP.

The ECC is developed in this study to address both spatial and temporal uncertainties in the food environment while accurately assessing individual exposures to that environment. It is designed to capture the complex dynamics of environmental contexts as well as individual exposures. Indeed, this extension of the space-time cube [79] is explicitly designed for use in environmental health research. The base of the space-time cube (or space-time aquarium), which is a time-geographic construct first introduced by Hägerstrand in the 1960s, represents the geographic contexts of the study area (x-axis and y-axis), with 3-D lines inside the cube representing an individual's movement trajectories. The cube's vertical dimension (z-axis) represents time. Figure A1 in the Appendix A illustrates a space-time cube that integrates geographic contexts and GPS trajectories. Note, however, that this representation visualizes only individual movement trajectories in 3-D, whereas the environmental context is represented on a 2-D plane. Constrained by the 2-D plane, the environmental context can be visualized and analyzed at only one time point using this space-time cube framework. In real-world contexts, however, environmental contexts and their influence on moving subjects may change over both space and time in highly complex ways. Representation of the environmental context should thus be also extended to capture and represent the dynamic features of the environment by integrating time as the third dimension.

By extending the traditional space-time cube, we propose the environmental context cube (ECC) as a new analytical framework for analyzing people's movement and their dynamic relationships with their environmental context (e.g., the food environment). The ECC is a collection of 3-D voxels arranged on a regular grid in 3-D space. The value of each voxel represents the environmental context at a specific geographic location (x- and y-coordinate) at a specific time (z-coordinate). Thus, spatial and temporal variations in the environmental context are rendered as the different values of the voxels in 3-D space at various locations and times. In the temporal dimension of the cube, layers of voxels constitute the ECC, with each layer representing the spatial configuration of the environmental context at a specific time of day. The size of the voxels in the 3-D space represents the spatial and temporal resolutions: The higher the spatial resolution, the more detailed the spatial variations represented; and the finer the temporal resolution, the more detailed is the representation of the temporal dynamics. Different spatiotemporal resolutions of the ECC may affect the accuracy with which variations in the environmental context can be captured. To thoroughly examine the ECC while exploring the effect of spatiotemporal resolutions (or scale effects) on measurement accuracy, we built ECCs featuring combinations of three different spatial resolutions (100 m × 100 m, 150 m × 150 m, 200 m × 200 m) and two temporal resolutions (30 min, 10 min), and then evaluated and compared their performance.

In this manner, we constructed a series of 3-D ECCs to represent the unhealthy food environment of the study area. We classified the food outlets in the study area into three categories as described by Rundle et al. [80]—BMI-healthy, BMI-unhealthy, BMI-neutral. Because exposure to BMI-unhealthy food outlets may be related to high BMI, as has been observed in many previous studies [41,45,46,81],

BMI-unhealthy food outlets were used in this study to generate 3-D ECCs for measuring individual exposure to unhealthy food environment. In Rundle et al.'s [80] classification system, BMI-unhealthy food outlets include fast-food restaurants, convenience stores, meat markets, pizzerias, bakeries, and candy and nut stores. Franklin County, the study area, contains 1645 BMI-unhealthy food outlets. All of them are included in the food environment analysis in this study. Figure 2 shows the location of these BMI-unhealthy food outlets.

In analyzing the business hours of the 1645 BMI-unhealthy food outlets included in the study, we found that many food outlets had different schedules on weekdays and weekends; some even had different schedules on Saturdays and Sundays. To give just one example, a restaurant might be open from 10 a.m. to 10 p.m. on weekdays, from 11 a.m. to 10 p.m. on Saturdays, and from 11 a.m. to 8 p.m. on Sundays. Accordingly, we generated three different environmental context cubes (ECCs) to better represent this dynamic food environment: one for weekdays, one for Saturdays, and the other for Sundays. To construct the ECC for one day, we first generated layers of the food environment at different times of the day. For ECCs with a temporal resolution of 30 min, we generated a food environment layer for each of the 48 half-hour time slots in the day. For each time slot, a food environment layer was created to estimate the extent and degree of environmental effects of BMI-unhealthy food outlets based on the locations of the outlets open at that specific time.

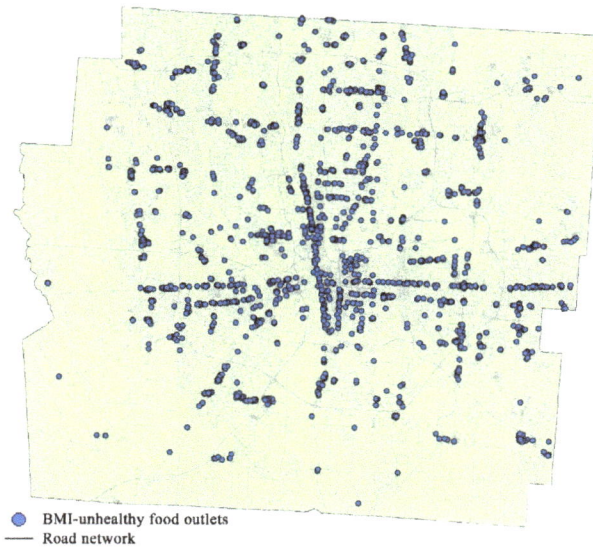

● BMI-unhealthy food outlets
—— Road network

Figure 2. The study area (Franklin County) and the location of BMI-unhealthy food outlets.

As already noted, any assessment of the environmental influence of food outlets should take into account the effects of distance decay. For this reason, based on the location of the food outlets operating during each of the 48 time slots of a day, we modeled the decline in each food outlet's influence using three distance-decay methods that were used in previous environmental health studies [30,72–77]: kernel density estimation (KD), an inverse-square distance-decay function (ISDD), and a negative-exponential distance-decay function (NEDD). The food environment at a specific time of day (a time slot) was thus represented as a raster layer created by estimating the extent and degree of the environmental effects of BMI-unhealthy food outlets based on the locations of food outlets operating at that time of day, using one of the three distance-decay functions. Figure 3 shows the food environment layers at three different time slots of the same day, as generated by the three distance-decay methods. Separate food environment layers were generated for the 48 time slots using each of these methods for three kinds of days (weekdays, Saturdays and Sundays). Then, for each kind of day, the 48 food environment raster layers were voxelized with the unit size of 30 min and mapped to the z-axis. In this way, a 3-D environmental context cube (ECC) was constructed by organizing the 48 voxelized layers chronologically using the assigned z-values (which represent the specific time corresponding to each layer). Because the ECCs were implemented using three distance-decay methods (KD, ISDD, NEDD) in three spatial resolutions (100 m × 100 m, 150 m × 150 m, 200 m × 200 m) for three kinds of day (weekdays, Saturdays, and Sundays), 27 ECCs were ultimately constructed with a temporal resolution of 30 min.

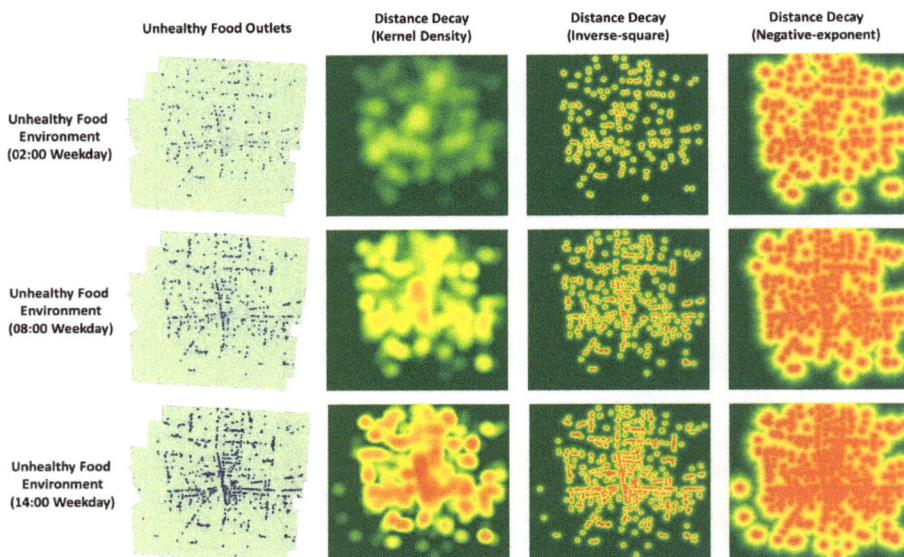

Figure 3. The food environment layers at different time of a day generated by the three different distance-decay methods (the food environment layers with spatial resolution of 100 m × 100 m are used in this figure to illustrate the three distance-decay methods).

To capture more details of the temporal variations in the food environment, another 27 environmental context cubes (ECCs) with a temporal resolution of 10 min were constructed using the same three distance-decay methods, three spatial resolutions, and three kinds of day. Each of these ECCs has 144 food environment layers, where each layer represents each of the 10-min slots that make up the 24 h of a day (e.g., 10:10 a.m., 10:20 a.m. and so on). These layers were calculated by raster algebra using linear interpolation, in which the pixel value of an additional layer (in addition to the original 48 layers at the resolution of 30 min) was calculated using linear polynomials based on the values of the corresponding pixels in the two temporally adjacent layers among the 48 30-min resolution layers. These 144 food environment layers were then voxelized, mapped to the z-axis, and organized chronologically to form the ECCs with a temporal resolution of 10 min. This higher temporal resolution allowed the temporal dynamics of the food environment in any particular day to be better represented. Figure 4 illustrates the process of the temporal interpolation as well as the generation of a 3-D ECC and its food environment layers.

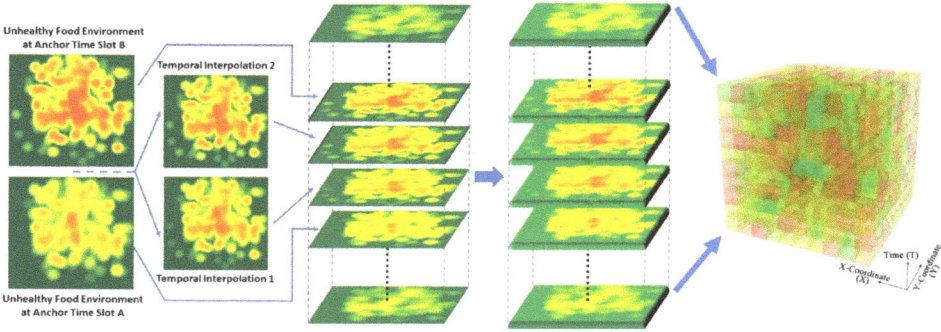

Figure 4. The process of the temporal interpolation and the generation of the 3-D environmental context cube with food environment layers.

To facilitate the implementation and computation of the 3-D environmental context cubes (ECCs), we converted each 3-D ECC to a 3-D point cloud, with each voxel in the cube represented by a point in the cloud at the centroid of the original voxel. As shown in Figure 5, the three dimensions of the points correspond to the x-coordinate (X), y-coordinate (Y), and time (T) seen in the original ECC. The values of the environmental factors were stored as an attribute table linked to each point in the 3-D point cloud.

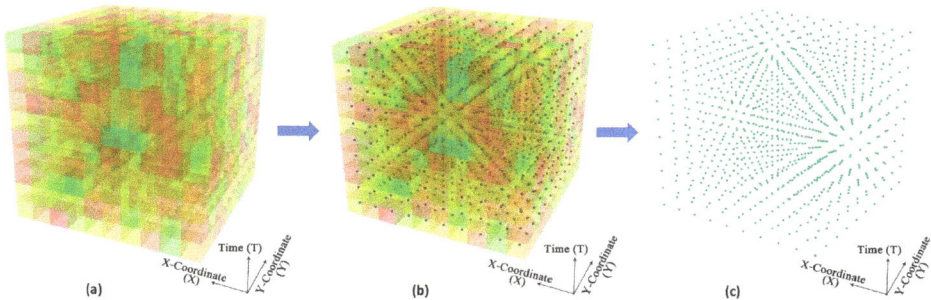

Figure 5. Implementation of the 3-D environmental context cube using a 3-D point cloud. (**a**): an environmental context cube, (**b**) voxels in the cube represented by points at the centroid of the original voxels, (**c**) the corresponding 3-D point cloud.

2.4. Capturing the Spatiotemporal Exposure Space with Individual Space-Time Tunnel

Using GPS trajectory data for individual exposure assessment could capture the daily movement of people and thus help mitigate the UGCoP to some degree. However, conventional methods capture only the spatial extents of individuals' activities using 2-D polygons that represent a person's activity space (e.g., GPS trajectory buffers, standard deviation ellipses, and minimum convex polygons) or, at most, weigh the accumulated time spent at different activity locations (e.g., kernel density surface, context-based crystal-growth activity space [68]), where environmental contexts were considered statically and the dynamics of the food environment ignored. Although these methods consider the accumulated time that an individual spends at different locations (e.g., person A spends 8 h at the workplace on weekdays), they ignore temporal variations in people's location of activity (e.g., person A stays at the workplace from 8 a.m. to 12 p.m. and from 1 p.m. to 5 p.m. on weekdays). Knowledge of the exact times when a person is at a location is essential for understanding the resulting level of exposure to the food environment. For example, consider a person who visits an area where many fast food restaurants may be found but does so at 1 a.m., when they are closed. Conventional activity space methods would include this occurrence in the environmental context exposure assessment even though the person was not actually exposed to fast food restaurants at that time. In this way, overlooking temporal variations in the food context and the exact times when people undertake their daily activities at various locations may introduce measurement error.

To help address the temporal uncertainty that is an essential element of the environmental context and the dynamics of people's daily activity, we propose the individual space-time tunnel (ISTT) as a way of representing the individual exposure space. The ISTT was generated by a 3-D buffer of an individual's GPS trajectory at a specific distance (e.g., 100 m) in a 3-D space. To generate the ISTT, GPS trajectories were projected into the ECC according to the geographic coordinates and timestamps of the GPS records. As shown in Figure 6a, the GPS trajectory of a subject is projected into the 3-D space of an ECC, much like the space-time paths inside a space-time aquarium. The voxels along a particular trajectory and its surrounding areas constitute the environmental context that influences the corresponding subject. Thus, environmental exposure should be derived using a 3-D buffer space of appropriate radius around people's movement trajectories, as shown in Figure 6b. The buffer radius B_r, a user-defined parameter that represents the effective range of a particular environmental influence, can vary for different population groups based on individual socio-demographic attributes (e.g., age). For example, older adults and children may have a smaller B_r than adolescents do, because they both tend to have lower mobility. We might also define B_r as a function of travel velocity. For example, we might associate higher velocity with smaller B_r, noting that higher velocity (i.e., quicker bypass) may allow for less influence on the subject from the environmental context around a location. For purpose of illustration, we set B_r to 100 m in this exploratory study.

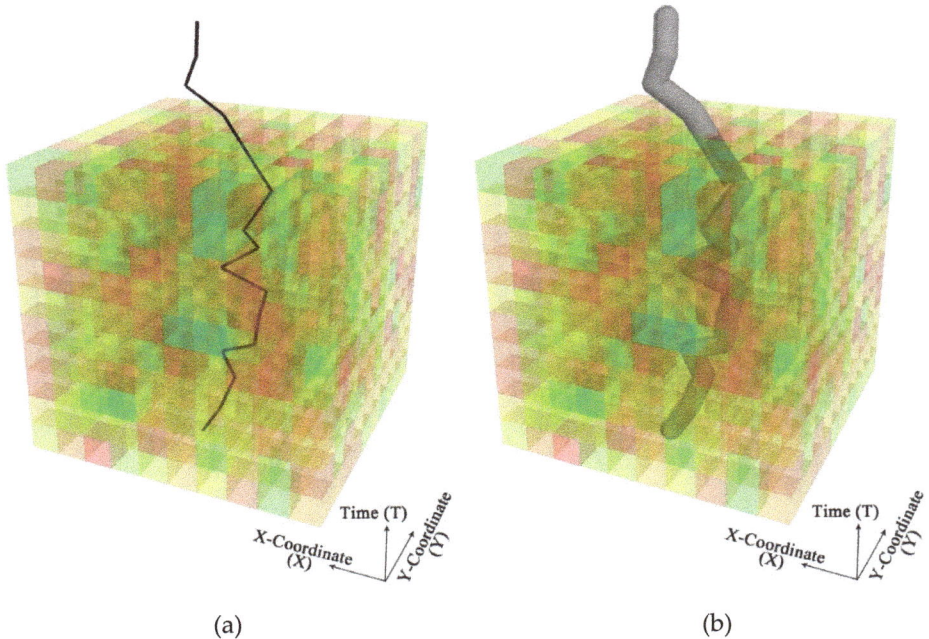

Figure 6. A GPS trajectory (**a**) and an individual space-time tunnel (**b**) projected into an environmental context cube.

2.5. Measuring Food Environment Exposure with the Environmental Context Exposure Index

The proposed 3-D environmental context cube (ECC) can capture the complexity and dynamics of the food environment, and the individual space-time tunnel (ISTT) can delineate the individual spatiotemporal exposure space by integrating spatial as well as temporal variations in a person's daily activities. As a result, individual exposures to the food environment can be derived by the 3-D intersection of the ECC and the ISTT: By projecting the 3-D ISTT into the corresponding point cloud of the ECC, as illustrated in Figure 7, we can link exposure to the food environment with all points located inside the ISTT in the 3-D space. The results of the 3-D intersection allow calculation of the environmental context exposure index (ECEI), which in turn allows the measurement of individual exposures to the environmental context. By capturing the extent to which a person is exposed to the relevant environmental context during each time unit throughout a day, the ECEI provides a new method for quantifying an individual's level of exposures to the food environment. In this study, the ECEI was used to analyze the association between individual exposure to the food environment and health outcomes.

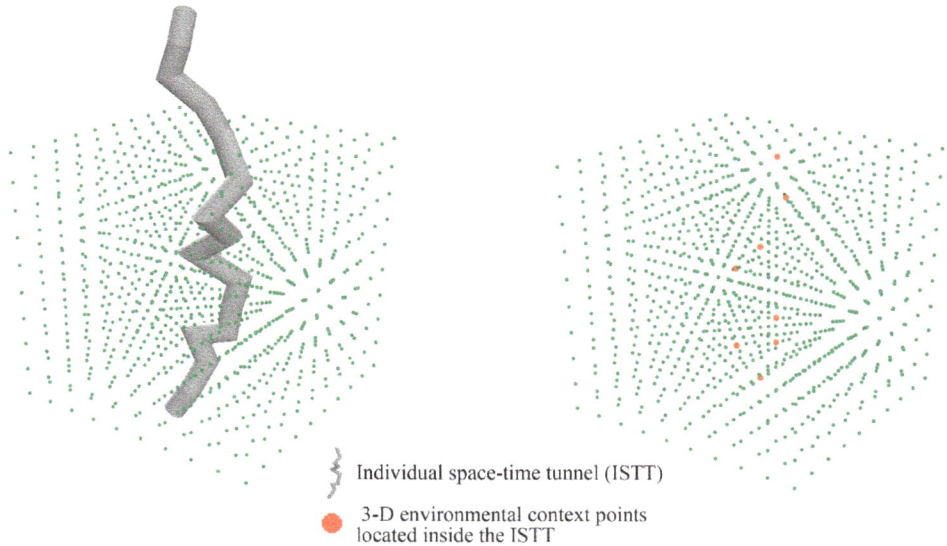

Individual space-time tunnel (ISTT)

3-D environmental context points located inside the ISTT

Figure 7. The 3-D intersection of the point cloud and individual space-time tunnel.

By identifying the 3-D intersection of the ISTT and the point cloud, subjects' exposures to the food environment can then be derived. After abstracting all intersected 3-D points from the ECC, the ECEI was evaluated as follows:

$$ECEI(j)(k) = \sum_{i=1}^{n} \frac{EC_{ij}W_i}{T} \quad (1 \leq i \leq n) \tag{1}$$

$$W_i = \begin{cases} 1 & if \ v_i = 0 \\ \left(\frac{1}{2}\right)^{v_i} & if \ v_i > 0 \end{cases} \quad (1 \leq i \leq n) \tag{2}$$

where $ECEI(j)(k)$ is the environmental context exposure index of environmental factor j for subject k, EC_{ij} is the value of environmental factor j for 3-D point i based on the intersection of the ISTT and the ECC, W_i is the weight for 3-D point i, T is the time span of the intersection (the time unit can be hour or day), and n is the total number of points derived by the 3-D intersection.

W_i is a user-defined parameter for calculating the environmental context exposure index (ECEI). In most cases, the point weight (W_i) can be set to 1, but it can also differ for different research questions. One possible method for assigning voxel weight is to use movement velocity, as shown in Equation (2), where v_i is the movement velocity of the subject when passing through voxel i: The higher the velocity, the smaller the weight should be, indicating less contextual influences. When speed equals 0, the subject is staying at that location, so weight is set to 1. A quickly moving subject, by contrast, may pass by a location quite rapidly; thus, the influence of the environmental factor at 3-D point *i* should be small and the weight less than 1. Again, for purpose of illustration, W_i was set to 1 globally for this exploratory study.

Using this method, we calculated an environmental context exposure index (ECEI) for each of the 54 environmental context cubes (ECCs) separately. Because the three distance-decay methods generate ECCs with different value ranges, we standardized the ECEI by using z-score to facilitate the comparison of the exposures measured by different ECCs.

2.6. Comparing the Individual Food Environment Exposure Measurement with Other Methods

To compare the proposed analytical framework for food environment exposure measurement with other methods, four widely used exposure assessment methods [52,81–86] were also implemented with the same dataset. The four methods are GPS trajectory buffers (GTBs), standard deviation ellipses with one or two standard deviation(s) (SDE1, SDE2) and minimum convex polygons (MCPs). Figure 8 illustrates these four methods based on one subject's GPS trajectory (note that the geographic coordinates of the GPS tracks shown in this figure have been modified for the purpose of human subjects' protection). The GTBs were created by a 100-meter 2-D buffer along the participant's GPS trajectories. The buffering area covered all the daily activity locations that this subject visited in the study period. The SDE is another widely-used method for exposure space delineation. Based on the transformed mean center and the rotated major and minor axes of all the GPS points of the subject, an ellipse was obtained based on either one or two standard deviation(s) of the distances between all pairs of GPS points. The SDEs represent the spatial distribution and directional trends of the subject's activity locations and normally does not include all of the GPS points. The MCP is the smallest convex polygon that contains all the GPS points of the subject, which covers all the daily activity locations. With the same data of BMI-unhealthy food outlets, exposure to BMI-unhealthy food environment was calculated as the density of BMI-unhealthy food outlets in these four delineations of exposure space. The results were standardized with z-score transformation and compared with those obtained using the ECCs and ECEIs.

2.7. Analytical Approach

To compare the performance of the environmental context cubes (ECCs) with different distance-decay methods at various spatial and temporal resolutions, as well as the exposure assessment results between the environmental context exposure index (ECEI) and other widely used food environment exposure measurements, we examined all these measurements and their relationship with participants' overweight status using binary logistic regression models, which are widely used in public health studies [44,46,87]. The response variable is individual overweight status (0: non-overweight; 1: overweight or obese) based on participants' BMI (non-overweight: BMI $< 25.0 \text{ kg/m}^2$; overweight or obese: BMI $\geq 25.0 \text{ kg/m}^2$), while the independent variable is individual food environment exposure. The models were controlled for subjects' age, gender, and education level. A total of 22 models were built with different measurements of BMI-unhealthy food environment exposure (18 measured by the ECEI based on various ECCs and 4 measured by other methods). The performance of these models was compared by the Akaike information criterion (AIC), Nagelkerke R^2, likelihood ratio chi-square (LR χ^2) and the corresponding *p*-value, which indicate the robustness of the model. The more robust a model is, the better exposure assessment will be obtained. In addition, the models were compared to see if a significant association existed between individual food environment exposure and overweight status.

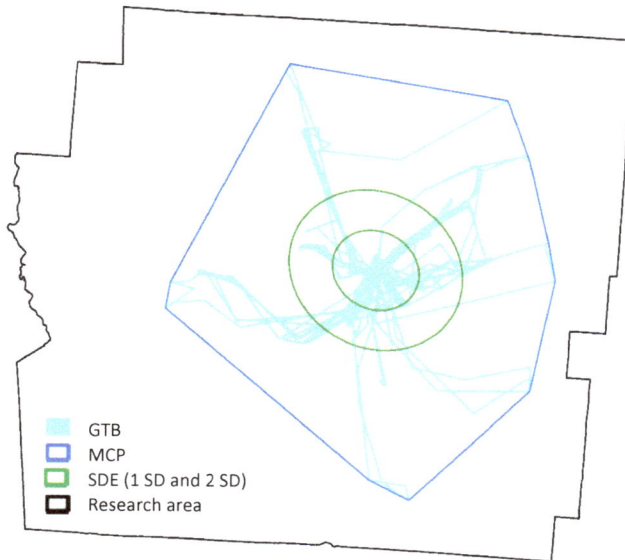

GTB
MCP
SDE (1 SD and 2 SD)
Research area

Figure 8. Four widely used methods for delineating individual exposure space based on one subject's GPS trajectory data.

3. Results

3.1. Variation in Food Environment Exposure Measurements with Different Methods

Individual food environment exposures were measured by the environmental context cubes (ECCs) and the environmental context exposure indexes (ECEIs) using three different distance-decay methods, three different spatial resolutions, and two different temporal resolutions, as well as other four widely used methods (GTB, MCP, SDE1, and SDE2). Figure 9 illustrates the standardized measures of these methods for each participant. In the figure, exposures measured by the ECCs with three distance-decay methods include only those with the highest spatial (100 m × 100 m) and temporal resolution (10 min), since they captured the finest detail of the spatial and temporal dynamics of the food environment. The measurement results of the ECCs with different spatial and temporal resolutions will be compared and discussed in the following sections. The horizontal axis of Figure 9 indicates the 46 participants in the study, while the vertical axis shows the food environment exposure measures. The figure indicates that different methods give considerably different exposure measures for the same participant.

To investigate the relationship among all the exposure measures obtained using different methods, we perform bivariate Pearson correlation analysis between each pair of the measures. Table A1 illustrates the results, which indicates that more than half of the pairs do not have significant correlations, including the pairs of ECC(KD)–MCP, ECC(ISDD)–MCP, ECC(ISDD)–SDE1, ECC(ISDD)–SDE2, ECC(NEDD)–GTB, ECC(NEDD)–MCP, ECC(NEDD)–SDE1, ECC(NEDD)–SDE2, GTB–SDE1, MCP–SDE1 and MCP–SDE2. Although the other pairs show significant correlations, most of the coefficients are smaller than 0.6, which indicate moderate to low associations. Only the pairs ECC(KD)–ECC(NEDD), ECC(ISDD)–ECC(NEDD), GTB–MCP and SDE1–SDE2 shows strong associations. It is reasonable that the results of the ECCs with different distance-decay methods are correlated with each other since they share the same model and concepts, while SDE1 and SDE2 are also the same methods with various parameters. The results show that individual exposures measured by different methods are mostly different from and not correlated with each other, which indicates the existence of the UGCoP. Therefore, it is worth comparing these measurements and exploring the accurate ways to assess individual food environment exposures.

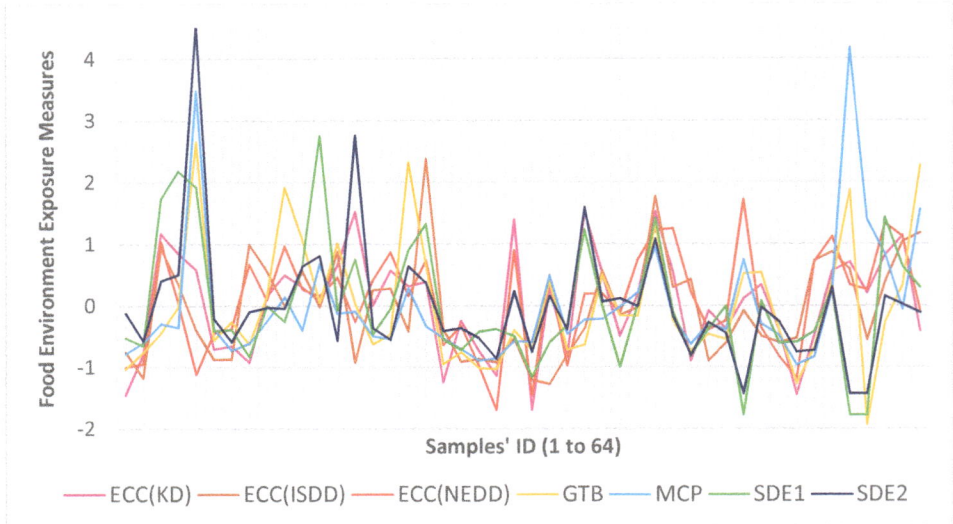

Figure 9. Comparison of the exposure measures obtained with different methods for each participant. (ECC: environmental context cube; KD: kernel density estimation; ISDD: inverse-square distance decay function; NEDD: negative-exponent distance decay function; GTB: GPS trajectory buffers; MCP: minimum convex polygons; SDE1: standard deviation ellipses with one standard deviation; SDE2: standard deviation ellipses with two standard deviations.)

3.2. Comparing the Performance of Food Environment Exposure Measurement Methods

Table A2 shows the results of the binary logistic regression models with different measurements of individual BMI-unhealthy food environment exposure on the relationships between food environment exposure and overweight status. In the table, models KD100T10, KD100T30, KD150T10, KD150T30, KD200T10, and KD200T30 use exposures measured based on ECCs with KD as the distance-decay function in different spatial and temporal resolutions. In addition, models ISDD100T10, ISDD100T30, ISDD150T10, ISDD150T30, ISDD200T10, and ISDD200T30 use the exposure assessed based on ECCs with ISDD in various spatial and temporal resolutions. Furthermore, models NEDD100T10, NEDD100T30, NEDD150T10, NEDD150T30, NEDD200T10, and NEDD200T30 use exposure evaluated based on ECCs with NEDD in different spatial and temporal resolutions. Lastly, models M-GTB, M-MCP, M-SDE1, M-SDE2 use the measurement of individual food environment exposure based on four widely used methods (GTB, MCP, SDE1, and SDE2). The table shows that all the logistic regression models are statistically significant with p-value < 0.001. The models explained at least 45% (Nagelkerke R^2) of the variance of participants' overweight status. Among these models, the most robust one is the ISDD100T10 with the smallest AIC (45.552), largest LR χ^2 (28.217), and p-value < 0.001. The model explained 61.13% (Nagelkerke R^2) of the variance of participants' overweight status. The least robust model is the KD150T10 (AIC = 54.240, LR χ^2 = 19.529), which only explained 46.12% of the variance.

Among the ECC models, the food environment exposures estimated by ISDD generates the best results, while the ones estimated by KD generate the worst results. Considering various spatial and temporal resolutions of the ECC, the finer the resolution, the better the results. For instance, among the ECC models with specific distance-decay function, the most robust model is always the one with the finest spatial resolution: KD100T30 (AIC = 53.879, Nagelkerke R^2 = 0.4681, LR χ^2 = 19.891) for ECC(KD); ISDD100T10 (AIC = 45.552, Nagelkerke R^2 = 0.6113, LR χ^2 = 28.217) for ECC(ISDD); NEDD100T10 (AIC = 49.769, Nagelkerke R^2 = 0.5420, LR χ^2 = 24.001) for ECC(NEDD). In addition, the table indicates that ECCs with a temporal resolution of 10 min normally generate better results compared to the ones with a temporal resolution of 30 min with several exceptions.

Regarding the four widely used exposure assessment methods, GTB performs the best with AIC = 51.462, Nagelkerke R^2 = 0.5124, LR χ^2 = 22.308. However, the models with ECC(ISDD) and ECC(NEDD) still perform much better than the GTB-based model. It is worth noting that the models with ECC(KD) have the worst performance when compared to all the other methods, which may indicate that the effects of food outlets may not follow the decay patterns as depicted by a kernel density estimation.

3.3. Association between Food Environment Exposure and Overweight Status

The associations between food environment exposure based on different ECCs and participants' overweight status are shown in Table A3. Almost all the models, except NEDD150T10, indicate that being female (compared to being male) is associated with higher odds of being overweight, while having a college degree and higher (compared high school degree and lower) is associated with lower odds of being overweight. However, significant association between BMI-unhealthy food environment exposure and overweight status is observed for only three of the models (ISDD100T10, ISDD100T30, and NEDD100T10). Higher unhealthy food environment exposure is found to be significantly associated with higher odds of being overweight in models ISDD100T10 (odds ratio (OR): 6.81; 95% confidential interval (CI): 1.76, 45.3; *p*-value < 0.01), ISDD100T30 (OR: 4.35; CI: 1.27, 22.62; *p*-value < 0.1) and NEDD100T10 (OR: 3.13; CI: 1.08, 11.47; *p*-value < 0.1). Referring to the performance of models discussed above, these three models are also the most robust models with the lowest AIC and highest LR χ^2, as well as the highest explanation rate of the variance in participants' overweight status.

Table A4 lists the results of the binary logistic regression models based on the other four widely used methods. The models M-GTP, M-MCP and M-SDE1 indicate that being female is associated with higher odds of being overweight while having a college degree and higher is associated with lower odds of being overweight. M-SDE2 is the only model that does not find an association between education level and overweight status. Interestingly, all these four models did not find any significant association between BMI-unhealthy food environment exposure and participants' overweight status.

The results indicate that the proposed framework generates better measurements of individual food environment exposures when compared to other widely used methods. This suggests the inconsistent findings in previous studies may be partly due to the methods used. Significant associations between BMI-unhealthy food environment exposures and overweight status were found in the three most robust models (ISDD100T10, ISDD100T30, and NEDD100T10). Being the most robust model, ISDD100T10 (explained 61.13% of the variance in participants' overweight status) found that higher unhealthy food environment exposure (OR: 6.81; CI: 1.76, 45.3; *p*-value < 0.01) is significantly associated with higher odds of being overweight.

4. Discussion

The proposed framework generated more reasonable and reliable results when compared to other methods, and thus obtained more accurate individual food environment exposures assessment. Regarding the distance-decay methods for generating the ECC, the ISDD represents the dynamic environmental contexts more accurately, and the ECC(ISDD) with a spatial resolution of 100 m × 100 m and a temporal resolution of 10 min performs best with the most robust regression models. Regarding the spatial and temporal resolution of the ECC, the finer the spatial and temporal resolution, the better the performance of the model. This suggests the existence of scale effects when using the ECC for measuring individual exposures. Thus, future application of the ECC may need to consider proper spatial and temporal resolution in order to generate reliable results.

The framework proposed in this study can help to mitigate the UGCoP. With respect to the spatial dimension, contextual units or areas in the study were not based on arbitrary pre-defined spatial boundaries (e.g., census tracts) but were delineated by ISTTs based on participants' actual movement trajectories (GPS tracks). This is significantly different from the methods used in most previous studies, which tended to measure contextual influences based on static residential neighborhoods that may not accurately represent the actual areas that exert contextual influences on individual behavior or health outcomes [59,88–90]. On the other hand, temporal variations in relevant environmental contexts were handled dynamically: The influence of the food outlets was measured with consideration of their business hours in order to more accurately capture their contextual effects. Taking into account the complex spatial and temporal configuration of individual contextual exposure, the proposed framework and methods help to mitigate UGCoP.

The ECEI based on the ECC and ISTT in the study is a quantitative measure of individual exposure to environmental contexts in unit time, which may be used as a standard measure of individual contextual exposure. It provides a useful standardized tool for environmental exposure assessment, while capturing the spatial and temporal variations in environmental contexts. It is also flexible to implement the ECEI for different research questions concerning different environmental contexts using the two user-defined parameters B_r and W_i. These two parameters can be explored in further studies to fit the research question. The index may be further used for comparative analysis of environmental exposures between different individuals or groups. In addition, the ECEI may be utilized to examine the relationships between environmental contexts and other health outcomes. The observed association may be used to investigate and identify high-risk environmental contexts and provide decision support for policy-making in public health.

Lastly, this research has several limitations that need to be addressed in future studies. First, this study implemented the proposed framework based on a relatively small sample of participants who live near parks. Larger GPS datasets with more subjects from different study sites are thus needed in future research to further evaluate the robustness of the framework. Second, this study only applied the framework to food environment exposures; further studies are needed to assess its effectiveness for addressing other health issues, such as physical activity and mental health. Third, we implemented the three distance-decay methods in Euclidean distance without considering transport modes and the configuration of road networks. More sophisticated methods [91] that incorporate transport modes in the ECC would help to further the application of the framework and has significant potential to better represent the environmental context. We will develop the ECC along this line in future studies. Fourth, since there is no data on participants' actual activities, there may be some uncertainty in the exposure measure. For instance, working and eating at a fast-food restaurant may mean different exposure and have different effects on a participant's body weight. If activity diary data are available, activity types can be integrated into the calculation of the ECEI by differentiating the contextual effects of different types of activity. Fifth, the proposed methodology can only explore the association between environmental exposures and health outcomes. Further investigations (e.g., controlled experiments or longitudinal studies) are still needed to validate any causal relationships.

5. Conclusions

This study developed and implemented an analytical framework to dynamically represent food environment and derive individual environmental exposures that effectively integrates human movement in space and time (e.g., GPS trajectories). The proposed framework incorporates the dynamics of the food environment into the environmental context cube (ECC), captures individual exposure space with the individual space-time tunnel (ISTT), and assesses the effects of individual exposure on people's overweight status with the environmental context exposure index (ECEI). The framework was designed to examine individual food environment exposure but can also be used in a wide range of environmental health studies.

Author Contributions: J.W. and M.P.K. conceived the idea; J.W. designed and performed the experiments and analyzed the data; J.W. wrote the paper; M.P.K. contributed to refining and revising the paper.

Acknowledgments: Jue Wang was supported by a Fred W. and Demetra Foster Fellowship. Mei-Po Kwan was supported by a grant from the National Natural Science Foundation of China (#41529101) and a John Simon Guggenheim Memorial Foundation Fellowship. The authors thank Deborah A. Cohen for her kind permission to use the data, which were collected in a study supported by a grant from the U.S. National Heart, Lung, and Blood Institute (NHLBI # R01HL092569). Please see [92,93] for details about the data collection process in the main study.

Conflicts of Interest: The authors declare no conflict of interest.

Appendix A

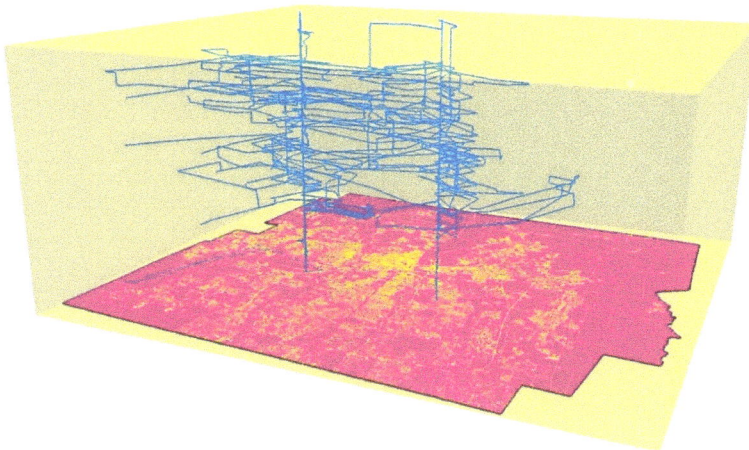

Figure A1. An example of the space-time cube (aquarium).

Table A1. The results of the bivariate Pearson correlation analysis between each pair of the methods for food environment exposure assessment.

Methods	ECC(KD)	ECC(ISDD)	ECC(NEDD)	GTB	MCP	SDE1	SDE2
ECC(KD)	-	0.407 *	0.658 *	0.438 *	0.364	0.508 *	0.476 *
ECC(ISDD)	-	-	0.642 *	0.396 *	0.198	0.358	0.057
ECC(NEDD)	-	-	-	0.269	0.180	0.168	−0.033
GTB	-	-	-	-	0.629 *	0.345	0.439 *
MCP	-	-	-	-	-	0.099	0.291
SDE1	-	-	-	-	-	-	0.699 *
SDE2	-	-	-	-	-	-	-

* *p*-value < 0.05.

Table A2. The results of binary logistic regression models with different measurements of individual BMI-unhealthy food environment exposure for relationships between food environment exposure and overweight status.

Model [a,b]	Method	Spatial Resolution	Temporal Resolution	AIC	Nagelkerke R^2	LR χ^2	*p*-Value
KD100T10		100 m × 100 m	10 min	53.898	0.4677	19.872	0.00053 ***
KD100T30			30 min	53.879	0.4681	19.891	0.00052 ***
KD150T10	ECC	150 m × 150 m	10 min	54.240	0.4612	19.529	0.00062 ***
KD150T30	(KD)		30 min	54.228	0.4615	19.542	0.00061 ***
KD200T10		200 m × 200 m	10 min	54.198	0.4620	19.571	0.00061 ***
KD200T30			30 min	54.223	0.4616	19.546	0.00061 ***

Table A2. *Cont.*

Model [a,b]	Method	Spatial Resolution	Temporal Resolution	AIC	Nagelkerke R^2	LR χ^2	*p*-Value
ISDD100T10		100 m × 100 m	10 min	45.552	0.6113	28.217	0.00001 ***
ISDD100T30			30 min	48.567	0.5624	25.202	0.00005 ***
ISDD150T10	ECC	150 m × 150 m	10 min	53.272	0.4794	20.498	0.00040 ***
ISDD150T30	(ISDD)		30 min	52.801	0.4881	20.969	0.00032 ***
ISDD200T10		200 m × 200 m	10 min	53.124	0.4822	20.645	0.00037 ***
ISDD200T30			30 min	54.073	0.4644	19.696	0.00057 ***
NEDD100T10		100 m × 100 m	10 min	49.769	0.5420	24.001	0.00008 ***
NEDD100T30			30 min	53.597	0.4734	20.172	0.00046 ***
NEDD150T10	ECC	150 m × 150 m	10 min	52.945	0.4855	20.825	0.00034 ***
NEDD150T30	(NEDD)		30 min	51.792	0.5064	21.977	0.00020 ***
NEDD200T10		200 m × 200 m	10 min	54.132	0.4633	19.638	0.00059 ***
NEDD200T30			30 min	54.199	0.4650	19.571	0.00061 ***
M-GTB	GTB	-	-	51.462	0.5124	22.308	0.00017 ***
M-MCP	MCP	-	-	52.390	0.4956	21.380	0.00027 ***
M-SDE1	SDE1	-	-	53.542	0.4744	20.228	0.00045 ***
M-SDE2	SDE2	-	-	51.753	0.5071	22.016	0.00020 ***

[a] N = 46 subjects, [b] Response variable: 0 non-overweight; 1 overweight, *** *p*-value < 0.001, AIC: Akaike information criterion (the smaller the value, the better the model fit), LR χ^2: likelihood ratio chi-square (the larger the value, the better the model fit).

Table A3. The association between food environment exposure and overweight status analyzed by binary logistic regression models with food environment exposure measured by different ECCs.

Variables	Model [a,b]	β (95% CI)	OR (95% CI)	Model [a,b]	β (95% CI)	OR (95%)
Gender (Female)		2.56 *** (0.97, 4.63)	12.97 *** (2.64, 102.57)		2.57 ** (0.97, 4.63)	13.01 ** (2.65, 102.77)
Age	KD100T10	0.05 (−0.02, 0.14)	1.05 (0.98, 1.14)	KD100T30	0.05 (−0.02, 0.14)	1.05 (0.98, 1.15)
Education (≥College Degree)		−2.37 ** (−4.46, −0.72)	0.09 ** (0.01, 0.49)		−2.37 ** (−4.47, −0.73)	0.09 ** (0.01, 0.48)
Env. Exp.		0.28 (−0.64, 1.27)	0.09 (0.01, 0.49)		0.29 (−0.64, 1.28)	1.34 (0.53, 3.60)
Gender (Female)		2.53 *** (0.91, 4.63)	12.62 *** (2.49, 102.72)		2.54 ** (0.92, 4.64)	12.73 ** (2.51, 103.68)
Age	KD150T10	0.05 (−0.02, 0.14)	1.05 (0.98, 1.15)	KD150T30	0.05 (−0.02, 0.14)	1.05 (0.98, 1.14)
Education (≥College Degree)		−2.43 *** (−4.56, −0.76)	0.09 *** (0.01, 0.47)		−2.42 ** (−4.55, −0.76)	0.09 ** (0.01, 0.47)
Env. Exp.		0.06 (−0.94, 1.04)	1.06 (0.39, 2.82)		0.08 (−0.90, 1.04)	1.08 (0.41, 2.83)
Gender (Female)		2.54 *** (0.94 4.62)	12.68 *** (2.56, 101.55)		2.53 ** (0.94, 4.61)	12.57 ** (2.56, 100.23)
Age	KD200T10	0.05 (−0.02, 0.13)	1.05 (0.98, 1.14)	KD200T30	0.05 (−0.02, 0.14)	1.05 (0.98, 1.14)
Education (≥College Degree)		−2.44 *** (−4.53, −0.83)	0.09 *** (0.01, 0.44)		−2.45 ** (−4.53, −0.83)	0.09 ** (0.01, 0.43)
Env. Exp.		0.11 (−0.84, 1.02)	1.12 (0.43, 2.77)		0.08 (−0.87, 0.99)	1.09 (0.42, 2.69)
Gender (Female)		3.61 *** (1.58, 6.37)	36.83 *** (4.87, 584.49)		3.30 ** (1.41, 5.84)	27.13 ** (4.10, 342.79)
Age	ISDD100T10	0.03 (−0.04, 0.12)	1.04 (0.96, 1.13)	ISDD100T30	0.03 (−0.05, 0.12)	1.03 (0.95, 1.12)
Education (≥College Degree)		−2.13 ** (−4.42, −0.31)	0.12 ** (0.01, 0.74)		−1.93 * (−4.09, −0.19)	0.14 * (0.02, 0.83)
Env. Exp.		1.92 ** (0.57, 3.81)	6.81 ** (1.76, 45.3)		1.47 * (0.24, 3.12)	4.35 * (1.27, 22.62)
Gender (Female)		2.90 *** (1.12, 5.23)	18.14 *** (3.06, 186.21)		2.92 ** (1.17, 5.21)	18.48 ** (3.21, 182.24)
Age	ISDD150T10	0.04 (−0.03, 0.13)	1.04 (0.97, 1.14)	ISDD150T30	0.04 (−0.03, 0.13)	1.05 (0.97, 1.14)
Education (≥College Degree)		−2.34 ** (−4.42, −0.71)	0.10 ** (0.01, 0.49)		−2.36 * (−4.45, −0.72)	0.09 * (0.01, 0.48)
Env. Exp.		0.45 (−0.44, 1.42)	1.57 (0.64, 4.12)		0.51 (−0.31, 1.47)	1.67 (0.73, 4.36)

Table A3. *Cont.*

Variables	Model [a,b]	β (95% CI)	OR (95% CI)	Model [a,b]	β (95% CI)	OR (95%)
Gender (Female)		2.68 *** (1.03, 4.86)	14.61 *** (2.80, 129.08)		2.57 ** (0.96, 4.68)	13.09 ** (2.62, 107.41)
Age	ISDD200T10	0.05 (−0.02, 0.13)	1.05 (0.98, 1.14)	ISDD200T30	0.05 (−0.02, 0.13)	1.05 (0.98, 1.14)
Education (≥College Degree)		−2.60 *** (−4.77, −0.94)	0.07 *** (0.01, 0.39)		−2.47 ** (−4.55, −0.85)	0.09 ** (0.01, 0.43)
Env. Exp.		0.49 (−0.41, 1.46)	1.63 (0.66, 4.31)		0.19 (−0.69, 1.11)	1.21 (0.50, 3.04)
Gender (Female)		2.81 *** (1.10, 5.04)	16.55 *** (3.02, 154.12)		2.57 ** (0.98, 4.64)	13.07 ** (2.66, 103.57)
Age	NEDD100T10	0.05 (−0.03, 0.13)	1.05 (0.97, 1.14)	NEDD100T30	0.05 (−0.02, 0.13)	1.05 (0.98, 1.14)
Education (≥College Degree)		−1.98 ** (−4.13, −0.26)	0.14 ** (0.02, 0.77)		−2.20 * (−4.35, +0.49)	0.11 * (0.01, 0.61)
Env. Exp.		1.14 * (0.08, 2.44)	3.13 * (1.08, 11.47)		0.37 (−0.51, 1.40)	1.44 (0.60, 4.06)
Gender (Female)		2.90 *** (1.15, 5.19)	18.25 *** (3.17, 180.20)		3.00 ** (1.25, 5.29)	20.09 ** (3.49, 199.09)
Age	NEDD150T10	0.04 (−0.04, 0.12)	1.04 (0.96, 1.13)	NEDD150T30	0.04 (−0.04, 0.12)	1.04 (0.96, 1.13)
Education (≥College Degree)		−2.19 (−2.29, −0.52)	0.11 (0.01, 0.59)		−2.21 * (−4.31, −0.55)	0.11 * (0.01, 0.58)
Env. Exp.		0.57 (−0.40, 1.62)	1.76 (0.67, 5.06)		0.72 (−0.17, 1.77)	2.06 (0.84, 5.81)
Gender (Female)		2.53 *** (0.94, 4.62)	12.64 *** (2.57, 101.77)		2.50 ** (0.92, 4.57)	12.22 ** (2.51, 96.49)
Age	NEDD200T10	0.05 (−0.02, 0.13)	1.05 (0.98, 1.14)	NEDD200T30	0.05 (−0.02, 0.14)	1.06 (0.98, 1.15)
Education (≥College Degree)		−2.46 *** (−4.54, −0.85)	0.09 *** (0.01, 0.43)		−2.48 ** (−4.57, −0.86)	0.08 ** (0.01, 0.42)
Env. Exp.		0.14 (−0.68, 0.93)	1.15 (0.51, 2.54)		−0.09 (−0.89, 0.67)	0.91 (0.41, 1.95)

[a] N = 46 subjects, [b] Response variable: 0 non-overweight; 1 overweight, * p-value < 0.1, ** p-value < 0.01, *** p-value < 0.001, Gender: 0-male, 1-female, Education: 0-without a college degree or higher; 1-with a college degree or higher, Env. Exp.: BMI-unhealthy food environment exposure measured by a specific method.

Table A4. The association between food environment exposure and overweight status analyzed by the binary logistic regression models with the food environment exposure measured by the other four widely used methods.

Variables.	Model [a,b]	β (95% CI)	OR (95% CI)
Gender (Female)		3.12 *** (1.29, 5.62)	22.68 *** (3.62, 275.66)
Age	M-GTP	0.08 (0.00, 0.17)	1.08 (10.00, 1.19)
Education (≥College Degree)		−2.48 ** (−4.72, −0.76)	0.08 ** (8.91, 0.47)
Env. Exp.		0.29 (−0.05, 0.69)	1.34 (9.52, 2.00)
Gender (Female)		2.57 *** (0.95, 4.70)	13.10 *** (2.60, 109.75)
Age	M-MCP	0.06 (−0.01, 0.15)	1.06 (0.99, 1.17)
Education (≥College Degree)		−2.53 *** (−4.70, −0.86)	0.08 *** (0.01, 0.42)
Env. Exp.		0.56 (−0.23, 1.53)	1.74 (0.79, 4.60)

Table A4. *Cont.*

Variables.	Model [a,b]	β (95% CI)	OR (95% CI)
Gender (Female)		2.32 ** (0.66, 4.43)	10.16 ** (1.93, 83.83)
Age	M-SDE1	0.06 (−0.02, 0.14)	1.06 (0.98, 1.15)
Education (≥College Degree)		−2.74 *** (−5.03, −0.99)	0.06 *** (0.01, 0.37)
Env. Exp.		−0.24 (−0.90, 0.31)	0.78 (0.40, 1.36)
Gender (Female)		2.33 ** (0.64, 4.51)	10.26 ** (1.90, 90.62)
Age	M-SDE2	0.04 (−0.03, 0.13)	1.05 (0.97, 1.14)
Education (≥College Degree)		−2.83 (−5.17, −1.07)	0.06 (0.01, 0.34)
Env. Exp.		−0.57 (−1.36, 0.12)	0.57 (0.26, 1.12)

[a] N = 46 subjects, [b] Response variable: 0 non-overweight; 1 overweight, ** *p*-value < 0.01, *** *p*-value < 0.001.

References

1. Prüss-Ustün, A.; Wolf, J.; Corvalán, C.; Bos, R.; Neira, M. *Preventing Disease Through Healthy Environments: A Global Assessment of the Burden of Disease from Environmental Risks*; WHO Press: Geneva, Switzerland, 2016.
2. Sallis, J.F.; Cerin, E.; Conway, T.L.; Adams, M.A.; Frank, L.D.; Pratt, M.; Salvo, D.; Schipperijn, J.; Smith, G.; Cain, K.L.; et al. Physical activity in relation to urban environments in 14 cities worldwide: A cross-sectional study. *Lancet* **2016**, *387*, 2207–2217. [CrossRef]
3. Mitchell, C.A.; Clark, A.F.; Gilliland, J.A. Built environment influences of children's physical activity: Examining differences by neighbourhood size and sex. *Int. J. Environ. Res. Public Health* **2016**, *13*. [CrossRef] [PubMed]
4. Browning, M.; Lee, K. Within what distance does "Greenness" best predict physical health? A systematic review of articles with GIS buffer analyses across the lifespan. *Int. J. Environ. Res. Public Health* **2017**, *14*, 675. [CrossRef] [PubMed]
5. Ta, N.; Chai, T.Y.; Kwan, M.P. Suburbanization, daily lifestyle and space-behavior interaction: A study of suburban residents in Beijing, China. *Acta Geogr. Sin.* **2015**, *70*, 1271–1280.
6. Eriksson, C.; Rosenlund, M.; Pershagen, G.; Hilding, A.; Östenson, C.G.; Bluhm, G. Aircraft Noise and Incidence of Hypertension. *Epidemiology* **2007**, *18*, 716–721. [CrossRef] [PubMed]
7. Park, Y.M.; Kwan, M.P. Individual exposure estimates may be erroneous when spatiotemporal variability of air pollution and human mobility are ignored. *Health Place* **2017**, *43*, 85–94. [CrossRef] [PubMed]
8. Ding, D.; Sallis, J.F.; Kerr, J.; Lee, S.; Rosenberg, D.E. Neighborhood environment and physical activity among youth: A review. *Am. J. Prev. Med.* **2011**, *41*, 442–455. [CrossRef] [PubMed]
9. Troped, P.J.; Wilson, J.S.; Matthews, C.E.; Cromley, E.K.; Melly, S.J. The Built Environment and Location-Based Physical Activity. *Am. J. Prev. Med.* **2010**, *38*, 429–438. [CrossRef] [PubMed]
10. Lytle, L.A.; Sokol, R.L. Measures of the food environment: A systematic review of the field, 2007–2015. *Health Place* **2017**, *44*, 18–34. [CrossRef] [PubMed]
11. Gamba, R.J.; Schuchter, J.; Rutt, C.; Seto, E.Y.W. Measuring the Food Environment and its Effects on Obesity in the United States: A Systematic Review of Methods and Results. *J. Community Health* **2015**, *40*, 464–475. [CrossRef] [PubMed]
12. Morland, K.B.; Evenson, K.R. Obesity prevalence and the local food environment. *Health Place* **2009**, *15*, 491–495. [CrossRef] [PubMed]
13. Cobb, L.K.; Appel, L.J.; Franco, M.; Jones-Smith, J.C.; Nur, A.; Anderson, C.A.M. The relationship of the local food environment with obesity: A systematic review of methods, study quality, and results. *Obesity* **2015**, *23*, 1331–1344. [CrossRef] [PubMed]

14. Caspi, C.E.; Sorensen, G.; Subramanian, S.V.; Kawachi, I. The local food environment and diet: A systematic review. *Health Place* **2012**, *18*, 1172–1187. [CrossRef] [PubMed]

15. Koohsari, M.J.; Mavoa, S.; Villianueva, K.; Sugiyama, T.; Badland, H.; Kaczynski, A.T.; Owen, N.; Giles-Corti, B. Public open space, physical activity, urban design and public health: Concepts, methods and research agenda. *Health Place* **2015**, *33*, 75–82. [CrossRef] [PubMed]

16. Lachowycz, K.; Jones, A.P.; Page, A.S.; Wheeler, B.W.; Cooper, A.R. What can global positioning systems tell us about the contribution of different types of urban greenspace to children's physical activity? *Health Place* **2012**, *18*, 586–594. [CrossRef] [PubMed]

17. Shareck, M.; Kestens, Y.; Vallée, J.; Datta, G.; Frohlich, K.L.; Vallee, J.; Datta, G.; Frohlich, K.L. The added value of accounting for activity space when examining the association between tobacco retailer availability and smoking among young adults. *Tob. Control* **2015**, *25*, 1–7. [CrossRef] [PubMed]

18. Lipperman-Kreda, S.; Morrison, C.; Grube, J.W.; Gaidus, A. Youth activity spaces and daily exposure to tobacco outlets. *Health Place* **2015**, *34*, 30–33. [CrossRef] [PubMed]

19. Kwan, M.P.; Kenda, L.L.; Wewers, M.E.; Ferketich, A.K.; Klein, E.G. Sociogeographic context, protobacco advertising, and smokeless tobacco usage in the Appalachian Region of Ohio (USA). In Proceedings of the International Medical Geography Symposium, Durham, UK, 11–15 July 2011.

20. Epstein, D.H.; Tyburski, M.; Craig, I.M.; Phillips, K.A.; Jobes, M.L.; Vahabzadeh, M.; Mezghanni, M.; Lin, J.L.; Furr-Holden, C.D.M.; Preston, K.L. Real-time tracking of neighborhood surroundings and mood in urban drug misusers: Application of a new method to study behavior in its geographical context. *Drug Alcohol Depend.* **2014**, *134*, 22–29. [CrossRef] [PubMed]

21. Seliske, L.M.; Pickett, W.; Boyce, W.F.; Janssen, I. Association between the food retail environment surrounding schools and overweight in Canadian youth. *Public Health Nutr.* **2009**, *12*, 1384. [CrossRef] [PubMed]

22. Oliver, L.N.; Hayes, M. V Effects of neighbourhood income on reported body mass index: An eight year longitudinal study of Canadian children. *BMC Public Health* **2008**, *8*, 16. [CrossRef]

23. Chaix, B. Geographic Life Environments and Coronary Heart Disease: A Literature Review, Theoretical Contributions, Methodological Updates, and a Research Agenda. *Annu. Rev. Public Health* **2009**, *30*, 81–105. [CrossRef] [PubMed]

24. Millstein, R.A.; Yeh, H.C.; Brancati, F.L.; Batts-Turner, M.; Gary, T.L. Food availability, neighborhood socioeconomic status, and dietary patterns among blacks with type 2 diabetes mellitus. *Medscape J. Med.* **2009**, *11*, 15. [PubMed]

25. Andersen, A.F.; Carson, C.; Watt, H.C.; Lawlor, D.A.; Avlund, K.; Ebrahim, S. Life-course socio-economic position, area deprivation and type 2 diabetes: Findings from the British women's heart and health study. *Diabet. Med.* **2008**, *25*, 1462–1468. [CrossRef] [PubMed]

26. Wheaton, B.; Clarke, P. Space Meets Time: Integrating Temporal and Contextual Influences on Mental Health in Early Adulthood. *Am. Sociol. Rev.* **2016**, *68*, 680–706. [CrossRef]

27. Curtis, S. *Space, Place and Mental Health*; Routledge: London, UK, 2010; ISBN 0754673316.

28. Stigsdotter, U.K.; Ekholm, O.; Schipperijn, J.; Toftager, M.; Kamper-Jorgensen, F.; Randrup, T.B. Health promoting outdoor environments-Associations between green space, and health, health-related quality of life and stress based on a Danish national representative survey. *Scand. J. Soc. Med.* **2010**, *38*, 411–417. [CrossRef] [PubMed]

29. Houle, J.N.; Light, M.T. The home foreclosure crisis and rising suicide rates, 2005 to 2010. *Am. J. Public Health* **2014**, *104*, 1073–1079. [CrossRef] [PubMed]

30. Kestens, Y.; Lebel, A.; Chaix, B.; Clary, C.; Daniel, M.; Pampalon, R.; Theriault, M.; Subramanian, S.V. Association between activity space exposure to food establishments and individual risk of overweight. *PLoS ONE* **2012**, *7*. [CrossRef] [PubMed]

31. Auchincloss, A.H. Neighborhood Resources for Physical Activity and Healthy Foods and Incidence of Type 2 Diabetes Mellitus. *Arch. Intern. Med.* **2009**, *169*, 1698. [CrossRef] [PubMed]

32. PAGAC Physical Activity Guidelines Advisory Committee Report. 2008. Available online: https://health. gov/paguidelines/report/pdf/CommitteeReport.pdf (accessed on 30 August 2018).

33. Ogden, C.L.; Carroll, M.D.; Kit, B.K.; Flegal, K.M. Prevalence of childhood and adult obesity in the United States, 2011–2012. *JAMA* **2014**, *311*, 806–814. [CrossRef] [PubMed]

34. Walker, R.E.; Keane, C.R.; Burke, J.G. Disparities and access to healthy food in the United States: A review of food deserts literature. *Health Place* **2010**, *16*, 876–884. [CrossRef] [PubMed]

35. Inagami, S.; Cohen, D.A.; Brown, A.F.; Asch, S.M. Body mass index, neighborhood fast food and restaurant concentration, and car ownership. *J. Urban Health* **2009**, *86*, 683–695. [CrossRef] [PubMed]

36. Vandevijvere, S.; Dominick, C.; Swinburn, B. The healthy food environment policy index: Findings of an expert panel in New Zealand. *Bull. World Health Organ.* **2015**, *93*, 294–302. [CrossRef] [PubMed]

37. Committee on Accelerating Progress in Obesity Prevention. *Accelerating Progress in Obesity Accelerating Progress in Obesity Prevention: Solving the Weight of the Nation*; National Academies Press: Washington, DC, USA, 2012; ISBN 0309221544.

38. Reisig, V.; Hobbiss, A. Food deserts and how to tackle them: A study of one city's approach. *Health Educ. J.* **2000**, *59*, 137–149. [CrossRef]

39. Chen, X.; Kwan, M.P. Contextual Uncertainties, Human Mobility, and Perceived Food Environment: The Uncertain Geographic Context Problem in Food Access Research. *Am. J. Public Health* **2015**, *105*, 1734–1737. [CrossRef] [PubMed]

40. Holsten, J.E. Obesity and the community food environment: A systematic review. *Public Health Nutr.* **2009**, *12*, 397–405. [CrossRef] [PubMed]

41. Maddock, J. The relationship between obesity and the prevalence of fast food restaurants: State-level analysis. *Am. J. Health Promot.* **2004**, *19*, 137–143. [CrossRef] [PubMed]

42. Lee, H. The role of local food availability in explaining obesity risk among young school-aged children. *Soc. Sci. Med.* **2012**, *74*, 1193–1203. [CrossRef] [PubMed]

43. Jilcott, S.B.; Wade, S.; McGuirt, J.T.; Wu, Q.; Lazorick, S.; Moore, J.B. The association between the food environment and weight status among eastern North Carolina youth. *Public Health Nutr.* **2011**, *14*, 1610–1617. [CrossRef] [PubMed]

44. Zick, C.D.; Smith, K.R.; Fan, J.X.; Brown, B.B.; Yamada, I.; Kowaleski-Jones, L. Running to the Store? The relationship between neighborhood environments and the risk of obesity. *Soc. Sci. Med.* **2009**, *69*, 1493–1500. [CrossRef] [PubMed]

45. Davis, B.; Carpenter, C. Proximity of fast-food restaurants to schools and adolescent obesity. *Am. J. Public Health* **2009**, *99*, 505–510. [CrossRef] [PubMed]

46. Li, F.; Harmer, P.; Cardinal, B.J.; Bosworth, M.; Johnson-Shelton, D. Obesity and the built environment: Does the density of neighborhood fast-food outlets matter? *Am. J. Health Promot.* **2009**, *23*, 203–209. [CrossRef] [PubMed]

47. Jeffery, R.W.; Baxter, J.; McGuire, M.; Linde, J. Are fast food restaurants an environmental risk factor for obesity? *Int. J. Behav. Nutr. Phys. Act.* **2006**, *3*, 1.

48. Dunn, R.A.; Sharkey, J.R.; Horel, S. The effect of fast-food availability on fast-food consumption and obesity among rural residents: An analysis by race/ethnicity. *Econ. Hum. Biol.* **2012**, *10*, 1–13. [CrossRef] [PubMed]

49. Black, J.L.; Macinko, J.; Dixon, L.B.; Fryer, G.E. Neighborhoods and obesity in New York City. *Health Place* **2010**, *16*, 489–499. [CrossRef] [PubMed]

50. Kwan, M.P. The Limits of the Neighborhood Effect: Contextual Uncertainties in Geographic, Environmental Health, and Social Science Research. *Ann. Am. Assoc. Geogr.* **2018**, 1–9. [CrossRef]

51. Wang, J.; Lee, K.; Kwan, M.P. Environmental Influences on Leisure-Time Physical Inactivity in the U.S.: An Exploration of Spatial Non-Stationarity. *ISPRS Int. J. Geo-Inf.* **2018**, *7*. [CrossRef]

52. Kwan, M.P.; Wang, J.; Tyburski, M.; Epstein, D.H.; Kowalczyk, W.J.; Preston, K.L. Uncertainties in the geographic context of health behaviors: A study of substance users' exposure to psychosocial stress using GPS data. *Int. J. Geogr. Inf. Sci.* **2018**, 1–20. [CrossRef]

53. Frank, L.D.; Schmid, T.L.; Sallis, J.F.; Chapman, J.; Saelens, B.E. Linking objectively measured physical activity with objectively measured urban form: Findings from SMARTRAQ. *Am. J. Prev. Med.* **2005**, *28*, 117–125. [CrossRef] [PubMed]

54. Clark, A.; Scott, D. Understanding the impact of the modifiable areal unit problem on the relationship between active travel and the built environment. *Urban Stud.* **2014**, *51*, 284–299. [CrossRef]

55. Feng, J.; Glass, T.A.; Curriero, F.C.; Stewart, W.F.; Schwartz, B.S. The built environment and obesity: A systematic review of the epidemiologic evidence. *Health Place* **2010**, *16*, 175–190. [CrossRef] [PubMed]

56. Leal, C.; Chaix, B. The influence of geographic life environments on cardiometabolic risk factors: A systematic review, a methodological assessment and a research agenda. *Obes. Rev.* **2011**, *12*, 217–230. [CrossRef] [PubMed]

57. Basta, L.A.; Richmond, T.S.; Wiebe, D.J. Neighborhoods, daily activities, and measuring health risks experienced in urban environments. *Soc. Sci. Med.* **2010**, *71*, 1943–1950. [CrossRef] [PubMed]

58. Wiehe, S.E.; Hoch, S.C.; Liu, G.C.; Carroll, A.E.; Wilson, J.S.; Fortenberry, J.D. Adolescent Travel Patterns: Pilot Data Indicating Distance from Home Varies by Time of Day and Day of Week. *J. Adolesc. Health* **2008**, *42*, 418–420. [CrossRef] [PubMed]

59. Kwan, M.P. From place-based to people-based exposure measures. *Soc. Sci. Med.* **2009**, *69*, 1311–1313. [CrossRef] [PubMed]

60. Kwan, M.P. Beyond space (as we knew it): Toward temporally integrated geographies of segregation, health, and accessibility: Space-time integration in geography and GIScience. *Ann. Assoc. Am. Geogr.* **2013**, *103*, 1078–1086. [CrossRef]

61. Cummins, S. Commentary: Investigating neighbourhood effects on health—Avoiding the 'local trap'. *Int. J. Epidemiol.* **2007**, *36*, 355–357. [CrossRef] [PubMed]

62. Kwan, M.P. The Uncertain Geographic Context Problem. *Ann. Assoc. Am. Geogr.* **2012**, *102*, 958–968. [CrossRef]

63. Kwan, M. How GIS can help address the uncertain geographic context problem in social science research. *Ann. GIS* **2012**, *18*, 245–255. [CrossRef]

64. Almanza, E.; Jerrett, M.; Dunton, G.; Seto, E.; Ann Pentz, M. A study of community design, greenness, and physical activity in children using satellite, GPS and accelerometer data. *Health Place* **2012**, *18*, 46–54. [CrossRef] [PubMed]

65. Chaix, B.; Méline, J.; Duncan, S.; Merrien, C.; Karusisi, N.; Perchoux, C.; Lewin, A.; Labadi, K.; Kestens, Y. GPS tracking in neighborhood and health studies: A step forward for environmental exposure assessment, A step backward for causal inference? *Health Place* **2013**, *21*, 46–51. [CrossRef] [PubMed]

66. Maddison, R.; Ni Mhurchu, C. Global positioning system: A new opportunity in physical activity measurement. *Int. J. Behav. Nutr. Phys. Act.* **2009**, *6*, 73. [CrossRef] [PubMed]

67. Laatikainen, T.E.; Hasanzadeh, K.; Kyttä, M. Capturing exposure in environmental health research: Challenges and opportunities of different activity space models. *Int. J. Health Geogr.* **2018**, *17*, 29. [CrossRef] [PubMed]

68. Wang, J.; Kwan, M.P.; Chai, Y. An Innovative Context-Based Crystal-Growth Activity Space Method for Environmental Exposure Assessment: A Study Using GIS and GPS Trajectory Data Collected in Chicago. *Int. J. Environ. Res. Public Health* **2018**, *15*, 703. [CrossRef] [PubMed]

69. Gulliver, J.; Briggs, D.J. Time-space modeling of journey-time exposure to traffic-related air pollution using GIS. *Environ. Res.* **2005**, *97*, 10–25. [CrossRef] [PubMed]

70. Franklin County Community Health Needs Assessment Steering Committee Franklin County Health Map 2013. 2013. Available online: https://www.columbus.gov/uploadedfiles%5CPublic_Health%5CContent_Editors%5CCenter_for_Assessment_and_Preparedness%5CAssessment_and_Surveillance%5CReports_and_Files%5CCPHHealthMap%20Revised_1.3.2013Final%20rev%2011713.pdf (accessed on 30 August 2018).

71. Wiehe, S.E.; Carroll, A.E.; Liu, G.C.; Haberkorn, K.L.; Hoch, S.C.; Wilson, J.S.; Fortenberry, J.D. Using GPS-enabled cell phones to track the travel patterns of adolescents. *Int. J. Health Geogr.* **2008**, *7*, 22. [CrossRef] [PubMed]

72. Dai, D.; Wang, F. Geographic disparities in accessibility to food stores in southwest Mississippi. *Environ. Plan. B Plan. Des.* **2011**, *38*, 659–678. [CrossRef]

73. Páez, A.; Mercado, R.G.; Farber, S.; Morency, C.; Roorda, M. Relative Accessibility Deprivation Indicators for Urban Settings: Definitions and Application to Food Deserts in Montreal. *Urban Stud.* **2010**, *47*, 1415–1438. [CrossRef]

74. Xu, Y.; Wen, M.; Wang, F. Multilevel built environment features and individual odds of overweight and obesity in Utah. *Appl. Geogr.* **2015**, *60*, 197–203. [CrossRef] [PubMed]

75. Lee, M.; Brown, A.; Goodchild, M. Does distance decay modelling of supermarket accessibility predict fruit and vegetable intake by individuals in a large metropolitan area? *J. Health Care Poor Underserved* **2013**, *24*, 172–185. [CrossRef]

76. Lamichhane, A.P.; Puett, R.; Porter, D.E.; Bottai, M.; Mayer-Davis, E.J.; Liese, A.D. Associations of built food environment with body mass index and waist circumference among youth with diabetes. *Int. J. Behav. Nutr. Phys. Act.* **2012**, *9*. [CrossRef] [PubMed]

77. Moore, K.; Roux, A.V.D.; Auchincloss, A.; Evenson, K.R.; Kaufman, J.; Mujahid, M.; Williams, K. Home and work neighbourhood environments in relation to body mass index: The Multi-Ethnic Study of Atherosclerosis (MESA). *J. Epidemiol. Community Health* **2013**, *67*, 846–853. [CrossRef] [PubMed]

78. Chen, X.; Clark, J. Measuring space-time access to food retailers: A case of temporal access disparity in Franklin County, Ohio. *Prof. Geogr.* **2016**, *68*, 175–188. [CrossRef]

79. Kwan, M.P. Interactive geovisualization of activity-travel patterns using three-dimensional geographical information systems: A methodological exploration with a large data set. *Transp. Res. Part C Emerg. Technol.* **2000**, *8*, 185–203. [CrossRef]

80. Rundle, A.; Neckerman, K.M.; Freeman, L.; Lovasi, G.S.; Purciel, M.; Quinn, J.; Richards, C.; Sircar, N.; Weiss, C. Neighborhood food environment and walkability predict obesity in New York City. *Environ. Health Perspect.* **2009**, *117*, 442–447. [CrossRef] [PubMed]

81. Rainham, D.; McDowell, I.; Krewski, D.; Sawada, M. Conceptualizing the healthscape: Contributions of time geography, location technologies and spatial ecology to place and health research. *Soc. Sci. Med.* **2010**, *70*, 668–676. [CrossRef] [PubMed]

82. Shannon, G.W.; Spurlock, C.W. Urban Ecological Containers, Environmental Risk Cells, and the Use of Medical Services. *Econ. Geogr.* **1976**, *52*, 171–180. [CrossRef]

83. Arcury, T.A.; Gesler, W.M.; Preisser, J.S.; Sherman, J.; Spencer, J.; Perin, J. The effects of geography and spatial behavior on health care utilization among the residents of a rual region. *Health Serv. Res.* **2005**, *40*, 135–155. [CrossRef] [PubMed]

84. Crawford, T.W.; Jilcott Pitts, S.B.; McGuirt, J.T.; Keyserling, T.C.; Ammerman, A.S. Conceptualizing and comparing neighborhood and activity space measures for food environment research. *Health Place* **2014**, *30*, 215–225. [CrossRef] [PubMed]

85. Zenk, S.N.; Schulz, A.J.; Matthews, S.A.; Odoms-Young, A.; Wilbur, J.E.; Wegrzyn, L.; Gibbs, K.; Braunschweig, C.; Stokes, C. Activity space environment and dietary and physical activity behaviors: A pilot study. *Health Place* **2011**, *17*, 1150–1161. [CrossRef] [PubMed]

86. Zhao, P.; Kwan, M.P.; Zhou, S. The uncertain geographic context problem in the analysis of the relationships between obesity and the built environment in Guangzhou. *Int. J. Environ. Res. Public Health* **2018**, *15*, 1–20. [CrossRef] [PubMed]

87. Mellor, J.M.; Dolan, C.B.; Rapoport, R.B. Child body mass index, obesity, and proximity to fast food restaurants. *Int. J. Pediatr. Obes.* **2011**, *6*, 60–68. [CrossRef] [PubMed]

88. Matthews, S.A. The salience of neighborhood: Some lessons from sociology. *Am. J. Prev. Med.* **2008**, *34*, 257–259. [CrossRef] [PubMed]

89. Chaix, B. Geographic life environments and coronary heart disease: A literature review, theoretical contributions, methodological updates, and a research agenda. *Annu. Rev. Public Health* **2009**, *30*, 81–105. [CrossRef] [PubMed]

90. Kwan, M.P. The Neighborhood Effect Averaging Problem (NEAP): An Elusive Confounder of the Neighborhood Effect. *Int. J. Environ. Res. Public Health* **2018**, *15*, 1841. [CrossRef] [PubMed]

91. Apparicio, P.; Gelb, J.; Dubé, A.S.; Kingham, S.; Gauvin, L.; Robitaille, É. The approaches to measuring the potential spatial access to urban health services revisited: Distance types and aggregation-error issues. *Int. J. Health Geogr.* **2017**, *16*, 1–24. [CrossRef] [PubMed]

92. Cohen, D.A.; Han, B.; Isacoff, J.; Shulaker, B.; Williamson, S.; Marsh, T.; McKenzie, T.L.; Weir, M.; Bhatia, R. Impact of park renovations on park use and park-based physical activity. *J. Phys. Act. Health* **2015**, *12*, 289–295. [CrossRef] [PubMed]

93. Evenson, K.R.; Wen, F.; Hillier, A.; Cohen, D.A. Assessing the contribution of parks to physical activity using GPS and accelerometry. *Med. Sci. Sports Exerc.* **2013**, *45*, 1981–1987. [CrossRef] [PubMed]

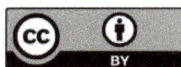

International Journal of
Environmental Research and Public Health

MDPI

Article

Evaluating the Accessibility of Healthcare Facilities Using an Integrated Catchment Area Approach

Xiaofang Pan [1,2], Mei-Po Kwan [3,4], Lin Yang [1,5,*], Shunping Zhou [1], Zejun Zuo [1] and Bo Wan [1]

[1]   Faculty of Information Engineering, China University of Geosciences, 388 Lumo Road,
     Wuhan 430074, China; xfpanem@163.com (X.P.); zhoushunping@mapgis.com (S.Z.);
     zuozejun@mapgis.com (Z.Z.); magicwan1105@163.com (B.W.)
[2]   School of Geographic Sciences, Xinyang Normal University, 237 Nanhu Road, Xinyang 464000, China
[3]   Department of Geography and Geographic Information Science, University of Illinois at Urbana-Champaign,
     Natural History Building, MC-150, 1301 W Green Street, Urbana, IL 61801, USA; mpk654@gmail.com
[4]   Department of Human Geography and Spatial Planning, Utrecht University, P.O. Box 80125,
     3508 TC Utrecht, The Netherlands
[5]   State Key Laboratory of Geo-information Engineering, Xi'an 710054, China
[*]   Correspondence: yanglin_2002_wh@163.com; Tel.: +86-159-2732-2600

Received: 23 July 2018; Accepted: 16 September 2018; Published: 19 September 2018

Abstract: Accessibility is a major method for evaluating the distribution of service facilities and identifying areas in shortage of service. Traditional accessibility methods, however, are largely model-based and do not consider the actual utilization of services, which may lead to results that are different from those obtained when people's actual behaviors are taken into account. Based on taxi GPS trajectory data, this paper proposed a novel integrated catchment area (ICA) that integrates actual human travel behavior to evaluate the accessibility to healthcare facilities in Shenzhen, China, using the enhanced two-step floating catchment area (E2SFCA) method. This method is called the E2SFCA-ICA method. First, access probability is proposed to depict the probability of visiting a healthcare facility. Then, integrated access probability (IAP), which integrates model-based access probability (MAP) and data-based access probability (DAP), is presented. Under the constraint of IAP, ICA is generated and divided into distinct subzones. Finally, the ICA and subzones are incorporated into the E2SFCA method to evaluate the accessibility of the top-tier hospitals in Shenzhen, China. The results show that the ICA not only reduces the differences between model-based catchment areas and data-based catchment areas, but also distinguishes the core catchment area, stable catchment area, uncertain catchment area and remote catchment area of healthcare facilities. The study also found that the accessibility of Shenzhen's top-tier hospitals obtained with traditional catchment areas tends to be overestimated and more unequally distributed in space when compared to the accessibility obtained with integrated catchment areas.

Keywords: healthcare accessibility; catchment areas; access probability; taxi GPS trajectories; E2SFCA

---

1. Introduction

Accessibility refers to the ease with which activity locations or urban services can be reached from a particular location or by an individual [1–5]. Location-based or place-based accessibility—which is conceptually different from individual-based accessibility—is widely used in assessing whether the spatial distribution of public facilities is optimal or not [6]. As an important component of public facilities, healthcare facilities provide residents with necessary medical services, and their distribution and accessibility affect residents' well-being directly. Good accessibility to healthcare facilities for every person is an essential goal for governments [7,8]. Thus, healthcare service planners need more accurate and reliable methods for finding deficiencies in the accessibility of health services [9,10].

Besides distance-based models, physician-to-population ratio-based models and gravity models, the two-step floating catchment area (2SFCA) method proposed by Luo and Wang [4] has grown in prominence in the last decade for evaluating the accessibility of healthcare [8]. In the 2SFCA method, a floating catchment area is used as a "window" in which residents may visit physicians, who in turn can serve those residents within the "window". Therefore, a physician-to-population ratio can be calculated for each health service, and then all the physician-to-population ratios can be summed up for each location within the catchment area and used as the accessibility of that location.

However, the 2SFCA method has two implicit limitations. One is that it uses dichotomies to deal with people's demands and another is that it does not consider distance decay within a catchment area [10]. In other words, people within a catchment area can access the physicians within it while people outside the catchment area cannot; besides, people within a catchment area have equal access to the physicians [10–13]. In real-world situations, distance from the health facilities within a catchment area may affect people's choice and behavior, and there are no hard boundaries that prevent people from using healthcare facilities in catchment areas outside of their own ones. To address these shortcomings, a distance-decay function has been used in recent studies as an additional component of the 2SFCA method [10,13,14] which includes, for example, the kernel density function [15] and the Gaussian function [16]. Luo and Qi [10] suggested that people would not mind a few minutes of difference in travel time to seek medical care, and proposed an enhanced two-step floating catchment area (E2SFCA) method which uses multiple distance decay weights that substitute the dichotomous scheme (zero and one) of the 2SFCA method. As an improvement of the 2SFCA method, a catchment area in the E2SFCA method is divided into several subzones according to the spatial barrier between residents and health services. For instance, a 30-min catchment area is divided into three subzones with breaks at 10 and 20 min [10,11], or a 180-min catchment area is divided into four subzones with breaks at 30, 60, and 120 min [12]. After that, the multiple distance decay weights are assigned to different subzones for calculating the physician-to-population ratio and accessibility.

Thus, in the enhanced two-step floating catchment area (E2SFCA) method, the catchments and subzones of healthcare facilities are artificially set according to the spatial barriers in different cases. To be consistent with the actual traffic conditions of different applications, travel time or travel distance based on the road network is often used as the spatial barrier or impedance [17]. Then accessibility is calculated based on the catchment areas generated based on the spatial barrier or impedance. However, in the real world, people who benefit from health services are affected by various factors in addition to spatial barriers, such as the effectiveness of services, attractiveness of the facility, and sociocultural or socioeconomic barriers [18–20]. For example, Dony et al. [20] proposed that the catchment area of a service facility is a function of its attractiveness. In a study that compares the potential and revealed access to healthcare facilities, Casas et al. [21] found that real travel time to the closest hospital is nearly six times longer than estimated travel time during the dengue fever outbreaks, which suggests that the healthcare facility where healthcare is received rarely coincides with the closest one. The study indicates that patients often prefer to visit healthcare facilities farther away from home instead of closer ones, and this is a common phenomenon. This bypass behavior [22] results in some users of the healthcare facilities in a catchment area not being included in it or some residents of a particular catchment area not visiting the facilities within it. In other words, the arbitrarily defined catchments and subzones, which are based on theoretical spatial barriers, may not represent the actual distribution of patients for the healthcare facilities in a study area. As Wang [23] suggested, any debate over the right size of catchment areas cannot be settled without analyzing real-world healthcare utilization patterns. Therefore, the catchments and subzones area in the E2SFCA method should be adjusted according to real healthcare access behavior.

Questionnaire data or patient information obtained from hospitals are often used as the data source for identifying actual catchment areas [24–27]. Nevertheless, large amounts of data about real patients are hard to obtain in many countries, including China, because of privacy concerns and commercial interests. In recent years, GPS trajectory data on the movement of taxis are increasingly used in social science and transportation studies [28–32]. As a common travel mode, especially in metropolitan areas, taxi travel accounts for a considerable proportion of total travel in China. For instance, from 2010 to 2016, the shares of taxi travel in total transport in Beijing, Shanghai, Guangzhou and Shenzhen (the top four metropolitan areas in China) were 8%, 16.5%, 13.8% and 12.2% respectively, according to statistical yearbooks data [33–36]. Similar to private cars, taxis are more convenient than other public transportation modes, so taxi becomes the first choice for people with medical emergencies or visiting hospitals when private cars are not available [37]. According to a report from the Didi Media Research Institute and CBNData (the biggest online taxi transaction platform in China), about 9.23% of taxi travel involves hospital visits [38]. This indicates that about 10% of taxi GPS tracks can be used to represent riders' actual visits to urban medical facilities.

To address the limitations of previous E2SFCA methods, this study uses taxi GPS trajectories to incorporate the access relationships between actual users and healthcare facilities in the assessment of the accessibility of these facilities. The catchment areas of medical facilities are adjusted by integrating actual access behaviors with theoretical catchments, and these adjusted catchment areas are then incorporated into the E2SFCA method to evaluate the accessibility of healthcare facilities. In comparison with previous studies, this study seeks to contribute to the literature in three main ways: (1) it proposes using access probability to depict people's access behaviors to healthcare facilities from the theoretical, actual, and integrated perspectives; (2) it formulates the notion of integrated catchment areas (ICA) to approximate the catchment areas of healthcare facilities through the constraint of integrated access probability instead of traditional spatial barriers; and (3) by introducing the ICA into the E2SFCA method and incorporating an actual access element in catchment area delineation, the resulting accessibility levels are more in line with people's actual behavior.

2. Method

2.1. Conceptual Framework

This study seeks to develop a method for delineating the catchment areas of healthcare facilities that takes into account people's actual hospital visit behaviors. As discussed earlier, a theoretical catchment area based on distance or travel time may not include some areas in which patients within the catchment area patronize physicians, or may contain some locations where no healthcare visits occur. Meanwhile, pertinent taxi trajectories can be used to identify the actual origins and destinations of real patients and thus address the limitations of traditional catchments to a certain extent. Theoretical (or model-based) catchments and trajectory data-based catchments are deployed in this study as two complementary perspectives. They are integrated to generate catchment areas that better reflect people's actual visits to healthcare facilities. The relationships between them are shown in Figure 1. A model-based catchment area (MCA) delineates the catchment area of a medical facility using theoretical distance. A data-based catchment area (DCA) is derived from a big taxi trajectory dataset. The MCA and DCA can be integrated to obtain the integrated catchment area (ICA), which adjusts the MCA to take into account actual hospital visit behavior. Through such integration, the ICA better reflects people's behavior and is used as the "window" in the E2SFCA method in this study.

In previous studies, if a location is within a spatial barrier threshold, it is regarded as inside the catchment area, and if a location is beyond this threshold, it is regarded as outside the catchment area. However, some residents within a catchment area may not utilize the healthcare facilities within it while some people living outside this catchment area may utilize these facilities. Therefore, in this paper, whether a location belongs to a catchment area or not depends on the probability of people who live at that location visiting the facilities within the catchment. In light of the flexibility of people's healthcare choices, every healthcare facility has a possibility of being visited by any patient. We thus define this possibility of visit as access probability. Access probability is in the range of zero to one and the value shows the likelihood of visiting a healthcare facility by people at a specified location.

Note that access probability generated from conventional models and actual data are not the same, which are defined as MAP (model-based access probability) and DAP (data-based access probability) respectively, while integrated access probability (IAP) refers to the likelihood of visiting a healthcare facility considering both model-based and data-based perspectives. In what follows, different access probability indexes are defined in detail.

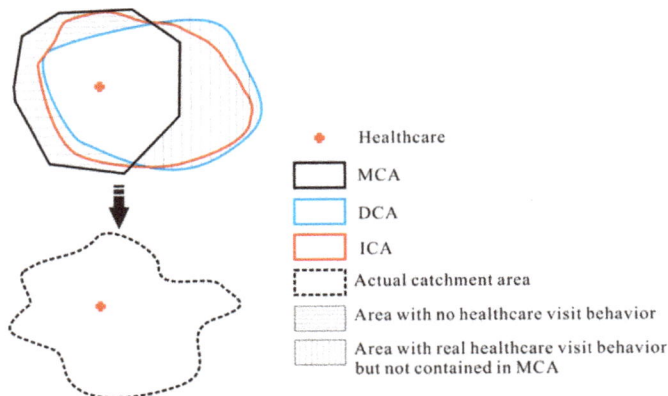

Figure 1. The relationship among model-based catchment area (MCA), data-based catchment area (DCA), integrated catchment area (ICA) and actual catchment area.

2.2. The Access Probability Indexes

Model-based access probability (MAP) is the access probability based on a spatial distance threshold. Ingram proposed an accessibility model and suggested that the shorter the distance from a specific location to a service facility, the higher the access probability of the location [39]. Furthermore, distance decay is an important notion in geography [40,41]. Therefore, according to the principles of least effort and distance decay, people tend to choose the nearest facility, and the probability of visiting a facility decreases as distance increases [27,42,43]. This means that the shorter the distance, the higher the MAP. Therefore, an inverted power function which is similar to a distance decay function is used in the MAP.

Suppose SA is the study area, let $F = \{f_1, f_2, \ldots, f_n\}$ be the set of healthcare facilities in SA, and k be any location within SA. The MAP of the resident at location k visiting a healthcare facility f_i can be expressed as Formula (1):

$$MAP(\alpha_k^{f_i}) = \frac{1/d_i}{\sum_{i=1}^{n} 1/d_i} \tag{1}$$

and Formula (1) satisfies the constraint of Formula (2):

$$MAP(\alpha_k^{f_1}) + MAP(\alpha_k^{f_2}) + \ldots + MAP(\alpha_k^{f_n}) = 1, \tag{2}$$

In Formula (1), d_i denotes the distance from k to f_i and n denotes the total number of facilities in the study area. For instance, as Figure 2 shows, the travel distance from location k to facilities f_1, f_2, f_3 are represented by the inverted power function weight (in parentheses on the line). The MAP of location k to the three healthcare facilities are: $MAP(\alpha_k^{f_1}) = \frac{0.3}{0.3+0.5+0.5} = 0.231$, $MAP(\alpha_k^{f_2}) = \frac{0.5}{0.3+0.5+0.5} = 0.385$, and $MAP(\alpha_k^{f_3}) = \frac{0.5}{0.3+0.5+0.5} = 0.385$.

However, data-based access probability (DAP), which denotes the actual visit probability based on taxi trajectory data, differs. It is defined by the number of passengers who get off at a healthcare facility. The more passengers that get off at a facility, the greater attractiveness and the higher actual access probability it has [6,44]. Therefore, the DAP of one location to a particular healthcare facility can be denoted as the percentage of patients who actually visited this facility among all patients that originated from that location. DAP is thus represented by Formula (3):

$$DAP(\alpha_k^{f_i}) = \frac{p_i}{\sum_{i=1}^{n} p_i} \tag{3}$$

Similarly, $DAP(\alpha_k^{f_i})$ satisfies Formula (4):

$$DAP(\alpha_k^{f_1}) + DAP(\alpha_k^{f_2}) + \ldots + DAP(\alpha_k^{f_n}) = 1 \tag{4}$$

In Formula (3), p_i denotes the number of residents who visit f_i from k and n denotes the total facilities number in the study area. As shown in Figure 2, the number of residents from k to f_1, f_2, f_3 are shown in parentheses below the line. Therefore, $DAP(\alpha_k^{f_1}) = \frac{80}{80+100+100} = 0.286$, $DAP(\alpha_k^{f_2}) = \frac{100}{80+100+100} = 0.357$, and $DAP(\alpha_k^{f_3}) = \frac{100}{80+100+100} = 0.357$.

MAP and DAP describe the access probability to a medical facility from two different perspectives. According to Section 2.1 above, integrated access probability (IAP) is defined as the combination of MAP and DAP. Obviously, an increase in both MAP and DAP leads to an increase in IAP (i.e., IAP is positively correlated with MAP and DAP). To ensure that the value of IAP is in the range of zero to one, IAP is formulated as a linear function of DAP and MAP with different weights. Therefore, the IAP of location k to healthcare f_i is expressed as Formula (5):

$$IAP(\alpha_k^{f_i}) = \lambda_1 MAP(\alpha_k^{f_i}) + \lambda_2 DAP(\alpha_k^{f_i}) \tag{5}$$

In Formula (5), λ_1, λ_2 denotes the weight of MAP and DAP respectively. If there are no residents visiting f_i, p_i is equal to zero and thus $DAP(\alpha_k^{f_i})$ is equal to zero. In this case, $IAP(\alpha_k^{f_i})$ is determined only by $MAP(\alpha_k^{f_i})$, which is the same as the traditional methods.

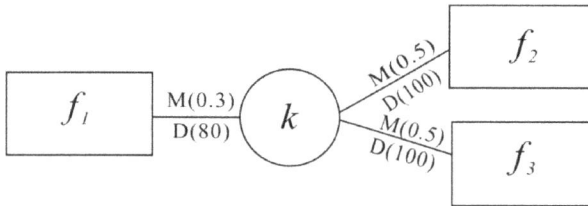

Figure 2. A scenario of model-based and data-based visiting probability to healthcare facilities.

2.3. The Integrated Catchment Area

The criterion for determining whether a location falls within the catchment area of a medical facility is the access probability of this location being greater than or equal to a certain threshold [45]. All the locations that satisfy the condition constitute the catchment area of this facility.

Assume δ is the access probability threshold, the catchment of the facility f_i under δ is the collection of location k whose access probability is greater than or equal to δ. Therefore, three catchment areas, MCA, DCA and ICA are formed as Formulas (6)–(8):

$$MCA(f_i, \delta) = \{k | MAP(\alpha_k^{f_i}) \geq \delta, k \in SA, f_i \in F, \delta \in [0,1]\}, \tag{6}$$

$$DCA(f_i, \delta) = \{k | DAP(\alpha_k^{f_i}) \geq \delta, k \in SA, f_i \in F, \delta \in [0,1]\}, \tag{7}$$

$$ICA(f_i, \delta) = \{k | IAP(\alpha_k^{f_i}) \geq \delta, k \in SA, f_i \in F, \delta \in [0,1]\}, \tag{8}$$

In Formulas (6)–(8), δ is the access probability threshold in the range of zero to one. $MCA(f_i, \delta)$, $DCA(f_i, \delta)$ and $ICA(f_i, \delta)$ denote the model-based, data-based, and integrated catchment areas of a healthcare facility that satisfy the constraint of δ. Due to the difference in access probability defined in Formulas (6)–(8), these three catchment areas are different at the same threshold. Moreover, different thresholds generate different results for each kind of catchment area, which means the catchment area varies with a change in the access probability threshold. In other words, if a set of continuous thresholds are given, a collection of catchment areas representing different access probabilities will be generated.

2.4. Accessibility Measurement Based on ICA

In order to differentiate the accessibility within a catchment area, multiple travel time zones within each catchment area are obtained and assigned with different weights in the E2SFCA method [10]. In this study, the integrated catchment area (ICA) is used in the E2SFCA method. Therefore, we name this method the E2SFCA-ICA method. In this method, the subzones are identified by different IAP thresholds. Given that the study area is covered by a grid structure and each grid represents a population unit, the E2SFCA-ICA method is implemented in two steps:

Step1: $ICA(f_i, \delta)$ is defined as the catchment area of facility f_i with IAP of δ. Then, each catchment area is divided into multiple subzones of $subzone_1, subzone_2, \ldots, subzone_r$ when the thresholds of IAP are $\delta_1, \delta_2, \ldots, \delta_r$, respectively. Search all population units (here, a grid cell) that are within $subzone_j$ from facility f_i and compute the weighted physician-to-population ratio R_i, which is represented by Formula (9):

$$R_i = \frac{S_i}{\sum_{k \in ICA(f_i, \delta_j)} pop_k w_j}$$
$$= \frac{S_i}{\sum_{k \in ICA(f_i, \delta_1)} pop_k w_1 + \sum_{k \in ICA(f_i, \delta_2)} pop_k w_2 + \ldots + \sum_{k \in ICA(f_i, \delta_r)} pop_k w_r} \tag{9}$$

where δ_j is the IAP threshold of $subzone_j$, $ICA(f_i, \delta_j)$ is the integrated catchment area (ICA) of f_i under δ_j, pop_k denotes the population unit of location k falling within $ICA(f_i, \delta_j)$ and S_i is the number of physicians in a healthcare facility f_i, and w_r is the distance weight for r_{th} subzone.

Step 2: For each location k, search all healthcare facilities that are within $ICA(f_i, \delta_j)$ and sum up all of the physician-to-population ratios as its accessibility, which is represented by Formula (10):

$$A_k = \sum_{i \in ICA(f_i, \delta_j)} R_i w_j$$
$$= \sum_{i \in ICA(f_i, \delta_1)} R_i w_1 + \sum_{i \in ICA(f_i, \delta_2)} R_i w_2 + \ldots + \sum_{i \in ICA(f_i, \delta_r)} R_i w_r, \tag{10}$$

where A_k represents the accessibility of location k, and R_i denotes the physician-to-population ratio of facility f_i that falls within the catchment area centered at population k. The same IAP threshold of subzone and distance weights in Step 1 are applied in Step 2.

The greater the value of A_k, the higher the accessibility of location k is to healthcare facilities. The smaller the differences in accessibility between different locations, the more equitable the distribution of healthcare facilities is, and vice versa. The advantage of this method is that the catchment areas and subzones are determined by the characteristics of the specific study area instead of an arbitrary value.

3. Case Study

3.1. Study Area

The study area for this research is Shenzhen, a metropolitan area in southern Guangdong Province in China. Shenzhen is comprised of six districts (Futian, Luohu, Nanshan, Yantian, Baoan, and Longgang) with a total area of 1996.85 km^2 and a permanent population of about 10.35 million in 2010 according to the Sixth National Census of China. The population of each sub-district is obtained from the Shenzhen statistical yearbook (http://www.sztj.gov.cn/). The year of the road network used in this study is 2010.

Taxis play an important role in public transportation in Shenzhen. According to a report from the Shenzhen Transportation Commission (http://www.sztb.gov.cn/), the number of taxi passengers exceeded 350 million each year from 2010 to 2017, which accounted for an average of 12.2% of travel by public transportation annually (Figure 3). In this study, the taxi trajectory dataset was collected from 12,448 taxis from 1 November to 7 November 2011. The weather in Shenzhen is comfortable in November, so passengers do not take taxis to protect themselves from storms or cold weather. Meanwhile, there are no holidays on these days, so taxis operated normally in this period.

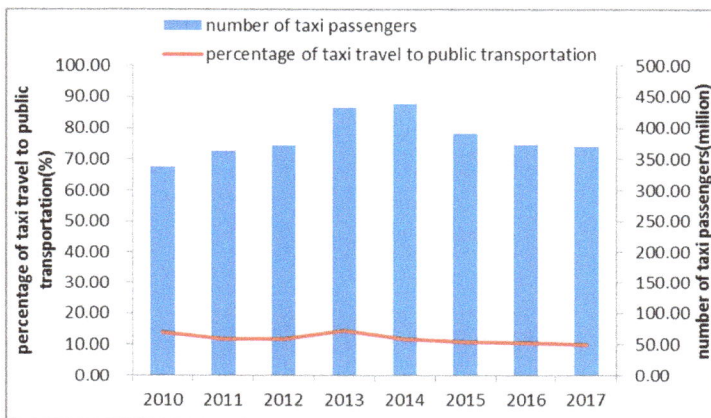

Figure 3. Taxi travel statistics of Shenzhen from 2010 to 2017.

In China, top-tier hospitals (3A-hospitals) are the highest level of hospitals according to the standard of classification. Eighty-eight percent of hospital visits by taxis are to top-tier hospitals, as reported by Didi Media Research Institute & CBNData [46]. This suggests that it is feasible to analyze the travel behavior of top-tier hospitals by taxi trajectory data. There were ten top-tier hospitals in Shenzhen by the end of 2014 according to Shenzhen Statistical Yearbook and all of them are the primary facilities covered by medical insurance (Table 1), which means that residents can choose any of these top-tier hospitals and get reimbursement for the same service at the same rate. The distribution of these ten top-tier hospitals and the population density of the study area are shown in Figure 4. The size of the yellow circle in Figure 4 denotes the number of physicians and the color of the sub-districts denotes their population density from low (light shades) to high (dark shades).

Table 1. The top-tier hospitals of Shenzhen.

Hospital Name	Abbreviation
Peking University Shenzhen Hospital	H1
Shenzhen People's Hospital	H2
The Second People's Hospital of Shenzhen	H3
The SIXTH people's Hospital of Shenzhen	H4
The Eighth People's Hospital of Shenzhen	H5
The Ninth People's Hospital of Shenzhen	H6
Shenzhen Traditional Chinese Medicine Hospital	H7
The Second Traditional Chinese Medicine Hospital of Shenzhen	H8
Shenzhen Maternity & Child Healthcare Hospital	H9
Shenzhen Pingle Orthopedic Hospital	H10

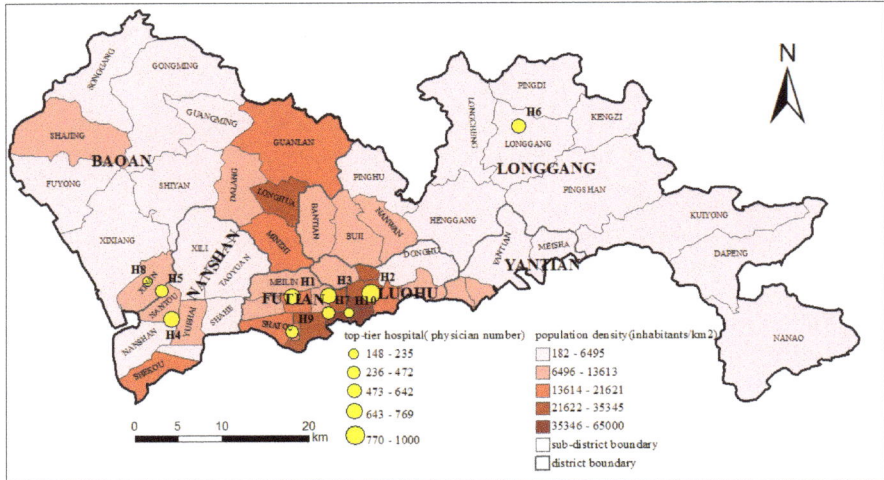

Figure 4. The top-tier hospitals and the population density of Shenzhen.

3.2. Data Processing

As Figure 5 shows, data processing in this study was performed in two phases: data preparation and data calculation. Data preparation preceded data calculation, which is composed of two steps.

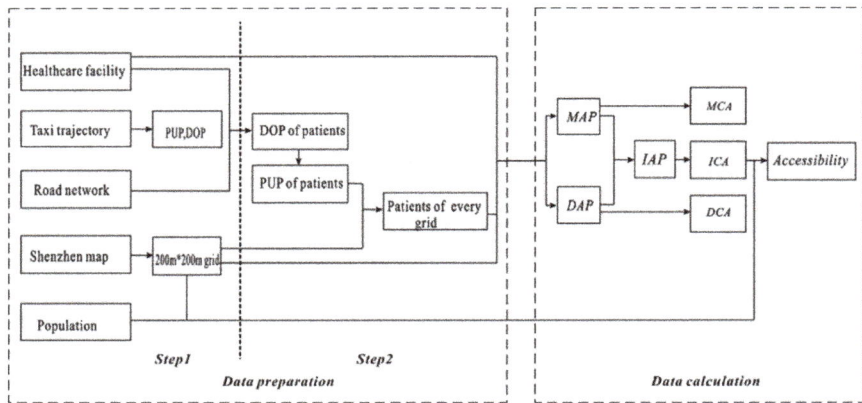

Figure 5. The flow of the accessibility evaluation.

Step 1 is data pre-processing. After the basic process of transforming coordinates, removing abnormal trajectories and map matching, the taxi trajectories used in this study included 75.94 million GPS points with an average sampling interval of 40 s. Then, the trajectory data were decomposed into individual trips which began with a pick-up point (PUP) and ended with a drop-off point (DOP) [47]. Meanwhile, the minimum geographic unit available to the public (which we can obtain) is the sub-district. However, this sub-district census unit is too large for capturing the details within it. To achieve higher spatial resolution, the study area was divided into grids of 200 × 200 m and each grid cell was taken as the basic population unit. Assuming that the population is uniformly distributed within each sub-district, the population of a grid cell can be calculated and the geographic centroid of the cell is considered the population demand center. A total of 47,779 grid cells or units cover the study area.

Step 2 is mainly for extracting the patients of each grid cell. First, a rectangular buffer at the gate of each hospital was constructed for identifying and extracting patient drop-offs at the hospital's entrance (drop-offs outside this buffer area are unlikely to be patient drop-offs from taxis; but note that one hospital seems to have several gates). The gates of the hospitals were located using Baidu map API (Application Programming Interface) tool (http://api.map.baidu.com/lbsapi/getpoint/index.html). Each buffer was set as a 100×20-m rectangle because we found that there are rarely other types of points of interest (POIs) within 50 m of the gates of the top-tier hospitals. Therefore, 100 m was used as the length of the rectangular buffer. Further, considering the interference of the facilities opposite a hospital, 20 m was set as the width of the rectangular buffer, which is usually smaller than the width of the road. Then, passengers with DOPs within the 100×20-m rectangular buffer at a hospital's gate were selected as the patients who visited the hospital and the corresponding PUPs were identified as the patients' home addresses. Finally, the patient number of each grid cell can be calculated by overlapping the PUPs of patients and the grid layer.

After this phase of data preparation, distances between the population units to the 10 hospitals were needed for the MAP calculation. It is important to note that, due to the nature of the raster (grid-based) spatial framework used in this study, it was normally not possible to take into account the effects of network topology and link/turn impedance between each hospital and each grid cell in the study area—since there is no obvious way in which variations in the distances among all the cells (representing network distance/time while taking topology and link/turn impedance into account) in a grid structure can be represented in ways that still allow for grid-based map algebra to operate (which operates on cell distance in the manner of "one cell, two cells or X cells apart" and thus allow for the calculation of distance based on the constant distance between any pair of cell centroids, but not on what the actual measured distance between two cells). This is a limitation all studies that examine catchment areas using a raster data structure would face and there is no satisfactory solution to the problem to date. In this case, a point-based topological network is an alternative choice to derive the distance.

Despite this limitation of the grid data structure used in our study, we implemented special procedures to utilize road network topology when estimating the MAP index. In this part of the analysis, we first constructed a topological network of the study area (which has 203,588 links and 73,515 nodes) that incorporates connectivity and directional restrictions (e.g., bidirectional or one-way roads), where road segment length was set as the link impedance. However, turn restrictions were not considered when constructing this topological network because such information was not available in the original digital road network. Using this topological road network of the study area, we mapped each of the 47,779 grid cells in the grid structure to the appropriate network node on the road network using the centroid of each grid cell. In order to derive the network-based distance matrix for estimating the MAP index, we used such mapping to transfer all cell-to-cell calculations to point-to-point network-based calculations, which was conducted using the shortest path algorithm and considering both network topology and link impedance between each hospital and each grid cell centroid. The $10 \times 47,779$ matrix (10 hospitals to 47,779 cells) of network travel distances was then calculated using ArcGIS. Therefore, the MAP index in this study was computed using a point-based network framework without involving any GPS trajectory data; while the DAP index was calculated using the grid-based framework using the large GPS trajectory dataset without using the topological road network because the taxi trajectories already reflect the effects of road connectivity and link impedance of the transport network in the study area. Meanwhile, the PUPs and DOPs obtained from Step 2 were used to calculate the DAP index matrix of $10 \times 47,779$.

Finally, in order to consider the effects of MAP and DAP equally, we set $\lambda_1 = \lambda_2 = 0.5$ in the following experiments to derive the ICAs of each hospital. These catchment areas thus reflect the link impedance of the transport network in the study area in many ways. The results and discussion of the ICA and accessibility are presented in Section 4 below.

4. Results and Discussion

4.1. Analysis of the Access Probability Threshold

Statistical results of the MAP, DAP, and IAP for each grid cell are shown in Table 2. The maximum MAP is only 0.31, which indicates that none of the hospitals has an absolute advantage in attracting patients because it is located geographically closer to them. However, the DAP ranges from zero to one, which indicates that people at the same location have similar behaviors when seeing a doctor because they may all visit a certain hospital (DAP = 1) without considering others. The minimum IAP is about half of the minimum DAP, and its maximum value of 0.66 suggests that any hospital has the probability of being visited but could not reach 100% attraction for the surrounding residents. For the convenience of comparing the results in a simpler classification, three values were selected respectively as high, middle and low levels of access probability for the MAP, DAP and IAP. That is, according to the different ranges of MAP, DAP and IAP, the high, middle and low levels of MAP were defined as 0.3, 0.2 and 0.1, the high, middle and low levels of DAP were defined as 0.9, 0.5 and 0.1, and the high, middle and low levels of IAP were defined as 0.5, 0.3 and 0.1, as Table 2 shows.

Table 2. The statistical results and levels of model-based access probability (MAP), data-based access probability (DAP) and integrated access probability (IAP).

	Min Value	Max Value	Std.	High Level	Middle Level	Low Level
MAP	0.000085	0.314345	0.038918	0.3	0.2	0.1
DAP	0	1	0.053472	0.9	0.5	0.1
IAP	0.000042	0.656681	0.036113	0.5	0.3	0.1

4.2. Analysis of the Differences among MCA, DCA, and ICA

MCA and DCA depict the catchment areas respectively from the conventional model and trajectory data. However, few studies discussed their differences and to what extent they differ from each other. In this section, we examine the differences between the MCA, DCA and ICA to explore the methodological issues concerning the measurement of accessibility.

Take hospital H1 as an example, the MCA at five different thresholds that represent different access probability levels (0.1, 0.15, 0.2, 0.25, 0.3) are shown in Figure 6a. Similarly, the DCA at five different thresholds (0.1, 0.3, 0.5, 0.7, 0.9) are shown in Figure 6b. The color changes from light blue to dark blue as access probability increases. At a high access probability level, the area of the MCA (H1, 0.3) is 18.34 km^2 and the area of the DCA (H1, 0.9) is 38.15 km^2, which means the DCA is about two times the size of the MCA. At a medium access probability level, the area of the MCA (H1, 0.2) is 83.32 km^2 and the area of the DCA (H1, 0.5) is 60.86 km^2, which means that the MCA is only slightly larger than the DCA. At a low access probability level, the area of the MCA (H1, 0.1) is 310.27 km^2 and the area of DCA (H1, 0.1) is 90.61 km^2, which indicates that the MCA is more than 3 times the size of the DCA. In addition to the large differences in size, the differences in shape between the MCA and DCA are also significant. Figure 6a shows that with the decrease in δ, the MCA mainly expands to the north of H1, which means that the users of this hospital are mainly distributed in areas in the north of H1 based on a largely conceptual understanding of accessibility (i.e., influenced mainly by distance). However, the DCA (Figure 6b) shows that distribution of the actual users of this hospital is extended in the east-west direction of H1, which is consistent with the distribution of the population in this region.

To further illustrate this gap, the difference in area between the MCA and DCA is represented as $\Delta area$ which can be obtained using Formula (11):

$$\Delta area = area_{MCA} - area_{DCA}, \tag{11}$$

In Formula (11), $area_{MCA}$ and $area_{DCA}$ denotes the area of the MCA and DCA respectively.

The Δ*area* of these 10 top-tier hospitals at low, middle and high levels of probability thresholds are shown in Figure 7a–c. Note that at the low probability level (Figure 7a), all of the ten Δ*area* are greater than zero, which means all of the MCA are larger than the DCA, and it also indicates that MCA tend to overestimate the catchment areas of healthcare facilities at low levels of probability thresholds. At the middle probability levels (Figure 7b), the Δ*area* value of more than half of the hospitals is above the horizontal axis, which indicates the MCA is slightly larger than the DCA at middle probability levels. At the high probability levels (Figure 7c), the Δ*area* value of nine hospitals is much less than zero, which indicates that MCA tends to underestimate the catchment areas of healthcare facilities at high levels of probability thresholds. The overestimation or underestimation indicates that catchment areas based on conventional accessibility models do tend to deviate considerably from the catchment areas that are delineated based on real hospital visit data and thus need adjustments in practical applications.

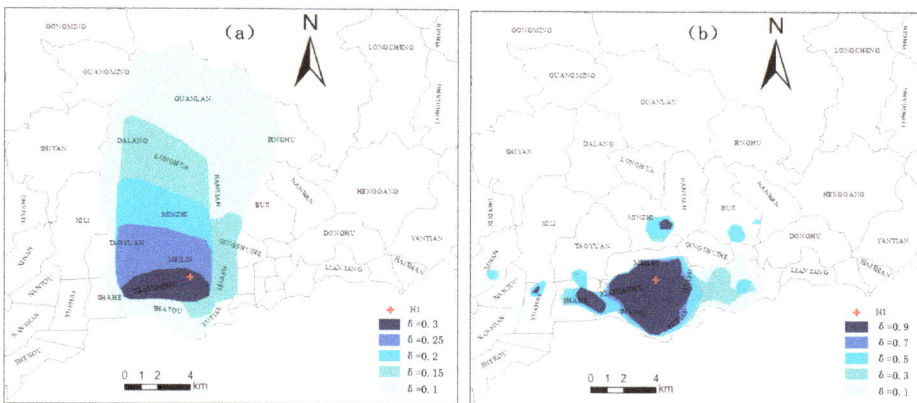

Figure 6. MCA and DCA of H1 under different thresholds (**a**) MCA (**b**) DCA.

The size of the ICA at low, middle and high levels of probability thresholds are shown in Figure 7d, which indicates that the size of the ICA varies across the 10 hospitals. This means that the size of the ICA varies by the location of a hospital. In the case of low levels of access probability, the area of H1 is the largest, followed by H2, H3 and H6, and then H4, H7, H8, H9 and H10. H1 is the most famous hospital in Shenzhen which can attract patients from far away. Therefore, its largest ICA corresponds well to the actual situation. This phenomenon also reveals that the more attractive a service facility is, the larger catchment area it has, which was proposed by Dony [20]. Similar reasons hold for H2 and H3. However, H6 is not as famous as H1, H2 and H3, but its ICA is approximately the same size as that of H3. This is mainly because H6 is the only top-tier hospital in Longgang district and it is far from other top-tier hospitals (see Figure 4). That is, people in Longgong district have few choices when seeking medical treatment. This also indicates that there is much less competition between H6 and other hospitals. For example, H4 (in Nanshan district) and H5 (in Baoan district) have similar reputations as H6 in their respective district, but H4 and H5 are close to each other and not far from Futian district which has four top-tier hospitals. Thus, the competition from the surrounding top-tier hospitals of H4 and H5 is more intense than the potential competitors of H6 which are located far away. Moreover, Longgang lies in the urban fringe and its urbanization level is lower than other districts. Therefore, a large ICA for H6, which is located in the urban fringe where medical resources are scarce, seems reasonable. This is also consistent with the findings of previous studies that healthcare facilities in the fringe of metropolitan areas or larger rural communities would frequently serve populations located well beyond the local community [8,14].

Therefore, our result shows that the size of the catchment areas varies by the location of a hospital. In addition, the attractiveness of the service facilities and the competition among them also affect the size of the service catchment areas.

The MCA (black line), DCA (blue line) and ICA (red line) of the 10 top-tier hospitals at three different access probability levels are shown in Figure 8. It can be seen that most of the MCA are more regular than the DCA in terms of shape. This is mainly because the MCA only considers distance but the DCA reflects complex human travel and activities. Furthermore, we find that at a high threshold level, the ICA are always at the intersection of the MCA and DCA. At a middle threshold level, the ICA are always similar to the DCA in shape. Moreover, at a low threshold level, the ICA is the result of the comprehensive adjustment of the MCA and DCA, but there are still many ICA (e.g., H2, H3, H4, H6, H7, and H10) that are very similar to the DCA in shape. This reflects two facts: (1) The ICA corrected the deviation of the MCA effectively, no matter what the access probability threshold is, the ICA can integrate the MCA and DCA in a way that obtains a shape and size that better reflect real hospital visit patterns; and (2) the DCA has a greater impact on the ICA than the MCA. In Section 4.1, the same weight ($\lambda_1 = \lambda_2$) is allocated to the MCA and DCA. In other words, the effects of the MCA and DCA on the ICA are given the same weight and considered equally in the experiment, but the ICA is still more similar to the DCA in shape, especially at a middle probability threshold level. This further illustrates the capability of the DCA in capturing more realistic catchment areas when compared to catchment areas based on conventional models of accessibility.

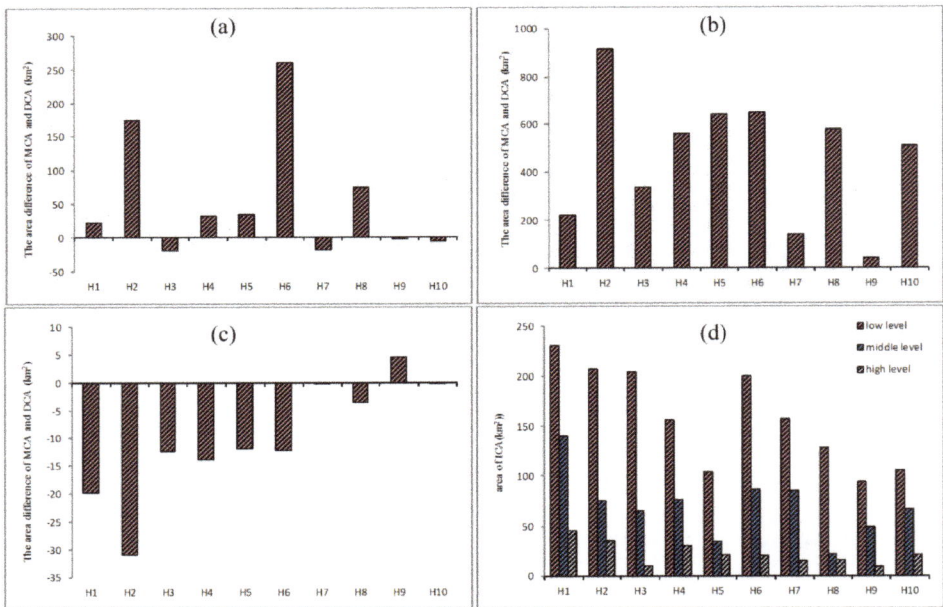

Figure 7. (**a**) Area differences of MCA and DCA at low level; (**b**) Area differences of MCA and DCA at middle level; (**c**) Area differences of MCA and DCA at high level; (**d**) The area of ICA at low, middle and high level.

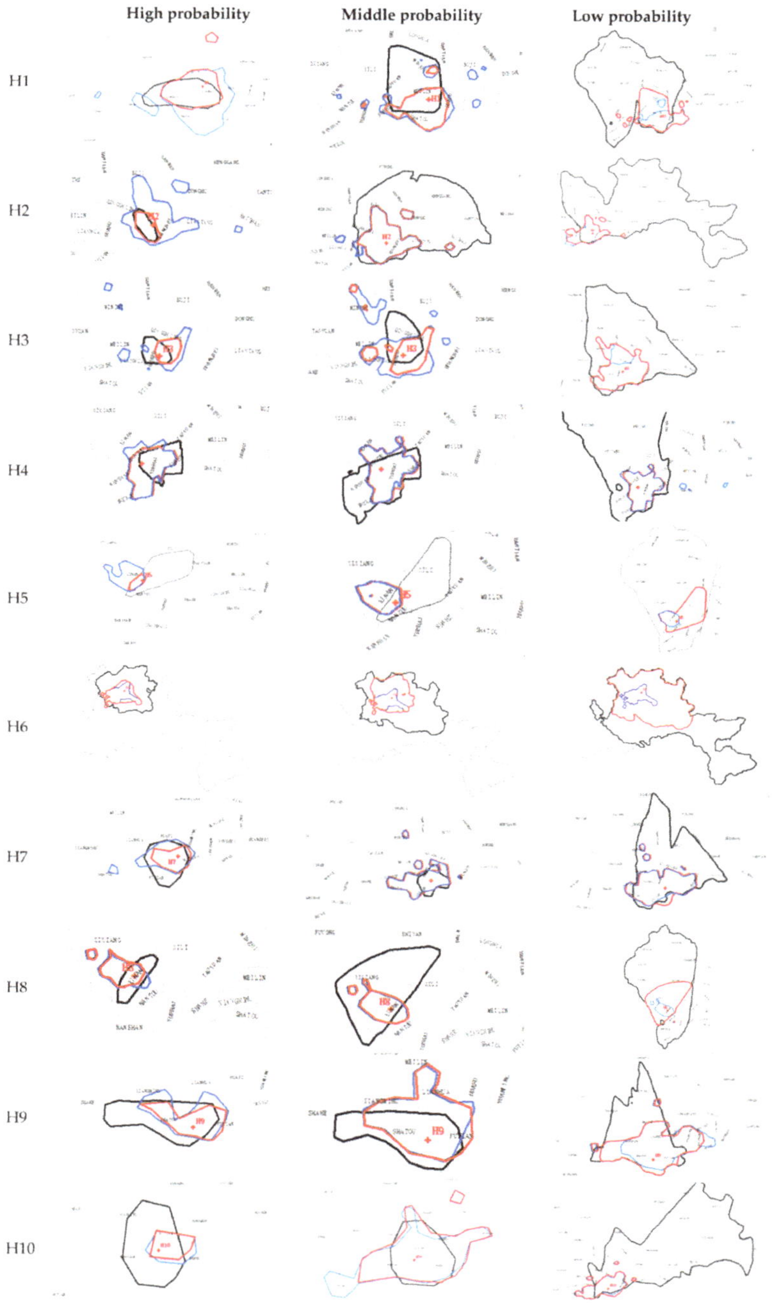

Figure 8. The boundary of the MCA, DCA and ICA at a high, middle and low level of probability threshold. (black line represents MCA boundary, blue line represents DCA boundary, red line represents ICA boundary).

4.3. Analysis of the Characteristics of the ICA

In this section, we further analyze the characteristics of the ICA. The ICA of the top-tier hospitals under six different access probability thresholds (0.1, 0.2, 0.3, 0.4, 0.5 and 0.6) are shown in Figure 9.

Three salient features stand out in Figure 9. First, when $\delta = 0.6$, six hospitals (H1, H2, H3, H4, H8 and H9) have completely independent ICA. This indicates that these hospitals have great influence and reputation because they have the highest access probability for patients. In other words, these are areas where loyal users of these healthcare facilities are located. With the prominence of these hospitals and their loyal users, these areas can be viewed as the core catchment areas of these six hospitals. Second, as δ decreases from 0.5 to 0.2, the ICA begin to overlap and two distinct regions appear (A and B region in Figure 9). Region A includes Nantou, Yuehai, Zhaoshang, Shekou, Nanshan, Shahe, Xixiang, and Xi'nan sub-districts, and Region B includes sub-districts of Guiyuan, Nanhu, Dongmen, Sungang, Cuizhu, Dongxiao, and Huangbei sub-districts. Further, the figure shows that the size and shape of these two regions change little when δ varies in the range of 0.5 to 0.2. This reveals that the two catchment areas remain stable with the change in access probability. Therefore, these two regions are the stable catchment areas of the six hospitals. Third, when δ decreases to 0.1, the catchment areas increase so rapidly that the ICA of the hospitals all overlap together to yield a fan-shaped area, which includes the south of Baoan district, Nanshan district, Futian district, and the west of Luohu district. In this large fan-shaped area, the low access probability suggests that residents are not sure which hospital they would access. So, this region is regarded as the uncertain catchment area of the healthcare facilities. Finally, when δ is less than 0.1, the catchment areas extend to the whole area of Shenzhen (the blank area of Figure 9). Due to the lowest access probability and remote distance from the top-tier hospitals, this big region is regarded as the remote catchment area of the top-tier hospitals.

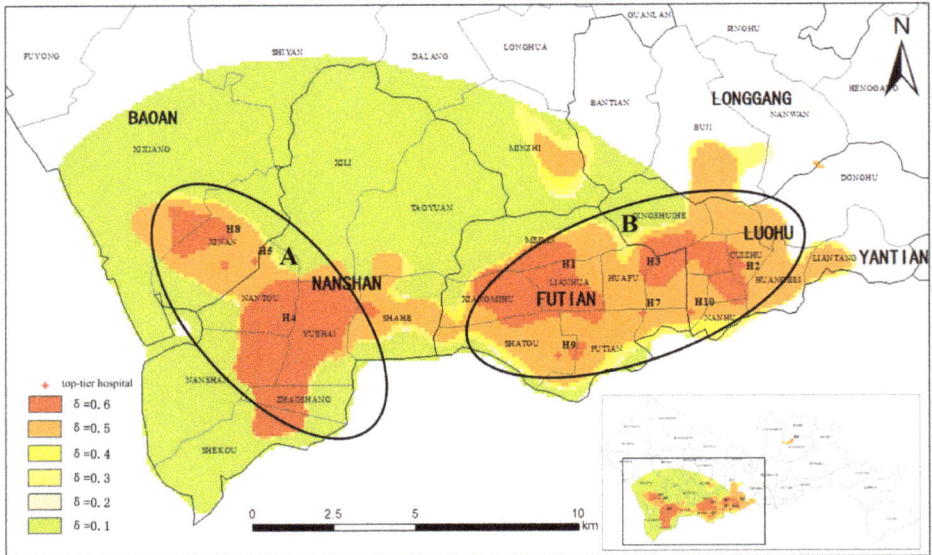

Figure 9. The ICA of the top-tier hospitals under different probability thresholds.

Therefore, we observe a core catchment area, a stable catchment area, an uncertain catchment area and a remote catchment area of the top-tier hospitals in the study area through three dividing points of the IAP thresholds, which are $\delta = 0.5$, $\delta = 0.2$ and $\delta = 0.1$. These three dividing points are more evident in Figure 10, which shows the percentage of the population and area of the ICA under different access probabilities (the percentage is the proportion of the population or area of the ICA of the population or area of the entire area of Shenzhen). The red line represents the percentage of population within the ICA at six IAP thresholds, and the blue line represents the percentage of areas of the ICA at six IAP thresholds. It can be seen that the two curves both drop sharply when δ is less than 0.1, then, their rates of descent become slower from $\delta = 0.1$ to $\delta = 0.2$, and then they almost become flat curves in the range of 0.2 to 0.5. Finally, the rate of decline accelerates again when δ is larger than 0.5.

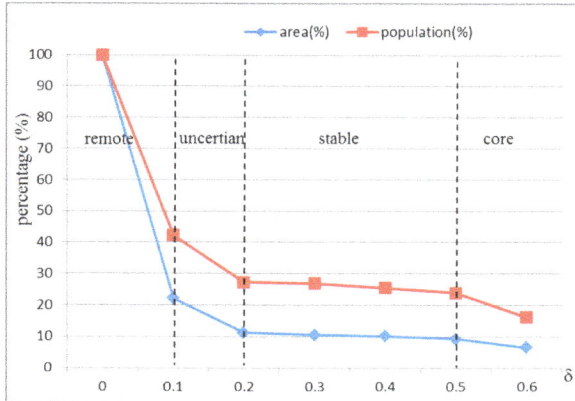

Figure 10. The population and area percentage of ICA under different access probabilities.

4.4. The Accessibility of the Top-Tier Hospitals

In this section, to compare our method with the traditional methods, the accessibility of the ten top-tier hospitals in the study area is calculated using the E2SFCA method based on the ICA, the E2SFCA method and the 2SFCA method. According to the results of Section 4.3, four regions are formed as the IAP decreases. Therefore, the catchment area can be divided into 4 subzones of $\delta > 0.5$, $0.2 \leq \delta < 0.5$, $0.1 \leq \delta < 0.2$ and $0 < \delta < 0.1$. In the traditional E2SFCA method, a 30-min driving zone divided into three subzones was often used as the catchment [10]. In later studies, a 60-min catchment area and four subzones were also used [48–51]. To correspond to the four subzones of ICA, a 60-min catchment area and four subzones of 0–10, 10–20, 20–30, and 30–60 min were used for the E2SFCA method, and 60-min catchment areas were used for the 2SFCA method. The Gaussian function, which has been shown to be superior to other functions, was adopted as the distance impedance function. Following McGrail [14], the distance decay weights of 1, 0.80, 0.55, and 0.15 were used for the four subzones. The accessibility based on the E2SFCA-ICA, the E2SFCA and the 2SFCA are shown in Figures 11–13.

As shown in Figures 11 and 12, and compared to using the E2SFCA method, high-accessibility areas shrink and the low-accessibility region increases when using the E2SFCA-ICA method. This indicates the travel time-based catchment areas used in the E2SFCA method tend to overestimate accessibility when compared to the ICA proposed in this study. This seems to suggest that 60-min catchment areas may lead to the overestimation of the number of accessible healthcare facilities. In traditional travel time-based catchment areas, all hospitals within a 60-min catchment area are lumped together as the supply of that catchment area. However, people actually have certain perceptions about the top-tier hospitals and the hospitals in the 60-min catchment area may not always be the final choice of the residents. As a result, the number of hospitals within the ICA is less than those found within the traditional 60-min catchment areas. The overestimation of hospital number with traditional methods thus tends to lead to the overestimation of the number of accessible healthcare facilities, which in turn results in the overestimation of the accessibility of these facilities. Accessibility scores are plotted in Figure 14 to compare the accessibility levels obtained when using the travel time-based E2SFCA method and the ICA-based E2SFCA method. The figure shows that most of the points fall above the 1:1 line, which further indicates that the E2SFCA method using the traditional catchment area tend to overestimate accessibility when compared to the ICA-based E2SFCA method.

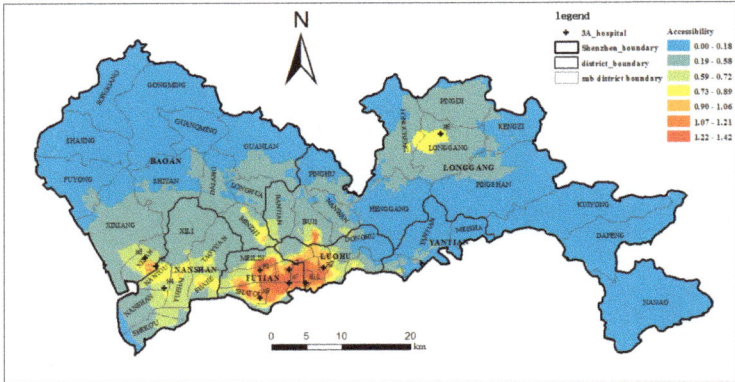

Figure 11. The accessibility of the top-tier hospitals (E2SFCA-ICA).

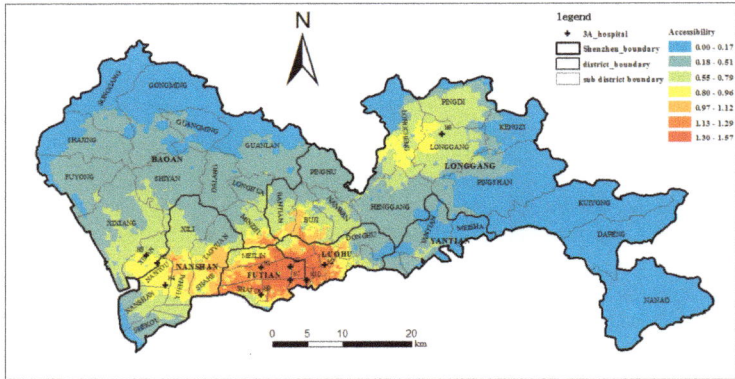

Figure 12. The accessibility of the top-tier hospitals (E2SFCA).

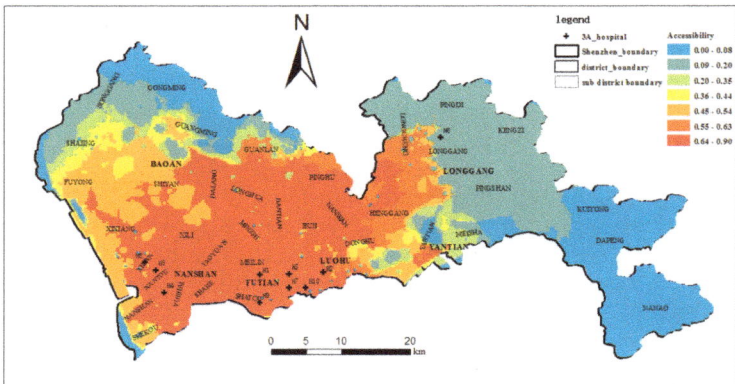

Figure 13. The accessibility of the top-tier hospitals (2SFCA).

Meanwhile, the accessibility of the top-tier hospitals is highly unequal over space. Figure 11 shows that high-accessibility areas are mainly concentrated in Luohu and Futian districts. The reason for this is that most of the top-tier hospitals are concentrated in these two districts (six out of ten hospitals), especially famous hospitals such as H1, H2, and H9. Great reputation, numerous physicians, and short distances lead to higher accessibility of this region. This also reveals how the unequal distribution of healthcare resources influences the unequal access to healthcare services in the study area [52]. Furthermore, we found substantial differences in the spatial distribution in areas with a shortage of top-tier hospitals when applying these two methods. Clearly, accessibility based on the ICA is more unequally distributed over space when compared to the spatial pattern obtained with the traditional method. This indicates that through integrating the actual visit behaviors of the residents, the uneven spatial distribution of accessibility to top-tier hospitals is aggravated. The percentages of the area and population with below-average accessibility were 62.4% and 42.2% with the traditional method, and 80.1% and 61.9% with the ICA method. This means that there are more people in a larger area with poor accessibility to the top-tier hospitals, and approximately 80% of the areas have below-average accessibility. This result is more consistent with our knowledge about the actual situation in Shenzhen, especially in sub-districts such as Shajing, Guanlan, and Longhua, whose population density is relatively high, but the accessibility to the top-tier hospitals is really low.

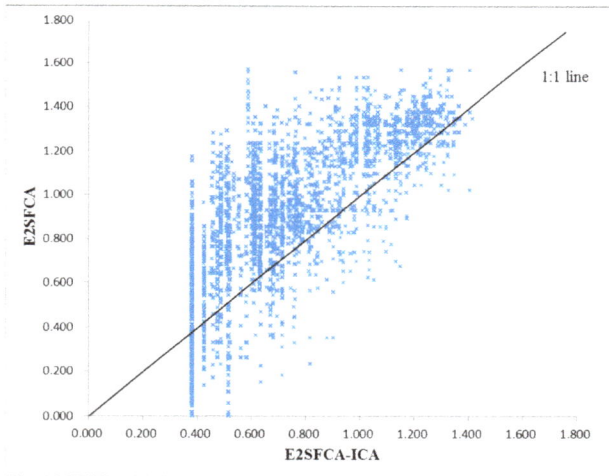

Figure 14. E2SFCA-ICA and E2SFCA comparison.

The unequal distribution of accessibility is more obvious when comparing the E2SFCA-ICA method with the 2SFCA method. As shown in Figure 13, the high accessibility region generated by the traditional 2SFCA method is much larger than that generated by the E2SFCA-ICA method. This is because not only real hospital visit behaviors but also distance decay are not considered in the 2SFCA method. In this case, detailed behavioral differences within the 60-min catchment area cannot be revealed and a large region of high accessibility is generated. Accordingly, the percentages of the area and population with below-average accessibility decreases to 48.9% and 24.4% when compared to the 80.1% and 61.9% obtained by the E2SFCA-ICA method. Further, comparing the sub-districts with high population density in Figure 4 with the regions with high accessibility in Figure 13, we can find that they almost completely overlap. That is to say, based on the traditional 2SFCA method, although the distribution of accessibility to top-tier hospitals is unbalanced, three-quarters of the people have above-average accessibility and the high-accessibility areas cover the high-population density regions well. However, the result by the E2SFCA-ICA method is not so optimistic. This demonstrates that the accessibility generated by the traditional 2SFCA method seems quite high throughout the city, while the accessibility that integrates real hospital visit behaviors reveals more uneven distribution. This is consistent with the results of Casas et al. [21] that "the potential access to a healthcare facility appears quite even throughout the city, the revealed access paints a very different picture."

5. Conclusions

Numerous previous studies focused on determining suitable catchment areas when evaluating the accessibility of healthcare facilities. However, few studies have explored the methodological issues concerning the measurement of accessibility using model-based and data-based methods. It is worth noting that, based on the results of this study, considerable differences may exist between catchment areas obtained with traditional models of accessibility and those derived from people's actual hospital visits. In this paper, the integrated accessibility probability (IAP) that integrates the access probability from the model-based approach and the data-based approach is presented to formulate integrated catchment areas and subzones for improving the assessment of healthcare accessibility. Some important conclusions of this paper are: (1) the proposed hybrid E2SFCA-ICA method can meaningfully divide the catchment area of a healthcare facility into four subzones (core catchment areas, stable catchment areas, uncertain catchment areas, and remote catchment areas), which are useful for understanding the distribution of healthcare visits in different regions of a study area; and (2) the traditional travel-time based catchment areas used in the E2SFCA method tend to overestimate healthcare accessibility. Furthermore, the accessibility of the top-tier hospitals in Shenzhen is more unequal over space when compared to the spatial pattern of the accessibility obtained with traditional methods.

Due to the difficulty in obtaining data about the overall utilization of public facilities, pertinent taxi trips were extracted from taxi GPS trajectories and used to represent people's visit to the high-level hospitals in the study area. In this manner, peoples' actual access behavior was taken into account based on the taxi trajectory data in this study, and then actual access probability was derived from the actual number of hospital visitors as a component of the integrated access probability. This is an attempt to evaluate accessibility using taxi GPS data in the absence of actual patient data. Although the patients who travel by taxi are part of the real patients of a hospital, the results reveal the effect of actual patient travel behaviors on hospital catchment areas. Previous studies found that evaluations based on different travel modes (e.g., bus, private car, biking, or walking) will lead to different accessibility results [20]. This is mainly because travel speed and travel time vary between different travel modes. So, if data of other travel modes used to visit the hospitals are available, the study can use the method to derive catchment areas using these multimodal travel data and provide a more complete picture of the service areas of the hospitals. Further, our method can be used to integrate hospital visit data based on different transport modes. In our method, the DAP index is denoted as the percentage of patients who actually visited a facility among all patients that originated from one location. It can be seen that the DAP index mainly focuses on the origin and destination of the actual patient and does not depend on a particular travel mode. Therefore, if other transport modes of actual patient data are available, the origin and destination of the patients can be extracted and then directly applied to the DAP index to enhance the accuracy and completeness of the results. This means that our approach can be adapted for evaluating the accessibility of healthcare facilities in areas with various multimodal trajectory datasets.

In addition, the ICA will have different sizes and characteristics in different applications, which is directly related to the spatial distribution of the service facilities and the specific behaviors of the people visiting these facilities. For example, with the decrease in the IAP, the ICA shows four distinct subzones at three turning points in this study. Accordingly, the ICA is divided into four subzones through these three turning points. In practical applications, the size of the ICA and the division between each subzone should be determined after analyzing the characteristics of the ICA. This is also consistent with previous views that the catchments in different areas should have different sizes [9,20,53].

Although the paper provides a novel method for integrating the model-based and data-based methods when evaluating the accessibility of healthcare facilities, several limitations should be addressed in future work. In particular, it is recognized that time is also an important factor that will influence people's use and visit behavior with respect to healthcare services [54]. For instance, people may have different choices of healthcare providers at different times (holidays or work days, peak or non-peak periods). Therefore, more studies should be carried out using an integrated space-time framework. Furthermore, the trajectory data were only used to derive the size of the catchment areas and subzones in this study. Further studies are needed to determine the proper data-based distance decay function within each subzone. Lastly, it is also important to note that, due to the nature of the raster (grid-based) spatial framework used in this study, it was not possible to take into account the effects of network topology and link/turn impedance between each hospital and each grid cell in the study—since there is no obvious way in which variations in the distances among all the cells (representing network distance/time while taking link/turn impedance into account) in a grid structure can be represented in ways that still allows for grid-based map algebra to operate (which operates on cell distance like one cell or two cells apart, not what the distance between two cells is). This is a limitation all studies that examine catchment areas would face and there is no satisfactory solution to the problem to date. Despite this limitation, our study used 75.94 million GPS points from 12,448 taxis in the study area to derive the E2SFCA-ICA catchment areas. These catchment areas thus reflect the link and turn impedance of the transport network in the study area in many ways, since they are real taxi trajectories that had been subject to real-world network impedance.

Author Contributions: Conceptualization, X.P., M.-P.K., L.Y., S.Z., Z.Z. and B.W.; Data curation, X.P. and L.Y.; Formal analysis, X.P. and L.Y.; Funding acquisition, M.-P.K., L.Y., S.Z. and Z.Z.; Methodology, X.P., M.-P.K. and L.Y.; Project administration, L.Y.; Supervision, M.-P.K., L.Y., S.Z., Z.Z. and B.W.; Validation, X.P.; Visualization, X.P.; Writing—original draft, X.P.; Writing—review & editing, M.-P.K., L.Y., S.Z., Z.Z. and B.W.

Funding: This research was supported by grants from the National Natural Science Foundation of China (grant numbers 41201385, 41301427, 41371422, and 41529101) and the State Key Laboratory of Geo-information Engineering (grant number SKLGIE2017-M-4-1). In addition, Mei-Po Kwan was supported by a John Simon Guggenheim Memorial Foundation Fellowship.

Acknowledgments: The authors would like to thank Songling Dai and Xuehua Han for their help in data processing during the experiment. They would also like to thank the anonymous reviewers for their helpful comments.

Conflicts of Interest: The authors declare no conflict of interest.

References

1. Hansen, W.G. How Accessibility Shapes Land Use. *J. Am. Inst. Plan.* **1959**, *25*, 73–76. [CrossRef]
2. Kwan, M.-P. Space-time and integral measures of individual accessibility: A comparative analysis using a point-based framework. *Geogr. Anal.* **1998**, *30*, 191–216. [CrossRef]
3. Kwan, M.-P. Gender and individual access to urban opportunities: A study using space-time measures. *Prof. Geogr.* **1999**, *51*, 210–227. [CrossRef]
4. Luo, W.; Wang, F. Measures of spatial accessibility to health care in a GIS environment: Synthesis and a case study in the Chicago region. *Environ. Plan. B Plan. Des.* **2003**, *30*, 865–884. [CrossRef]
5. Kwan, M.-P.; Weber, J. Scale and accessibility: Implications for the analysis of land use-travel interaction. *Appl. Geogr.* **2008**, *28*, 110–123. [CrossRef]
6. Wang, H.D.; Yue, Y.; Li, Y.G.; Huang, L. Spatial Correlation Analysis of Attractiveness of Commercial Facilities. *Geomat. Inf. Sci. Wuhan Univ.* **2011**, *36*, 1102–1106.
7. Dussault, G.; Franceschini, M.C. Not enough there, too many here: Understanding geographical imbalances in the distribution of the health workforce. *Hum. Resour. Health* **2006**, *4*, 12. [CrossRef] [PubMed]
8. McGrail, M.R.; Humphreys, J.S. Measuring spatial accessibility to primary health care services: Utilising dynamic catchment sizes. *Appl. Geogr.* **2014**, *54*, 182–188. [CrossRef]
9. McGrail, M.R.; Humphreys, J.S. Measuring spatial accessibility to primary care in rural areas: Improving the effectiveness of the two-step floating catchment area method. *Appl. Geogr.* **2009**, *29*, 533–541. [CrossRef]

10. Luo, W.; Qi, Y. An enhanced two-step floating catchment area (E2SFCA) method for measuring spatial accessibility to primary care physicians. *Health Place* **2009**, *15*, 1100–1107. [CrossRef] [PubMed]
11. Hu, R.; Dong, S.; Zhao, Y.; Hu, H.; Li, Z. Assessing potential spatial accessibility of health services in rural China: A case study of Donghai county. *Int. J. Equity Health* **2013**, *12*, 35. [CrossRef] [PubMed]
12. Wan, N.; Zhan, F.B.; Zou, B.; Chow, E. A relative spatial access assessment approach for analyzing potential spatial access to colorectal cancer services in Texas. *Appl. Geogr.* **2012**, *32*, 291–299. [CrossRef]
13. Delamater, P.L. Spatial accessibility in suboptimally configured health care systems: A modified two-step floating catchment area (M2SFCA) metric. *Health Place* **2013**, *24*, 30–43. [CrossRef] [PubMed]
14. McGrail, M.R. Spatial accessibility of primary health care utilising the two step floating catchment area method: An assessment of recent improvements. *Int. J. Health Geogr.* **2012**, *11*, 50. [CrossRef] [PubMed]
15. Guagliardo, M.F. Spatial accessibility of primary care: Concepts, methods and challenges. *Int. J. Health Geogr.* **2004**, *3*, 3. [CrossRef] [PubMed]
16. Dai, D. Racial/ethnic and socioeconomic disparities in urban green space accessibility: Where to intervene? *Landsc. Urban Plan.* **2011**, *102*, 234–244. [CrossRef]
17. Delmelle, E.M.; Cassell, C.H.; Dony, C.; Radcliff, E.; Tanner, J.P.; Siffel, C.; Kirby, R.S. Modeling travel impedance to medical care for children with birth defects using geographic information systems. *Birth Defects Res. Part A Clin. Mol. Teratol.* **2013**, *97*, 673–684. [CrossRef] [PubMed]
18. Wang, F.; Luo, W. Assessing spatial and nonspatial factors for healthcare access: Towards an integrated approach to defining health professional shortage areas. *Health Place* **2005**, *11*, 131–146. [CrossRef] [PubMed]
19. Hyndman, J.C.; D'Arcy, C.; Holman, J.; Pritchard, D.A. The influence of attractiveness factors and distance to general practice surgeries by level of social disadvantage and global access in Perth, Western Australia. *Soc. Sci. Med.* **2003**, *56*, 387–403. [CrossRef]
20. Dony, C.C.; Delmelle, E.M.; Delmelle, E.C. Re-conceptualizing accessibility to parks in multi-modal cities: A variable-width floating catchment area (vfca) method. *Landsc. Urban Plan.* **2015**, *143*, 90–99. [CrossRef]
21. Casas, I.; Delmelle, E.; Delmelle, E.C. Potential versus revealed access to care during a dengue fever outbreak. *J. Transp. Health* **2016**, *4*, 18–29. [CrossRef]
22. Yang, G.; Song, C.; Shu, H.; Zhang, J.; Pei, T.; Zhou, C. Assessing patient bypass behavior using taxi trip origin-destination (OD) data. *ISPRS Int. J. Geo-Inf.* **2016**, *5*, 157. [CrossRef]
23. Wang, F.H. Measurement, optimization, and impact of health care accessibility: A methodological review. *Ann. Assoc. Am. Geogr.* **2012**, *102*, 1104–1112. [CrossRef] [PubMed]
24. Zinszer, K.; Charland, K.; Kigozi, R.; Dorsey, G.; Kamya, M.R.; Buckeridge, D.L. Determining health-care facility catchment areas in Uganda using data on malaria-related visits. *Bull. World Health Organ.* **2014**, *92*, 178–186. [CrossRef] [PubMed]
25. Shortt, N.K.; Moore, A.; Coombes, M.; Wymer, C. Defining regions for locality health care planning: A multidimensional approach. *Soc. Sci. Med.* **2005**, *60*, 2715–2727. [CrossRef] [PubMed]
26. Lovett, A.; Haynes, R.; Sünnenberg, G.; Gale, S. Car travel time and accessibility by bus to general practitioner services: A study using patient registers and GIS. *Soc. Sci. Med.* **2002**, *55*, 97–111. [CrossRef]
27. Parker, E.B.; Campbell, J.L. Measuring access to primary medical care: Some examples of the use of geographical information systems. *Health Place* **1998**, *4*, 183–193. [CrossRef]
28. Kwan, M.-P. The uncertain geographic context problem. *Ann. Assoc. Am. Geogr.* **2012**, *102*, 958–968. [CrossRef]
29. Shen, Y.; Kwan, M.P.; Chai, Y. Investigating commuting flexibility with GPS data and 3D geovisualization: A case study of Beijing, China. *J. Transp. Geogr.* **2013**, *32*, 1–11. [CrossRef]
30. Song, C.; Qu, Z.; Blumm, N.; Barabási, A.L. Limits of predictability in human mobility. *Science* **2010**, *327*, 1018–1021. [CrossRef] [PubMed]
31. González, M.C.; Hidalgo, C.A.; Barabási, A.L. Understanding individual human mobility patterns. *Nature* **2008**, *453*, 779–782. [CrossRef] [PubMed]
32. Lazer, D.; Pentland, A.; Adamic, L.; Aral, S.; Barabasi, A.L.; Brewer, D.; Christakis, N.; Contractor, N.; Fowler, J.; Gutmann, M. Life in the network: The coming age of computational social science. *Science* **2009**, *323*, 721–723. [CrossRef] [PubMed]
33. Beijing Statistical Yearbook. Available online: http://www.bjstats.gov.cn/tjsj/ (accessed on 23 July 2018).
34. Shanghai Urban Transportation Administrative Dept. Available online: http://www.shygc.net/pageHome.do?page=init (accessed on 23 July 2018).
35. Guangzhou Statistical Yearbook. Available online: www.gzstats.gov.cn (accessed on 23 July 2018).

36. Shenzhen Transportation Commission. Available online: http://www.sztb.gov.cn/ (accessed on 23 July 2018).

37. Li, L.; Wang, S.; Li, M.; Tan, J. Comparison of travel mode choice between taxi and subway regarding traveling convenience. *Tsinghua Sci. Technol.* **2018**, *2*, 135–144. [CrossRef]

38. Didi Media Research Institute & CBNData. 2016 Intelligent Travel Big Data Report. 2017. Available online: http://www.imxdata.com/archives/20017 (accessed on 12 April 2017).

39. Ingram, D.R. The concept of accessibility: A search for an operational form. *Reg. Stud. J. Reg. Stud. Assoc.* **1971**, *5*, 101–107. [CrossRef]

40. Zhou, Y.; Fang, Z.; Thill, J.C.; Li, Q.; Li, Y. Functionally critical locations in an urban transportation network: Identification and space-time analysis using taxi trajectories. *Comput. Environ. Urban Syst.* **2015**, *52*, 34–47. [CrossRef]

41. Joseph, A.E.; Bantock, P.R. Measuring potential physical accessibility to general practitioners in rural areas: A method and case study. *Soc. Sci. Med.* **1982**, *16*, 85–90. [CrossRef]

42. Kwan, M.-P. Beyond space (as we knew it): Toward temporally integrated geographies of segregation, health, and accessibility. *Ann. Assoc. Am. Geogr.* **2013**, *103*, 1078–1086. [CrossRef]

43. Alford-Teaster, J.; Lange, J.M.; Hubbard, R.A.; Lee, C.I.; Haas, J.S.; Shi, X.; Carlos, H.A.; Henderson, L.; Hill, D.; Tosteson, A.N.A.; et al. Is the closest facility the one actually used? An assessment of travel time estimation based on mammography facilities. *Int. J. Health Geogr.* **2016**, *15*, 8. [CrossRef] [PubMed]

44. Qi, L.L.; Zhou, S.H.; Yan, X.P. Endpoint Attractive Factors of Medical Facilities' Accessibility: Based on GPS Floating Car Data in Guangzhou. *Sci. Geogr. Sin.* **2014**, *34*, 580–586.

45. Chen, B.Y.; Yuan, H.; Li, Q.; Wang, D.; Shaw, S.L.; Chen, H.P.; Lam, W.H. Measuring place-based accessibility under travel time uncertainty. *Int. J. Geogr. Inf. Sci.* **2016**, *31*, 783–804. [CrossRef]

46. Didi Media Research Institute & CBNData. 2016 Smart Travel Data and Medical Reports. Available online: http://www.sohu.com/a/79676781_355066 (accessed on 12 June 2017).

47. Yang, L.; Kwan, M.-P.; Pan, X.; Wan, B.; Zhou, S. Scalable space-time trajectory cube for path-finding: A study using big taxi trajectory data. *Transp. Res. Part B* **2017**, *101*, 1–27. [CrossRef]

48. Wang, X.; Pan, J. Assessing the disparity in spatial access to hospital care in ethnic minority region in sichuan province, china. *BMC Health Serv. Res.* **2016**, *16*, 399. [CrossRef] [PubMed]

49. Vadrevu, L.; Kanjilal, B. Measuring spatial equity and access to maternal health services using enhanced two step floating catchment area method (e2sfca)—A case study of the Indian sundarbans. *Int. J. Equity Health* **2016**, *15*, 87. [CrossRef] [PubMed]

50. Dewulf, B.; Neutens, T.; Weerdt, Y.D.; Weghe, N.V.D. Accessibility to primary health care in Belgium: An evaluation of policies awarding financial assistance in shortage areas. *BMC Fam. Pract.* **2013**, *14*, 122. [CrossRef] [PubMed]

51. Wan, N.; Zou, B.; Sternberg, T. A three-step floating catchment area method for analyzing spatial access to health services. *Int. J. Geogr. Inf. Sci.* **2012**, *6*, 1073–1089. [CrossRef]

52. Ursulica, T.E. The relationship between health care needs and accessibility to health care services in Botosani County-Romania. *Procedia Environ. Sci.* **2016**, *32*, 300–310. [CrossRef]

53. Luo, W.; Whippo, T. Variable catchment sizes for the two-step floating catchment area (2SFCA) method. *Health Place* **2012**, *18*, 789–795. [CrossRef] [PubMed]

54. Ren, F.; Tong, D.; Kwan, M.-P. Space-time measures of demand for service: Bridging location modeling and accessibility studies through a time-geographic framework. *Geografiska Annaler B* **2014**, *96*, 329–344. [CrossRef]

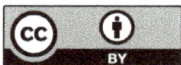

International Journal of
*Environmental Research
and Public Health*

MDPI

Article

Impacts of Individual Daily Greenspace Exposure on Health Based on Individual Activity Space and Structural Equation Modeling

Lin Zhang [1,2], Suhong Zhou [1,2,*], Mei-Po Kwan [3,4], Fei Chen [1,2] and Rongping Lin [1,2]

[1] School of Geography and Planning, Sun Yat-sen University, Guangzhou 510275, China;
     zhanglin8@mail2.sysu.edu.cn (L.Z.); FeiFei17213454@163.com (F.C.); linrp3@mail2.sysu.edu.cn (R.L.)
[2] Guangdong Provincial Engineering Research Center for Public Security and Disaster,
     Guangzhou 510275, China
[3] Department of Geography and Geographic Information Science, Natural History Building,
     1301 W Green Street, University of Illinois at Urbana-Champaign, Urbana, IL 61801, USA;
     mpk654@gmail.com
[4] Department of Human Geography and Spatial Planning, Utrecht University,
     3584 CB Utrecht, The Netherlands
*   Correspondence: eeszsh@mail.sysu.edu.cn; Tel.: +86-138-2504-4799

Received: 30 September 2018; Accepted: 16 October 2018; Published: 22 October 2018

Abstract: Previous studies on the effects of greenspace exposure on health are largely based on static contextual units, such as residential neighborhoods, and other administrative units. They tend to ignore the spatiotemporal dynamics of individual daily greenspace exposure and the mediating effects of specific activity type (such as physical activity). Therefore, this study examines individual daily greenspace exposure while taking into account people's daily mobility and the mediating role of physical activity between greenspace exposure and health. Specifically, using survey data collected in Guangzhou, China, and high-resolution remote sensing images, individual activity space for a weekday is delineated and used to measure participants' daily greenspace exposure. Structural equation modeling is then applied to analyze the direct effects of individual daily greenspace exposure on health and its indirect effects through the mediating variable of physical activity. The results show that daily greenspace exposure directly influences individual health and also indirectly affects participants' health status through physical activity. With respect to the total effects, daily greenspace exposure helps improve participants' mental health and contributes to promoting their social health. It also helps improve participants' physical health, although to a lesser extent. In general, the higher the daily greenspace exposure, the higher the physical activity level and the better the overall health (including physical, mental, and social health).

Keywords: greenspace exposure; health; human mobility; physical activity; structural equation modeling; Guangzhou

---

1. Introduction

Economic growth and urbanization can bring better living conditions, various opportunities (e.g., rapid development of the tertiary industry, employment opportunities, education and health care opportunities), and challenges (e.g., resource destruction, environmental pollution and frequent disasters). In the process, however, environmental problems are becoming increasingly serious, including a dramatic decrease in greenspace. Many urban dwellers today do not have easy access to and contact with various forms of greenspace (e.g., parks, green corridors, and functional green structures), including natural and artificial greenspace, which has negative impacts on human health and sustainable development in urban areas [1]. A report by the World Health Organization

(WHO) showed that nearly 25% of the world's diseases were caused by environmental factors. With the faster-than-ever pace of modern life, an increasing number of urban residents experience unfavorable environmental exposures that adversely affect their mental health and often lead to negative emotions [2,3]. In addition, the modern living environment often leads to the separation between individuals and families, as well as the reduction in social cohesion and interaction. Therefore, countries around the world have formulated the National Environment and Health Action Plan (NEHAP) [4,5], which emphasizes environmental benefits that help counteract these urban threats and improve people's health outcomes [6,7]. Coincidentally, China has put forward the "Healthy China" initiative and highlighted the role of the environment in promoting national health and quality of life.

Urban greenspace has been associated with a wide range of health benefits. Decades of research has examined the direct effects of greenspace on people's physical and mental health based on fixed contextual or areal units (e.g., census tracts, postcode areas and street network buffers). Some researchers suggested that residential green environment can help to regulate microclimate [8], purify the air [9], reduce noise pollution [10], and promote the quality of the residential environment [11,12]. All of these ecological benefits contributed to reducing the risk of obesity [13] and high blood pressure and diabetes [14], thereby improving physical health in general [15,16]. Meanwhile, a rapidly expanding literature showed that exposures to greenspace help to strengthen individual attention [17], enhance intelligence and inspiration [18,19], and promote self-awareness and ability to reinvent oneself [20,21]. Availability of ample greenspace has been found to have restorative [18] and stress-relieving qualities [22,23], and is recommended as an effective way to decrease violence and crime [24]. Wood et al. [25] and Akpinar et al. [26] indicated that better psychosocial status was not only associated with the quantity and accessibility of greenspace, but also with the functions and types of the greenspace people are exposed to. Berg et al. [27] found that the time spent on visits to greenspace should be considered individually, since it is a mediator in the relationship between greenspace and mental health.

Previous research mainly focuses on the direct effects of greenspace on physical and mental health. Recently, the literature on greenspace and individual health has expanded to consider its effects on people's physical activity. Although urban inhabitants typically benefit from superior access to medical technology, health care, and other services, these benefits are offset by their sedentary lifestyle and lack of physical activity [28,29]. Inadequate physical activity has been identified as a major risk factor of human health. Urban greenspace is now recognized as a suitable setting for physical activity and for its potential for promoting health outcomes. Some studies sought to examine the association between objectively measured greenspace, physical activity, and physical health. The results suggested that the provision of abundant urban greenspace may reduce the risk of obesity and promote physical health by increasing people's physical activity level [30,31]. A series of studies on the relationship between greenspace and individual mental health outcomes showed that physical activity is likely to be a mediating factor in this relationship: Namely, residents with higher levels of access to greenspace, and thus more opportunities for physical activity, reported better stress-relieving effects, mental health, and well-being [30,32–34].

However, previous studies have rarely paid attention to the influence of daily greenspace exposure on social health and social interaction. Generally, the above studies analyzed the effects of greenspace on one or two dimension(s) of health (e.g., physical health, mental health, or social health) through the mediator of physical activity, but the different effects of greenspace on different dimensions of health were ignored. Thus, this paper focuses on the direct and indirect effects of objectively measured greenspace on three dimensions of health (physical health, mental health, and social health), and compares the different effects of greenspace on these health dimensions. Considering the definition of "greenspace" in previous studies that only includes "vegetation coverage" as too narrow, this paper extends the concept of "greenspace" to the broader notion of "greenspace exposure" by adding an activity dimension according to the concept of "environmental exposure science." Greenspace exposure in this study encompasses the quantity, quality, and accessibility of greenspace for a person to meet the needs for a better urban environment and recreational activities in the actual geographic areas of his or her daily life. Among the indicators of greenspace selected in this paper, green vegetation contributes to improving the natural environment. Physical activity sites can provide more structured environments for social interactions and physical activity [35]. In addition, accessibility to greenspace also has an impact on physical activity and social interactions.

In addition, some qualitative and quantitative studies examined the relationship between the environment and health using fixed geographic or contextual units based on buffer areas around individuals' residences [36–38] or administrative units, such as census tracts, postcode areas and street network buffers [39–41]. These studies presupposed that the most relevant areas affecting health were residential neighborhoods or residence-based buffer zones delimited in a variety of ways. This presupposition entails the view that people who live in the same contextual unit experience the same environmental impacts, regardless of where they actually work or undertake their daily activities. However, it is inappropriate to use static geographic units like census tracts to represent people's true activity space that exerts contextual influence on their health, since there are considerable differences in people's daily spatiotemporal behaviors, which may lead to their exposures to different areas beyond their residential neighborhoods [42–44]. Static geographic units cannot accurately represent people's activity space, since they ignore human mobility and daily spatiotemporal behaviors [45–47]. Thus, human mobility cannot be neglected and it is essential to look beyond residential neighborhoods to take into account people's environmental exposure in their daily activity space. Recently, Kwan [45,46,48] called our attention to the crucial role of human mobility and daily activity space in accurately assessing people's environmental exposure through the notion of the uncertain geographic context problem (UGCoP). Several studies have provided important evidence on how the UGCoP may affect research findings in environmental health studies and the need to use geographic units or methods that capture people's spatiotemporal activities [49–52]. For example, Zhao et al. [47] suggested that researchers should try to estimate the influence of various environmental exposure on individual health more accurately using contextual units that can capture people's daily activities and travel. Therefore, this study seeks to identify and delineate residents' activity space during the 24 h of a weekday to capture the real contextual areas that people are exposed to and interact with, in order to advance the analysis of how true environmental exposure level in people's daily activity space affect their health. The reason for choosing only weekdays to study is that participants in this research are between 19 and 59 years of age and are employed (e.g., employees, employers) (note that students are excluded from the study), which may lead to routine and similar activities during weekdays. However, there may be considerable variations and irregularity in their activities in weekend days. Therefore, we selected to focus on participants' daily activities in a weekday as their usual behaviors in this research, since they have more regular and frequent activities in weekdays, which took up most of their individual life when compared with weekends. In addition, given that where and when people spend their time differ from individual to individual, the spatiotemporal features of daily activities and their cumulative effects are also considered in this article. These features include activity types, activity locations and actual time spent in different areas.

Based on such considerations, this study takes advantage of the methods of human mobility research and constructs a conceptual framework for modeling the health benefit of individual daily greenspace exposure. A structural equation model is used to analyze the causal mechanisms among daily greenspace exposure, physical activity, and individual health based on questionnaire survey data and objectively measured data (e.g., deriving vegetation coverage using remote sensing images). Meanwhile, individual activity space is considered when analyzing how greenspace exposure influence people's health behaviors and outcomes. Specifically, the article seeks to address the following questions: Is there any relationship among daily greenspace exposure, physical activity and individual health from the perspective of human mobility and the uncertain geographic context problem? Does individual daily greenspace exposure directly affect health, and does it also indirectly affect health through the mediating role of physical activity? How do specific elements of daily greenspace exposure and physical activity influence the different dimensions of individual health? This paper seeks to enrich and deepen our knowledge of health geography and spatiotemporal behaviors. Moreover, it has theoretical and practical value for urban planning, informing greenspace construction programs and strategies for achieving global environmental health.

2. Study Design

2.1. Conceptual Framework and Hypotheses

Recent studies have examined the relationship among greenspace, physical activity and health, indicating that physical activity may play a partly intermediate role in this relationship [33,53,54]. Thus, the conceptual framework for this study focuses on the impacts of daily greenspace exposure and physical activity on individual health and is presented in Figure 1. As shown in the figure, the framework illustrates the interactions among daily greenspace exposure, physical activity, and individual health (physical health, mental health, and social health). On the one hand, daily greenspace exposure has a direct and important impact on health. On the other hand, it contributes to improving people's overall health status indirectly through promoting physical activity, which plays a mediating role in the relationship between daily greenspace exposure and health outcomes. Thus, the following hypotheses are proposed based on this conceptual framework (Table 1). The paper will employ structural equation modeling to test these hypotheses.

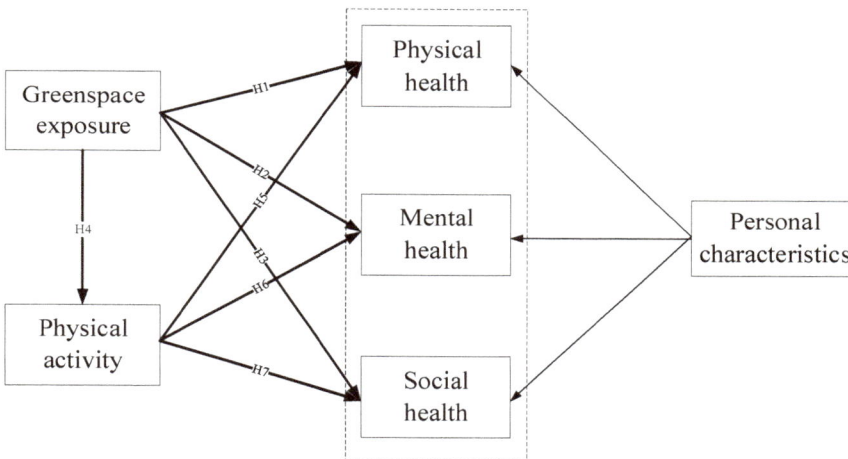

Figure 1. Conceptual framework.

Table 1. Hypotheses for this study.

Hypotheses
H1 Daily greenspace exposure has a significant positive effect on physical health.
H2 Daily greenspace exposure has a significant positive effect on mental health.
H3 Daily greenspace exposure has a significant positive effect on social health.
H4 Daily greenspace exposure has a significant positive effect on physical activity, which plays a mediating role in the relationship between daily greenspace exposure and individual health.
H5 Physical activity has a significant positive effect on physical health.
H6 Physical activity has a significant positive effect on mental health.
H7 Physical activity has a significant positive effect on social health.

2.2. Study Area

The study area for this research is Guangzhou, China. As the capital of Guangdong Province, Guangzhou is one of the four megacities in China and has a total area of 7434.4 km^2. The urbanization rate of Guangzhou reached 86.14% with a permanent population of about 14.5 million and a gross domestic product (GDP) of 2150.315 billion RMB in 2017 [55]. Increasing urbanization has resulted in a great proportion of the megacity's population being exposed to environmental threats. This study thus selected Guangzhou as a representative megacity of China and investigated 11 typical residential blocks in it (Liurong, Jianshe, Yuancun, Shipai, Tianhenan, Tangxia, Tongde, Xingang, Ruibao, Longjin and Nancunzhen). Each of these residential blocks is nearly 1 km^2 in area, and they include historical blocks, *danwei* communities, commercial housing, affordable housing and informal housing. These residential blocks are located in seven of the central, transitional and marginal districts of the city, which include Liwan, Yuexiu, Tianhe, Haizhu, Baiyun, Panyu and Huangpu Districts (Figure 2).

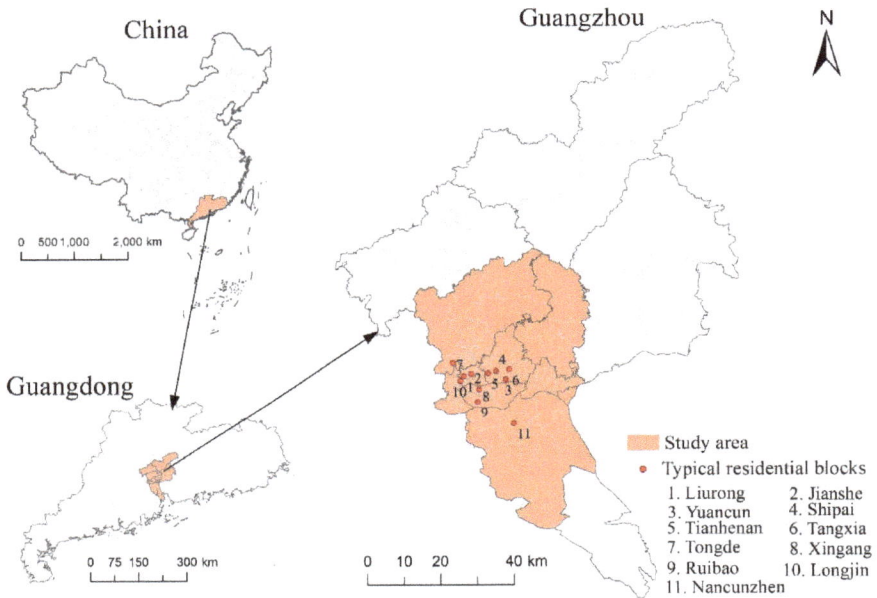

Figure 2. Study area.

2.3. Data

2.3.1. Data Collection and Participants' Data

Data for this study were collected in August 2017 through a questionnaire survey called the "Survey of Residents' Daily Activity and Community Integration in Guangzhou". Specifically, the questionnaire survey ran from March 2017, and lasted about five months. During this period, some trained interviewers who were experienced employees of a professional survey research company in Guangzhou were hired. These interviewers received training through our detailed explanation of the questionnaire and the reasons for asking those questions in the context of the study, undertaking formal investigation and then collecting final questionnaire data in August 2017. The questionnaire survey was approved by Sun Yat-sen University (SYSU), and supported by grants from the National Natural Science Foundation of China (41522104), and all participants gave informed consent. Respondents in the survey were proportionally selected from the adult residents in the 11 selected residential blocks in Guangzhou based on the size of the permanent population of each block reported in the Sixth National

Census of China. Each questionnaire was administered by a trained interviewer in a face-to-face interview with a participant, and it took about 30–40 min to fill out. A total of 1003 valid and usable questionnaires were finally obtained.

Individual-level data items solicited through the questionnaires include personal characteristic (demographic and socioeconomic characteristics), residential and employment information, physical activity, self-reported health conditions, social interactions, and activity logs.

(i) Demographic and socioeconomic characteristics—Demographic indicators solicited through the questionnaires include gender, age, and marital status. The proportions of males and females in the sample are quite balanced. The proportion of young people (between the age of 19 and 44) is noticeably higher (75.37%; note that juveniles under 19 and elderly people over 59 were excluded from the study). In addition, education level and personal monthly income, which are highly related to socioeconomic status, were also obtained from the participants.

(ii) Physical activity indicators—Physical activity level was assessed mainly by their duration, frequency, and intensity [33,37]. The duration and frequency of physical activity over the past week were self-reported by participants and include three types of physical activity (PA): Brisk walking (for recreational and transportation purposes), moderate PA (dancing, playing bowling/ping-pong/badminton, and so on) and vigorous PA (aerobic exercise, running, fast cycling, swimming, playing basketball/football, and so on). The intensity of weekly physical activity is measured by metabolic equivalents (METs). Metabolic equivalents are equal to total brisk walking minutes × 3.5 + total moderate PA minutes × 4.0 + total vigorous PA minutes × 8.0 (International Physical Activity Questionnaire, IPAQ) [37,56,57]. Weekly metabolic equivalents (METs) are used to assess whether the participants have met the physical activity recommendation (>600 MET-min/week). Low-level PA (0–600 MET-min/week) is defined as not meeting the recommendation, intermediate-level PA (600–1500 MET-min/week) and high-level PA (>1500 MET-min/week) are defined as meeting the recommendation and exceeding the recommendation respectively [58]. Specifically, this recommendation (>600 MET-min/week) could be regarded as a standard for an individual to engage in his or her physical activity. For example, low-level PA that doesn't meet the recommendation chronically may lead to adverse individual health outcomes. Conversely, people's morbidity and mortality will drop significantly as they increase their physical activity from a low level to an intermediate level or a high level.

(iii) Health indicators—The definition of health by the WHO in 1948 is "A state of complete physical, mental and social well-being and not merely the absence of disease or infirmity." Thus, this study focuses on the three dimensions of physical health, mental health, and social health [59]. Physical health refers to the state that people has a strong and healthy physique, as well as a better self-protection ability to reduce harm and restore an (adapted) equilibrium [59]. Information about participants' individual subjective feeling of physical health status was obtained in the survey using the *MOS 36-Item Short-Form Health Survey (SF-36, items 1, 4, and 7)* [60], which has been widely used in previous studies. Mental health is defined as a state of emotional well-being, in which individual can recognize his or her own potential, cope with stressful situations effectively, work productively and fruitfully, and make a contribution to her or his community. The *World Health Organization's Five Well-Being Indexes (WHO-5)* [61], which has short and positively worded items, is one of the most widely used instruments for assessing people's subjective mental health. Social health refers to the ability of an individual to have a good interpersonal relationship and social adaptation. For this research, the five questions on social health used in the survey were derived from the scales used in previous studies (*Social Cohesion and Trust Scale* [62], *Social Wellbeing Scale* [63] and *Social Support List-Interactions (SSL-I)* [64]), and their reliability and validity have been confirmed to be excellent [39,65]. All of these self-evaluation indicators are described qualitatively through a 5-point Likert scale ranging from "poor" to "excellent."

2.3.2. Activity Space of Participants

Activity space, which is the area containing all locations where an individual undertakes his or her daily activities [52,66], is used to delineate individual contextual units in this study. In the survey, 1003 participants were interviewed and a total of 14,439 items were recorded in their activity logs for a weekday, so there are approximately 14.4 activities recorded for each participant. These items include activity locations or stay points (residences, workplaces, restaurants, shopping places, fitness places, entertainment places and so on) and travel characteristics like origin, destination, transportation mode and time spent. Among these activity spaces, the top three where participants spent most time were residence (54.99%), workplace (32.88%) and travel (8.64%) (Table 2). Based on these detailed activity log data, the activity space for each participant was delineated using actual individual trajectory reported by participants. Note that Kwan et al. [52] have compared seven different methods for delineating people's activity space and found that different methods may lead to different individual exposure level and health outcomes. Since different methods for delineating activity space have different strengths and weaknesses, we used a hybrid method in this study to integrate two elements of participants' daily activities and mobility to assess their greenspace exposure: The activity space of each participant was constructed using two types of buffers based on their activity locations or stay points and travel behaviors, respectively. According to the buffer sizes used in previous studies [67–69], a 1000 m-buffer was used around each stay point and a 500 m-buffer was used for travel routes (Figure 3). Due to the different durations that each participant spent at different activity locations, the person's exposure to greenspace would also change over time. Therefore, the effect of time on greenspace exposure also needs to be considered when constructing the activity space. In this research, individual daily greenspace exposure was more accurately assessed based on the proportion of time spent at different activity locations. The formulae and computing steps are given in Section 2.3.3 below.

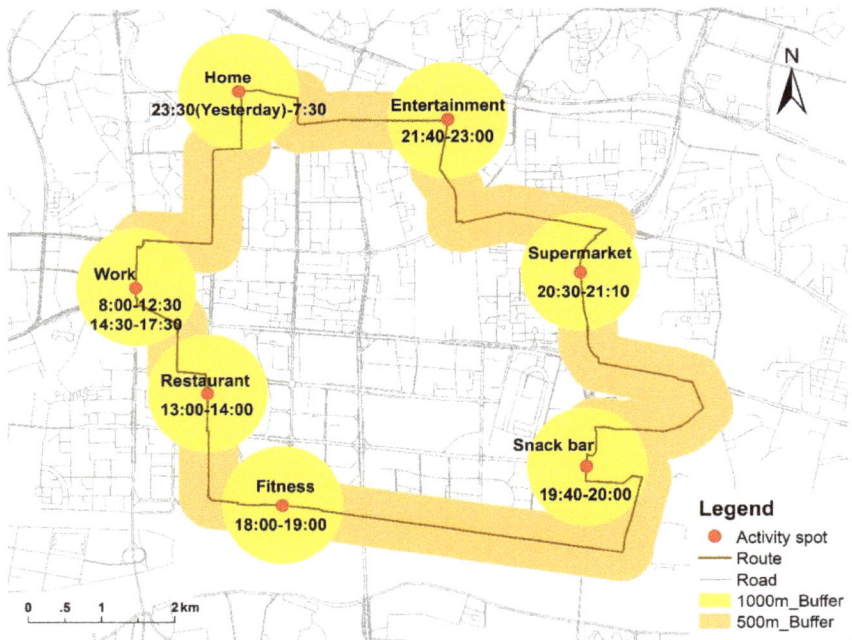

Figure 3. Construction of individual activity space using two types of buffer areas.

Table 2. Time spent of the study participants on daily activity (N = 1003).

Daily Activity	Time Spent (h)	Per Capita Time Spent (h)	Percentage in a Weekday
Residence	13,236.08	13.20	54.99%
Work	7914.25	7.89	32.88%
Dining (in restaurant)	364.17	0.36	1.51%
Shopping	106.87	0.11	0.44%
Fitness (in fitness place)	86.93	0.09	0.36%
Entertainment	98.53	0.10	0.41%
Travel	2079.67	2.07	8.64%
Other	183.67	0.18	0.76%
Total	24,070.17	24.00	100.00%

2.3.3. Greenspace Data and Exposure Assessment

Greenspace data used in this study were automatically extracted and calculated from remote sensing images covering Guangzhou in November 2015 using ENVI 5.2 (Palm Bay, FL, USA) and ArcGIS 10.3 (Redlands, CA, USA). These remote sensing images, with a spatial resolution of 2 m, are obtained from the Gao Fen-1 (GF-1) satellite, the first satellite of China's High-Resolution Earth Observation System (CHEOS). Using these remote sensing images, three objective indicators (vegetation coverage, physical activity site coverage, and accessibility to the nearest greenspace) used in previous studies [36,37] were selected for measuring participants' exposure to greenspace in the study area. Among these indicators, vegetation coverage and physical activity site coverage were calculated based on the time-weighted average method [70,71]. The three objective indicators are described as follows.

(1) Vegetation coverage: This is the time-weighted proportion of the area of vegetation that is within the activity space buffers of a participant.

$$Vegetation\ coverage = \left(\frac{S_{v1}}{S_{b1000}} \times \frac{t_1}{24} + \frac{S_{v2}}{S_{b1000}} \times \frac{t_2}{24} + \ldots + \frac{S_{vn}}{S_{b1000}} \times \frac{t_n}{24} \right) + \left(\frac{S_{vt}}{S_{b500}} \times \frac{t_t}{24} \right), \quad (1)$$

$$t_1 + t_2 + \ldots + t_n + t_t = 24(h), \quad (2)$$

where S_{b1000} is the area of 1000 m-buffer; S_{v1} is the area of vegetation coverage in the first activity space buffer, S_{vn} is the area of vegetation coverage in the nth activity space buffer, and so on; t_1 is the time the participant spent in the first activity space, t_n is the time the participant spent in the nth activity space, and so on; S_{b500} is the area of 500 m-buffer; S_{vt} is the area of the vegetation coverage in the travel route buffer; t_t is the time the participant spent in the travel route.

(2) Physical activity site coverage: This is the time-weighted proportion of the area of physical activity sites (parks, squares, outdoor playgrounds, and so on) that can be accessed within a participant's activity space buffers.

$$Physical\ activity\ site\ coverage$$
$$= \left(\frac{S_{pas1}}{S_{b1000}} \times \frac{t_1}{24} + \frac{S_{pas2}}{S_{b1000}} \times \frac{t_2}{24} + \ldots + \frac{S_{pasn}}{S_{b1000}} \times \frac{t_n}{24} \right) + \left(\frac{S_{past}}{S_{b500}} \times \frac{t_t}{24} \right), \quad (3)$$

where S_{pas1} is the area of physical activity site in the first activity space buffer, S_{pasn} is the area of physical activity site in the nth activity space buffer, and so on; S_{past} is the area of physical activity site in the travel route buffer.

(3) Accessibility to the nearest greenspace: This is the average of the sum of the distances between each activity site of a participant to the nearest greenspace in the respective activity space buffers.

$$Accessibility\ to\ the\ nearest\ greenspace = \left(\frac{D_1 + D_2 + \ldots + D_n}{n} \right), \quad (4)$$

where D_1 is the distance from the first activity site to its nearest greenspace in the first activity space buffer, D_n is the distance from the nth activity site to its nearest greenspace in the nth activity space buffer, and so on; n is the number of activity space buffer. These three greenspace exposure indicators were used in this study to capture various forms of greenspace exposure for the participants.

2.4. Structural Equation Modeling

As a powerful method for examining the causal relationships among a set of variables, structural equation modeling has been widely used in the literature of health geography [72,73]. It can be used to estimate abstract concepts (such as health status) using measured variables, examine the complex causal relationships among variables using feedback loops, and improve the accuracy and credibility of model results by considering the influence of measurement error. Structural equation modeling is suitable for identifying the mediating effects of variables and thus was used in this study.

Before constructing the structural equation model (SEM), the reliability and validity of the variables were verified by using Cronbach's Alpha and factor analysis in order to make the model results more convincing. The results suggest that variables selected in this study have a relatively high reliability (Cronbach's Alpha is 0.726 ($\geq$0.700)) and validity (Kaiser-Meyer-Olkin (KMO) is 0.779 (>0.700) and Sig. is 0.000 (<0.05)).

Given that this study focuses mainly on the direct effects of greenspace exposure on health and the indirect effects of greenspace exposure on health through physical activity, personal characteristics are taken mainly as control variables in the SEM (Table 3). Greenspace exposure, physical activity, and health status are the exogenous variable, mediator variable, and endogenous variable respectively in the model (Table 4).

Table 3. Demographic and socioeconomic characteristics of the study participants (N = 1003).

Personal Characteristic	Code	Variable	Percent (%)
Gender	PC1	Male	49.95
		Female	50.05
Age (years)	PC2	Young people (19–44)	75.37
		Middle-aged people (45–59)	24.63
Marital status	PC3	Married	80.06
		Single	19.94
Education	PC4	Primary school or lower	0.10
		Junior high school degree	6.28
		Senior high school degree	27.52
		Bachelor degree	65.20
		Master degree or higher	0.90
Personal monthly income (RMB)	PC5	$\leq$2999 Yuan	1.20
		3000–4999 Yuan	32.10
		5000–8999 Yuan	48.55
		9000–11,999 Yuan	7.48
		$\geq$12,000 Yuan	10.67

Table 4. Variables of the structural equation model.

Type	Latent Variable	Measured Variable	Code
Exogenous variable	Greenspace exposure	Vegetation coverage	GE1
		Physical activity site coverage	GE2
		Accessibility to the nearest greenspace	GE3
Mediator variable	Physical activity	Duration	PA1
		Frequency	PA2
		Intensity	PA3
Endogenous variable	Physical health	How much bodily pain have you had during the past four weeks?	PH1
		During the past four weeks, have you had any problems with your work or other regular daily activities as a result of your physical health?	PH2
		In general, what would you say your physical health is?	PH3
	Mental health	I have felt cheerful and in good spirits	MH1
		I have felt calm and relaxed	MH2
		I have felt active and vigorous	MH3
		I woke up feeling fresh and rested	MH4
		My daily life has been filled with things that interested me	MH5
	Social health	People around here are willing to help their neighbors	SH1
		This is a close-knit neighborhood	SH2
		People in this neighborhood can be trusted	SH3
		People in this neighborhood get along well with each other	SH4
		People in this neighborhood can handle questions together	SH5

3. Results

3.1. Model Testing

The SEM is constructed and revised using AMOS 21.0. It is found that the SEM presented in Figure 4 is an ideal research model with high goodness-of-fit and stability through the analysis of the structural equation model's matching degree (Table 5). Besides, the measuring results of the SEM's paths suggest that five paths in the hypotheses are verified (C.R. > 1.96, $p < 0.05$). As shown in Table 6, these verified paths indicate that greenspace exposure has a significant positive effect on mental health, social health, and physical activity, thus retaining H2, H3, and H4, respectively. Meanwhile, the paths from physical activity to physical health and mental health are significant, respectively, retaining the hypotheses (H5 and H6) that physical activity has a positive effect on physical health and mental health. Although greenspace exposure has an effect on physical health, and physical activity has a positive influence on social health, the effects of these two paths are not statistically significant ($p > 0.05$; H1 and H7 are invalid). Thus, the effect of greenspace exposure on physical health and the effect of physical activity on social health are both considered 0.00 in further analysis. The specific effect relationships between the latent variables are shown in Table 7.

Table 5. Analysis of the structural equation model's matching degree.

	CMIN/DF	GFI	RMR	RMSEA	AGFI	PNFI	PCFI
Suggested values	≤5	>0.90	<0.05	<0.08	>0.90	>0.50	>0.50
Correction model	4.790	0.913	0.035	0.061	0.892	0.694	0.723

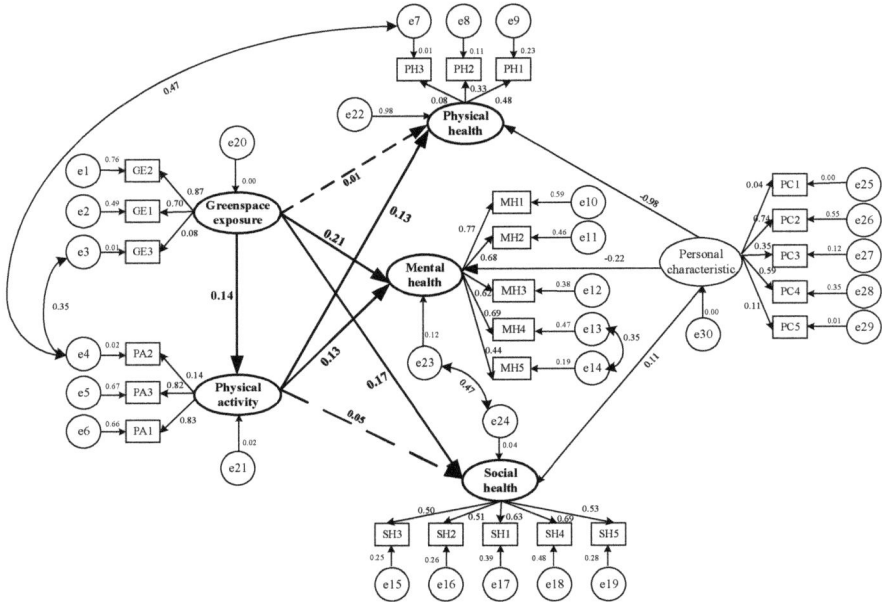

Figure 4. Effects of daily greenspace exposure on health.

Table 6. Test results of the causal paths of the SEM.

Relationship between Variables	Path Coefficient [a]	C.R.	p	Consequence
Greenspace exposure → Physical health	-	-	-	H1 Invalid
Greenspace exposure → Mental health	0.21	5.344	***	H2 Valid
Greenspace exposure → Social health	0.17	3.968	***	H3 Valid
Greenspace exposure → Physical activity	0.14	3.213	**	H4 Valid
Physical activity → Physical health	0.13	2.156	*	H5 Valid
Physical activity → Mental health	0.13	3.457	***	H6 Valid
Physical activity → Social health	-	-	-	H7 Invalid

$***\ p < 0.001$, $**\ p < 0.01$, $*\ p < 0.05$; [a] Standardized path coefficients.

Table 7. Effect relationships between the latent variables of the SEM.

Total Effect	Direct Effect	Indirect Effect
Greenspace exposure → Physical health	Greenspace exposure → Physical health	Greenspace exposure → Physical activity → Physical health
(0.018)	(0.00)	(0.018)
Greenspace exposure → Mental health	Greenspace exposure → Mental health	Greenspace exposure → Physical activity → Mental health
(0.228)	(0.21)	(0.018)
Greenspace exposure → Social health	Greenspace exposure → Social health	Greenspace exposure → Physical activity → Social health
(0.17)	(0.17)	(0.00)

Greenspace exposure → Physical activity → Physical health: It is a path that greenspace exposure affects physical health indirectly by affecting physical activity. In this indirect path, there are two direct paths: "Greenspace exposure → Physical activity" (0.14) and "Physical activity → Physical health" (0.13), which means that physical activity as a mediator connects the other two variables (greenspace exposure and physical health) and drives this indirect path. Thus, the indirect effect of greenspace exposure on physical health is $0.14 \times 0.13 \approx 0.018$ (three decimal places).

3.2. Effects of Daily Greenspace Exposure on Health

3.2.1. Direct Effects

The correlation coefficients between greenspace exposure and its measured variables (vegetation coverage [GE1], physical activity site coverage [GE2] and accessibility to the nearest greenspace [GE3]) are 0.70, 0.87 and 0.08 respectively (Figure 4), suggesting that "vegetation coverage (GE1)" and "physical activity site coverage (GE2)" are more closely related to participant's daily greenspace exposures. As shown in Table 7, greenspace exposure has a direct positive effect on mental health (0.21) and social health (0.17). However, greenspace exposure is not associated with physical health (0.00). These direct effects on the three dimensions of health indicate that participants' psychological condition and social interactions are significantly better for participants who were exposed to more greenspace than those who were exposed to more greenspace-poor areas. In addition, the impact of greenspace exposure on mental health is more obvious than its impact on social health.

3.2.2. Indirect Effects

The indirect effects of daily greenspace exposure on individual health are realized through physical activity, the mediator variable. The correlation coefficients between physical activity and its measured variables (duration [PA1], frequency [PA2] and intensity [PA3]) are 0.83, 0.14, and 0.82, respectively (Figure 4), suggesting that "duration (PA1)" and "intensity (PA3)" of physical activity have great influences on the level of physical activity undertaken by participants. Daily greenspace exposure level has a strong relationship with physical activity level ($p < 0.01$) (Table 6). It is similar to what was found in previous studies that greenspace provides the beautiful environment and comfortable space for physical activity and could effectively alleviate the decline in physical activity level, due to a lack of venues [74,75]. Besides, the correlation between "accessibility to the nearest greenspace (e3)" and "frequency (e4)" shows that an increase in the accessibility of greenspace may enhance the frequency of people's physical activity (Figure 4). Physical activity has a significant positive effect on physical health (0.13) and mental health (0.13), as shown in Table 6. In particular, the correlation between "frequency (e4)" and "self-rated physical health (e7)" indicates that the higher the frequency of a participant's physical activity, the better is her or his physical health (Figure 4). However, physical activity is not associated with social health (0.00), so this outcome is excluded from further analysis.

As shown in Table 7, the indirect effects of daily greenspace exposure on participants' physical health and mental health through physical activity are 0.018 and 0.018, respectively. The results indicate that the indirect effect of daily greenspace exposure on mental health (0.018) is equal to that on physical health (0.018), but is greater than that on social health (0.00). In contrast, the direct effect of daily greenspace exposure on social health (0.17) is less than that on mental health (0.21), but is greater than that on physical health (0.00). By comparing the results of indirect effects and direct effects of daily greenspace exposure on health, it can be observed that the effects of daily greenspace exposure on physical health and social health changed greatly after adding the mediating variable of physical activity, indicating that physical activity plays a mediating role in the relationship between greenspace exposure and health.

3.2.3. Total Effects

The total effects (direct effects + indirect effects) of daily greenspace exposure on physical health, mental health, and social health are 0.018, 0.228, and 0.17, respectively (Table 7), all of which have increased when compared with the direct effects.

Among the three dimensions of health, daily greenspace exposure level has the most obvious effect on mental health. This indicates that daily greenspace exposure plays a primary role in improving participants' mental health, likely through an increase in the quantity and quality of greenspace in their activity space. Specifically, people could release stress and tension, mitigate negative emotions and create a relaxed and pleasant mental state through frequent contact with greenspace.

Although daily greenspace exposure has the lowest indirect effect on social health, its total effect on social health is second, due to its higher direct effect. This suggests that natural environment provides more opportunities for people to engage in physical activity with families and neighbors, which promotes interpersonal relationships, fosters social interactions, strengthens community cohesion, and enhances individual well-being.

Notably, daily greenspace exposure has the lowest total effect on physical health, due to the fact that its direct effect on physical health is the lowest. The main reason resulting in its lowest direct effect on physical health is that this study only considers the coverage of greenspace and ignores other factors, such as the diversity of plant species, landscaping design and layout, and so on. In contrast, the indirect effect of daily greenspace exposure on physical health is higher, indicating that promoting physical health through physical activity may yield better outcomes than relying on the direct effects. For instance, greenspace with high accessibility and attractive surroundings can help stimulate people's interest in physical activity, which in turn reduces the incidence of diseases and helps maintain health through higher levels of physical activity.

4. Discussion

Urban greenspace planning is a crucial issue in the context of rapid urbanization and sustainable development, as greenspace helps to support physical activity and improve individual health outcomes. Recent research has underlined the importance of planning and management of greenspace, especially in megacities, due to the huge populations and scarcity of space [76–78].

4.1. Urban Greenspace Planning Implications

Urban greenspace exposure makes a great contribution to counteracting people's sedentary lifestyle, increasing their physical activity and improving their health status. However, there is a general underestimation of the value of daily greenspace exposure in urban planning and park management in China. Therefore, conducting research in this area and applying the findings to improve the planning and design of greenspace in urban areas has great significance to urban sustainability and healthy living. In order to further promote the beneficial influence of greenspace on health outcomes, residents should be advised to heighten their environmental protection consciousness and increase their utilization rate of greenspace. In addition, urban planners should take more measures in constructing greenspace and building ecological cities so as to increase people's greenspace exposure. These specific measures include increasing the proportion of greenspace in urban areas, and promoting supporting facilities and services like seats and outdoor exercise or fitness equipment. Finally, relevant government departments should establish and improve laws and regulations to protect public health through constructing a green environment for promoting health and formulating and implementing health education action plan.

4.2. Limitations

One limitation of this research is that greenspace exposure indicators included only objectively measured variables, which precluded the ability to draw conclusions about the influence of subjective assessment of greenspace exposure on health. Subjective assessment should be coupled with objectively measured data in future studies, such as the evaluation of the quantity and quality of one's activity space, the utilization rate of greenspace and subjective assessment of sanitary condition.

Another limitation of this study relates to the survey of mental health, which only reflects the overall state of mind in the recent period. However, mental state (pleasant, stressful, anxious, and so on) and emotions (positive feelings, negative feelings, and so on) will also change momentarily depending on different events that people experience in their daily life. Future research may shed new light on the moderating effects of greenspace exposure on changes in people's mental states that are affected by the stressful events or daily emergencies they experience. For instance, respondents may be asked to wear global positioning systems (GPS) to track their movement patterns in a more objective manner and list all activities they are engaged in and how they felt during each activity through responding to real-time prompts based on ecological momentary assessment (EMA) methods. In future work, conducting studies with these additional components has potential to help improve research results.

5. Conclusions

The objective of this study is to examine the relationship between daily greenspace exposure and individual health from the point of view of human mobility and the uncertain geographic context problem. The results indicate that daily greenspace exposure directly influences participants' health and indirectly affects their health status through the mediating effect of physical activity. Specifically, the direct effect of daily greenspace exposure on mental health is more significant than its direct effect on social health, while such direct effect on physical health is not obvious. The indirect effect of daily greenspace exposure on mental health is similar to that on physical health, but such indirect effect on social health is not remarkable. In addition, the total effect of daily greenspace exposure on mental health is more obvious than its total effect on social health. However, the total effect of daily greenspace exposure on physical health is not significant. On the whole, a higher level of individual daily greenspace exposure in the study area is related to better physical activity and overall health. Daily greenspace exposure primarily helps to improve participants' mental health and relieve their negative feelings, and then promote their social health and strengthen social cohesion, and enhance their physical health and reduce the incidence of diseases to a lesser extent.

Author Contributions: Conceptualization, L.Z. and S.Z.; Data curation, L.Z.; Formal analysis, L.Z. and M.-P.K.; Funding acquisition, L.Z., S.Z. and M.-P.K.; Investigation, F.C. and R.L.; Methodology, L.Z.; Resources, F.C.; Software, R.L.; Writing—original draft, L.Z.; Writing—revising and editing, S.Z. and M.-P.K.

Funding: This research was supported by grants from the National Natural Science Foundation of China (41522104, 41871148, 41529101). In addition, L.Z. was supported by the International Program for Ph.D. Candidates of Sun Yat-Sen University, and M.-P.K. was supported by a John Simon Guggenheim Memorial Foundation Fellowship.

Acknowledgments: The authors thank Jinpei Ou, the editor and the anonymous reviewers for their helpful comments and suggestions.

Conflicts of Interest: The authors declare no conflict of interest.

References

1. Wolf, K.L.; Robbins, A.S. Metro nature, environmental health, and economic value. *Environ. Health Perspect.* **2015**, *123*, 390–398. [CrossRef] [PubMed]
2. Lederbogen, F.; Kirsch, P.; Haddad, L.; Streit, F.; Tost, H.; Schuch, P.; Wüst, S.; Pruessner, J.C.; Rietschel, M.; Deuschle, M. City living and urban upbringing affect neural social stress processing in humans. *Nature* **2011**, *474*, 498. [CrossRef] [PubMed]
3. Peen, J.; Schoevers, R.A.; Beekman, A.T.; Dekker, J. The current status of urban-rural differences in psychiatric disorders. *Acta Psychiatr. Scand.* **2010**, *121*, 84–93. [CrossRef] [PubMed]
4. Kahlmeier, S.; Künzli, N.; Braunfahrländer, C. The first years of implementation of the Swiss National Environment and Health Action Plan (NEHAP): Lessons for environmental health promotion. *Soz. Präventivmed.* **2002**, *47*, 67–73. [CrossRef] [PubMed]
5. Karr, G.; Pecassou, B.; Boudet, C.; Ramel, M. Assistance for selecting the priority substances of the future French national environment and health action plan (Plan national santé environment—PNSE3): Developing and implementing a collective risk indicator. *Environ. Risques Santé* **2014**, *13*, 232–243.
6. Hartig, T.; Mitchell, R.; De Vries, S.; Frumkin, H. Nature and health. *Annu. Rev. Public Health* **2014**, *35*, 207–228. [CrossRef] [PubMed]
7. Largo-Wight, E. Cultivating healthy places and communities: Evidenced-based nature contact recommendations. *Int. J. Environ. Health Res.* **2011**, *21*, 41–61. [CrossRef] [PubMed]
8. Hsiao, L.L.; Yu, S.S. The Impact of Green Space Changes on Air Pollution and Microclimates: A Case Study of the Taipei Metropolitan Area. *Sustainability* **2014**, *6*, 8827–8855.
9. Selmi, W.; Weber, C.; Rivière, E.; Blond, N.; Mehdi, L.; Nowak, D. Air pollution removal by trees in public green spaces in Strasbourg city, France. *Urban For. Urban Green.* **2016**, *17*, 192–201. [CrossRef]

10. Dzhambov, A.M.; Dimitrova, D.D. Green spaces and environmental noise perception. *Urban For. Urban Green.* **2015**, *14*, 1000–1008. [CrossRef]

11. Bolund, P.; Hunhammar, S. Ecosystem services in urban areas. *Ecol. Econ.* **1999**, *29*, 293–301. [CrossRef]

12. Langner, M.; Kull, M.; Endlicher, W.R. Determination of PM_{10} deposition based on antimony flux to selected urban surfaces. *Environ. Pollut.* **2011**, *159*, 2028–2034. [CrossRef] [PubMed]

13. Ghimire, R.; Ferreira, S.; Green, G.T.; Poudyal, N.C.; Cordell, H.K.; Thapa, J.R. Green Space and Adult Obesity in the United States. *Ecol. Econ.* **2017**, *136*, 201–212. [CrossRef]

14. Groenewegen, P.P.; Zock, J.P.; Spreeuwenberg, P.; Helbich, M.; Hoek, G.; Ruijsbroek, A.; Strak, M.; Verheij, R.; Volker, B.; Waverijn, G.; et al. Neighbourhood social and physical environment and general practitioner assessed morbidity. *Health Place* **2017**, *49*, 68–84. [CrossRef] [PubMed]

15. Lachowycz, K.; Jones, A.P. Towards a better understanding of the relationship between greenspace and health: Development of a theoretical framework. *Landsc. Urban Plan.* **2013**, *118*, 62–69. [CrossRef]

16. Feng, J.; Glass, T.A.; Curriero, F.C.; Stewart, W.F.; Schwartz, B.S. The built environment and obesity: A systematic review of the epidemiologic evidence. *Health Place* **2010**, *16*, 175–190. [CrossRef] [PubMed]

17. De Vries, S. Nearby nature and human health: Looking at the mechanisms and their implications. In *Innovative Approaches in Researching Landscape and Health*; Ward Thompson, C., Bell, S., Aspinall, P., Eds.; Routledge: Oxon, UK, 2010; pp. 77–96.

18. Kaplan, S. The restorative benefits of nature: Toward an integrative framework. *J. Environ. Psychol.* **1995**, *15*, 169–182. [CrossRef]

19. Kaplan, R.; Kaplan, S. *The Experience of Nature: A Psychological Perspective*; Cambridge University Press: Cambridge, UK, 1989.

20. Bowler, D.E.; Buyung-Ali, L.M.; Knight, T.M.; Pullin, A.S. A systematic review of evidence for the added benefits to health of exposure to natural environments. *BMC Public Health* **2010**, *10*, 456. [CrossRef] [PubMed]

21. Bratman, G.N.; Hamilton, J.P.; Daily, G.C. The impacts of nature experience on human cognitive function and mental health. *Ann. N. Y. Acad. Sci.* **2012**, *1249*, 118–136. [CrossRef] [PubMed]

22. Wells, N.M.; Evans, G.W. Nearby nature a buffer of life stress among rural children. *Environ. Behav.* **2003**, *35*, 311–330. [CrossRef]

23. Van den Berg, A.E.; Maas, J.; Verheij, R.A.; Groenewegen, P.P. Green space as a buffer between stressful life events and health. *Soc. Sci. Med.* **2010**, *70*, 1203–1210. [CrossRef] [PubMed]

24. Bogar, S.; Beyer, K.M. Green Space, Violence, and Crime: A Systematic Review. *Trauma Violence Abus.* **2016**, *17*, 160–171. [CrossRef] [PubMed]

25. Wood, L.; Hooper, P.; Foster, S.; Bull, F. Public green spaces and positive mental health-investigating the relationship between access, quantity and types of parks and mental wellbeing. *Health Place* **2017**, *48*, 63–71. [CrossRef] [PubMed]

26. Akpinar, A.; Barbosa-Leiker, C.; Brooks, K.R. Does green space matter? Exploring relationships between green space type and health indicators. *Urban For. Urban Green.* **2016**, *20*, 407–418. [CrossRef]

27. Berg, M.V.D.; Poppel, M.V.; Smith, G.; Triguero-Mas, M.; Andrusaityte, S.; Kamp, I.V.; Mechelen, W.V.; Gidlow, C.; Gražulevičiene, R.; Nieuwenhuijsen, M.J.; et al. Does time spent on visits to green space mediate the associations between the level of residential greenness and mental health? *Urban For. Urban Green.* **2017**, *25*, 94–102. [CrossRef]

28. Choi, J.Y.; Chang, A.K.; Choi, E.J. Effects of a Physical Activity and Sedentary Behavior Program on Activity Levels, Stress, Body Size, and Sleep in Sedentary Korean College Students. *Holist. Nurs. Pract.* **2018**, *32*, 287–295. [CrossRef] [PubMed]

29. Ng, S.W.; Popkin, B.M. Time use and physical activity: A shift away from movement across the globe. *Obes. Rev.* **2012**, *13*, 659–680. [CrossRef] [PubMed]

30. Akpinar, A. How is quality of urban green spaces associated with physical activity and health? *Urban For. Urban Green.* **2016**, *16*, 76–83. [CrossRef]

31. Coombes, E.; Jones, A.P.; Hillsdon, M. The relationship of physical activity and overweight to objectively measured green space accessibility and use. *Soc. Sci. Med.* **2010**, *70*, 816–822. [CrossRef] [PubMed]

32. Cohen-Cline, H.; Turkheimer, E.; Duncan, G.E. Access to green space, physical activity and mental health: A twin study. *J. Epidemiol. Community Health* **2015**, *69*, 523–529. [CrossRef] [PubMed]

33. Richardson, E.A.; Pearce, J.; Mitchell, R.; Kingham, S. Role of physical activity in the relationship between urban green space and health. *Public Health* **2013**, *127*, 318–324. [CrossRef] [PubMed]

34. Ambrey, C.L. Urban greenspace, physical activity and wellbeing: The moderating role of perceptions of neighbourhood affability and incivility. *Land Use Policy* **2016**, *57*, 638–644. [CrossRef]
35. Godbey, G.C.; Caldwell, L.L.; Floyd, M.; Payne, L.L. Contributions of leisure studies and recreation and park management research to the active living agenda. *Am. J. Prev. Med.* **2005**, *28*, 150–158. [CrossRef] [PubMed]
36. Fan, Y.L.; Das, K.V.; Chen, Q. Neighborhood green, social support, physical activity, and stress: Assessing the cumulative impact. *Health Place* **2011**, *17*, 1202–1211. [CrossRef] [PubMed]
37. Ulmer, J.M.; Wolf, K.L.; Backman, D.R.; Tretheway, R.L.; Blain, C.J.; O'Neil-Dunne, J.P.; Frank, L.D. Multiple health benefits of urban tree canopy: The mounting evidence for a green prescription. *Health Place* **2016**, *42*, 54–62. [CrossRef] [PubMed]
38. Browning, M.; Lee, K. Within what distance does "greenness" best predict physical health? A systematic review of articles with GIS buffer analyses across the Lifespan. *Int. J. Environ. Res. Public Health* **2017**, *14*, 675. [CrossRef] [PubMed]
39. De Vries, S.; van Dillen, S.M.E.; Groenewegen, P.P.; Spreeuwenberg, P. Streetscape greenery and health: Stress, social cohesion and physical activity as mediators. *Soc. Sci. Med.* **2013**, *94*, 26–33. [CrossRef] [PubMed]
40. Maas, J.; van Dillen, S.M.E.; Verheij, R.A.; Groenewegen, P.P. Social contacts as a possible mechanism behind the relation between green space and health. *Health Place* **2009**, *15*, 586–595. [CrossRef] [PubMed]
41. Richardson, E.A.; Mitchell, R. Gender differences in relationships between urban green space and health in the United Kingdom. *Soc. Sci. Med.* **2010**, *71*, 568–575. [CrossRef] [PubMed]
42. Matthews, S.A. The Salience of Neighborhood: Some Lessons from Sociology. *Am. J. Prev. Med.* **2008**, *34*, 257–259. [CrossRef] [PubMed]
43. Kwan, M.-P. From place-based to people-based exposure measures. *Soc. Sci. Med.* **2009**, *69*, 1311–1313. [CrossRef] [PubMed]
44. Kwan, M.-P. Beyond space (as we knew it): Toward temporally integrated geographies of segregation, health, and accessibility. *Ann. Assn. Am. Geogr.* **2013**, *103*, 1078–1086. [CrossRef]
45. Kwan, M.-P. The neighborhood effect averaging problem (NEAP): An elusive confounder of the neighborhood effect. *Int. J. Environ. Res. Public Health* **2018**, *15*, 1841. [CrossRef] [PubMed]
46. Kwan, M.-P. The limits of the neighborhood effect: Contextual uncertainties in geographic, environmental health, and social science research. *Ann. Assn. Am. Geogr.* **2018**. [CrossRef]
47. Zhao, P.X.; Kwan, M.-P.; Zhou, S.H. The uncertain geographic context problem in the analysis of the relationships between obesity and the built environment in Guangzhou. *Int. J. Environ. Res. Public Health* **2018**, *15*, 308. [CrossRef] [PubMed]
48. Kwan, M.-P. The uncertain geographic context problem. *Ann. Assn. Am. Geogr.* **2012**, *102*, 958–968. [CrossRef]
49. James, P.; Berrigan, D.; Hart, J.E.; Hipp, A.; Hoehner, C.M.; Kerr, J.; Major, J.M.; Oka, M.; Laden, F. Effects of buffer size and shape on associations between the built environment and energy balance. *Health Place* **2014**, *27*, 162–170. [CrossRef] [PubMed]
50. Park, Y.M.; Kwan, M.-P. Individual exposure estimates may be erroneous when spatiotemporal variability of air pollution and human mobility are ignored. *Health Place* **2017**, *43*, 85–94. [CrossRef] [PubMed]
51. Laatikainen, T.E.; Hasanzadeh, K.; Kyttä, M. Capturing exposure in environmental health research: Challenges and opportunities of different activity space models. *Int. J. Health Geogr.* **2018**, *17*, 29. [CrossRef] [PubMed]
52. Kwan, M.-P.; Wang, J.; Tyburski, M.; Epstein, D.H.; Kowalczyk, W.J.; Preston, K.L. Uncertainties in the geographic context of health behaviors: A study of substance users' exposure to psychosocial stress using GPS data. *Int. J. Geogr. Inf. Sci.* **2018**. [CrossRef]
53. Han, K.T. The Effect of Nature and Physical Activity on Emotions and Attention while Engaging in Green Exercise. *Urban For. Urban Green.* **2017**, *24*, 5–13. [CrossRef]
54. Mitchell, R. Is physical activity in natural environments better for mental health than physical activity in other environments? *Soc. Sci. Med.* **2013**, *91*, 130–134. [CrossRef] [PubMed]
55. Statistical Communique of the Guangzhou on the 2017 National Economic and Social Development. Available online: http://www.gz.gov.cn/gzgov/gysy2/201804/19a6eb2090a542c78afc520d792c9208.shtml (accessed on 1 April 2018).
56. Craig, C.L.; Marshall, A.L.; Sjorstrom, M.; Bauman, A.E.; Booth, M.L.; Ainsworth, B.E.; Pratt, M.; Ekelund, U.; Yngve, A.; Sallis, J.F.; et al. International physical activity questionnaire: 12-country reliability and validity. *Med. Sci. Sports Exerc.* **2003**, *35*, 1381–1395. [CrossRef] [PubMed]

57. Ainsworth, B.E.; Haskell, W.L.; Herrmann, S.D.; Meckes, N.; Bassett, D.R., Jr.; Tudor-Locke, C.; Greer, J.L.; Vezina, J.; Whitt-Glover, M.C.; Leon, A.S. 2011 compendium of physical activities: A second update of codes and MET values. *Med. Sci. Sports Exerc.* **2011**, *43*, 1575–1581. [CrossRef] [PubMed]

58. Haskell, W.L.; Lee, I.-M.; Pate, R.R.; Powell, K.E.; Blair, S.N.; Franklin, B.A.; Macera, C.A.; Heath, G.W.; Thompson, P.D.; Bauman, A. Physical activity and public health: Updated recommendation for adults from the American College of Sports Medicine and the American Heart Association. *Circulation* **2007**, *116*, 1081–1093. [CrossRef] [PubMed]

59. Huber, M.; Knottnerus, J.A.; Green, L.; van der Horst, H.; Jadad, A.R.; Kromhout, D.; Leonard, B.; Lorig, K.; Loureiro, M.I.; van der Meer, J.W.M.; et al. How should we define health? *BMJ* **2011**, *343*, d4163. [CrossRef] [PubMed]

60. McHorney, C.A.; Ware, J.E.; Raczek, A.E. The MOS 36-Item Short-Form Health Survey (SF-36): II. Psychometric and Clinical Tests of Validity in Measuring Physical and Mental Health Constructs. *Med. Care* **1993**, *31*, 247–263. [CrossRef] [PubMed]

61. Bech, P.; Olsen, L.R.; Kjoller, M.; Rasmussen, N.K. Measuring well-being rather than the absence of distress symptoms: A comparison of the SF-36 Mental Health subscale and the WHO-Five Well-Being Scale. *Int. J. Meth. Psychiatr. Res.* **2003**, *12*, 85–91. [CrossRef]

62. Sampson, R.J.; Raudenbush, S.W.; Earls, F. Neighborhoods and violent crime: A multilevel study of collective efficacy. *Science* **1997**, *277*, 918–924. [CrossRef] [PubMed]

63. Völker, B.; Flap, H.; Lindenberg, S. When Are Neighbourhoods Communities? Community in Dutch Neighbourhoods. *Eur. Sociol. Rev.* **2007**, *23*, 99–114. [CrossRef]

64. Kempen, G.I.J.M.; Van Eijk, L.M. The psychometric properties of the SSL12-I, a short scale for measuring social support in the elderly. *Soc. Indic. Res.* **1995**, *35*, 303–312. [CrossRef]

65. Robinson, D.; Wilkinson, D. Sense of community in a remote mining town: Validating a Neighborhood Cohesion scale. *Am. J. Community Psychol.* **1995**, *23*, 137–148. [CrossRef]

66. Rainham, D.; McDowell, I.; Krewski, D.; Sawada, M. Conceptualizing the healthscape: Contributions of time geography, location technologies and spatial ecology to place and health research. *Soc. Sci. Med.* **2010**, *70*, 668–676. [CrossRef] [PubMed]

67. Sallis, J.F.; Cerin, E.; Conway, T.L.; Adams, M.A.; Frank, L.D.; Pratt, M.; Salvo, D.; Schipperijn, J.; Smith, G.; Cain, K.L.; et al. Physical activity in relation to urban environments in 14 cities worldwide: A cross-sectional study. *Lancet* **2016**, *387*, 2207–2217. [CrossRef]

68. Berke, E.M.; Koepsell, T.D.; Moudon, A.V.; Hoskins, R.E.; Larson, E.B. Association of the built environment with physical activity and obesity in older persons. *Am. J. Public Health* **2011**, *97*, 486–492. [CrossRef] [PubMed]

69. Frank, L.D.; Schmid, T.L.; Sallis, J.F.; Chapman, J.; Saelens, B.E. Linking objectively measured physical activity with objectively measured urban form: Findings from SMARTRAQ. *Am. J. Prev. Med.* **2005**, *28*, 117–125. [CrossRef] [PubMed]

70. Phillips, M.L.; Esmen, N.A. Computational method for ranking task-specific exposures using multi-task time-weighted average samples. *Ann. Occup. Hyg.* **1999**, *43*, 201–213. [CrossRef]

71. Evanoff, B.; Zeringue, A.; Franzblau, A.; Dale, A.M. Using job-title-based physical exposures from O*NET in an epidemiological study of carpal tunnel syndrome. *Hum. Factors* **2014**, *56*, 166–177. [CrossRef] [PubMed]

72. Weden, M.M.; Carpiano, R.M.; Robert, S.A. Subjective and objective neighborhood characteristics and adult health. *Soc. Sci. Med.* **2008**, *66*, 1256–1270. [CrossRef] [PubMed]

73. Mohamadian, H.; Eftekhar, H.; Rahimi, A.; Mohamad, H.T.; Shojaiezade, D.; Montazeri, A. Predicting health-related quality of life by using a health promotion model among iranian adolescent girls: A structural equation modeling approach. *Nurs. Health Sci.* **2011**, *13*, 141–148. [CrossRef] [PubMed]

74. Mytton, O.T.; Townsend, N.; Rutter, H.; Foster, C. Green space and physical activity: An observational study using health survey for England data. *Health Place* **2012**, *18*, 1034–1041. [CrossRef] [PubMed]

75. Hillsdon, M.; Panter, J.; Foster, C.; Jones, A. The relationship between access and quality of urban green space with population physical activity. *Public Health* **2006**, *120*, 1127–1132. [CrossRef] [PubMed]

76. Standish, R.J.; Hobbs, R.J.; Miller, J.R. Improving city life: Options for ecological restoration in urban landscapes and how these might influence interactions between people and nature. *Landsc. Ecol.* **2013**, *28*, 1213–1221. [CrossRef]

77. Haaland, C.; Bosch, C.K.V.D. Challenges and strategies for urban green-space planning in cities undergoing densification: A review. *Urban For. Urban Green.* **2015**, *14*, 760–771. [CrossRef]

78. Tan, P.Y.; Wang, J.; Sia, A. Perspectives on five decades of the urban greening of Singapore. *Cities* **2013**, *32*, 24–32. [CrossRef]

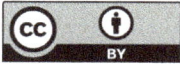

International Journal of
*Environmental Research
and Public Health*

MDPI

Article

An Improved Healthcare Accessibility Measure Considering the Temporal Dimension and Population Demand of Different Ages

Lan Ma [1], Nianxue Luo [1,*], Taili Wan [1], Chunchun Hu [1] and Mingjun Peng [2]

[1] School of Geodesy and Geomatics, Wuhan University, Wuhan 430079, China;
    lanma_sgg@whu.edu.cn (L.M.); wantaili@whu.edu.cn (T.W.); chchhu@sgg.whu.edu.cn (C.H.)
[2] Wuhan Land Resources and Planning Bureau, Wuhan 430014, China; Pmj@wpl.gov.cn
*   Correspondence: nxluo@sgg.whu.edu.cn; Tel.: +86-133-1712-3688

Received: 10 September 2018; Accepted: 29 October 2018; Published: 31 October 2018

Abstract: Healthcare accessibility has become an issue of social equity. An accurate estimation of existing healthcare accessibility is vital to plan and allocate health resources. Healthcare capacity, population demand, and geographic impedance are three essential factors to measure spatial accessibility. Additionally, geographic impedance is usually represented with a function of travel time. In this paper, the three-step floating catchment area (3SFCA) method is improved from the perspectives of the temporal dimension and population demand. Specifically, the travel time from the population location to the service site is precisely calculated by introducing real-time traffic conditions instead of utilizing empirical speed in previous studies. Additionally, with the utilization of real-time traffic, a dynamic result of healthcare accessibility is derived during different time periods. In addition, since the medical needs of the elderly are higher than that of the young, a demand weight index of demand is introduced to adjust the population demand. A case study of healthcare accessibility in Wuhan shows that the proposed method is effective to measure healthcare accessibility during different time periods. The spatial accessibility disparities of communities and crowdedness of hospitals are identified as an important reference for the balance between the supply and demand of medical resources.

Keywords: healthcare accessibility; population demand; geographic impedance; the elderly; urban planning; 3SFCA; real-time traffic; crowdedness

1. Introduction

Healthcare accessibility is the relative convenience of achieving healthcare services at a certain location [1]. By studying the disparities of spatial distribution between medical resources and inhabitants, areas lacking medical resources are revealed. Thus, an accurate estimation of existing healthcare accessibility is of great significance for government departments to make scientific decisions on urban planning so as to guarantee the proper allocation of medical resources.

The concept of access to healthcare has evolved during the last decades. Penchansky and Thomas [2] conceptualized access into five specific dimensions to describe the fit between the patient and the healthcare system. Additionally, these dimensions are availability, accessibility, accommodation, affordability, and acceptability. In recent studies, this concept was introduced by describing broad dimensions. As described by Levesque et al. [3], access encompassed five dimensions: approachability, acceptability, availability and accommodation, affordability, and appropriateness. Saurman [4] argued that awareness should be another dimension of access and modified Penchansky and Thomas's Theory of access. Access to healthcare is decided by the spatial accessibility of healthcare services, which is a primary deciding factor of healthcare utilization [5].

As to measure and evaluate healthcare accessibility, three factors are essential: healthcare capacity, population demand, and geographic impedance [6–8]. Healthcare capacity is the supply of healthcare services. Additionally, it can be represented by using the amount of specific facilities, physicians, or sickbeds. Population demand means the number of people who may need the services. Geographic impedance indicates to what extent the 'distance' between service location and population demand will affect accessibility. The 'distance' is usually characterized by travel time.

For patients, especially with acute diseases, an accurate estimation of travel time from the population location to hospitals is of crucial importance. In previous research, the classic method of simulating travel time to assign each road an empirical speed and then conduct a road network analysis [9–11]. However, with the development of urbanization, tidal transportation is a common phenomenon nowadays and road congestion varies during different time periods (e.g., at rush hours or at non-peak periods). Without considering traffic conditions, the theoretical travel time given by the classic approach is usually inaccurate. Healthcare accessibility is a static result by given travel time in previous studies. However, when considering traffic conditions, accessibility is dynamic. In addition, the elderly are mostly valetudinarian and need more frequent communications with healthcare providers [12]. Given the same population, a community with a higher proportion of the elderly will need more medical resources than that with a lower proportion. However, existing studies rarely consider the impact of different ages on medical needs. Additionally, as a result, the population demand is underestimated, especially in areas where there are more old people.

With the popularization of low-cost GPS devices and the development of Location Based Services (LBS), commercial map companies such as Google, Baidu, and AutoNavi, can obtain the location of floating vehicles or public users. With the help of big data mining technology, real-time traffic conditions are derived and provided to the public for route planning. Nowadays, people prefer to select a route with the help of real-time traffic conditions to reduce travel time, e.g., searching for medical treatment.

The paper improves the three-step floating catchment area (3SFCA) method, a recent method to measure healthcare accessibility. Specifically, the travel time is precisely calculated by introducing real-time traffic conditions from AutoNavi. Additionally, with the utilization of real-time traffic, dynamic results of healthcare accessibility are derived during different time periods. Besides, the population demand is adjusted by a demand weight index that characterizes the difference in medical needs between the elderly and the young. This improved method is illustrated and validated by a case study of healthcare accessibility in Wuhan. Results show that this study is of great significance in guiding how to better plan urban medical facilities.

2. A Methodological Review

Numerous measures have been utilized to estimate spatial accessibility, including the regional availability model [13], the gravity model [14], and the two-step floating catchment area (2SFCA) [15] method. The regional availability method is simply the ratio of supply (the capacity of service site) and demand (population) within a given area (e.g., administrative boundary). However, this method has been criticized because of its unreasonable assumptions: people do not go beyond the given area to seek medical services and all individuals within the given area have equal access regardless of the distance decay. The gravity model assumes that one's spatial access to medical services decreases with the increase of its distance to nearby medical sites in a gravitational way [14], which is theoretically sounder. However, it requires more computation and the result is not intuitive to interpret [16]. The 2SFCA is a special case of the gravity model but intuitive to interpret.

2.1. The Basic Two-Step Floating Catchment Area Method

Luo and Wang [15] developed the 2SFCA method and this method is conducted in two steps:

Step 1: Generate a zone (or catchment) with a threshold travel cost (d_0) for each service site j and search all population locations within the catchment. The supply-to-demand ratio R_j for each service site j is calculated according to the site's capacity and population demand with the following equation:

$$R_j = \frac{S_j}{\sum_{k \in \{Dist(k,j) \le d_0\}} P_k},$$

(1)

where $Dist(i, j)$ is travel cost from i to j, S_j is the supply capacity of service site j, P_k is the number of people in population location k, respectively.

Step 2: Generate a catchment with d_0 as threshold travel cost for each population location i and search all service sites within the catchment. Additionally, the spatial access index (SPAI) of i, A_i^F, is derived by summing the ratios of service sites within the catchment area of population location i:

$$A_i^F = \sum_{j \in \{Dist(i,j) \le d_0\}} R_j$$

(2)

The 2SFCA method has provided a widely accepted model to estimate healthcare accessibility since it was proposed [7,17–19]. Despite its popularity, the 2SFCA method has two major limitations. One limitation is that it assumes all locations within the given catchment area have equal access without a distance decay. In fact, people's willingness to travel decreases with increasing distance. The other limitation of the 2SFCA method is that it utilizes fixed catchment size. For example, the catchment sizes of rural and urban areas should be different because people in rural areas are willing to travel further to seek medical services than those in urban areas. The subsequent research mainly aims at overcoming above two limitations.

2.2. Major Extensions of 2SFCA

Most existing pieces of literature extends the basic 2SFCA method from three aspects: the introduction of impedance function, the calculation of catchment sizes, and the competition effect of supply and demand.

2.2.1. Extension on Introduction of the Impedance Function

It is generally accepted that the 2SFCA method is insufficient without the addition of impedance function [20–23]. Luo and Qi [22] presented an enhanced 2SFCA (E2SFCA) method by introducing Gaussian weights when calculating the supply-to-demand ratio. The Gaussian weights are calculated from the Gaussian function and utilized to reveal that people's willingness to travel decreases with the increasing distance. This E2SFCA method works in two steps. First, a 30-min catchment around each service site j is generated and the catchment is divided into three subzones with a 10-min interval. The method of dividing the catchment area into several sub-areas is called the zonal method. Additionally, the supply-to-demand ratio R_j is calculated by

$$R_j = \frac{S_j}{\sum_{r=1,2,3} \sum_{k \in D_r} P_k W_r}$$

(3)

where W_r is a Gaussian weight defined beforehand for the rth subzone D_r. The spatial access index is then calculated by

$$A_i^F = \sum_{r=1,2,3} \sum_{j \in D_r} R_j W_r$$

(4)

Some researchers have suggested that a sudden drop occurs at the edge of each zone when the zonal method is applied to large geographical areas [20,21]. Hence, some continuous impedance functions were developed. Mcgrail and Humphreys [23] proposed a continuous impedance function.

In this function, a weight was assigned the value 1 for the first 10 min, the value 0 for more than 60 min, and a gradual decay for the time between 10 and 60 min. More continuous impedance functions, such as the Gaussian function [24,25], the kernel density function [20,26] and the gravity-based function (e.g., the power function, exponential function) [27–29] were subsequently introduced to model the distance decay effect. By generalizing the impedance function as a term $f(d)$ [1], all measures in the 2SFCA method can be integrated as follows:

$$A_i^F = \sum_{j \in \{Dist(i,j) \le d_0\}} R_j f(d_{ij}) = \sum_{j \in \{Dist(i,j) \le d_0\}} (S_j f(d_{ij}) / \sum_{k \in \{Dist(k,j) \le d_0\}} P_k f(d_{kj})), \tag{5}$$

where the impedance function, $f(d)$, indicating how travel cost influences accessibility, can be a piecewise function or a continuous function.

The nature of this extension is to add an additional impedance function within the catchment area of 2SFCA. All references above are based on the extension of the impedance function and the difference between them mainly lies in the decay trend of impedance functions.

2.2.2. The Extension on the Calculation of Catchment Sizes

The other limitation of the 2SFCA method is that it utilizes fixed catchment size. Luo and Whippo [30] proposed a new method named Variable 2SFCA(V2SFCA) to define the catchment sizes dynamically by increasing the catchment size progressively till a base population and a ratio of physician-to-population were met. This V2SFCA method can determine the appropriate catchment sizes effectively. However, the determination of the base population and the physician-to-population ratio is somewhat subjective, which is due to a lack of an adequate basis. McGrail and Humphreys [21] divided the catchment area into five levels based on population density to measure healthcare accessibility. Additionally, this extension is called Dynamic 2SFCA(D2SFCA). The D2SFCA has a strong practical significance, especially suitable for the case studies in areas where urban and rural areas are mixed. Tao et al. [27] demonstrated that different facilities may have different search radius and generally large-scaled facilities have large search radii. So different catchment sizes were assigned to each healthcare site according to its capacity. The results show that the multi-radius is superior to single search radius utilized in the basic 2SFCA when calculating accessibility. Jamtsho et al. [31] proposed a nearest-neighbor two-step floating catchment area (NN-2SFCA) model. This method assumes that the demand points only select a certain number of closest facilities within the search radius.

2.2.3. The Extension Based on the Competition Effect of Supply and Demand

In addition to the above extensions for the two major limitations of 2SFCA, the competition effect between facilities is also considered by some scholars. Wan et al. [32] demonstrated that the potential competition between service sites would affect the population demand on sites and the population demand might be overestimated in the E2SFCA method. A three-step floating catchment area(3SFCA) method was proposed to minimize this overestimation. It assumed that people's demand for a healthcare site is affected by the availability of other nearby sites. Specifically, a selection weight for each pair of demand-supply sites was introduced into this method, thus adjusting the population demand. This method is implemented in three steps. It first divides the catchment into 4 sub-zones (i.e., 10, 20, 30, and 60 min, respectively) and assigns a Gaussian weight to each service site based on the sub-zone in which it lies. Additionally, the selection weight G_{ij} is computed by

$$G_{ij} = \frac{T_{ij}}{\sum_{k \in \{Dist(i,k) \le d_0\}} T_{ik}} \tag{6}$$

where G_{ij} indicates the probability of selection on a service site, T_{ij} and T_{ik} are the predefined Gaussian weights for service site j and k, respectively. The second step is to calculate the adjusted supply-to-demand ratio R_j:

$$R_j = \frac{S_j}{\sum\limits_{r=1,2,3,4} \sum\limits_{k \in D_r} G_{kj} P_k W_r} \tag{7}$$

The third step is to calculate the SPAI of population location i by summing up the physician-to-population ratios of service site j within the catchment area of population location i:

$$A_i^F = \sum\limits_{r=1,2,3,4} \sum\limits_{j \in D_r} G_{ij} R_j W_r \tag{8}$$

The 3SFCA method effectively minimizes the overestimation of the healthcare demand. However, the selection weight utilized in this method was just based on the travel time. In real life, people's selection on a service site was not only related to travel time, but also affected by the capacity of the site. The Huff model is a gravity-based model proposed by Huff to survey the scale of retail stores [33]. The core idea of the Huff model is that consumers' purchase probabilities are positively related to the attractiveness/capacity of stores and inversely related to its distance from consumers. So, the Huff model is commonly utilized to quantify the probability of people's choice of a service site out of other nearby available ones. Luo [34] integrated the original Huff model and floating catchment area method to express population selection of services. The negative power distance impedance function is utilized in the original Huff model and the probability of the population location i in choosing service site j, $Prob_{ij}$, is calculated by

$$Prob_{ij} = \frac{S_j d_{ij}^{-\beta}}{\sum\limits_{s \in D_0} S_s d_{is}^{-\beta}} \tag{9}$$

where d_{ij} is the travel cost from i to j, β is a distance impedance coefficient indicating the extent of the distance decay, respectively. Luo [35] proposed an enhanced three-step floating catchment area (E3SFCA) method by modifying this negative power function with a Gaussian function. The modified Huff model is overwritten as follows:

$$Prob_{ij} = \frac{S_j e^{-d_{ij}^2/\beta}}{\sum\limits_{s \in D_0} S_s e^{-d_{is}^2/\beta}} \tag{10}$$

Instead of the predefined subzone-based Gaussian weight in previous studies, a continuous Gaussian weight is utilized to model the spatial interactions between the demand and supplies. Additionally, the adjusted supply-to-demand ratio R_j and the SPAI of the population location i are computed respectively according to

$$R_j = \frac{S_j}{\sum\limits_{k \in D_0} Prob_{kj} P_k W_{kj}} \tag{11}$$

and

$$A_i^F = \sum\limits_{j \in D_0} Prob_{ij} R_j W_{ij} \tag{12}$$

The E3SFCA method can better adjust the population demand to overcome the overestimation and underestimation problems and, therefore, generate more reliable measures of spatial access to healthcare services.

3. An Improved 3SFCA Method

Despite many achievements in developing the 2SFCA method, problems remain. In previous studies, a common calculation method of travel time is to assign each road an empirical speed and then a conduct road network analysis [9–11], which ignores complicated traffic conditions in reality. Meanwhile, the individual healthcare demand of different age groups is considered equally, disregarding that the elderly usually have a higher healthcare demand than the young and thus the population demand is underestimated. To overcome the limitations of estimating travel cost and population demand, this paper improves the 3SFCA method. The improved method is based on more reasonable assumptions about the patient's medical seeking behavior and medical needs for medical services.

When seeking medical care, especially in emergencies, patients are more likely to use taxis or private cars than buses or rail transit. An accurate estimation of driving time from the population location to hospitals is of crucial importance. In this paper, the driving time is precisely calculated by introducing real-time traffic conditions from AutoNavi. The AutoNavi distance measurement API is a travel distance calculation interface provided in the form of HTTP and the query data is returned in JSON or XML. Its strategy aims to avoid traffic jams, but it may take longer because of the possibility of a detour. People's travel behavior of searching for medical care is highly consistent with this strategy. Given an origin (i.e., population location) and a destination (i.e., service site), the driving time between two points is achieved with the API. Thus, the AutoNavi API is utilized to estimate the driving time at different periods by programming in Asp.net.

In general, people tend to go to neighboring hospitals that are rich in medical resources when seeking medical care. This health-seeking behavior is consistent with the core idea of the Huff model. So, the Huff model is utilized to calculate the probability of people seeking a service site. The key of the Huff model is the determination of the impedance function. So far, the most common forms of impedance functions are the negative power function ($f(d_{ij}) = d_{ij}^{-\beta}$), the exponential function ($f(d_{ij}) = e^{-\beta d_{ij}}$), and the Gaussian function ($f(d_{ij}) = e^{-d_{ij}^2/\beta}$). As shown in Figure 1, the power function and the exponential function are convex functions. The convex function tends to decay too sharply near the origin when compared with the empirical evidence. However, the decay curve of the Gaussian function is S-shaped, and its decay rate increases first and then slows down with the increase of the distance. Since the Gaussian function relatively has a slow decline rate close to the origin, it is superior and can better reveal the effect of distance decay [36,37]. Therefore, the Gaussian function is utilized in this method as the impedance function. In general, 10 min is treated as an initial impedance with no decay [23]. Thus, the Gaussian function is revised as

$$f(d_{ij}) = \begin{cases} 1 & d_{ij} \leq 10 \\ e^{-(d_{ij}-10)^2/\beta} & 10 < d_{ij} \leq d_0 \\ 0 & d_{ij} > d_0 \end{cases} \tag{13}$$

where d_{ij} is the travel time obtained in real-time traffic.

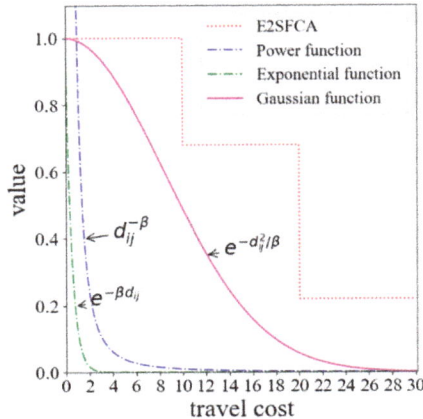

Figure 1. Major forms of impedance functions.

Both experience and statistics indicate that the elderly are at high risk of chronic diseases (e.g., heart disease, stroke, cancer, diabetes and lung disorders). Early literature has suggested that the prevalence of chronic diseases in the elderly is 2 to 3 times that of the general population [38,39]. According to the statistics, the prevalence ratio of chronic diseases among the aged is 53.8% and among which the urban aged is 77.7%. The prevalence ratio in cities is higher than that in rural areas. Moreover, the prevalence ratio varies according to the level of the city and the high-level cities have a high prevalence ratio [40]. In the latest research, a report entitled "China's Pension Industry Development Strategy Research (2014)" released by China's Center for Information Industry Development (CCID) Consulting pointed out that 80% to 90% of the aged are in the chronic and sub-healthy group and their demands for medical care are 3–5 times that of the young in China. Therefore, a demand weight index (DW) is introduced in this improved method to reveal the differences in the medical needs between the elderly and the young. The improved method is implemented in three steps:

Step 1: The probability of the population location i choosing service site j, $Prob_{ij}$, is calculated by

$$Prob_{ij} = \frac{C_j f(d_{ij})}{\sum\limits_{s \in D_0} C_s f(d_{is})} \tag{14}$$

where $f(d_{ij})$ is the revised Gaussian function (see Equation (13)).

Step 2: We assume that the medical needs of the elderly are DW times as big as the young. Thus, the adjusted population demand in location k, P_k, is revised as follows:

$$
\begin{aligned}
P_k &= DW * Pop_{oldk} + Pop_{elsek} \\
&= DW * Pop_{oldk} + Pop_{allk} - Pop_{oldk} \\
&= Pop_{allk} + (DW - 1) * Pop_{oldk}
\end{aligned} \tag{15}
$$

where Pop_{allk} is the total number of people in the population location k, Pop_{oldk} is the count of the elderly in the population location k, DW is a demand weight index revealing the differences in the medical needs between the elderly and the young. With the adjusted population demand P_k, the supply-to-demand R_j is implemented by

$$R_j = \frac{S_j}{\sum\limits_{k \in D_0} Prob_{kj} P_k f(d_{kj})} \tag{16}$$

Step 3: Compute the spatial access index of population site *i* by

$$A_i^F = \sum_{j \in D_0} Prob_{ij} R_j f(d_{ij}) \tag{17}$$

This improved method considers real-time traffic when calculating travel time, and thus dynamic results of accessibility are derived, which is conducive to a more comprehensive understanding of the accessibility in different time periods. Besides, it assumes that the elderly have a higher demand for medical resources than the young, which is a logical assumption in accordance with reality. Hence, the population demand has increased compared with previous methods assuming that the medical needs of the elderly and the young are the same.

4. A Case Study

4.1. Study Area and Data

Wuhan is the provincial capital of Hubei in central China. It has abundant water resources. This city has 13 municipal districts with a total area of 8494.41 square kilometers and has 10,914 thousand permanent residents in 2017. As shown in Figure 2, the study area is the main urban area of Wuhan as well as the core functional area.

The study area mainly covers 7 districts (i.e., the Jiang'an, Jianghan, Qiaokou, Hanyang, Wuchang, Hongshan and Qingshan Districts), which consists of 926 communities. Figure 3a,b show the distribution of the population and the elderly, respectively. The elderly mainly inhabit the Wuchang and Jianghan Districts.

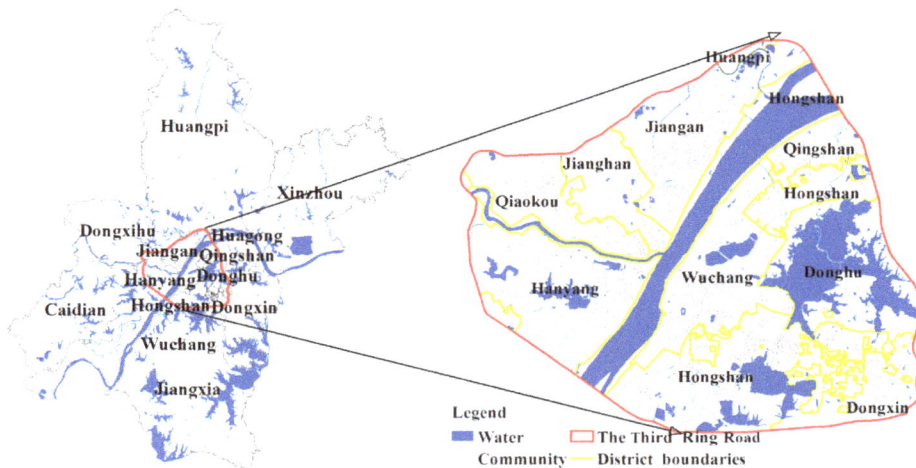

Figure 2. The study area.

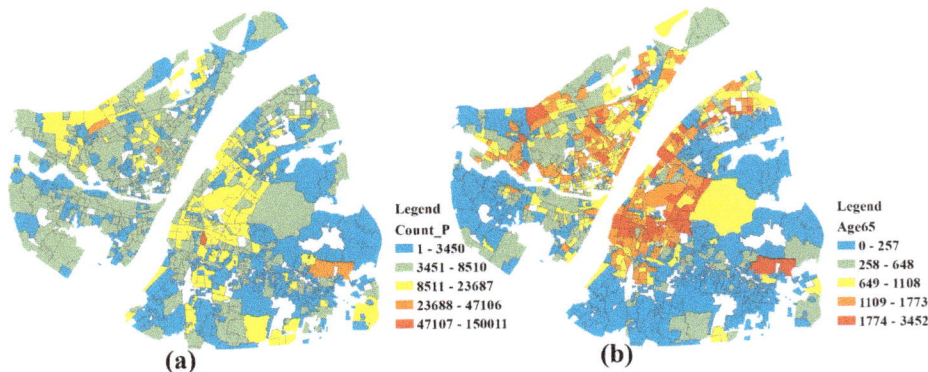

Figure 3. (**a**) The population distribution map; (**b**) the elderly distribution map.

Hospitals are divided into 3 levels (first-, second- and third-class hospitals) in the Chinese healthcare system. The third-class hospitals are superior while the first-class hospitals are inferior in terms of function, facilities, and technical strength, and the second-class hospitals are in between. Some researchers have indicated that the patients' willingness to travel is closely related to the healthcare provider [41,42]. In general, patients tend to choose hospitals that are professional and have a good reputation (e.g., the second- or third-class hospitals in China) [43–45]. This study focuses on the second- and third-class hospitals which represent the major medical resources of the city. A total of 88 hospitals are included in this paper. The number of beds and health technicians are obtained from the corresponding official websites of the hospitals. The distribution of hospitals and the number of beds in each hospital are shown in Figure 4a,b. Most medical resources are concentrated in the Wuchang and Jianghan Districts.

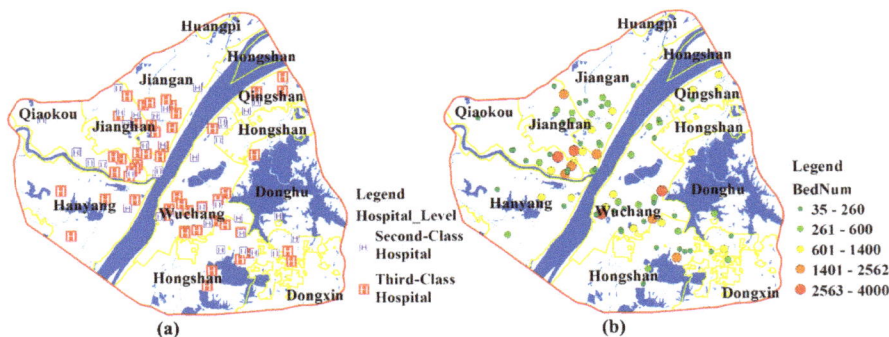

Figure 4. (**a**) A distribution map of the hospitals; (**b**) the distribution of the number of beds.

4.2. Data Preprocessing

4.2.1. Estimation of Population Locations

Previous studies usually utilize the geometry center of the research unit to represent population location when calculating the travel time to healthcare services. However, this method is not applicable in communities with imbalanced population distributions. Many communities in Wuhan contain some areas of water, where few people reside. As shown in Figure 5a, the community, named East Lake Road Community, is largely occupied by water and people here basically live in the western part of the community. As a result, the geometry center and population location are obviously inconsistent.

However, the median center is a central trend measure and its total Euclidean distance to all elements in the data set is minimal. Therefore, the median centers of buildings are regarded as the population location of each community in this paper. The population locations of communities in Wuhan is illustrated in Figure 5b.

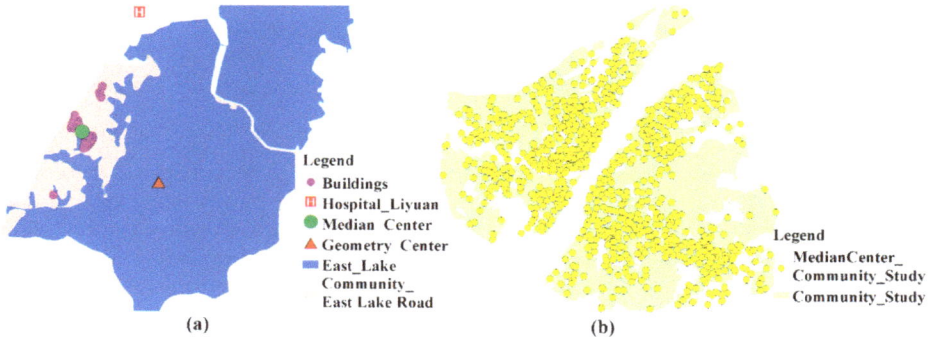

Figure 5. (**a**) The geometry center and median center of East Lake Road Community; (**b**) median centers of the study communities.

4.2.2. Estimation of Hospital's Beds

The number of beds and health technicians is obtained from the corresponding official websites of hospitals. For some reasons, there may be data missing. Data missing generally occurs in the following 2 scenarios and the corresponding solutions are as follows:

Scenario 1: The number of beds is missing while the number of health technicians is available;

Solution 1: Calculate the missing data according to the standard for the classification of hospitals shown in Table 1. For example, if the number of health technicians of a third-class hospital is 550 while the number of beds is missing, the number of beds can be calculated by 550/1.03 with a result of 534.

Scenario 2: The number of beds and the number of health technicians are both missing.

Solution 2: Mean completer method is a widely used imputation method [46]. The number of beds is numerical, so the missing values are filled with the average number of beds in other hospitals of that class. For example, given that a hospital is a second-class hospital and the data of the number of beds and health technicians are both missing if the average number of beds in other second-class hospitals is 350, the number of beds in this hospital can be assigned the value 350.

Table 1. The standard for classification of hospitals.

Level	Number of Beds	Technician Number
first-class	≤ 100	0.7 * Number of beds
second-class	100–500	0.88 * Number of beds
third-class	>500	1.03 * Number of beds

* refers to a multiplication sign.

4.3. Evaluation Procedure

The evaluation procedure is composed of three steps. Firstly, the sensitivity of SPAI is assessed for the improved method. Secondly, healthcare accessibility results during different time periods are implemented. Thirdly, the crowdedness of hospitals is calculated and hospital beds shortage areas are identified.

As mentioned in Section 3, the demand for medical care among the elderly is 3–5 times that of the young in China and the high-level cities have a high prevalence ratio. As one of the biggest cities in China, the DW of Wuhan is set to 5 in this paper.

4.3.1. Sensitive Assessment

No matter the 2SFCA method or its developments, the choice of the impedance coefficient is arbitrary. Since the impedance coefficient reflects the extent to which people's willingness to travel decays over time, it should be determined based on actual surveys of healthcare utilization behavior. However, this takes a lot of manpower and capital investment, and the findings of specific case areas may not be extended to other areas, so they are not highly operational. Thus, with the lack of a sufficient basis for parameter setting of the impedance function, more comprehensive results should be provided as references through multi-scenario analysis, and sensitivity assessment should be conducted for the setting of the key parameter β.

Thirty minutes has been considered an appropriate catchment size to analyze the healthcare accessibility [15,47]. Kwan [48] suggested that value 0.01 is a critical value for the Gaussian function approaching 0. As shown in Figure 6, for travel cost (i.e., 30 min), the β value of 90 corresponds to the Gaussian value of 0.01. Therefore, the minimum value of β is set to 90 so that the Gaussian value is always greater than 0.01. The maximum value is set to 590 because the curve is relatively 'flat' at this point [49]. Six impedance coefficients, which range from 90 to 590 with an increment of 100, are used to evaluate the stability of SPAI.

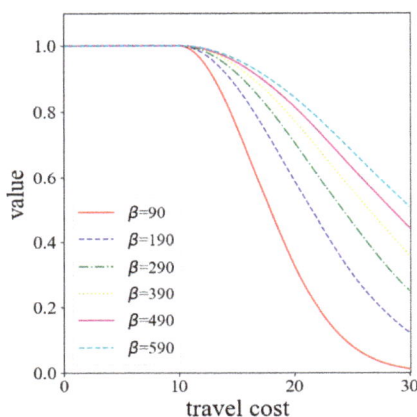

Figure 6. The revised Gaussian function with different impedance coefficients (β).

4.3.2. Healthcare Accessibility Analysis During Different Time Periods

As indicated in Section 3, it is inaccurate to evaluate travel time without considering an actual traffic situation. Comparing the accessibility during different time periods (e.g., at rush hours or at non-peak periods) helps to understand the accessibility more comprehensively as the traffic situation changes, and thus providing a basis for policy-makers to make relevant policies.

Road congestion varies during different time periods. Generally, the morning peak is from 7:00 a.m. to 9:00 a.m. and the evening peak is from 5:00 p.m. to 7:00 p.m. During rush hours, some major roads are regularly choked with traffic and the travel cost will increase dramatically. Thus, based on the traffic condition, the consulting hours of hospitals (i.e., generally from 7:00 a.m. to 6:00 p.m.) are divided into 5 time periods. These 5 time periods are 7:00 a.m. to 9:00 a.m., 9:00 a.m. to 12:00 p.m., 12:00 p.m. to 2:30 p.m., 2:30 p.m. to 5:00 p.m., and 5:00 p.m. to 6:00 p.m. respectively. By dividing consulting hours, a dynamic accessibility result is obtained. Specifically, this study mainly obtained the travel time from community to healthcare site at following 5 time points: 07:40 a.m., 10:40 a.m., 12:40 p.m., 3:20 p.m., and 5: 20 p.m. Besides, in consideration of the extent to which travel time affects people's travel choices, a strong distance impedance is utilized in this study, namely, β is set to 90.

4.3.3. Calculating the Crowdedness of Hospitals and Identifying Shortage Areas

An important goal of calculating spatial accessibility is to identify shortage areas of healthcare services and then take measures to minimize inequities. In the latest study, an inverted two-step floating catchment area (i2SFCA) method is introduced to capture the "crowdedness" (scarcity of resources or intensity of competition) for facilities [50]. The i2SFCA method is an extension of the classic Huff model. The crowdedness is a ratio of population served to supply capacity (e.g., patients per sickbed). Specifically, it is calculated as

$$C_j = V_j/S_j = \sum_{i=1}^{m} [D_i f(d_{ij}) / \sum_{l=1}^{n} (S_l f(d_{il}))] \tag{18}$$

where C_j is the demand-to-supply ratio at service site j, V_j is the total number of population attracted by site j, S_j is the capacity of site j, D_i is the population size at population location i, m and n are the number of population locations and service sites, respectively, and $f(d)$ is a generalized impedance function and its specific form utilized in this paper is the Gaussian function. A high crowdedness value means that the facility is crowded with patients. The crowdedness of hospitals in the study area is calculated based on the i2SFCA method.

According to the Norm for the Urban Public Facilities Planning (GB50442-2008), which is utilized as a guide to make urban public facilities planning more scientific, the city scale and the number of beds per thousand people are determined. Table 2 shows the relationship between population size and city scale. Table 3 is the standard of number of beds per thousand people. Since the population size of Wuhan is larger than 2 million, the number of beds per thousand people should be larger than 7. In this paper, the number of beds is used as the capacity of hospitals, and thus the actual indicator of accessibility is the number of beds available per people. Thus, 0.007 is a reasonable threshold value to identify areas where medical resources are scarce.

Table 2. The city scale standard.

City Scale	Small City	Middle City	Large City		
			I	II	III
Population Size (ten thousand)	<20	20–50	50–100	100–200	≥200

Table 3. The standard of the number of beds per thousand people.

City Size	Small City	Middle City	Large City		
			I	II	III
Number of beds per thousand people	4–5	4–5	4–6	6–7	≥7

5. Results

5.1. Results of Sensitivity Assessment

Table 4 shows the minimum, maximum, mean, standard deviation (SD), and coefficient of variation (CV) values of SPAI with different distance impedance coefficients β. CV is a statistic to measure the variation degree of each observation and calculated by the ratio of SD to mean. As shown in Table 4, the mean value remains almost unchanged while the CVs decrease sharply with the increase of β. Since the increase of β indicates the weakening of distance impedance effect, the decrease of CVs implies that a weaker distance impedance results in a lesser extent of the variance of spatial accessibility. The statistical values are further illustrated in Figure 7. With the increasing of β, the values of SPAI become more concentrated. In other words, the difference in spatial accessibility between communities is narrowed.

Table 4. The descriptive statistics of the results.

Distance Impedance Coefficient (β)	Minimum	Maximum	Mean	SD	CV
90	0.00134	0.01534	0.00811	0.00278	0.34245
190	0.00331	0.01213	0.00816	0.00172	0.21049
290	0.00431	0.01111	0.00820	0.00126	0.15365
390	0.00494	0.01059	0.00822	0.00102	0.12416
490	0.00535	0.01026	0.00823	0.00088	0.10705
590	0.00564	0.01003	0.00824	0.00079	0.09632

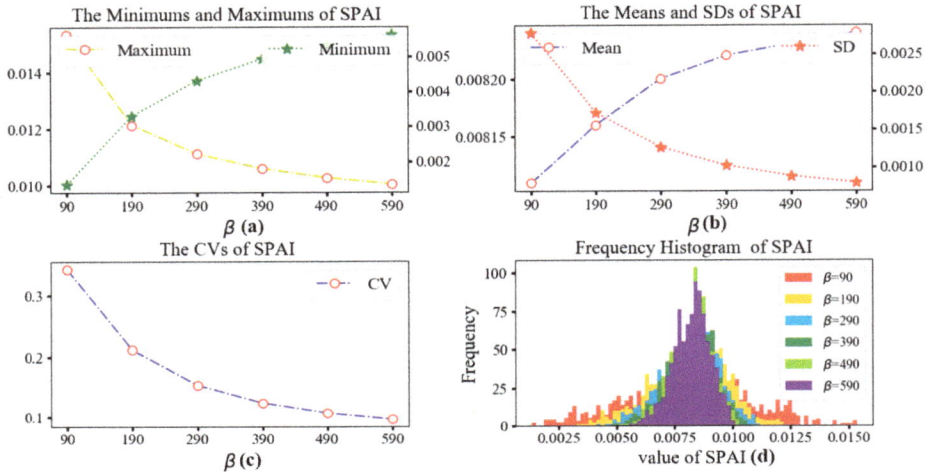

Figure 7. (**a**) The minimums and maximums of SPAI; (**b**) The means and SDs of SPAI; (**c**) The CVs of SPAI; (**d**) The frequency histogram of SPAI.

The geographic patterns of SPAI for different extents of distance impedance coefficients are shown in Figure 8. For the purpose of comparison, the values of SPAI are categorized into the same intervals (i.e., <=0.005, 0.0051–0.0065, 0.0066–0.0080, 0.0081–0.0095, 0.0096–0.0110, and >0.011). It can be observed that the geographic patterns of SPAI change significantly among the first three impedance coefficients. For example, the SPAI values of almost all communities in Luonan Street and Zhuodaoquan Street are greater than 0.011 when β is 90. However, only one community has large SPAIs (e.g., SPAI > 0.011) when β is 290. Besides, the geographic patterns of SPAI remain unchanged when β is bigger than 290. It can be concluded that a faster decay speed will lead to a greater difference in accessibility between communities. Therefore, the SPAI values of hospital adjacent areas are significantly higher than that of other regions which are away from the hospital.

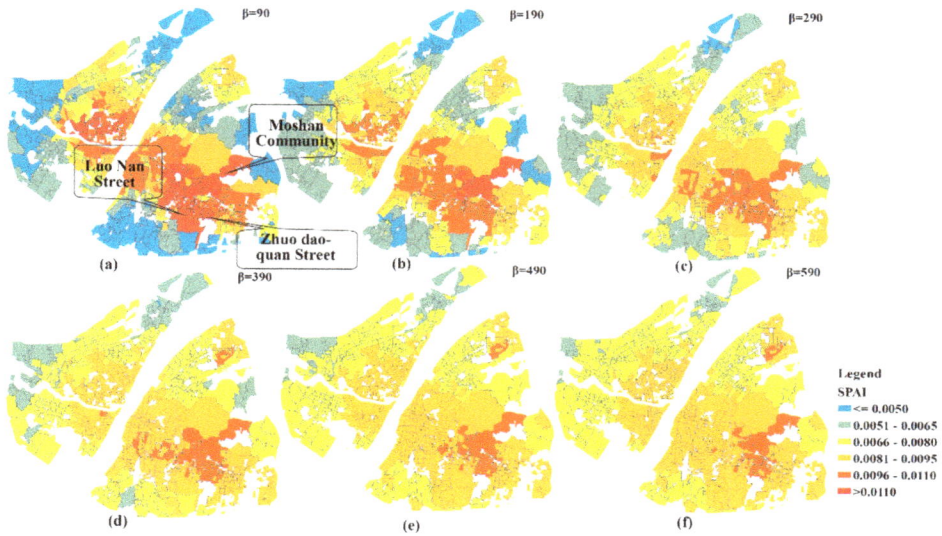

Figure 8. The geographic patterns of SPAI with different β values. (**a**) β = 90; (**b**) β = 190; (**c**) β = 290; (**d**) β = 390; (**e**) β = 490; (**f**) β = 590.

5.2. Dynamic Healthcare Accessibility Analysis

The geographic patterns of SPAI during different time periods are shown in Figure 9. During the rush hours (e.g., 07:40 and 17:20), the number of communities characterized by a large SPAIs is significantly higher than that of other times in this study. Additionally, during the flat hump period (e.g., at 12:40), almost all communities have no large SPAIs and the difference in accessibility between communities is narrowed.

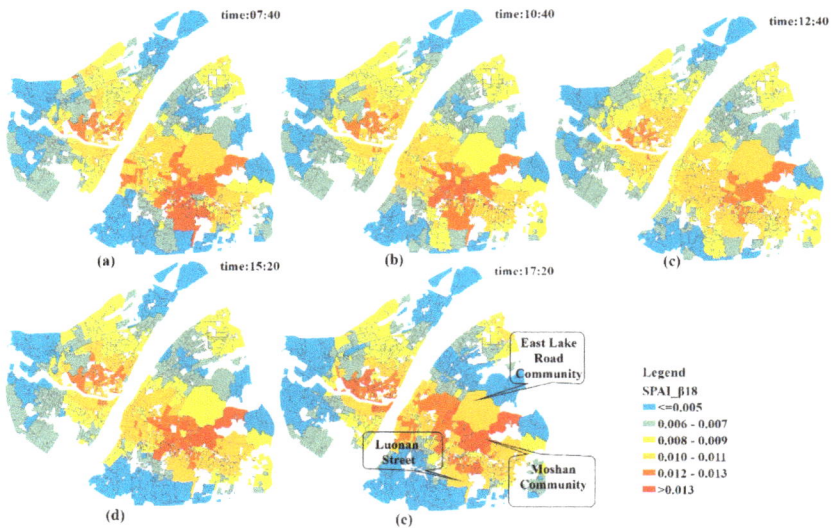

Figure 9. The geographic patterns of SPAI at different points-in-time. (**a**) 07:40; (**b**) 10:40; (**c**) 12:40; (**d**) 15:20; (**e**) 17:20.

As for the local analysis, the SPAIs of communities around the East Lake Road Community, Moshan Community and Luonan Street present the biggest change. When coupled with the information in Table 5 and Figure 10, it can be concluded that traffic congestion has significantly increased the accessibility of the communities near hospitals, and the difference in spatial accessibility to healthcare services between communities is enlarged. That is, worse traffic conditions lead to a greater distance impedance effect between hospitals and the communities far from hospitals. As a result, the competition between communities near hospitals and those relatively far away from hospitals is decreasing, and the spatial accessibility of communities near hospitals which are less affected by traffic is dramatically increasing.

Table 5. The top ten congestion road sections in rush hour provided by the Wuhan Traffic Management Bureau.

Rank	Road Name (a.m.)	Road Name (p.m.)
1	Donghu Road	Luoshi Road
2	Luoshi Road	Minzu Avenue
3	Tangxunhu North Road	Auxiliary Road of Wuluo
4	Daxueyuan Road	Daxueyuan Road
5	Auxiliary Road of Donghu	Shucheng Road
6	Wuhan Avenue	Wuluo Road
7	Minzu Avenue	Huquan Street
8	Nanhu Avenue	Guanggu Avenue
9	Jianshe No1 Road	Julong Avenue
10	Auxiliary Road of Luoshi	Jianshe No1 Road

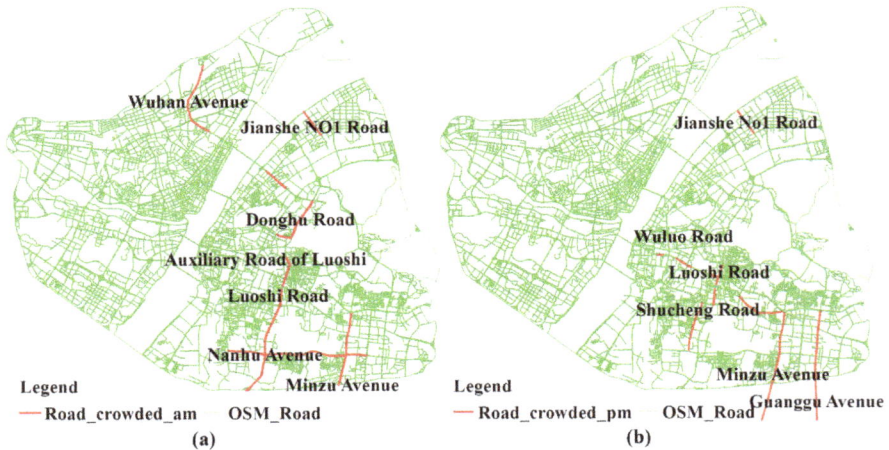

Figure 10. The congestion road sections in rush hour. (a) morning peak; (b) evening peak.

5.3. Results of Hospitals Crowdedness and Identifying Shortage Areas

The crowdedness of hospitals is shown in Figure 11. The hospitals within the Inner Ring Road or outside the Second Ring Road are less crowded while those between them are relatively more crowded. Besides, the hospitals in the Jiang'an District generally have higher crowdedness values. The high value of crowdedness indicates that hospitals are in short supply and the number of beds in these hospitals needs to increase. Additionally, the hospitals at the boundary of the Third Ring Road are less crowded. However, since the population demand of areas outside the boundary is not considered, the crowdedness values of hospitals at the boundary might be inaccurate.

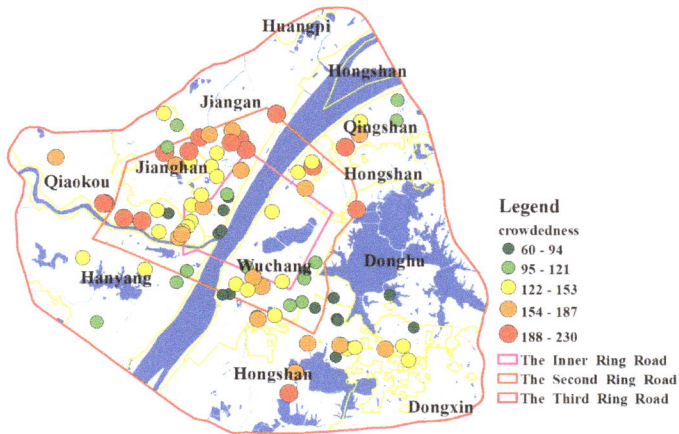

Figure 11. The crowdedness of hospitals.

A concentric geographic pattern of SPAI is shown in Figure 12. The healthcare accessibility declines as the distance to the core of the study area increases. As indicated in Section 4.3.3, the shortage areas are determined as areas whose spatial access index is smaller than 0.007. There are 330 communities that are identified as shortage areas. The demand for beds in most communities of the study area is met. Additionally, most of these shortage areas are in the suburbs, which implies that the medical infrastructure in suburban areas needs to be strengthened. The SPAIs near the boundary in the study area are not referenced because hospitals outside the boundary are not considered, which is likely to affect the calculation of supply in the catchment of population locations.

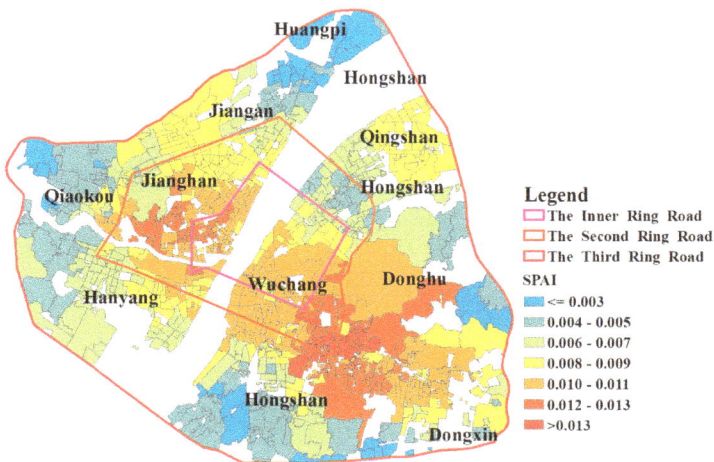

Figure 12. The geographic pattern of SPAI.

6. Discussion and Conclusions

In this paper, two important variables (travel cost and population demand) of measuring healthcare accessibility are improved. Specifically, real-time traffic information is introduced to calculate the travel time and a demand weight index is used to adjust the population demand.

By changing the distance impedance coefficient β, the sensitivity assessment of accessibility is carried out in this study. The comparison result shows that a strong distance impedance will enlarge the accessibility difference between communities. Besides, traffic congestion has significantly increased the accessibility of communities near hospitals by keeping distant communities from accessing healthcare services. As a result, the difference in spatial accessibility between communities is enlarged. Based on the i2SFCA method, the crowdedness of hospitals in the study area is calculated. The results show that hospitals within the Inner Ring Road or outside the Second Ring Road of Wuhan are less crowded while those between them are more crowded. Notably, hospitals in the Jiang'an District generally have a higher crowdedness, which implies that hospitals in this area are in short supply and the number of beds in these hospitals needs to be increased. Finally, 0.007 is used as a threshold value for designating hospital beds shortage areas and the result shows that most of these shortage areas are in the suburbs, which implies that the medical infrastructure in suburban areas needs to be strengthened.

The major advantage of this improved method compared to previous models lies in its reasonable assumptions about patient's medical seeking behavior and medical needs for medical services. With the utilization of real-time traffic, the travel time is accurately estimated. Additionally, dynamic results of healthcare accessibility are derived during different time periods, which helps to understand the accessibility more comprehensively. Using a demand weight index, the differences between the elderly and the young in the needs of medical facilities are clearly reflected and one can, therefore, better adjust the population demand.

Despite the notable advantage, several issues deserve particular attention when implementing this method in healthcare accessibility studies. First, the determination of the impedance coefficient β is somewhat arbitrary. As suggested by Huff and McCallum [51], it should be determined based on actual surveys of healthcare utilization behavior. Future researches may focus on exploring the health-seeking behavior of patients by utilizing taxi GPS trajectory data or pedestrian-based trajectory data collected by mobile phones, which will help to calibrate the impedance coefficient. Second, a fixed 30-min catchment size is utilized since the study area of this paper is the main urban area of Wuhan city, which is a relatively small area. However, if the study area is expanded to an entire city or a larger area, a variable or a dynamic catchment size is required. Third, the utilization of the AutoNavi API plays an important role when calculating travel time. Although AutoNavi proves to be a very powerful tool in the field of route planning, its calculation process remains a black box and cannot be controlled by the researchers.

In conclusion, this improved method provides a new perspective for analyzing healthcare accessibility and shows great potential in the allocation works of healthcare resources.

Author Contributions: Methodology, L.M.; Software, L.M.; Validation, L.M.; Formal Analysis, L.M.; Investigation, L.M.; Resources, M.P.; Writing-Original Draft Preparation, L.M.; Writing-Review & Editing, L.M. and T.W. and C.H.; Visualization, L.M.; Supervision, N.L.; Project Administration, N.L. and L.M.

Funding: This research was funded by National Key R&D Program of China under grant number 2017YFC1405304; The Fundamental Research Funds for Central Universities under grant number 2042017kf0224.

Conflicts of Interest: The authors declare no conflict of interest. Authors ensure that there are no personal circumstances, interest or sponsors that may be perceived as inappropriately influencing the representation or interpretation of reported research results.

References

1. Wang, F. Measurement, Optimization, and Impact of Health Care Accessibility: A Methodological Review. *Ann. Assoc. Am. Geogr.* **2012**, *102*, 1104–1112. [CrossRef] [PubMed]

2. Penchansky, R.; Thomas, J.W. The concept of access: Definition and relationship to consumer satisfaction. *Med. Care* **1981**, *19*, 127. [CrossRef] [PubMed]

3. Levesque, J.F.; Harris, M.F.; Russell, G. Patient-centred access to health care: Conceptualising access at the interface of health systems and populations. *Int. J. Equity Health* **2013**, *12*, 18. [CrossRef] [PubMed]

4. Saurman, E. Improving access: Modifying Penchansky and Thomas's Theory of Access. *J. Health Serv. Res. Policy* **2016**, *21*, 36–39. [CrossRef] [PubMed]

5. Siegel, M.; Koller, D.; Vogt, V.; Sundmacher, L. Developing a composite index of spatial accessibility across different health care sectors: A German example. *Health Policy* **2016**, *120*, 205–212. [CrossRef] [PubMed]

6. Kleinman, J.C.; Makuc, D. Travel for ambulatory medical care. *Med. Care* **1983**, *21*, 543–557. [CrossRef] [PubMed]

7. Luo, W. Using a GIS-based floating catchment method to assess areas with shortage of physicians. *Health Place* **2004**, *10*, 1–11. [CrossRef]

8. Wing, P.; Reynolds, C. The availability of physician services: A geographic analysis. *Health Serv. Res.* **1988**, *23*, 649–667. [PubMed]

9. Luo, J.; Chen, G.; Li, C.; Xia, B.; Sun, X.; Chen, S. Use of an E2SFCA Method to Measure and Analyse Spatial Accessibility to Medical Services for Elderly People in Wuhan, China. *Int. J. Environ. Res. Public Health* **2018**, *15*, 1503. [CrossRef] [PubMed]

10. Ni, J.; Wang, J.; Rui, Y.; Qian, T.; Wang, J. An Enhanced Variable Two-Step Floating Catchment Area Method for Measuring Spatial Accessibility to Residential Care Facilities in Nanjing. *Int. J. Environ. Res. Public Health* **2015**, *12*, 14490–14504. [CrossRef] [PubMed]

11. Tao, Z.L.; Cheng, Y.; Dai, T.Q.; Rosenberg, M.W. Spatial optimization of residential care facility locations in Beijing, China: Maximum equity in accessibility. *Int. J. Health Geogr.* **2014**, *13*, 33. [CrossRef] [PubMed]

12. Shrivastava, S.R.; Shrivastava, P.S.; Ramasamy, J. Health-care of Elderly: Determinants, Needs and Services. *Int. J. Prev. Med.* **2013**, *4*, 1224–1225. [PubMed]

13. Khan, A.A. An Integrated Approach to Measuring Potential Spatial Access to Health Care Services. *Socio-Econ. Plan. Sci.* **1992**, *26*, 275–287. [CrossRef]

14. Joseph, A.E.; Bantock, P.R. Measuring Potential Physical Accessibility to General Practitioners in Rural Areas: A Method and Case Study. *Soc. Sci. Med.* **1982**, *16*, 85–90. [CrossRef]

15. Luo, W.; Wang, F. Measures of Spatial Accessibility to Health Care in a GIS Environment: Synthesis and a Case Study in the Chicago Region. *Environ. Plan. B Plan. Des.* **2003**, *30*, 865–884. [CrossRef]

16. Joseph, A.E.; Phillips, D.R. *Accessibility and Utilization: Geographical Perspectives on Health Care Delivery*; Harper & Row: New York, NY, USA, 9780063182769.

17. Guagliardo, M.F. Spatial accessibility of primary care: Concepts, methods and challenges. *Int. J. Health Geogr.* **2004**, *3*, 3. [CrossRef] [PubMed]

18. Wang, F.; Luo, W. Assessing spatial and nonspatial factors for healthcare access: Towards an integrated approach to defining health professional shortage areas. *Health Place* **2005**, *11*, 131–146. [CrossRef] [PubMed]

19. Yang, D.H.; Goerge, R.; Mullner, R. Comparing GIS-based methods of measuring spatial accessibility to health services. *J. Med. Syst.* **2006**, *30*, 23. [CrossRef] [PubMed]

20. Dai, D.; Wang, F. Geographic disparities in accessibility to food stores in southwest Mississippi. *Environ. Plan. B Plan. Des.* **2011**, *38*, 659–677. [CrossRef]

21. Langford, M.; Fry, R.; Higgs, G. Measuring transit system accessibility using a modified two-step floating catchment technique. *Int. J. Geogr. Inf. Sci.* **2012**, *26*, 193–214. [CrossRef]

22. Luo, W.; Qi, Y. An enhanced two-step floating catchment area (E2SFCA) method for measuring spatial accessibility to primary care physicians. *Health Place* **2009**, *15*, 1100–1107. [CrossRef] [PubMed]

23. Mcgrail, M.R.; Humphreys, J.S. The index of rural access: An innovative integrated approach for measuring primary care access. *BMC Health Serv. Res.* **2009**, *9*, 124. [CrossRef] [PubMed]

24. Dai, D. Black residential segregation, disparities in spatial access to health care facilities, and late-stage breast cancer diagnosis in metropolitan Detroit. *Health Place* **2010**, *16*, 1038–1052. [CrossRef] [PubMed]

25. Dai, D. Racial/ethnic and socioeconomic disparities in urban green space accessibility: Where to intervene? *Landsc. Urban Plan.* **2011**, *102*, 234–244. [CrossRef]

26. Schuurman, N.; Bérubé, M.; Crooks, V.A. Measuring potential spatial access to primary health care physicians using a modified gravity model. *Can. Geogr.* **2010**, *54*, 29–45. [CrossRef]

27. Tao, Z.; Cheng, Y.; Dai, T. Measuring spatial accessibility to residential care facilities in Beijing. *Prog. Geogr.* **2014**, *33*, 616–624.

28. Wang, C.J. Function simulation and regularity of distance decay of inter-urban traffic flow in China. *Prog. Geogr.* **2009**, *28*, 690–696.

29. Wang, F.; Tang, Q. Planning toward Equal Accessibility to Services: A Quadratic Programming Approach. *Environ. Plan. B Plan. Des.* **2013**, *40*, 195–212. [CrossRef]

30. Luo, W.; Whippo, T. Variable catchment sizes for the two-step floating catchment area (2SFCA) method. *Health Place* **2012**, *18*, 789–795. [CrossRef] [PubMed]

31. Jamtsho, S.; Corner, R.; Dewan, A. Spatio-Temporal Analysis of Spatial Accessibility to Primary Health Care in Bhutan. *ISPRS Int. Geo-Inf.* **2015**, *4*, 1584–1604. [CrossRef]

32. Wan, N.; Zou, B.; Sternberg, T. A 3-step floating catchment area method for analyzing spatial access to health services. *Int. J. Geogr. Inf. Sci.* **2012**, *26*, 1073–1089. [CrossRef]

33. Huff, D.L. A Probabilistic Analysis of Shopping Center Trade Areas. *Land Econ.* **1963**, *39*, 81–90. [CrossRef]

34. Luo, J. Integrating the Huff Model and Floating Catchment Area Methods to Analyze Spatial Access to Healthcare Services. *Trans. GIS* **2014**, *18*, 436–448. [CrossRef]

35. Luo, J. Analyzing Potential Spatial Access to Primary Care Services with an Enhanced Floating Catchment Area Method. *Cartogr. Int. J. Geogr. Inf. Geovis.* **2016**, *51*, 12–24. [CrossRef]

36. Wang, L. Immigration, ethnicity, and accessibility to culturally diverse family physicians. *Health Place* **2007**, *13*, 656–671. [CrossRef] [PubMed]

37. Ingram, D.R. The concept of accessibility: A search for an operational form. *Reg. Stud.* **1971**, *5*, 101–107. [CrossRef]

38. Feng, X.S.; Wang, D.Y. Demand analysis of medical services for the elderly in China. *China Health Stat.* **1999**, *16*, 287–289.

39. Liu, G.E.; Cai, C.G.; Li, L. An empirical analysis of China's elderly medical security and medical service demand. *Econ. Res.* **2011**, *46*, 95–107.

40. Jiang, H.D.; Yan, L. Intelligent Care in China. *J. Chin. Inf.* **2013**, *16*, 48–51.

41. Groux, P.; Anchisi, S.; Szucs, T. Are Cancer Patients Willing to Travel More or Further Away for a Slightly More Efficient Therapy? *Cancer Clin. Oncol.* **2014**, *3*, 36. [CrossRef]

42. Exworthy, M.; Peckham, S. Access, Choice and Travel: Implications for Health Policy. *Soc. Policy Adm.* **2006**, *40*, 267–287. [CrossRef]

43. Liu, S.; Griffiths, S.M. From economic development to public health improvement: China faces equity challenges. *Public Health* **2011**, *125*, 669–674. [CrossRef] [PubMed]

44. Mathers, N.; Huang, Y.C. The future of general practice in China: From 'barefoot doctors' to GPs? *Br. J. Gen. Pract.* **2014**, *64*, 270–271. [CrossRef] [PubMed]

45. Wang, H.H.; Wang, J.J.; Wong, S.Y.; Wong, M.C.; Li, F.J.; Wang, P.X.; Zhou, Z.H.; Zhu, C.Y.; Griffiths, S.M.; Mercer, S.W. Epidemiology of multimorbidity in China and implications for the healthcare system: Cross-sectional survey among 162,464 community household residents in southern China. *BMC Med.* **2014**, *12*, 188. [CrossRef] [PubMed]

46. Dou, D.Y.; Zhao, Y.K. Research on data imputation based on rough sets. In Proceedings of the China Grain Computing Joint Conference, Taiyuan, China, 1 August 2007.

47. Lee, R.C. Current approaches to shortage area designation. *J. Rural Health* **1991**, *7*, 437. [PubMed]

48. Kwan, M.P. Space-Time and Integral Measures of Individual Accessibility: A Comparative Analysis Using a Point-based Framework. *Geogr. Anal.* **1998**, *30*, 191–216. [CrossRef]

49. Wan, N.; Zhan, F.B.; Zou, B.; Chow, E. A relative spatial access assessment approach for analyzing potential spatial access to colorectal cancer services in Texas. *Appl. Geogr.* **2012**, *32*, 291–299. [CrossRef]

50. Wang, F. Inverted Two-Step Floating Catchment Area Method for Measuring Facility Crowdedness. *Prof. Geogr.* **2018**, *70*, 251–260. [CrossRef]

51. Huff, D.; McCallum, B.M. Calibrating the Huff Model Using ArcGIS Business Analyst. Available online: http://www.esri.com/library/whitepapers/pdfs/calibrating-huff-model.pdf (accessed on 29 May 2018).

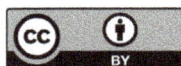

International Journal of
*Environmental Research
and Public Health*

MDPI

Article

Perceived Environmental, Individual and Social Factors of Long-Distance Collective Walking in Cities

Peng Yang [1], Shanshan Dai [1,*], Honggang Xu [1] and Peng Ju [2]

[1]   School of Tourism Management, Sun Yat-sen University, Zhuhai 519000, China;
      yangp55@mail2.sysu.edu.cn (P.Y.); xuhongg@mail.sysu.edu.cn (H.X.)
[2]   Shenzhen Tourism College, Jinan University, Shenzhen 518053, China; jupeng@sz.jnu.edu.cn
*   Correspondence: daishsh3@mail.sysu.edu.cn; Tel.: +86-135-8032-1551

Received: 11 September 2018; Accepted: 1 November 2018; Published: 4 November 2018

Abstract: Long-distance collective walking is a popular activity in cities across China. However, related research is limited, creating a research gap to explore participants' dynamic experience and related influential factors. Therapeutic mobilities theory explores the relationships among walking, health, and well-being from a qualitative perspective. Based on therapeutic mobilities theory, following a systematic process, this study develops a scale to quantitatively estimate the perceived environmental, personal, and social factors that may influence health and well-being. By applying construal level theory, this paper further hypothesizes that personality traits and familiarity moderate environmental, personal, and social perceptions. Data were collected with a paper survey (n = 926) from the "Shenzhen 100 km Walking" event. The findings highlight that long-distance collective walkers have comparatively greater experiences of health and well-being in three aspects: positive social interaction, individual development, and environmental understanding. Personality traits, familiarity, and gender moderate this well-being experience. Theoretical and managerial implications are discussed.

Keywords: well-being experience; long-distance walking; collective leisure activity; walking event; urban leisure

1. Introduction

Walking is diverse and dynamic [1]. In the past two centuries, walking has shifted from a central mode of transport to a leisure activity [2]. In recent years in China, walking has become a popular daily leisure activity for urban residents. The number of people aged 20 and older who regularly participate in "fitness walking" reached 54.6% in 2014, an increase of 12.8% compared to 2007 [3].

Previous research has investigated diverse styles of walking, including wandering, strolling, trail-walking, trekking, hiking, and hiking-walking. Organized long-distance collective walking (LDCW) is a newly developed walking event that has spread widely in Chinese cities. Previous researchers have focused on the emotional experience and health function of walking [2,4–7]. However, as long-distance collective walking is a walking event, physical health factors may not be the main concern. The impact of walking on well-being, as an emerging research direction, provides a new perspective to understand why people engage in long-distance walking [8,9].

Gatrell (2013) proposed the therapeutic mobilities theory to map the relationships between walking and well-being and health from a qualitative approach. Based on the therapeutic mobilities theory, this study develops and validates a scale to estimate the subjective health and well-being experiences of long-distance walkers. To our knowledge, this study is the first attempt to examine empirically the participants' experience within a walking event context.

By applying construal level theory [10–13], this paper investigates the factors that influence the experience. The moderating roles of adventurous personality traits, familiarity, and gender are explored. Data from the "Shenzhen 100 km Walking" event, which is a well-known LDCW activity in China, were collected and used in this empirical study. This study will provide managerial insights for walking event managers and urban planning officials to design walkable environments and target different population segments.

2. Literature Review

2.1. Walking, Experience, and Well-Being

Exploring comprehensive experiences provides a foundation for understanding complex tourism and walking activity [14–17]. Donald and Vesna (2009), through hiking and walking in Mountain Nature Park, identified three main experiences: (1) affinity with nature and the outdoors, (2) mental and physical benefits, and (3) interaction with others and development of self-knowledge [18]. Their findings are supported by various studies [19].

Specifically, Gatrell's (2013) framework for walking components serves as a foundation for structuring the relationship between walking experiences and well-being [20]. Based on his idea that movement itself can be conducive to well-being and health, and a literature review, he argued that walking contributes to well-being through three aspects: It improves physical fitness and mental health, it cements existing or develops new friendships and social interactions, and it permits an engagement with places and environments as encountered on the move. He named these three aspects the active body, the social body, and the walking context, respectively.

Engaging in physical activity, walkers may have individual physical and psychological experiences. Walking is generally acknowledged as the most common form of exercise. Regular walking of moderate to vigorous intensity is the traditional research focus in the walking field [21,22]. Regular walking is among the most effective interventions when used to promote physical activity and adherence to exercise [21]. Morgan, Tobar, and Snyder's (2010) comparative study of walkers indicated that walking can benefit both cardiovascular and psychological health [22]. Psychological benefits include improved sense of well-being, more positive (i.e., vigor) and less negative (i.e., tension, depression) feelings and mood states, and enhanced self-esteem [23,24].

Walking is inherently a social activity [25]; different types of social relations are identified as arising from the walk experience [26]. For example, many walkers share a social experience which is similar to a festival experience [27]. Walking helps to develop social connections with other people. Walking is a way "to go out to be energized by different people" [28]. In the city, walking improves the levels of social interaction and participation in neighborhood life. If the environment is perceived as safe and friendly, people are more likely to engage with others, including volunteering and attending activities in local community centers [29].

Walking also provides an opportunity to be aware of one's surroundings [20]. The environment has an important impact on walking [30]. Walking activities usually happen in specific environment settings, such as, for example, natural areas [31,32], the countryside [2]), the urban environment [5,33,34], and trails in parks [18], as well as other areas [31]. Some studies have highlighted the experience with nature, such as a wilderness experience. The wilderness experience embodies such aspects as autonomy, spontaneity, solitude, freedom of action, challenge, risk, spiritual values, and aesthetic appreciation [35,36]. Other studies have explored the effective potential of walking in the full range of typically encountered non-natural built settings, specifically, urban settings. Bornioli, Parkhurst, and Morgan (2018) showed that walking in high-quality urban settings can have positive outcomes. However, the walking environment of LDCW is complicated and includes not only urban and rural areas, but also natural areas.

Consumers' feelings affect their quality of life [37] and the environment critically influences the health and well-being of a city's inhabitants [38]. Recent studies have explicitly linked walking and well-being [9,20,28,39,40]. Morgan, Tobar, and Snyder's (2010) research indicated that continuous walking positively influenced a number of variables that are indicators of physical and psychological well-being [22]. Doughty's (2013) ethnographic study investigated the social dynamics of embodied movement in a walking group and found therapeutic outcomes [39]. Furthermore, because the act of walking includes interaction with the physical landscape and social surroundings (whether intended or unintended), studies have encouraged the mobilization of the "therapeutic landscapes" concept to better grasp the interconnections of walking, well-being, and place [20,39]. Walking is a kind of therapeutic mobility step to well-being.

2.2. Long-Distance Collective Walking

Few studies have explored the experience of long-distance walkers [14,15]. Long-distance walking refers to either single-day walks of 20 mi (about 32.2 km) or more or multi-day walks that typically follow designated long-distance footpaths [1].These activities have the following features: recreational and long-distance walking in multiple environments including urban and natural environments, organized by volunteers or non-governmental organizations (NGOs), and generally in small groups but with overall numbers reaching more than 10,000. The meaning of long-distance walking goes far beyond the physical and psychological. The long-distance route transforms recreational walking into a multi-day holiday.

Related research has highlighted the happiness experience, such as enjoyment and engagement [14–16]. Seven experience items have been identified, including enjoy meeting fellow walkers, experience of solitude, experience of freedom, having time to think and relax, enjoy the scenery, and feeling closeness with nature [14]. Rather than decreasing in intensity, the enjoyment of long-distance walking finishes on an upward trend. Saunders, Laing, and Weiler (2013) interviewed 25 long-distance walkers reporting personally significant experiences on multi-day hikes, suggesting increased self-confidence and other enduring changes which enhance well-being [41]. Crust, Keegan, Piggott, and Swann (2011) aimed to understand walkers' positive psychological movement from three aspects: life of enjoyment, life of engagement, and life of affiliation. This study was conducted in a natural space away from the urban environment [15]. Based on his investigation with six long-distance walkers, the essence of long-distance walking is described as a "journey of self-discovery" that occurs within a world detached from the stresses of modern life. Compared to regular walking or a sport event, long-distance walking might come with higher intensity and greater mental challenge and result in a flow experience and engagement.

While researchers have found that social interaction is a vital and enjoyable aspect of shared experience [15], the social interaction of long-distance collective walkers has not been fully discussed. In the Western context, many walkers walk alone. Walking is often regarded as an individual activity and demonstrates its effectiveness as a physical and psychological treatment activity [21,22,32,42,43]. Some studies have examined solitary walkers [32,42–44] or small group walking practices [45]. Some walkers prefer to enjoy an individual solitary experience. For them, the walking environment just provides a bubble for a "journey of self-discovery" [15]. Wylie (2005) added that walking alone allowed "a close visual, tactile, and sonorous relationship with the earth, the ground, mud, stinging vegetation" [43]. Since collective walking is a particular walking style, walking group studies have thus far shown evidence that group walks provide an excellent milieu in which social networks can be generated and strengthened [46]. Outdoor group walks also have the potential to be a useful health intervention as they increase physical activity and are cost effective [47]. Walking provides opportunities for stimulation, restoration, contemplation [40], and in the case of collective walks, a sense of pleasure from the shared experience [48]. Furthermore, in the Eastern context, people may prefer walking in a group because the collective preference may be more important; this will be tested in our study.

Research has documented the different kinds of walking experiences in different contexts. A substantial body of research on walking exists and there are many types of walking and many areas and environmental conditions in which walking is, or can be, performed. Among these studies, relatively few have focused specifically on walking as a collective activity. At the present time, no single theory seems capable of explaining the experience of LDCW and the links between the walkers' experience and their well-being. Thus, the argument goes that it is not so much the inherent and perceived properties of walking that matter, but rather the experiences walkers get from LDCW in the Eastern context and how the experiences contribute to the walkers' well-being.

Gartrell's therapeutic mobilities theory has been extensively employed in exploring casual walkers' experience. Therapeutic mobilities theory maps the relations between walking and well-being and health using a qualitative approach. The core of the theory is that walking is therapeutic in the active body, social body, and walking context [20]. These three aspects shape the characteristics of walking. The number of participants in long-distance collective walking events is relatively high. Empirically estimating LDCW participants' experience may provide an opportunity to understand why LDCW is popular. On the basis of Gartrell's theoretical framework, walking is therapeutic in that the active body provides a physical and emotional aspect experience, walking is therapeutic in that the social body provides a social experience, and the walking context provides an environmental experience. Thus, we propose the following hypothesis.

Hypothesis 1 (H1) *The experience of long-distance collective walkers includes three aspect of well-being experiences: physical and emotional experience, social experience, and environmental experience.*

2.3. The Moderating Effect of Personal Traits and Familiarity Based on Construal Level Theory

Construal level theory is a social psychology theory that describes how the context, such as the psychological distance, shapes mental representations [10–12]. Researchers have shown that different dimensions of psychological distance affect mental construals [49]. According to the theory, peoples' temporal perspectives influence how they evaluate an event [11] and therefore might affect their experience. An individual will likely view a far-distant event in abstract terms, consider general issues, and describe the event using dream-like words. In contrast, a near-distant event is viewed in more concrete terms and in greater detail, with more practical issues being considered [13].

Construal level theory is powerful in explaining consumer behavior and perception. However, it has received limited attention in walking and well-being research. Walking participants are heterogeneous, and different walkers have different experiences [1]. Within the context of LDCW, participants' sensation-seeking personality and familiarity with LDCW represent their psychological distance [50].

Personality traits determine the tendency to seek various experiences and sensations and the willingness to obtain stimulation [51]. Personality may influence destination choices, leisure activities, and other travel-related decisions [52]. Based on construal level theory, people's psychological experience of something is egocentric, specifically influenced by the level of mental construal. This egocentric mental construal is characterized by personality traits in this study. In the specific case of long-distance walking, which is a kind of adventure activity, participants with adventure-seeking tendencies may seek novel, varying, and stimulating experiences. Adventure-seeking is an often recognized and studied sub-dimension of personality traits [53]. Accordingly, we propose the following hypothesis.

Hypothesis 2 (H2) *In the context of LDCW, walkers with higher adventure-seeking tendencies have more well-being experiences.*

Hypothesis 3 (H3) *In the context of LDCW, walkers with higher adventure-seeking tendencies have more environmental experiences.*

Hypothesis 4 (H4) *In the context of LDCW, walkers with higher adventure-seeking tendencies have stronger individual experiences.*

Hypothesis 5 (H5) *In the context of LDCW, walkers with higher adventure-seeking tendencies have stronger social experiences.*

Well-being effects derived from a walking environment may depend on personal characteristics such as age, gender, and physical condition [40]. Social factors or socio-demographic attributes are significant covariates of urban residents' mental health [54]; thus, gender is another factor that may moderate the LDCW well-being experience. Because of their longstanding social roles and social identities, men and women have different physical activity behaviors [55,56]. Overall, women spend considerably more time walking than men [57] and more women than men walk for errands and leisure, in line with a general trend for women to devote more time and make more trips than men to serve their household [58]. The level of physical activity also differs by gender, with women being less active than men [59]. In addition, men often outperform women in physical activities, but women's emotional and psychological experiences in leisure activities are more intense. Women tend to be more sensitive to their environment [60]. Within the LDCW context, we propose the following hypothesis.

Hypothesis 6 (H6) *In the context of LDCW, walkers' gender affects the experiences of well-being.*

Hypothesis 7 (H7) *In the context of LDCW, female walkers have stronger environmental experiences.*

Hypothesis 8 (H8) *In the context of LDCW, female walkers havefewer individual experiences.*

Hypothesis 9 (H9) *In the context of LDCW, female walkers have fewer social experiences.*

Construal level theory also points out that psychological experience is determined by time, space, and social and hypothetical distance [13]. When people have high familiarity with a particular activity, the time distance between them is shorter, the space distance is closer, and the social distance is closer. As to LDCW, some researchers have pointed out that walking in unfamiliar environments may result in negative emotional experiences, such as feelings of solitude [61], fear [32], depression, tension, isolation, or being confined [31], and the familiarity that walkers have with the environment and activity has an impact on their experience. Familiarity in a commercial sense usually refers to the cumulative number of times a consumer experiences a product and is related to the number of times consumers use the product [62,63]. Accordingly, we propose the following hypothesis:

Hypothesis 10 (H10) *Walkers' familiarity with LDCW moderates their well-being experiences.*

Hypothesis 11 (H11) *Walkers who have higher familiarity with LDCW have lower environmental experiences.*

Hypothesis 12 (H12) *Walkers who have higher familiarity with LDCW have higher individual experiences.*

Hypothesis 13 (H13) *Walkers who have higher familiarity with LDCW havefewer social experiences.*

3. Method

3.1. Shenzhen 100 km Walking

The "Shenzhen 100 km Walking" event is held by MoFang Forum, a famous outdoor network platform in China. The "Shenzhen 100 km Walking" event is one of the most representative of many large-scale walking events in China and was one of the first walking events in China. The first event was held in 2001, and Jin (2012) pointed out that from the beginning of 1998, walking events only emerged in Beijing, Guangzhou, Kunming, Shanghai, and other large cities, and various walking events organized by governments only began to emerge on a large scale after 2005 [64]. The "Shenzhen 100 km Walking" event has been held 16 times, and it has a broad social impact. The number of participants in the first session was 52, and in 2016, the number of participators formally signed up was 60,723; the actual number of participators was more than 100,000. The walking trajectory of the 2016 event is shown in Figure 1. The walking trajectory is along the southern border of Shenzhen.

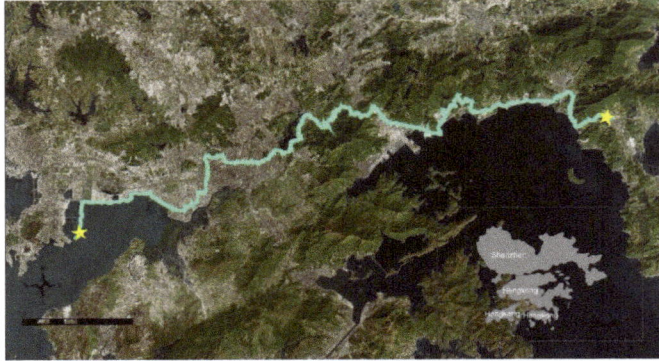

Figure 1. The walking trajectory of the 2016 "Shenzhen 100 km Walking" event.

First, the "Shenzhen 100 km Walking" is a non-competitive long-distance walking event in which participants walk about 100 km within one day, with the hiking routes set up by organizers within the multiple environments of Shenzhen city. The typical walking environments are shown in Figure 2. Not everyone is required to complete the whole 100 km; the organizers believe that participants should choose the distance to walk based on their own abilities. Most of the participants are hiking enthusiasts and some just want to feel the atmosphere of the event. Organizers have stressed that participants enjoy the event as it eases the pressures of life and promotes a healthy and environmentally friendly way of life.

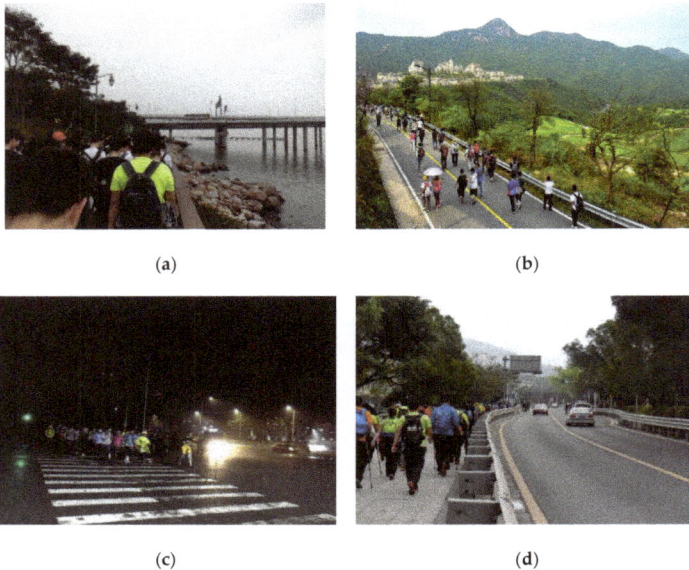

(a)

(b)

(c)

(d)

Figure 2. The typical walking environment of the 2016 "Shenzhen 100 km Walking" event [65]: (a): Ocean Bay; (b): mountain area; (c): urban area (walking in the night); (d): rural area.

Second, it is a collective activity. It is a large event initiated by tour pals (travel enthusiasts) [66] in the network platform MoFang. MoFang users themselves set up the organizing committee, organize activities, and organize this event. Formal participants need to join a team of 5–6 people to complete the registration, and many informal participants join the walking teams during the event. The participants are not only citizens of Shenzhen, but people from all parts of China. Some media have called it a "folk organization's walking event [67]."

Third, it is a meaningful human mobility event. Each session of the "100 km" event has a clear theme. For example, the first session is themed "Feet Measured Shenzhen," the thirteenth session is themed "Walk without Leaving a Trace," and the sixteenth session is themed "Let's Go," which reflects the cultural theme of these outdoor activities and the main form of this event, which is a kind of human mobility. This event has become a "very influential business card of Shenzhen" [68] and has even "become a side of the cultural banner of Shenzhen" [69].

3.2. Questionnaire Development

As the development and validation of a questionnaire require a systematic process [70] and no established measurements existed for a walking event, measures for the experience and relevance of an LDCW were developed specifically for this study.

Rigorous procedures for scale development were followed [71,72]. The first step was specifying the construct domain of the "LDCW experience." In this stage, a focus group consisting of three experts and two PhD students majoring in leisure and event research was established to discuss and define the characteristics of a walking experience. Discussions combined with an extensive literature review helped us identify the physical aspect, emotional aspect, environmental aspect, and social aspect as four dimensions of a walking experience. After the construct domains were specified, both deductive and inductive approaches were used to generate an item pool to measure each dimension [73]. Four dimensions relating to the walking experience were collected and adapted from the literature to generate the initial items. This process resulted in the identification of 16 items: 3 in physical activity aspects, 6 in emotional aspects, 5 in environmental aspects, and 2 in social aspects.

Thereafter, semi-structured interviews with people who had participated in related activities were carried out. Based on the participants' descriptions of their LDCW experiences, corresponding items were added or dropped in the questionnaire. Specifically, two items were added and two were dropped in emotional aspects, four items were added and two dropped in the environmental aspect, and two of the environmental aspects were divided into four items. Interviewees were also invited to assess the content validity of these items, asked to provide comments on the content and understandability of the items, and asked to edit and improve the items to enhance their clarity and readability.

To test the hypothesis that personality traits and familiarity affect the experience, the questionnaire also included adventure-seeking scales to measure participants' self-cognitive assessments of personality characteristics. Adventure-seeking scales had two items (I like to do frightening things, and I would like to try bungee jumping) [74]. These two items were revised to I like outdoor activities", according to a revised Chinese version developed by Chen et al. [53]. The second item was having adventures always makes me happy. Within the LDCW context, we used two questions to evaluate personality traits: I am a person who likes to participate in outdoor activities and I am a person who likes to challenge myself.

The participants' familiarity with walking events was assessed by this question: "Have you enrolled in the event in advance?" As the route of a long-distance walking event changes every year, familiarity in the context of LDCW is defined by whether the participant has engaged in pre-trip planning [75]. In LDCW, not all participants are required to enroll in advance, but if the participants do enroll in advance, they need to be involved more in pre-walk planning, such as becoming familiar with the route, the check-in point, and the event theme.

The specific items are shown in Table 1. The initial set of 19 items was developed, and 5-point Likert scales ranging from 1 (strongly disagree) to 3 (neither agree nor disagree) to 5 (strongly agree) were used.

Table 1. Walking experience scales.

Construct and Items	Sources
Physical and Emotional aspects	
bring health and fitness	[22]
to achieve a reflexive awareness of the self	[2]
overcoming physical challenge	[15]
get psychological benefits	[15]
overcoming psychological challenge	[15]
get a new vision of life	interview
embrace trade-offs and compromise	interview
gain achievement	[76]
stress release	[14,18]
Environmental aspects	
get to know new places	[76]
feeling a closeness with nature	[14]
enjoy beautiful scenery	[14,76]
experience city culture	interview
to understand city condition	interview
perceived meaning of environmental protection	interview
Social aspects	
get help from volunteer	[18]
support within the team member	[18]
encouragement among participants	[14,76]
interaction with others/huts	[18]

3.3. Pilot Study

After the content adequacy and validity were ensured, an initial questionnaire was designed and a small-scale pretest was conducted. The purpose of the pilot study was to determine whether our planned measures for the variables were meaningful to the respondents. The test was conducted on a group of participants (n = 105) who had attended the "2015 Shenzhen 100 km Walking" event and who were recruited through an online survey by snowball sampling. The participants were asked to rate the validated set of items.

This step was to explore the structure of the meaning of the experience and to test the concurrent validity. An exploratory factor analysis (EFA) was conducted using the data from the pretest, and the results are presented in Table 2. Before performing the EFA, the appropriateness of the 105 responses was examined. The normality was judged by estimating the skewness and kurtosis of each item. The slightly non-normal distribution is not likely to influence the final results [77].

Principal component analysis with varimax rotation was used for the exploratory analysis, and the structure was determined by the rotated component matrix. The number of factors was identified using the eigenvalue greater than 1.0 criterion [78]. The eigenvalue indicated that three common factors reflect the data characteristics well. Physical experience and emotional experience merged into one factor, and further reduction of items was performed. Items with high cross-loadings (>0.5) and low factor loadings (<0.5) were deleted one at a time to ensure accuracy. After each deletion, the Kaiser-Meyer-Olkin (KMO) value and commonalities were re-examined. After no item failed to meet the criteria, there were 16 measurement variables which were entered in the factor analysis (Table 2). In this step, three items were excluded: "bring health and fitness," "stress release," and "embrace trade-offs and compromise." The internal validity was assessed. The KMO value was 0.858, which was close to 1, indicating sampling adequacy, and Bartlett's test of sphericity was 965.578 (df = 120, p = 0.00 < 0.05), supporting the factorability of the data. Three factors explained 66.188% of the total variance (>cutoff value 60%). Cronbach's alpha values ranged from 0.843 to 0.878 (>0.80), and the reliability of the questionnaire scale was established.

Table 2. Exploratory factor analysis for walking event participants.

Factor	Skewness	Kurtosis	MV(SD)	Factor Loading	Cronbach's α
Environmental experience				25.196% [a]	0.878
3.4 experience city culture of Shenzhen	−1.136	1.698	4.17 (0.884)	0.861	
3.6 perceived meaning of environmental protection	−1.292	1.542	4.18 (0.829)	0.832	
3.2 enjoy beautiful scenery	−0.676	0.031	3.98 (0.98)	0.754	
3.3 feeling a closeness with nature	−0.882	0.901	4.09 (1.05)	0.718	
3.5 to understand city condition of Shenzhen	−0.363	−0.6	3.9 (0.954)	0.71	
3.1 get to know new places	−1.589	2.369	4.26 (1.016)	0.512	
Activity experience				20.672% [a]	0.843
2.3 overcoming psychological challenge	−1.351	1.947	4.38 (0.823)	0.844	
1.3 overcoming physical Challenge	−1.704	2.296	4.5 (0.82)	0.803	
2.1 get psychological benefits	−1.053	0.53	4.45 (0.7)	0.699	
1.2 to achieve a reflexive awareness of the self	−0.668	−0.734	4.2 (0.883)	0.602	
2.2 get a new vision of life	−0.952	−0.071	4.57 (0.572)	0.594	
2.4 gain achievement	−0.597	−0.884	4.17 (0.895)	0.564	
Social interaction experience				20.32% [a]	0.869
4.3 encouragement among participants	−1.691	2.345	4.61 (0.663)	0.921	
4.2 support within the team member	−1.801	2.529	4.63 (0.674)	0.873	
4.4 interaction with others/huts	−1.287	0.324	4.56 (0.684)	0.789	
4.1 get help from volunteer	−1.692	1.978	4.57 (0.753)	0.706	
Cumulative validity				66.188% [a]	

[a] Denotes for variance contribution rate.

The pilot study showed three factors of the LDCW experience. Factor 1 involved items measuring environmental experiences (three items). The experience dimension is the most important factor (variance contribution rate is 25.196%). Factor 2 focused on the five items measuring individual experience, emphasis on physical cognition, and perceptions of positive mental experiences. The variance contribution rate of Factor 2 was 20.672%. Factor 3 contained the four items measuring the social interaction experience (Table 2).

3.4. Investigation Procedure

After discussing and resolving any discrepancies, the survey was considered to be appropriate for data collection. Formal research was conducted on 20 March 2016, during the "Shenzhen 100 km Walking" event, and 22 research assistants were sent to collect the questionnaires from the participants. As some participants might choose to withdraw halfway through, we chose two points, at the middle (Dongbei) and the end (Dapeng square) of the walking route to collect the data. Hard-copy questionnaires were used. Questionnaires were distributed face-to-face. A total of 1000 questionnaires was distributed with 926 valid questionnaires recovered, for a recovery rate of 92.6%; 328 valid questionnaires were collected in Dongbei and 598 valid questionnaires in Dapeng square.

4. Results

4.1. Respondents' Profiles

To gain a preliminary understanding of the respondents, descriptive statistics were gathered, and the results are presented in Table 3. The profiles of the respondents showed that most walking event participants in this study were well educated (e.g., bachelor's degree and above, 54.0%), young (under 35, 76.0%), and male (72.3%). This group of people also reflected the typical characteristics of the new generation in China which has a good education and the wealth to seek new experiences to complement and fit into their busy daily routines [23].

Table 3. The demographic characteristics of the respondents.

Items	Sample Size	Proportion (%)
Gender		
Male	666	72.3
Female	255	27.7
Age		
26 and under	324	34.0
27–35	393	42.5
36–45	141	15.2
46–59	61	6.6
60 and above	6	0.6
Education		
Primary school and below	8	0.9
Junior middle school	26	2.8
High school	128	12.8
Training school	263	28.4
Bachelor degree and above	500	54.0
Occupation		
Government/institution	68	7.4
State-owned enterprise	130	14.1
Private enterprise	497	53.8
Self-employed person	46	5.0
Student	55	6.0
Retired	5	0.5
Agriculture	5	0.5
Other	118	12.8

4.2. Model Evaluation and Scale Reliability

Confirmatory factor analysis (CFA) was used to verify factorial structures and items identified from the EFA. Before conducting the CFA, the data were screened to see if they violated multivariate normality by Holling's T test [77]. Confirmatory factor analysis was conducted with the software AMOS 21.0, and the measurement properties of the 16-item scale were assessed by examining the overall model fit.

First, the overall model fit was evaluated. The goodness-of-fit indices include the overall fit index $\chi 2(101) = 224.083$, absolute goodness-of-fit index (GFI) = 0.923, value-added goodness-of-fit index (AGFI) = 0.889, normed fit index (NFI) = 0.910, comparative fit index (CFI) = 0.971, and incremental fit index (IFI) = 0.923, all of which were higher than the cutoff value 0.9; the root mean square error of approximation (RMSEA) = 0.075 was less than the ideal value of 0.1 [79]. The overall model fit indicated that the model fit the data adequately.

Subsequently, we assessed the reliability and validity of the identified scale. The standardized factor loadings of all factors were higher than 0.6, with the Cronbach's α coefficients and combination reliability (CR) value of each factor being greater than 0.8 and average variance extracted (AVE) values higher than or close to 0.5 [79], indicating acceptable internal consistency. The final results are presented in Table 4. Discriminant validity is confirmed when the square root of the AVE exceeds the inter-correlations of the construct with other constructs in the measurement model [80]. Discriminant validity is assessed by the confidence interval test, which involves calculating the 95% confidence interval around the correlation between the factors. If the 95% confidence interval is not higher than the square root of the AVE, discriminant validity is demonstrated. The results of each pair of dimensions in this study are shown in Table 4. Discriminant validity for these constructs is supported. The assessment of the measurement model supported the reliability and validity.

Table 4. Discriminant validity test of constructs (95% confidence interval of correlates).

	Environmental		Activity	
	Lower Bound	Upper Bound	Lower Bound	Upper Bound
Activity	0.452	0.559		
Social	0.402	0.522	0.333	0.467

4.3. Experience of LDCW

The CFA results are reported in Table 5. The experience of long-distance collective walkers includes three aspects of the well-being experiences: physical and emotional experience, social experience, and environmental experience. Tests of Hypothesis 1 showed that compared to individual or small-group walking activities, long-distance outdoor walkers had more intense experiences [5,14,81]. In particular, the social interaction experience was the strongest (mean = 4.502, SD = 0.594), and the standard deviation was minimal. Following was the individual experience (mean = 4.237; SD = 0.637). The environmental experience was the lowest, but still relatively high (mean = 3.990; SD = 0.689). A paired sample T-test was used to assess statistical differences between the three scales [82]. The results suggest that the mean value of the social experience is significantly higher than the mean value of the environmental experience ($t = 7.162$, $p < 0.01$), and the mean value of the social experience is significantly higher than the mean value of the individual experience ($t = 6.667$, $p < 0.01$). There is no significant difference between the mean value of the environmental experience and the mean value of the individual experience.

Compared to general walking activities, the empirical data from the LDCW participants show a highly positive experience in social relationships. Walking is useful in helping develop social interaction, producing additional social capital through pleasant conversation with people, walking with dogs [20], meeting fellow walkers [14], and interacting with others [18]. In comparison, in competitive events such as marathons, social interaction generally only manifests between teammates [83]. LDCW participants gain support from group members, volunteers, and other participants, and the social interactions among them are more profound. In the "Shenzhen 100 km Walking" event, the participants are organized in small teams during the whole process, and the participants feel the support and encouragement from their teammates. Some participants do not participate in a team, but interact with walkers through greeting and encouraging them, sharing supplies, or supporting the volunteers and, thus, the walking event provides a social space. Participants escape from their daily environments and gain a rare social experience with friends, colleagues, and strangers just by walking. During the interviews, participants stated things like: "In the city, we usually work like a stranger, but this activity involves everyone, whether the walkers, volunteers or people around, we all seemed more cordial" and "The opportunity was provided by our company, there is little chance for colleagues to walk together like this and talk about all kinds of topics while walking."

The second experience dimension is the individual experience. Previous studies have shown that walking generally improves physical fitness and mental health [20,84,85]. People who participate in LDCW events are more likely to challenge their physical and mental limits and achieve a sense of accomplishment, resulting in positive emotions. Furthermore, daily walking and professional events emphasize the physical experience [22], while long-distance walking emphasizes the spiritual experience [5,14]. Our study has reached similar conclusions.

Walking also provides an opportunity for walkers to engage with the environment. Environment "walkability" is a key concept influencing the feelings of well-being that arise from walking [20]. For individual long-distance walkers, the walking environment provides a bubble for a "journey of self-discovery" [15]. In LDCW events, people are not just concerned about environmental walkability, and the connections with multiple environments provide a meaningful environmental experience for participants, including the intrinsic value of both city life [1,86] and rural nature [2]. People move through the walking environment to deepen their understanding of the living environment, think about the meaning of walking in the city they live in, and thereby achieve a sense of well-being.

Table 5. Confirmatory factor analysis for walking event participants.

Factor	MV (SD)	Factor Loading	Std. Factor Loading	CR	Average Extracted Variance
Environmental experience	3.99 (0.69)		0.870 [b]	0.871	0.530
3.4 experience city culture of Shenzhen	3.98 (0.925)	0.781	0.798		
3.3 feeling a closeness with nature	3.96 (0.886)	0.772	0.755		
3.5 to understand city condition of Shenzhen	3.92 (0.903)	0.754	0.741		
3.2 enjoy beautiful scenery	4.05 (0.856)	0.704	0.670		
3.1 get to know new places	3.84 (0.891)	0.683	0.681		
3.6 perceived meaning of environmental protection	4.19 (0.862)	0.672	0.717		
Individual experience	4.23 (0.68)		0.843 [b]	0.847	0.480
2.3 overcoming psychological challenge	4.26 (0.879)	0.821	0.761		
1.3 overcoming physical Challenge	4.38 (0.846)	0.775	0.674		
2.1 get psychological benefits	4.35 (0.787)	0.728	0.756		
2.4 gain achievement	4.09 (0.951)	0.661	0.628		
1.2 to achieve a reflexive awareness of the self	4.27 (0.800)	0.598	0.621		
2.2 get a new vision of life	4.08 (0.855)	0.593	0.706		
Social interaction experience	4.50 (0.60)		0.855 [b]	0.858	0.603
4.3 encouragement among participants	4.54 (0.708)	0.832	0.842		
4.2 support within the team member	4.46 (0.740)	0.808	0.815		
4.4 interaction with others/huts	4.51 (0.690)	0.784	0.764		
4.1 get help from volunteer	4.50 (0.716)	0.712	0.676		

CR: Composite Reliability; Factor loadings of items on factors to which they belong; [b] Cronbach alpha.

4.4. The Moderating Effect of Personality Traits and Familiarity

The third objective of the study was to test the moderating effect of personality traits and familiarity. The participants were categorized into two types: highly adventurous and less adventurous. Participants agreed that both enjoying outdoor activities and self-challenges are defined as highly adventurous. In terms of familiarity, the participants were clustered into two types: high familiarity and low familiarity. The high familiarity participants were defined by whether they had enrolled for the LDCW in advance.

To examine whether personality traits and familiarity influenced the LDCW experience, multivariable analysis of variance (MANOVA) was used [87]. Tables 6 and 7 show the summary of the multivariate and univariate results. MANOVA results suggest that the main effects of all three moderators on the three experiential dimensions are significant ($F = 22.435$, $p < 0.01$; $F = 3.736$, $p < 0.01$; $F = 2.250$, $p < 0.05$). The interaction effect of familiarity and gender on experience is significant ($F = 2.538$, $p < 0.01$). This partly supports Hypotheses 2–4.

Table 6. MANOVA results for experience differences under the influence of personal traits and familiarity.

Dependent Variable	Source	Type III Sum of Squares	df	Mean Square	F	Sig.
	adventurous		3		22.435	0.000
	Familiarity		6		3.736	0.001
	Gender		9		2.250	0.017
Multivariate Statistics	adventurous * Familiarity		3		0.385	0.764
	adventurous * Gender		3		0.234	0.872
	Familiarity * Gender		3		2.538	0.055
	adventurous * Familiarity * Gender		3		0.220	0.882
Univariate Statistics						
	Model	14,023.821 [a]	11	1274.893	2926.739	0.000
	adventurous	16.023	1	16.023	36.785	0.000
	Familiarity	7.145	2	3.572	8.201	0.000
Environmental	Gender	6.052	3	2.017	4.631	0.003
experience	adventurous * Familiarity	0.000	1	0.000	0.001	0.978
	adventurous * Gender	0.059	1	0.059	0.137	0.712
	Familiarity * Gender	1.958	1	1.958	4.494	0.034
	adventurous * Familiarity * Gender	0.008	1	0.008	0.019	0.890
	Model	15,879.146 [b]	11	1443.559	3935.115	0.000
	adventurous	19.214	1	19.214	52.376	0.000
	Familiarity	0.618	2	0.309	0.843	0.431
Individual experience	Gender	0.965	3	0.322	0.877	0.453
	adventurous * Familiarity	0.158	1	0.158	0.430	0.512
	adventurous * Gender	0.049	1	0.049	0.134	0.714
	Familiarity * Gender	0.534	1	0.534	1.455	0.228
	adventurous * Familiarity * Gender	0.073	1	0.073	0.199	0.656
	Model	17,894.661 [c]	11	1626.787	5058.896	0.000
	adventurous	12.403	1	12.403	38.569	0.000
	Familiarity	1.558	2	0.779	2.423	0.089
Social interaction	Gender	3.858	3	1.286	3.999	0.008
experience	adventurous* Familiarity	0.201	1	0.201	0.625	0.430
	adventurous * Gender	0.030	1	0.030	0.094	0.759
	Familiarity * Gender	2.098	1	2.098	6.525	0.010
	adventurous * Familiarity * Gender	0.051	1	0.051	0.158	0.691

[a]. R Squared = 0.974 (Adjusted R Squared = 0.973); [b]. R Squared = 0.980 (Adjusted R Squared = 0.980); [c]. R Squared = 0.985 (Adjusted R Squared = 0.984)

Table 7. MANOVA summary statistics.

	Higher Familiarity				Lower Familiarity			
	Male		Female		Male		Female	
Environmental experience	3.925	(0.702)	3.998	(0.685)	4.024	(0.654)	4.358	(0.566)
higher adventurous	4.134	(0.728)	4.205	(0.671)	4.256	(0.630)	4.565	(0.596)
lower adventurous	3.760	(0.635)	3.861	(0.662)	3.861	(0.625)	4.232	(0.515)
Individual experience	4.242	(0.648)	4.246	(0.640)	4.205	(0.612)	4.328	(0.606)
higher adventurous	4.486	(0.588)	4.505	(0.555)	4.382	(0.514)	4.580	(0.495)
lower adventurous	4.050	(0.628)	4.075	(0.637)	4.081	(0.647)	4.175	(0.621)
Social interaction experience	4.497	(0.609)	4.507	(0.595)	4.444	(0.581)	4.721	(0.377)
higher adventurous	4.677	(0.552)	4.738	(0.428)	4.599	(0.466)	4.891	(0.224)
lower adventurous	4.355	(0.615)	4.354	(0.641)	4.336	(0.630)	4.618	(0.414)

Standard deviations are shown within parentheses.

Environmental experience. A univariate analysis indicated that all three factors had significant effects on the environmental experience. The F values are 36.785, 8.201, and 4.631, respectively, for the factors of adventurous, familiarity, and gender, and the p-values are all lower than 0.01. There is a significant mean difference between high adventurous and low adventurous (mean difference = 0.366, $t(924) = 8.273$, $p < 0.01$). Hypothesis 3 was then tested. Female participants' environmental experience is significantly higher than male participants' environmental experience (mean difference = 0.138, $t(880) = -2.682$, $p < 0.01$). Hypothesis 7 testing showed that participants who were less familiar with LDCW had a significantly higher environmental experience than participants who were more familiar with LDCW (mean difference = -0.178, $t(881) = -3.241$, $p < 0.05$). When hypothesis 11 was tested, the interaction effect of familiarity and sex on the environmental experience was significant

(F = 1.958, p < 0.05). Female participants with lower familiarity (M = 4.565) had a significantly higher environmental experience than other participants. This interaction effect is further illustrated in Figure 3.

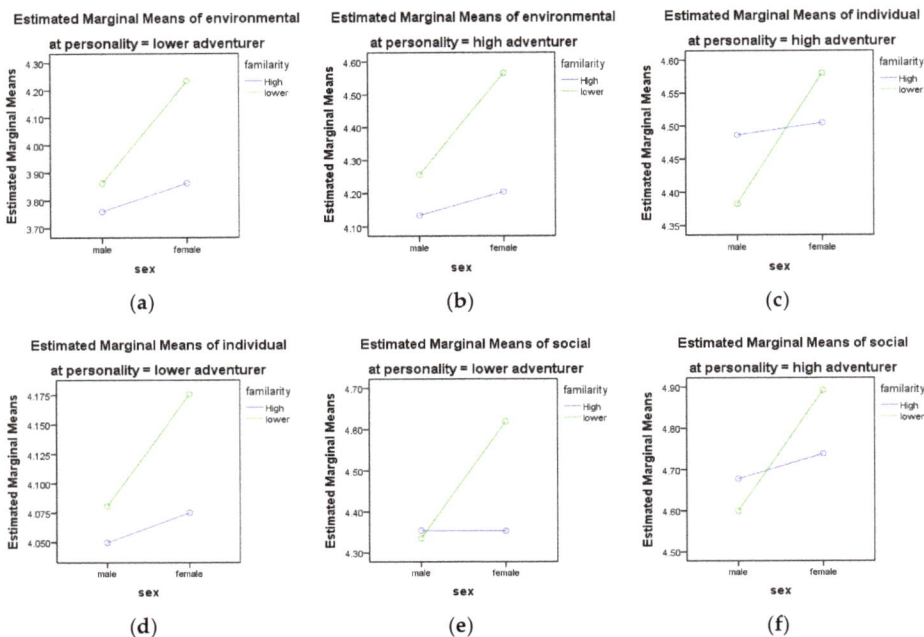

Figure 3. Interactive influence of personal traits and familiarity to walking experience.

Individual experience. A univariate analysis indicated that the factor adventurous had significant effects on the individual experience (F = 52.376, p < 0.01). There is a significant mean difference between high adventurous and low adventurous. Participants with higher adventurousness (M = 0.201) had a significantly higher individual experience than the participants with lower adventurousness (M = 3.843). Hypothesis 4 was also supported. The mean difference was −0.426 (t(924) = −10.628, p < 0.01). There was no interaction effect.

Social interaction experience. A univariate analysis indicated that all three factors had significant effects on the social interaction experience. The F values are 38.569 (p < 0.01), 2.432 (p < 0.1), and 3.99 (p < 0.01). There is a significant mean difference between high adventurous and low adventurous (mean difference = 0.324, t(924) = 8.499, p < 0.01). Hypothesis 5 was then confirmed. Female participants' social interaction experience was significantly higher than male participants' social interaction experience (mean difference = −0.07, t(880) = −1.659, p < 0.1). Tests of Hypothesis 9 showed that the interaction effect of familiarity and sex on the social interaction experience was significant (F = 6.525, p < 0.01). Female participants with lower familiarity (M = 4.891) had a significantly higher social interaction experience than others. This interaction effect is further illustrated in Figure 3.

The results support these hypotheses; higher adventurous participants have a higher experience in each dimension. These results show that personality traits are not just a factor in decision-making processes [52,88], but they also influence the overall experience when participating in a leisure activity.

These results support the hypothesis that walkers' gender affects the experiences of well-being. Specifically, female walkers obtain well-being from social interaction and individual development more than male walkers. Such results may be due to the historical perception of walking and the different cognitions of LDCW. Walking has also been considered an acceptable form of physical activity for women as it was perceived to be consistent with femininity [57]. However, LDCW was seen as a competitive sport for men, which is more in line with their need for physical activity or mental health. At the same time, women walk more as a leisure (or recreational) activity to gain well-being through contact with new environments and different people.

Furthermore, participants with lower familiarity had intense environmental and social experiences. Generally, familiarity can be treated as a kind of positive and active prior accumulated experience [63]. However, according to construal level theory, familiarity may just increase customers' perception of the core value provided by a product's or service's quality [62]. A study from the perspective of destination image attributes showed that pre-trip planning would turn a destination from fantasy to reality [75]. For walking event participants, the social interaction experience as the periphery experience is high when participants are less familiar with LDCW. This is the typical character of collective physical activity in China. People do not need to engage in a lot of pre-planning behavior, and they may have high well-being experiences.

5. Conclusions

5.1. Summary of Findings

The traditional focus of walking promotion campaigns has involved beliefs about the benefits of walking on physical health [48], but walking is now more regarded as a recreational activity which may enhance well-being [20,89]. LDCW, as a booming walking activity in China, has scarcely been explored. The current study has the strength of being the first quantitative exploration of well-being experiences and related influential factors of LDCW in the context of China framed by the theory of therapeutic mobilities and construal level theory. Therapeutic mobilities theory provides a base for developing experience scales. Construal level theory is applied to examine the influential factors. Therapeutic mobilities theory posits that the walking experience helps participants in walking toward well-being. Construal level theory asserts that the walking experience is filled with dynamics. This finding provides an empirical demonstration of Gatrell's (2013) therapeutic mobilities theory, which suggests that walking improves health and well-being through the active body, social body, and walking contexts [20]. The finding is consistent with construal level theory.

Based on the "Shenzhen 100 km Walking" event, the following conclusions are obtained:

(1) The participants gain well-being from three dimensions: social interaction experience, individual experience, and environmental experience.
(2) In LDCW, walkers with higher adventure-seeking personality traits have more well-being experiences in each dimension.
(3) Gender has a significant influence on both the environmental experience and the social interaction experience, and female walkers obtain well-being from social interaction and individual development more than male walkers while males have more experience of individual development.
(4) Familiarity has a significant influence on both the environmental experience and the social interaction experience, and participants with less familiarity have significantly more environmental experiences.
(5) Gender and familiarity also have a significant interaction influence on both the environmental experience dimension and the social interaction experience dimension. Female participants with lower familiarity have stronger environmental experience and social experience.

This study provides several theoretical contributions, including on the walking experience, well-being, and event management.

First, this paper provides a new perspective to understand a walking event based on the participants' experience. Following systematic scale development procedures, this paper developed and validated a measurement scale to identify LDCW participants' social interaction, individual development, and environmental understanding experiences. Although walking experience research has been a hot topic in recent years [90,91], a limitation of former research is the lack of quantitative measurements of walkers' experience from the perspective of well-being and therapeutic benefits. This study bridges this research gap by validating that walking participants generally have rich experiences that enhance their well-being.

Second, this paper contributes to construal level theory by testing the experiences' influential factors, such as adventure-seeking personality, familiarity, and gender. According to construal level theory, different dimensions of psychological distance affect mental construals [49]. This paper is the first attempt to test multilevel influential factors in experience research. The findings suggest that experiences are affected by multiple psychological dimensions; this provides a new perspective to explore complex mental construals.

5.2. Implications

Several practical implications can be derived from this study. Contemporary Chinese are keen for group leisure and fitness activities, and long-distance walking is an effective way to achieve the goal of national fitness. This is a topic that has important policy implications for public health domains. Participants are motivated to engage in more physical exercise, while obtaining happiness and health. Therefore, proactive policies should be formulated to encourage and manage these activities. Based on the findings, the following implications can be provided for event organizers: First, they should be mindful to provide a diverse walking environment, opportunities for social interaction, physical exercise, and mental challenges, so that participants can gain well-being and events can attract more people to participate. Second, they should focus more on participants' social interaction rather than competition. Also, organizers can promote participants' environmental experiences and enhance their urban identities by arranging different routes, designing different themes, and creating different activities. Third, event organizers should cater to the needs of different people with different personality traits. For example, female participants should be given more opportunities to communicate in the group, while male participants should be challenged more in the routes. Participants with high familiarity should maintain consistency in the innate character of the event while innovating in other dimensions.

5.3. Limitations and Future Research

This research also has some limitations. First, the study collected data only from the "Shenzhen 100 km Walking" event, and whether the conclusions of this study can be extended to other walking events such as the official organization of competitive long-distance walking events needs further examination. Second, the survey sample was mostly well educated, young individuals, so the results might not be generalizable to other populations. In the meantime, having more than half the questionnaires collected at the end of the walk might have led to a more expert sample of walkers, who actually managed to finish the walk. Third, diverse psychological dimensions might affect participants' experience. The influential factors, such as familiarity, also need more detailed exploration.

The dynamics and experiences gained during the walking process are worth additional investigation [14]. Further quantitative and/or qualitative (including mixed methods) research can explore more details of the relationships between walking and well-being. Future research is also warranted on the different types of LDCW activities that can support health and well-being, while looking at different cultural contexts and different socio-economic groups.

Author Contributions: P.Y. co-developed the questionnaire, performed the investigation and statistical analysis, and wrote the major part of the paper; S.D. contributed to the research design, literature review, performed the statistical analysis and wrote the methodology and result parts; H.X. contributed to the research design, literature review, co-developed the questionnaire and the refinement of the questionnaire and approved the final manuscript; P.J. contributed to the research background, data collection and research design.

Funding: This research is funding by National Nature Science Foundation of China in full, Grant Reference (41771145, 41601611), and the special construction funds of Jinan University for high-level university.

Conflicts of Interest: The authors declare no conflict of interest. The founding sponsors had no role in the design of the study; in the collection, analyses, or interpretation of data; in the writing of the manuscript, and in the decision to publish the results.

References

1. Kay, G.; Moxham, N. Paths for whom? Countryside access for recreational walking. *Leis. Stud.* **1996**, *15*, 171–183. [CrossRef]
2. Edensor, T. Walking in the British Countryside: Reflexivity, Embodied Practices and Ways to Escape. *Body Soc.* **2000**, *6*, 81–106. [CrossRef]
3. 2014 National Fitness Activities Survey Bulletin. Available online: http://www.sport.gov.cn/n16/n1077/n1422/7300210.html (accessed on 1 November 2018).
4. Johansson, M.; Sternudd, C.; Kärrholm, M. Perceived urban design qualities and affective experiences of walking. *J. Urban Des.* **2016**, *21*, 256–275. [CrossRef]
5. Middleton, J. Sense and the city: Exploring the embodied geographies of urban walking. *Soc. Cult. Geogr.* **2010**, *11*, 575–596. [CrossRef]
6. Urry, J. *Sociology Beyond Societies: Mobilities for the Twenty-First Century*; Routledge: London, UK, 2012.
7. Amato, J.A. *On Foot: A History of Walking*; NYU Press: New York, NY, USA, 2004.
8. Balter, O.; Hedin, B.; Tobiasson, H.; Toivanen, S. Walking Outdoors during Seminars Improved Perceived Seminar Quality and Sense of Well-Being among Participants. *Int. J. Environ. Res. Public Health* **2018**, *15*, 303. [CrossRef] [PubMed]
9. Marselle, M.R.; Irvine, K.N.; Warber, S.L. Walking for well-being: Are group walks in certain types of natural environments better for well-being than group walks in urban environments? *Int. J. Environ. Res. Public Health* **2013**, *10*, 5603–5628. [CrossRef] [PubMed]
10. Trope, Y.; Liberman, N. Construal-level theory of psychological distance. *Psychol. Rev.* **2010**, *117*, 440. [CrossRef] [PubMed]
11. Liberman, N.; Trope, Y. The role of feasibility and desirability considerations in near and distant future decisions: A test of temporal construal theory. *J. Pers. Soc. Psychol.* **1998**, *75*, 5–18. [CrossRef]
12. Liberman, N.; Trope, Y. The Psychology of Transcending the Here and Now. *Science* **2008**, *322*, 1201–1205. [CrossRef] [PubMed]
13. Narayan, J.; Ordóñez, L. Effect of effort and deadlines on consumer product returns. *J. Consum. Psychol.* **2012**, *22*, 260–271. [CrossRef]
14. Breejen, L.D. The experiences of long distance walking: A case study of the West Highland Way in Scotland. *Tour. Manag.* **2007**, *28*, 1417–1427. [CrossRef]
15. Crust, L.; Keegan, R.; Piggott, D.; Swann, C. Walking the Walk: A Phenomenological Study of Long Distance Walking. *J. Appl. Sport Psychol.* **2011**, *23*, 243–262. [CrossRef]
16. Ratna, A. Walking for leisure: The translocal lives of first generation Gujarati Indian men and women. *Leis. Stud.* **2017**, *36*, 1–15. [CrossRef]
17. Yan, B.J.; Zhang, J.; Zhang, H.L.; Lu, S.J.; Guo, Y.R. Investigating the motivation—Experience relationship in a dark tourism space: A case study of the Beichuan earthquake relics, China. *Tour. Manag.* **2016**, *53*, 108–121. [CrossRef]
18. Roberson, D.N.; Babic, V. Remedy for modernity: Experiences of walkers and hikers on Medvednica Mountain. *Leis. Stud.* **2009**, *28*, 105–112. [CrossRef]
19. Chhetri, P. A GIS methodology for modelling hiking experiences in the Grampians National Park, Australia. *Tour. Geogr.* **2015**, *17*, 795–814. [CrossRef]
20. Gatrell, A.C. Therapeutic mobilities: Walking and 'steps' to wellbeing and health. *Health Place* **2013**, *22*, 98–106. [CrossRef] [PubMed]
21. Agency, N.H.D. *The Effectiveness of Public Health Interventions for Increasing Physical Activity Among Adults: A Review of Reviews*; Health Development Agency: London, UK, 2004.

22. Morgan, A.L.; Tobar, D.A.; Snyder, L. Walking toward a new me: The impact of prescribed walking 10,000 steps/day on physical and psychological well-being. *J. Phys. Act. Health* **2010**, *7*, 299–307. [CrossRef] [PubMed]

23. Barton, J.; Hine, R.; Pretty, J. The health benefits of walking in greenspaces of high natural and heritage value. *J. Integr. Environ. Sci.* **2009**, *6*, 261–278. [CrossRef]

24. Biddle, S.; Mutrie, N.; Gorely, T. *Psychology of Physical Activity: Determinants, Well-Being and Interventions*, 3rd ed.; Routledge: New York, NY, USA, 2015.

25. Bean, C.E.; Kearns, R.; Collins, D. Exploring social mobilities: Narratives of walking and driving in Auckland, New Zealand. *Urban Stud.* **2008**, *45*, 2829–2848. [CrossRef]

26. Grant, G.; Pollard, N.; Allmark, P.; Machaczek, K.; Ramcharan, P. The social relations of a health walk group: An ethnographic study. *Qual. Health Res.* **2017**, *27*, 1701–1712. [CrossRef] [PubMed]

27. Li, Y.; Wood, E.H.; Thomas, R. Innovation implementation: Harmony and conflict in Chinese modern music festivals. *Tour. Manag.* **2017**, *63*, 87–99. [CrossRef]

28. Ziegler, F.; Schwanen, T. I like to go out to be energised by different people: An exploratory analysis of mobility and wellbeing in later life. *Ageing Soc.* **2011**, *31*, 758–781. [CrossRef]

29. Leyden, K.M. Social capital and the built environment: The importance of walkable neighborhoods. *Am. J. Public Health* **2003**, *93*, 1546–1551. [CrossRef] [PubMed]

30. Dadpour, S.; Pakzad, J.; Khankeh, H. Understanding the Influence of Environment on Adults' Walking Experiences: A Meta-Synthesis Study. *Int. J. Environ. Res. Public Health* **2016**, *13*, 731. [CrossRef] [PubMed]

31. Chhetri, P.; Arrowsmith, C.; Jackson, M. Determining hiking experiences in nature-based tourist destinations. *Tour. Manag.* **2004**, *25*, 31–43. [CrossRef]

32. Coble, T.G.; Selin, S.W.; Erickson, B.B. Hiking alone: Understanding fear, negotiation strategies and leisure experience. *J. Leis. Res.* **2003**, *35*, 1–22. [CrossRef]

33. Boddy, T. Underground and overhead: Building the analogous city. *Var. A Theme Park* **1992**, *53*, 123.

34. Mattias, K.; Johansson, M.; Lindelöw, D.; Ferreira, I.A. Interseriality and different sorts of walking: Suggestions for a relational approach to urban walking. *Mobilities* **2017**, *12*, 20–35. [CrossRef]

35. Kliskey, A.D. Linking the wilderness perception mapping concept to the recreation opportunity spectrum. *Environ. Manag.* **1998**, *22*, 79–88. [CrossRef]

36. Brown, P.J.; Haas, G.E. Wilderness Recreation Experiences: The Rawah Case. *J. Leis. Res.* **1980**, *12*, 229–241. [CrossRef]

37. Lee, S.; Manthiou, A.; Jeong, M.; Tang, L.; Chiang, L. Does consumers' feeling affect their quality of life? roles of consumption emotion and its consequences. *Int. J. Tour. Res.* **2015**, *17*, 409–416. [CrossRef]

38. Li, H.; Chen, W.; He, W. Planning of Green Space Ecological Network in Urban Areas: An Example of Nanchang, China. *Int. J. Environ. Res. Public Health* **2015**, *12*, 12889–12904. [CrossRef] [PubMed]

39. Doughty, K. Walking together: The embodied and mobile production of a therapeutic landscape. *Health Place* **2013**, *24*, 140–146. [CrossRef] [PubMed]

40. Ettema, D.; Smajic, I. Walking, places and wellbeing. *Geogr. J.* **2015**, *181*, 102–109. [CrossRef]

41. Saunders, R.E.; Laing, J.; Weiler, B. Personal Transformation through Long-Distance Walking. In *Tourist Experience and Fulfilment: Insights from Positive Psychology*; Felip, S., Pearce, P., Eds.; Routledge: London, UK; pp. 127–146.

42. Booth, F. *The Independent Walker's Guide to Great Britain*; Interlink Pub Group Inc.: New York, NY, USA, 1998.

43. Wylie, J. A single day's walking: Narrating self and landscape on the South West Coast Path. *Trans. Inst. Br. Geogr.* **2005**, *30*, 234–247. [CrossRef]

44. Jarvis, R. *Romantic Writing and Pedestrian Travel*; Palgrave Macmillan Press: New York, NY, USA, 1997.

45. Holt, K.G.; Jeng, S.F.; Ratcliffe, R.; Hamill, J. Energetic cost and stability during human walking at the preferred stride frequency. *J. Mot. Behav.* **1995**, *27*, 164–178. [CrossRef] [PubMed]

46. South, J.; Giuntoli, G.; Kinsella, K. *An Evaluation of the Walking for Wellness Project and the Befriender Role*; Institute for Health & Wellbeing, Centre for Health Promotion Research, Leeds Metropolitan University: Leeds, UK, 2013.

47. Hanson, S. Towards an Understanding of Walking Groups as a Health Promoting Intervention. Ph.D. Thesis, University of East Anglia, Norwich, UK, 2016.

48. Darker, C.D.; Larkin, M.; French, D.P. An exploration of walking behaviour–an interpretative phenomenological approach. *Soc. Sci. Med.* **2007**, *65*, 2172–2183. [CrossRef] [PubMed]

49. Trope, Y.; Liberman, N.; Wakslak, C. Construal levels and psychological distance: Effects on representation, prediction, evaluation, and behavior. *J. Consum. Psychol.* **2007**, *17*, 83–95. [CrossRef]

50. Zuckerman, M.; Neeb, M. Sensation seeking and psychopathology. *Psychiatry Res.* **1979**, *1*, 255–264. [CrossRef]

51. Bornioli, A.; Graham, P.; Morgan, P.L. The psychological wellbeing benefits of place engagement during walking in urban environments: A qualitative photo-elicitation study. *Health Place* **2018**, *53*, 228–236. [CrossRef] [PubMed]

52. Yoo, K.H.; Gretzel, U. Antecedents and impacts of trust in travel-related consumer-generated media. *Inf. Technol. Tour.* **2010**, *12*, 139–152. [CrossRef]

53. Chen, X.; Fang, L.; Nydegger, L.; Jie, G.; Ren, Y.; Dinaj-Koci, V.; Sun, H.; Stanton, B. Brief Sensation Seeking Scale for Chinese—Cultural adaptation and psychometric assessment. *Pers. Individ. Dif.* **2013**, *54*, 604–609. [CrossRef] [PubMed]

54. Ma, J.; Li, C.; Kwan, M.P.; Chai, Y. A Multilevel Analysis of Perceived Noise Pollution, Geographic Contexts and Mental Health in Beijing. *Int. J. Environ. Res. Public Health* **2018**, *15*, 1479. [CrossRef] [PubMed]

55. Chau, J.; Smith, B.; Bauman, A.; Merom, D.; Eyeson-Annan, M.; Chey, T.; Farrell, L. Recent trends in physical activity in New South Wales. Is the tide of inactivity turning? *Aust. N. Z. J. Public Health* **2010**, *32*, 82–85. [CrossRef] [PubMed]

56. Langea, D.; Koring, M.B.; Parschau, L.B.; Lippke, S.; Knolla, N.; Schwarzer, R. Sex differential mediation effects of planning within the health behavior change process. *Soc. Sci. Med.* **2018**, *211*, 137–146. [CrossRef] [PubMed]

57. Kavanagh, A.M.; Bentley, R. Walking: A Gender Issue? *Aust. J. Soc. Issues* **2008**, *43*, 45–64. [CrossRef]

58. Pollard, T.M.; Wagnild, J.M. Gender differences in walking (for leisure, transport and in total) across adult life: A systematic review. *BMC Public Health* **2017**, *17*, 341. [CrossRef] [PubMed]

59. Webb, T.L.; Sheeran, P. Does changing behavioral intentions engender behavior change? A meta-analysis of the experimental evidence. *Psychol. Bull.* **2006**, *132*, 249–268. [CrossRef] [PubMed]

60. Jackson, V.; Stoel, L.; Brantley, A. Mall attributes and shopping value: Differences by gender and generational cohort. *J. Retail. Consum. Serv.* **2011**, *18*, 1–9. [CrossRef]

61. Lynn, N.A.; Brown, R.D. Effects of recreational use impacts on hiking experiences in natural areas. *Landsc. Urban Plan.* **2003**, *64*, 77–87. [CrossRef]

62. Alba, J.W.; Hutchinson, J.W. Dimensions of Consumer Expertise. *J. Consum. Res.* **1987**, *13*, 411–454. [CrossRef]

63. Huang, L.; Gursoy, D.; Xu, H. Impact of personality traits and involvement on prior knowledge. *Ann. Tour. Res.* **2014**, *48*, 42–57. [CrossRef]

64. Jin, Q.; Fang, J.; Li, T. *The Occurrence, Development and Prospect of Hiking Tourism in China*; Social Sciences Literature Press: Beijing, China, 2012; pp. 323–336. (In Chinese)

65. The Glory of a City. Available online: http://www.doyouhike.net/forum/sz100km/sz100km16/2361188,0, 0,1.html (accessed on 18 July 2017). (In Chinese)

66. Interpretation of "Tour Pal". Available online: http://sh.eastday.com/qtmt/20090817/u1a616462.html (accessed on 18 July 2017). (In Chinese)

67. "Shenzhen 100 km" Event—Stem from Folk Spontaneously. *Jing Newspaper*, 4 May 2017. (In Chinese)

68. 2016 Shenzhen 100 km End. Available online: http://news.xinhuanet.com/sports/2016-03/25/c_128834491. htm (accessed on 18 July 2017). (In Chinese)

69. New Departure of 2017 "Shenzhen 100 km". *Shenzhen Special Zone Daily*, 23 April 2017. (In Chinese)

70. MacKenzie, S.B.; Podsakoff, P.M.; Rich, G.A. Transformational and transactional leadership and salesperson performance. *J. Acad. Mark. Sci.* **2001**, *29*, 115. [CrossRef]

71. Churchill, G.A. A paradigm for developing better measures of marketing constructs. *J. Mark. Res.* **1979**. [CrossRef]

72. DeVellis, R.F. *Scale Development: Theory and applications*; Sage publications: Thousand Oaks, CA, USA, 2016.

73. Liang, J.; Fan, J.; Chen, Z. Theoretical Construct and Its Measurement. In *Empirical Methods in Organization and Management Research*; Chen, X., Shen, W., Eds.; Peking University Press: Beijing, China, 2018; pp. 323–325. (In Chinese)

74. Hoyle, R.H.; Stephenson, M.T.; Palmgreen, P.; Pugzles Lorch, E.; Donohew, R.L. Reliability and validity of a brief measure of sensation seeking. *Pers. Individ. Differ.* **2002**, *32*, 401–414. [CrossRef]

75. Tan, W.K. From fantasy to reality: A study of pre-trip planning from the perspective of destination image attributes and temporal psychological distance. *Serv. Bus.* **2018**, *12*, 1–20. [CrossRef]

76. Kaplanidou, K.; Christine, V. The meaning and measurement of a sport event experience among active sport tourists. *J. Sport Manage.* **2010**, *24*, 544–566. [CrossRef]

77. Hair, J.; Black, W.; Babin, B.; Anderson, R.; Tatham, R. *Multivariate Data Analysis*; Prentice Hall: Upper Saddle River, NJ, USA, 1998.

78. Kaiser, H.F. The Application of Electronic Computers to Factor Analysis. *Educ. Psychol. Meas.* **1960**, *20*, 141–151. [CrossRef]

79. Byrne, B.M. *Structural Equation Modeling With AMOS: Basic Concepts, Applications, and Programming*; Routledge: London, UK, 2016.

80. Fornell, C.; Larcker, D.F. Structural equation models with unobservable variables and measurement error: Algebra and statistics. *J. Mark. Res.* **1981**. [CrossRef]

81. Chhetri, P.; Arrowsmith, C. Developing A Spatial Model Of Probable Hiking Experiences Through Natural Landscapes. *Surveyor* 2002, *31*, 87–102. [CrossRef]

82. Berenson, M.; Levine, D.; Szabat, K.A.; Krehbiel, T.C. *Basic Business Statistics: Concepts and Applications*; Prentice Hall: Upper Saddle River, NJ, USA, 2012.

83. Bach, G.R. Marathon group dynamics. I. Some functions of the professional group facilitator. *Psychol. Rep.* **1967**, *20*, 229–233. [CrossRef] [PubMed]

84. Fisher, K.J.; Li, F. A community-based walking trial to improve neighborhood quality of life in older adults: A multilevel analysis. *Ann. Behav. Med.* **2004**, *28*, 186–194. [CrossRef] [PubMed]

85. Temple, V.A.; Frey, G.C.; Stanish, H.I. Physical activity of adults with mental retardation: Review and research needs. *Am. J. Health Promot. Ajhp* **2006**, *21*, 2. [CrossRef] [PubMed]

86. De Certeau, M. Walking in the City. In *Everyday Life*; University of California Press: Berkeley, CA, USA, 1984.

87. Sharpe, N.R.; Veaux, R.D.D.; Velleman, P.F. *Business Statistics: A First Course*; Prentice Hall: Upper Saddle River NJ, USA, 2012.

88. Zhang, L.Y. Unusual Environment: The Core Concept of Tourism Research-A New Framework for Tourism Research. *Tour. Trib.* **2008**, *23*, 12–16. (In Chinese) [CrossRef]

89. Hall, C.M.; Ram, Y.; Shoval, N. (Eds.) *The Routledge International Handbook of Walking*; Routledge: Abingdon, UK, 2017.

90. Kim, H.; Yang, S. Neighborhood Walking and Social Capital: The Correlation between Walking Experience and Individual Perception of Social Capital. *Sustainability* **2017**, *9*, 680. [CrossRef]

91. Murata, H.; Bouzarte, Y.; Kanebako, J.; Minamizawa, K. Walk-In Music: Walking Experience with Synchronized Music and Its Effect of Pseudo-gravity. In Proceedings of the Adjunct Publication of the 30th Annual ACM Symposium on User Interface Software and Technology, Quebec City, QC, Canada, 22–25 October 2017; pp. 177–179.

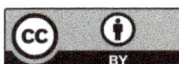

International Journal of
*Environmental Research
and Public Health*

MDPI

Article

Geographic Imputation of Missing Activity Space Data from Ecological Momentary Assessment (EMA) GPS Positions

Jeremy Mennis [1,*], **Michael Mason** [2], **Donna L. Coffman** [3] **and Kevin Henry** [1]

[1] Department of Geography and Urban Studies, Temple University, Philadelphia, PA 19122, USA;
    kevinahenry@temple.edu
[2] Center for Behavioral Health Research, University of Tennessee, Knoxville, TN 37996, USA;
    mmason29@utk.edu
[3] Department of Epidemiology and Biostatistics, Temple University, Philadelphia, PA 19122, USA;
    donna.coffman@temple.edu
*   Correspondence: jmennis@temple.edu; Tel.: +01-215-204-4748

Received: 25 October 2018; Accepted: 30 November 2018; Published: 4 December 2018

Abstract: This research presents a pilot study to develop and compare methods of geographic imputation for estimating the location of missing activity space data collected using geographic ecological momentary assessment (GEMA). As a demonstration, we use data from a previously published analysis of the effect of neighborhood disadvantage, captured at the U.S. Census Bureau tract level, on momentary psychological stress among a sample of 137 urban adolescents. We investigate the impact of listwise deletion on model results and test two geographic imputation techniques adapted for activity space data from hot deck and centroid imputation approaches. Our results indicate that listwise deletion can bias estimates of place effects on health, and that these impacts are mitigated by the use of geographic imputation, particularly regarding inflation of the standard errors. These geographic imputation techniques may be extended in future research by incorporating approaches from the non-spatial imputation literature as well as from conventional geographic imputation and spatial interpolation research that focus on non-activity space data.

Keywords: missing data; spatial data; imputation; geographic imputation; activity space; ecological momentary assessment; EMA

1. Introduction

The role of space and place in shaping health has received increasing attention in the health and medical research community [1–3]. Researchers have argued, however, that investigating the influence of place on health should focus not simply on an individual's residential neighborhood, but on the environmental exposures that occur throughout an individual's activity space [4–6]—the routine locations an individual visits throughout his or her daily life, such as places of work or school, recreation and leisure, social interaction with friends and family, and so on [7]. Activity space is recognized as a key construct in investigations of substance use, physical activity, stress, healthy eating, exposure to air pollution, and other place-related health outcomes [8–12]. Research on activity space and health has been facilitated by the development and adoption of geospatial technologies, such as global positioning systems (GPS), which allows for the tracking and encoding of individual mobility, and geographic information systems (GIS), which facilitates the integration of mobility data with other spatial data capturing exposures to environmental health hazards or amenities [13,14].

One novel approach to capturing activity space data for studies of place and health behaviors combines GPS with ecological momentary assessment (EMA), a technique where individuals complete brief surveys concerning their moods, behaviors, and social interactions, typically via a mobile phone. EMA has the advantage of capturing 'momentary' health data in real-time and in individuals' natural environments, thus helping to reduce bias associated with survey recall [15]. GPS can be used to simultaneously capture location at the moment of EMA survey response, thus yielding a set of georeferenced EMA observations, each with a precise location and time-stamp. In sum, these EMA location data can be considered an expression of an individual's activity space and can be combined with other spatial data within GIS [16], an approach termed geographic EMA (GEMA).

GEMA has been used to investigate a variety of health behaviors, but perhaps most prominently for studies of place effects on substance use, where activity space data are typically used to assess individuals' exposures to environmental risk, such as neighborhood disadvantage, neighborhood disorder, or the locations of stores selling alcohol or tobacco, to develop statistical models of the effect of such exposures on substance use and related outcomes [17–20]. One particular challenge with the use of GEMA concerns the occurrence of missing activity space data, i.e., situations in which an EMA survey response is recorded, but a corresponding geographic coordinate position is not captured. GPS-derived coordinate positions may be unobtainable due to a variety of reasons: Atmospheric refraction of the signal from the satellite to the receiver; the presence of tree canopy, buildings, or other features, which can serve to block or attenuate communication between the satellite and receiver; the GPS signal may reflect off buildings or other features in the environment, generating multiple paths from the satellite to the receiver; error in the synchronization of the satellite and receiver clocks; error in the ephemeris information concerning the satellite orbital position; and the geometric dilution of precision (GDOP) regarding the geometric relationships that occur between the receiver and satellites, where a coordinate position is more difficult to obtain when satellites cluster together in the sky, and which is typically encoded during GPS data capture using National Marine Electronics Association (NMEA) data standards [21,22]. Consequently, missing or inaccurate activity space data in GEMA studies is a common occurrence [21,23].

The simplest approach to treating missing activity space data in GEMA is listwise deletion (i.e., complete case analysis)—the simple elimination of any EMA observation (i.e., an individual EMA response) with missing location data from the analysis. Unfortunately, this approach has the effect of reducing statistical power as well as introducing potential bias in geographic cluster detection and into measures of environmental exposure, and can result in biased regression parameter estimates and standard errors [24–27].

An alternative approach is to impute the missing activity space locations. Conventional statistical imputation for non-spatial data includes approaches that estimate missing data values using the mean of the known values or by replacing the missing value with a randomly selected known value [28,29]. Model-based approaches have employed regression or the expectation-maximization (EM) algorithm to estimate missing values [30,31]. More recently, multiple imputation methods have become more accessible and prominent, whereby model-based approaches are used to generate a distribution of missing data values, which can be employed in a series of analytical models and where parameter estimates are pooled [32,33].

Geographic imputation [34] departs somewhat from the statistical imputation literature and refers generally to estimating missing location data. It is typically applied to estimating residential locations for individuals from administrative health data in the case when address geocoding fails due to a missing or incorrect street address, or for other reasons [35–37]. Often this involves a situation where the residential municipality or zip code for an individual is known, and the analyst is attempting to estimate the residential location more precisely within that spatial unit, for instance, by estimating the location as the centroid (geometric center) of the unit or through an aerial interpolation technique that incorporates ancillary data to enhance the accuracy of the estimation [34,38–42].

Geographic imputation of missing activity space data, in the context of GEMA or similar data collection designs, differs from this previous geographic imputation research in several important ways: (1) For each individual, there are a set of activity space points (not just a single missing residential location); (2) the activity space data are not missing due to a failure of geocoding (i.e., there are no address data available); and (3) there is no spatial unit, such as a zip code, that constrains where the activity space point is to be estimated. Some researchers have also sought to impute missing GPS tracking data, i.e., a continuous stream of coordinate positions captured at regular time intervals, say, every 30 s, by taking a moving average of the known GPS locations [43], but this also differs from many conventional EMA study designs, which aim to sample at random, discrete moments in time, not continuously.

The aim of the present research is to develop and compare methods of geographic imputation for estimating the location of missing activity space data collected using GEMA. We consider this a pilot study that investigates the feasibility of adapting relatively simple geographic and conventional statistical (i.e., non-geographic) imputation methods to missing GEMA activity space data, and thus paves the way for the development of more sophisticated GEMA geographic imputation research in the future. The significance of this research lies in its ability to establish a baseline approach and comparative framework for geographic imputation of activity space data, which, to our knowledge, has not been addressed in the geographic imputation or statistical imputation literatures. The present research can also shed light on related domains of activity space data analysis other than GEMA methods where missing data may be problematic.

To this end, we use data from a previously published GEMA analysis of the effect of neighborhood disadvantage, captured at the U.S. Census Bureau tract level, on momentary psychological stress among a sample of urban adolescents [17]. Here, we aim to use geographic imputation to estimate the neighborhood disadvantage for EMA observations where momentary stress is recorded, but there is no associated geographic coordinate, and thus the neighborhood disadvantage at that EMA location is unknown. By holding out portions of the original data set, we investigate the impact of listwise deletion, as well as of two different geographic imputation methods we develop, on the direct and moderated effect estimates of neighborhood disadvantage on stress.

2. Materials and Methods

2.1. Study Setting

Data are derived from the Social-Spatial Adolescent Study, a two-year longitudinal study of peer and environmental effects on substance use among an urban, primarily African American population of adolescents. The study follows 248 adolescents who were recruited primarily from a public adolescent medicine clinic in Richmond, Virginia between 2012 and 2014. Written informed assent was obtained from adolescents and consent was obtained from their parents prior to commencing any research activities. The Temple University, Virginia Commonwealth University, and the Richmond City Health Department's institutional review boards approved the research protocol. All participants were given a mobile phone with embedded GPS for the duration of the study. Full battery assessments collecting home address, demographic information, substance use involvement, and other measures were completed in-person at baseline and every six months thereafter. In addition, every two months following enrollment, subjects received 3–6 EMA surveys per day over a four-day period via an embedded URL link to the survey sent as a text message to their mobile phone. The EMA survey asked questions about momentary moods, behaviors, and social interactions. During the moment of the EMA survey response, their location in the form of a geographic coordinate position was collected with GPS. The data set thus comprises a set of discrete activity space locations interspersed over one year for each subject (i.e., as opposed to, say, a GPS 'track' of individual movement taken over a smaller time frame). Further details on the study and the data can be found in [44,45].

2.2. Measures

The present research investigates geographic imputation using the data and analyses from previously published research focusing on the association between exposure to neighborhood disadvantage and psychological stress [17]. These data were gathered in the first year of the study data collection. Of the 3882 EMA responses completed outside the home (as indicated by the subject in the EMA response), we used the 1617 for which coordinate location data were available and which occurred in the Richmond, Virginia study region, for 137 subjects (twelve EMA observations for two subjects were missing values of the stress outcome variable in the 1629 EMA observations reported in [17]). Figure 1 shows a map of the EMA locations located in and around the city of Richmond, with location randomized within each tract to preserve privacy. The use of this data set allows us to compare various imputation techniques in the context of a published, theoretically derived statistical model of a place association with a health outcome.

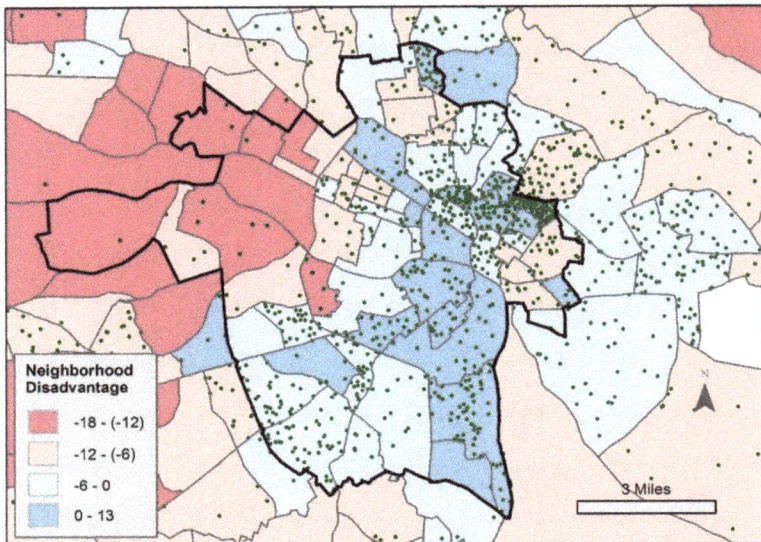

Figure 1. Map of the ecological momentary assessment (EMA) locations (green points) overlain on neighborhood disadvantage by census tract in the Richmond, Virginia area, where greater disadvantage is shown in blue. The city of Richmond is outlined in bold. The coordinate position of each EMA location is randomized within each tract for privacy protection. Note that some EMA locations occur outside the area of the map.

We focus on two particular statistical models presented in [17]. The first employs generalized estimating equations (GEE) to estimate the effect of neighborhood disadvantage on momentary stress (from the EMA) while controlling for age at enrollment (13 or 14 years), sex (male or female), race (white, African American, or other race), and substance use. Substance use was measured using the Adolescent Alcohol and Drug Involvement Scale (AADIS) [46], a continuous scale where higher values indicate greater substance use involvement. The AADIS has favorable internal consistency (Cronbach's alpha = 0.94) and correlates highly with self-report and clinical measures of substance use ($r = 0.72$ and $r = 0.75$, respectively), and with subjects' perceptions of the severity of their own substance use problem ($r = 0.79$). Age, sex, race, and substance use are taken from the full battery assessment collected at baseline. Stress is measured according to the EMA survey item "How stressed out are you right now?" with possible integer values of 1 ("Not at all stressed out") through to 9 ("Very stressed out").

Neighborhood disadvantage is conceptualized as a multidimensional measure incorporating aspects of income, educational attainment, residential stability, and family composition, as has been used in previous research [17,47]. For each EMA observation, neighborhood disadvantage is calculated based on the U.S. Census Bureau tract within which that EMA observation occurs. Tract disadvantage is calculated as $((a/10) + (b/10)) - ((c/10) + (d/10))$, where a is the poverty rate, b is the percentage of female-headed households with children, c is the percentage of adults with a bachelor's degree or higher, and d is the percentage of owner-occupied housing [47]. Higher values indicate greater neighborhood disadvantage (Figure 1). We calculate a measure, which we call 'relative disadvantage', which indicates whether the subject has traveled to an EMA location relatively more, or less, disadvantaged as compared to the tract where they reside. Relative disadvantage is calculated by subtracting the disadvantage measured at the subject's home location (indicated at baseline) from the momentary disadvantage (disadvantage at the EMA location). The GEE model adjusts for subject and tract level clustering using an exchangeable correlation structure. Table 1 (Model 1) shows the results of the model reported in [17], where higher relative disadvantage is significantly associated with higher stress.

Table 1. Generalized estimating equations (GEE) models of momentary stress ($n = 1617$). Model 1 shows the direct effect of relative disadvantage and Model 2 shows the moderation of that effect by substance use.

Independent Variable	Model 1	Model 2
Intercept	1.872 *** (1.648–2.096)	1.753 *** (1.534–1.973)
Age 14 (Ref = Age 13)	0.094 (−0.197–0.384)	0.090 (−0.196–0.376)
Male (Ref = Female)	−0.168 (−0.449–0.113)	−0.184 (−0.460–0.091)
White (Ref = Af. American)	−0.569 *** (−0.959–(−0.188))	−0.422 * (−0.789–(−0.056))
Other Race (Ref = Af. American)	0.169 (−0.286–0.624)	0.316 (−0.146–0.778)
Substance Use	0.027 *** (0.017–0.037)	0.001 (−0.020–0.017)
Relative Disadvantage	0.030 *** (0.013–0.047)	0.031 *** (0.021–0.041)
Sub. Use X Rel. Disadvantage		0.002 *** (0.001–0.003)

*** $p < 0.005$, * $p < 0.05$.

We also investigate a second GEE model, which includes a test of moderation. Here, we consider whether substance use involvement moderates the association of relative disadvantage with stress, where we expect the relationship to be stronger among subjects with greater substance use. For this purpose, we add an interaction term to Model 1 composed of the product of the substance use and relative disadvantage variables. The results are reported in Table 1 (Model 2), where the effect of relative disadvantage on stress is significantly greater for subjects with higher substance use involvement [17].

2.3. Analytic Plan

To support our analysis, we create three new data sets in which we retain a certain percentage of the original data set's neighborhood disadvantage values and remove the rest, i.e., we 'pretend' the disadvantage values for the non-retained EMA observations are missing. For this purpose, we assigned each EMA observation a random number between 0 and 1, and then sorted them in ascending order. For the first new data set, we retained the first 50% ($n = 808$) of the disadvantage values, and for the second and third data sets, we retained the first 70% ($n = 1131$) and the first 90% ($n = 1455$), respectively. Thus, 50% of the disadvantage values are missing for the first data set, 30% are missing for the second data set, and 10% are missing for the third data set. The values that are set to missing are missing completely at random (MCAR) [48].

We use these data sets to test two geographic imputation methods. Note that our aim is not necessarily to impute a specific point location for each EMA observation with a missing location value, but rather to estimate a specific census tract location, which can serve as the basis for calculating a relative disadvantage value that can then be entered into the model of stress. The first imputation method is an adaptation of the hot deck (HD) imputation technique developed for non-geographic data [49] and is somewhat similar conceptually to the random property allocation technique described in [38]. In the conventional HD approach, a random value from the known values in the data set is used to replace a missing data value. We adapt this for GEMA activity space data by replacing a missing tract value for an EMA observation with a random tract, and thus a neighborhood disadvantage value, extracted from the retained (i.e., non-missing) values in the data set. Unlike with conventional HD imputation, however, the tract drawn from the retained values is extracted from an EMA observation for the same subject, rather than a random observation from the entire data set, i.e., the activity space location is imputed using another, previously visited activity space location. The neighborhood disadvantage value for the imputed tract is then used as an estimate for all the missing neighborhood disadvantage values for that subject.

We refer to the second geographic imputation method as activity space centroid (ASC) imputation. For each subject, the centroid (point location) of the known activity space locations for that subject is calculated as the mean of the X and Y geographic coordinates from the retained, non-missing, values in the data set, such that the centroid falls in the geometric center of the subject's known EMA locations. We then retrieve the neighborhood disadvantage value of the census tract that contains that centroid, and use that as the imputed disadvantage value for all the missing disadvantage values for that subject. Note that the activity space centroid may be in a census tract for which an observed activity space location occurs in the retained values, or it may be in an entirely new tract. Thus, unlike the HD imputation, the imputed neighborhood disadvantage value may be different than any of the observed disadvantage values contained in the data. Each of the two imputation procedures, HD and ASC, is applied to the 50% retained, 70% retained, and 90% retained data sets, resulting in six imputed data sets for analysis. Finally, using the simplest approach to deal with the missing data—listwise deletion—we use only the subsets of EMA observations that were non-missing in the 50%, 70%, and 90% retained data sets.

We report descriptive statistics for the neighborhood disadvantage variable for the original data set and for each of each of the six imputed data sets. We then report the Pearson correlation between the imputed disadvantage values and the observed disadvantage values from the original data set for the imputed observations (not including the retained observations) within each data set (50% imputed, 30% imputed, and 10% imputed). Because the data are clustered by subject, we also report the association between the imputed and original observed disadvantage values using GEE (clustered by subject) by regressing the original disadvantage value on the imputed value for the six data sets of imputed observations. The original disadvantage variable coefficient indicates the degree of association after controlling for subject-level clustering.

Using the imputed disadvantage values for each of the six imputed data sets, we recalculate the relative disadvantage variable values for the imputed EMA observations, and then re-fit Model 1. We also re-fit Model 1 to each of the three listwise-deleted data sets. We compare the resulting coefficients of the relative disadvantage variable derived using the six imputed and three listwise-deleted data sets to those from the original data set presented in Model 1 (Table 1). We then repeat the procedure applied to Model 1 to compare the coefficients of the moderating variable to those presented in Model 2 (Table 1). All procedures were carried out in ArcGIS (ESRI, Inc., Redlands, CA, USA) and SPSS (IBM, Inc., Armonk, NY, USA).

3. Results

3.1. Descriptive Statistics

The original data set contains 1617 EMA observations for 137 subjects, with a mean of 12 EMA observations per subject. However, the number of EMA observations varies widely among subjects, from 1 to 54. Table 2 shows the descriptive statistics for the original observed neighborhood disadvantage variable and the imputed disadvantage variable in each of the six imputed data sets. Note that the minimum and maximum values are identical for all data sets, but the mean and standard deviation vary. The number of valid N (number of EMA observations) and number of subjects also varies. This is because for a handful of subjects with low numbers of EMA observations available, there are not any EMA observations in the retained portion of the data set that can be used in the HD or ASC imputation procedures. This is the case for 10 subjects with 16 EMA observations in the 50% retained data set, and for five subjects with eight EMA observations in the 70% retained data subset. In addition, the ASC imputation resulted in one imputed activity space location in a census tract with a zero population; thus, the disadvantage value for this EMA observation could not be imputed. Not surprisingly, the mean values for the 50% retained data set depart the most from the original observed disadvantage mean due to the larger percentage of missingness. The HD imputations maintain standard deviation values more similar to that of the original data as compared to the ASC imputations, particularly for data sets with a greater proportion of missing data.

Table 2. Descriptive statistics for observed and imputed neighborhood disadvantage using different imputation methods and for different data sets (HD = hot deck imputation; ASC = activity space centroid imputation; and 50%, 70%, and 90% refer to the percentage of the data retained versus imputed).

Variable	Valid N (# Subjects)	Minimum	Maximum	Mean (SD)
Original Disadvantage	1617 (137)	−18.54	13.47	−1.68 (7.30)
HD 50% Disadvantage	1601 (127)	−18.54	13.47	−2.77 (7.10)
ASC 50% Disadvantage	1601 (127)	−18.54	13.47	−1.97 (6.93)
HD 70% Disadvantage	1609 (132)	−18.54	13.47	−1.60 (7.33)
ASC 70% Disadvantage	1608 (132)	−18.54	13.47	−1.85 (6.96)
HD 90% Disadvantage	1614 (135)	−18.54	13.47	−1.89 (7.36)
ASC 90% Disadvantage	1613 (135)	−18.54	13.47	−1.62 (7.21)

3.2. Correlation of Observed and Imputed Neighborhood Disadvantage for Different Imputation Methods

Here, we report Pearson r correlations of the original, observed disadvantage with the imputed disadvantage values for subsets of the data that were imputed (not including the retained data). For the 50% imputed data subset, $r = 0.25$ and $r = 0.34$ for the HD ($n = 793$) and ASC ($n = 793$) imputation methods, respectively. For the 30% imputed data subset, $r = 0.38$ ($n = 478$) and $r = 0.33$ ($n = 477$), for HD and ASC respectively. For the 10% imputed data subset, $r = 0.32$ ($n = 159$) and $r = 0.53$ ($n = 158$), for HD and ASC respectively. All correlations are significant at $p < 0.005$. Results of the GEE of observed disadvantage regressed on imputed disadvantage, controlling for clustering by subject, are reported in Figure 2. When adjusted by subject-level clustering, ASC tends to outperform HD imputation across all three imputed data sets, though the difference is modest for the 50% and 30% imputed data sets.

3.3. Comparison of Model 1 GEE Relative Disadvantage Coefficients between the Original Data Set and the Listwise Deletion and Imputed Data Sets

Figure 3 shows the results of Model 1 applied to the original data compared to the listwise deletion approach, in which the model is applied to 50%, 70%, and 90% of the EMA observations retained from the original data set. The relative disadvantage coefficient value is shown, along with 95% confidence intervals. Not surprisingly, a greater percentage of missing data results in larger departures of the coefficient value from that derived from the original data set. When 50% of the values are missing, the resulting estimate departs from the original coefficient estimate by approximately one third.

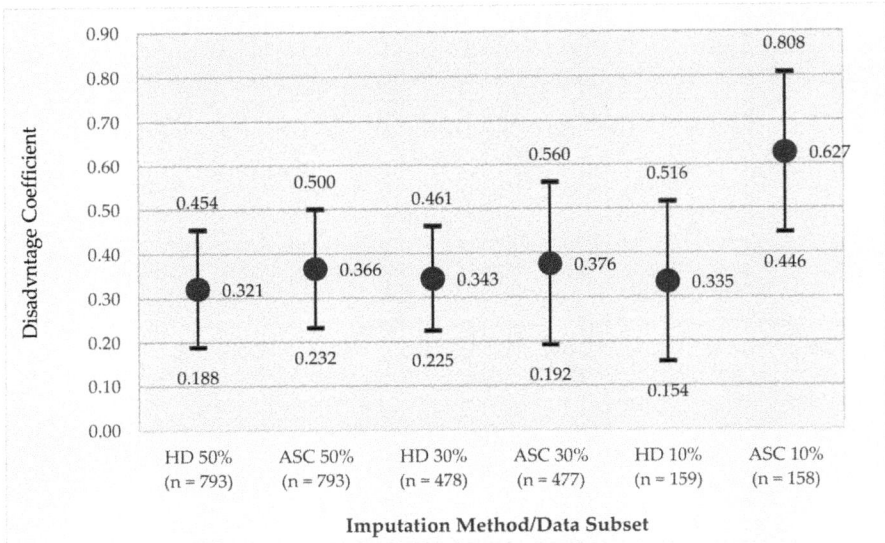

Figure 2. Generalized estimating equations (GEE) coefficients of observed disadvantage (clustered by subject) regressed on imputed disadvantage values. Coefficients are reported for each combination of imputation technique (hot deck (HD) or activity space centroid (ASC)) applied to different subsets of the imputed data (50% imputed, 30% imputed, and 10% imputed). Circle markers represent coefficient values; whiskers represent 95% confidence intervals. All coefficients are significant at $p < 0.005$.

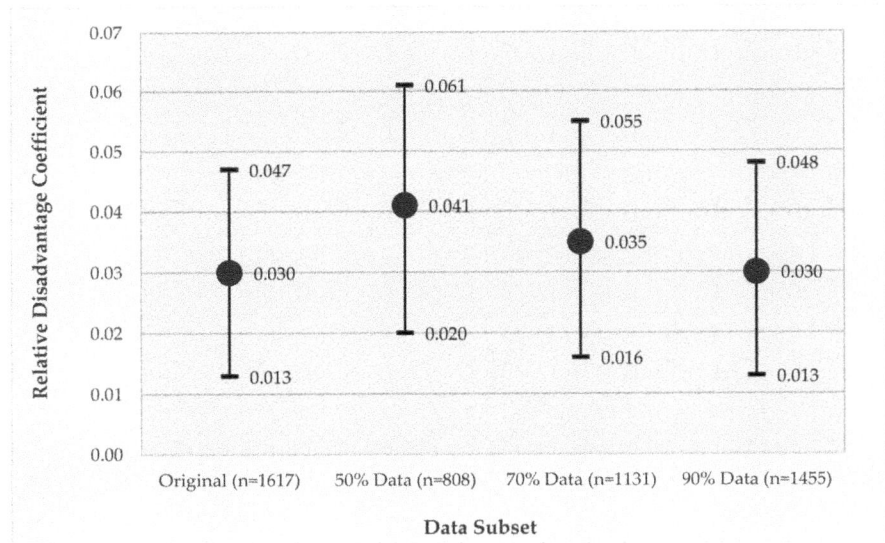

Figure 3. Results for the listwise deletion data sets for Model 1, GEE coefficients of the effect of relative disadvantage on momentary stress. Coefficients are reported for the original data set (100% retained) and each data subset—50% retained, 70% retained, and 90% retained subsets of the original data set. Circle markers represent coefficient values; whiskers represent 95% confidence intervals. All coefficients are significant at $p < 0.005$.

Figure 4 shows an analogous graph of the results of Model 1 comparing the original data set with different imputed data sets using the two imputation techniques and the different percentage of observations retained versus imputed. Departures from the original relative disadvantage coefficient value are modest, with the 50% retained data sets departing the most from the original coefficient value.

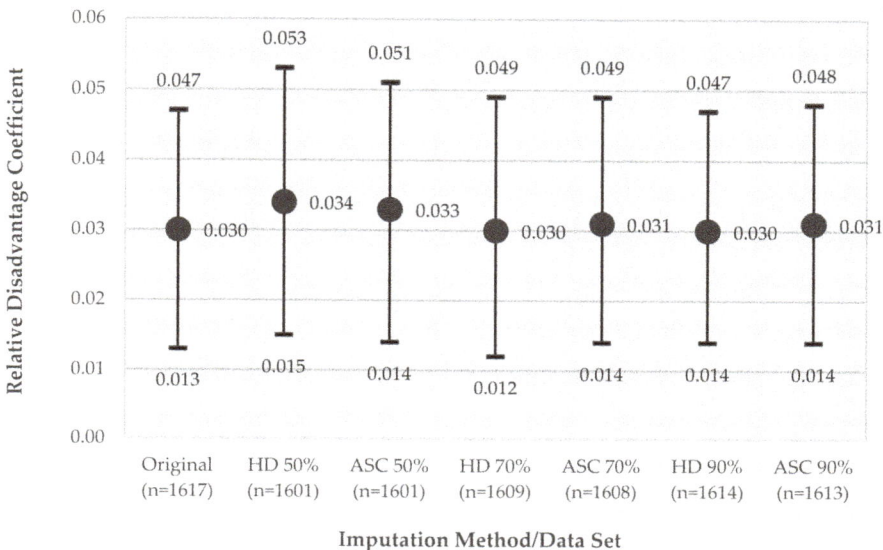

Figure 4. Results for the imputed data sets for Model 1, GEE coefficients of the effect of relative disadvantage on momentary stress. Coefficients are reported for the original data set (100% retained) and for each imputation technique (hot deck (HD) or activity space centroid (ASC)) applied to different percentages of the retained observations (50% retained (50% imputed), 70% retained (30% imputed), and 90% retained (10% imputed)). Circle markers represent coefficient values; whiskers represent 95% confidence intervals. All coefficients are significant at $p < 0.005$.

3.4. Comparison of Model 2 GEE Moderator Coefficients between the Original Data Set and the Listwise Deletion and Imputed Data Sets

Figures 5 and 6 present results analogous to those presented in Figures 3 and 4, but for the coefficient estimate for the moderator variable (substance use X relative disadvantage) in Model 2. In the results for the listwise deletion comparisons (Figure 5), the coefficient values are relatively stable across the different data subsets, but the coefficient for the 50% data subset changes in significance from $p < 0.005$ to $p < 0.01$ and, notably, the confidence intervals are substantially larger due to the substantial reduction in sample size.

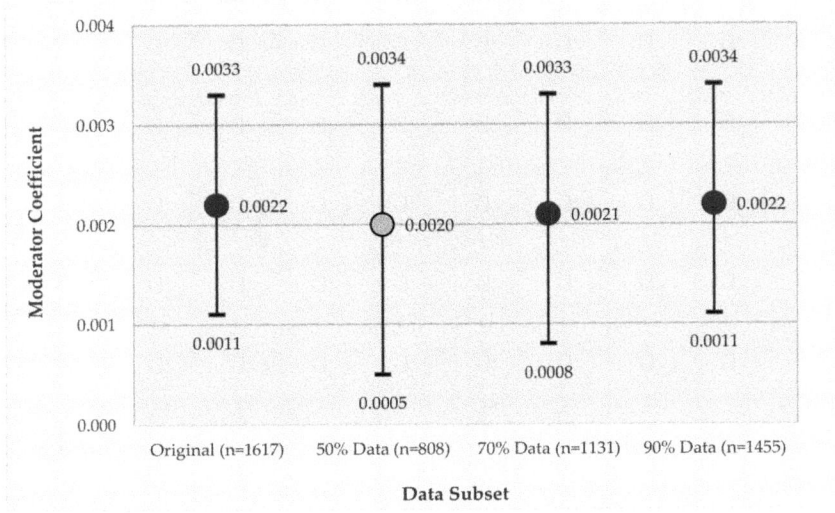

Figure 5. Results for the listwise deletion data sets for Model 2, GEE coefficients of the effect of the moderator variable (relative disadvantage X substance use) on momentary stress. Coefficients are reported for the original data set (100% retained) and for each data subset—50% retained, 70% retained, and 90% retained subsets of the original data set. Circle markers represent coefficient values; whiskers represent 95% confidence intervals. Marker fill indicates coefficient significance, where dark gray is $p < 0.005$ and light gray is $p < 0.01$.

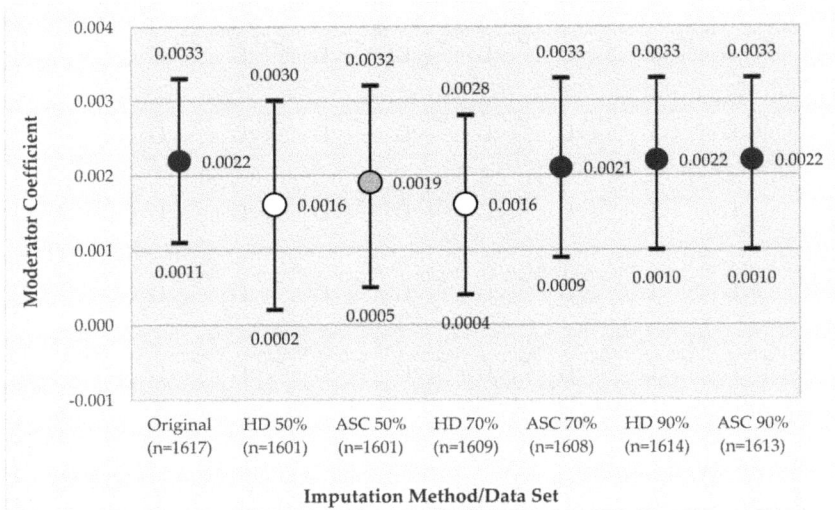

Figure 6. Results for the imputed data for Model 2, GEE coefficients of the effect of the moderator variable (relative disadvantage X substance use) on momentary stress. Coefficients are reported for the original data set (100% retained) and for each combination of imputation technique (hot deck (HD) or activity space centroid (ASC)) applied to different percentage retained data sets (50% retained (50% imputed), 70% retained (30% imputed), and 90% retained (10% imputed)). Circle markers represent coefficient values; whiskers represent 95% confidence intervals. Marker fill indicates coefficient significance, where dark gray is $p < 0.005$, light gray is $p < 0.01$, and white is $p < 0.05$.

In Figure 6, which compares results across the six different imputed data sets, substantial differences are observed. The coefficient significance is reduced to $p < 0.05$ for the 50% retained and 70% retained HD imputed data sets, and to $p < 0.01$ for the 50% retained ASC imputed data set due to the wider confidence intervals. For both the 50% and 70% retained data sets, the ASC imputed coefficient value is nearer to the original coefficient value as compared to the HD imputation. When only 10% of the data are missing, both imputation methods recover the estimate and its variability from the original data.

4. Discussion

To the best of our knowledge, this research represents the first study to develop and compare methods for geographic imputation of missing activity space data derived from GEMA. While we consider this a pilot study that implements relatively simple imputation techniques on a single empirical data set, this research provides a proof of concept for how geographic imputation methods can be adapted for GEMA activity space data and other activity space data generated from similar study designs. Our results suggest that geographic imputation can be used effectively to estimate the location of missing GEMA activity space data in studies of place effects on health.

In our analyses, we found that listwise deletion of missing activity space data, particularly at levels of 50% and 30% missing data, can bias estimates of place effects on health, in the present case, the effect of relative disadvantage on momentary stress. Listwise deletion changed the magnitude, significance, and/or standard errors of the relative disadvantage coefficient, particularly for 50% missingness and when estimating the significance and standard errors of the moderated effect. These impacts were ameliorated to some extent by using geographic imputation, particularly in mitigating the inflation of the standard errors, though results were more variable regarding the moderation effects. We found that ASC imputation generally outperformed HD imputation, though the difference was relatively modest.

We acknowledge several limitations. Our analysis focused on a single empirical GEMA data set gathered from a study of neighborhood disadvantage, substance use, and psychological stress among a sample of urban adolescents. The generalizability of our findings to other data sets and analytical contexts is unknown. We also used only one random draw to distinguish between retained and deleted observations to test our imputation methods. A more robust approach would repeat the analysis multiple times using different randomly drawn retained and deleted observations. Further, we note that our description focuses on the imputation of the census tracts that contain the missing EMA locations, rather than the imputed activity space points themselves. However, this is for the purpose of testing the effects of imputation on the regression models; the HD and ASC imputation methods could just as easily be used to estimate the missing EMA locations at the point level by selecting the coordinate positions from the known EMA locations rather than the tract identifier.

We also acknowledge that there may be bias regarding which observations are missing. Many simple imputation procedures, including the ones developed in the present research, are themselves susceptible to bias when observations are not missing completely at random (MCAR) or missing at random (MAR) [48]. While this issue is germane to any study employing survey data, it is likely to be particularly problematic in GEMA, where individuals may be hesitant to reveal their location in studies of sensitive health behaviors, such as substance use or sexual behavior [50,51]. Indeed, individuals may purposively hide their location in certain situations. We should also note that the original EMA data contains extensive missing data; thus, the data set used to test the sensitivity of the listwise deletion and geographic imputation methods is itself potentially prone to these same issues of missing data.

It is also possible that missing location data may occur more often in certain environments, such as densely developed urban areas or indoors, where the GPS signal is more likely to be physically blocked. Notably, the limited research on this topic, including our own, has not found any substantial associations between the demographic characteristics of the subject or the environmental conditions of the location of data capture with the spatial accuracy or missingness of the EMA location data [21,42], though further research is certainly warranted. In future geographic imputation research, it may be useful to stratify the deleted observations by the environmental characteristics (e.g., by land use or degree of urbanization) of where the EMA location occurs, to investigate consequences of excluding EMA locations from certain types of environments.

The HD and ASC geographic imputation methods we developed for this pilot study are relatively simple and may be improved. First, the methods are 'fixed' or deterministic in the sense that they assign a single location to all missing activity space observations for each subject. This has the result of clustering all missing data at one location for each subject. One could introduce a stochastic element to geographic imputation [34,37,40], where, for instance, for each of a subject's missing activity space locations, the HD imputation would randomly draw a new imputed location from the subject's set of known locations, rather than 'reuse' a single imputed location. With this approach, locations visited more often would be more likely to be selected. Or, for the ASC imputation, instead of estimating all of a subject's missing activity space locations to occur at the centroid of the known EMA locations, one could model the likelihood of the missing location occurring at a given location as a function of the distance to the centroid, generating a point cloud of estimated locations for missing activity space data dispersed around the centroid. This may address the issue of the centroid occurring in a tract outside the sample of known EMA locations. It may also be useful to exclude subjects with low numbers of known EMA locations to begin with, for instance, those subjects with less than five known EMA locations, thus ensuring an adequate sample of locations from which to base the imputation.

The geographic imputation methods described here could also be extended to model-based and multiple imputation approaches [30–33]. For example, a regression equation could be developed for each subject that estimates the likelihood that a particular tract (or other spatial encoding) contains a missing activity space point based on the distance of the tract to the subject's home, the age and sex of the subject, and other characteristics of the individual. It may also be useful to incorporate the temporal component of the EMA data, such as the time of day or day of the week that the EMA response occurred, as the daily and weekly rhythms of life make it more likely for individuals to travel to certain locations on, say, weekdays versus weekends or mornings versus evenings. Such a model could also be improved by incorporating spatial and temporal dasymetric methods [52], where spatial partitions, such as land use or neighborhood socioeconomic characteristics, and temporal partitions, such as weekday/weekend divisions, can be used to further refine the model, as has been used with spatial data in previous geographic imputations of residential addresses [34,41,42]. This approach would yield a surface of the spatial distribution of the likelihood of a particular missing activity space location occurring, which could be used to stochastically generate a set of imputed values for each missing activity space location, which could in turn be used to generate a distribution of model coefficients that could then be pooled, as in conventional multiple imputation.

5. Conclusions

Health researchers utilizing GEMA or related approaches to collecting activity space data should be aware of the issue of missing location data and its impact on statistical analyses of place effects on health behaviors and outcomes. Geographic imputation can be used to estimate missing activity space locations and thus maintain statistical power and reduce bias in estimates of coefficients and standard errors in models of direct and moderated effects. The present pilot study provides an empirical example of both the impact of listwise deletion on analytical results and the implementation of two simple geographic imputation techniques adapted for GEMA activity space data. These geographic imputation techniques may be extended in future research by incorporating approaches from the non-geographic imputation literature as well as from conventional geographic imputation and spatial interpolation research that focus on non-activity space data.

Author Contributions: Conceptualization, J.M. and M.M.; methodology, J.M., M.M. and D.L.C., and K.H.; formal analysis, J.M.; investigation, M.M and J.M..; resources, M.M.; writing—original draft preparation, J.M.; writing—review and editing, J.M., M.M., D.L.C. and K.H.; visualization, J.M.; project administration, M.M. and J.M; funding acquisition, M.M. and J.M.

Funding: This research was supported by National Institutes of Health (NIH) National Institute on Drug Abuse (NIDA), grant number R01DA031724-06, by NIH National Cancer Institute (NCI) and the Office of Behavioral and Social Science Research (OBSSR), grant number 1R01CA229542-01, and by Temple University. The content is solely the responsibility of the authors and does not necessarily represent the official views of NIH, NIDA, NCI, or OBSSR.

Acknowledgments: Thank you to Mei-Po Kwan for guest editing this special issue and for the invitation to submit this article.

Conflicts of Interest: The authors declare no conflict of interest. The funders had no role in the design of the study; in the collection, analyses, or interpretation of data; in the writing of the manuscript, or in the decision to publish the results.

References

1. Richardson, D.B.; Volkow, N.D.; Kwan, M.-P.; Kaplan, R.M.; Goodchild, M.F.; Croyle, R.T. Spatial turn in health research. *Science* **2013**, *339*, 1390–1392. [CrossRef] [PubMed]

2. Wild, C.P. The exposome: From concept to utility. *Int. J. Epidemiol.* **2012**, *41*, 24–32. [CrossRef] [PubMed]

3. Diez Roux, A.; Mair, C. Neighborhoods and health. *Ann. N. Y. Acad. Sci.* **2010**, *1186*, 125–145. [CrossRef]

4. Browning, C.R.; Soller, B. Moving beyond neighborhood: Activity spaces and ecological networks as contexts for youth development. *Cityscape* **2014**, *16*, 165–196. [PubMed]

5. Kwan, M.-P. The limits of the neighborhood effect: Contextual uncertainties in geographic, environmental, health, and social science research. *Ann. Am. Assoc. Geogr.* **2018**. [CrossRef]

6. Mennis, J.; Yoo, E.-H.E. Geographic information science and the analysis of place and health. *Trans. GIS* **2018**, *22*, 842–854. [CrossRef]

7. Golledge, R.G.; Stimson, R.J. *Spatial Behavior: A Geographic Perspective*; Guilford Press: New York, NY, USA, 1997.

8. Mennis, J.; Mason, M.; Ambrus, A. Urban greenspace is associated with reduced psychological stress among adolescents: A geographic ecological momentary assessment (GEMA) analysis of activity space. *Landsc. Urban Plan.* **2018**, *174*, 1–9. [CrossRef]

9. Mennis, J.; Mason, M.J. People, places, and adolescent substance use: Integrating activity space and social network data for analyzing health behavior. *Ann. Assoc. Am. Geogr.* **2011**, *101*, 272–291. [CrossRef]

10. Zenk, S.N.; Schulz, A.J.; Matthews, S.A.; Odoms-Young, A.; Wilbur, J.; Wegrzyn, L.; Gibbs, K.; Braunschweig, C.; Stokes, C. Activity space environment and dietary and physical activity behaviors: A pilot study. *Health Place* **2011**, *17*, 1150–1161. [CrossRef]

11. Yoo, E.; Rudra, C.; Glasgow, M.; Mu, L. Geospatial estimation of individual exposure to air pollutants: Moving from static monitoring to activity-based dynamic exposure assessment. *Ann. Assoc. Am. Geogr.* **2015**, *105*, 915–926. [CrossRef]

12. Helbich, M.; van Emmichoven, M.J.Z.; Dijst, M.J.; Kwan, M.-P.; Pierik, F.H.; de Vries, S.I. Natural and built environmental exposures on children's active school travel: A Dutch global positioning system-based cross-sectional study. *Health Place* **2016**, *39*, 101–109. [CrossRef] [PubMed]

13. Stahler, G.J.; Mennis, J.; Baron, D. Geospatial technology and the exposome: New perspectives on addiction. *Am. J. Public Health* **2013**, *103*, 1354–1356. [CrossRef] [PubMed]

14. Kwan, M.-K. GIS methods in time-geographic research: Geocomputation and geovisualization of human activity patterns. *Geogr. Ann. Ser. B Hum. Geogr.* **2005**, *86*, 267–280. [CrossRef]

15. Shiffman, S.; Stone, A.A.; Hufford, M.R. Ecological momentary assessment. *Ann. Rev. Clin. Psychol.* **2008**, *4*, 1–32. [CrossRef]

16. Kirchner, T.R.; Shiffman, S. Spatio-temporal determinants of mental health and well-being: Advances in geographically-explicit ecological momentary assessment (GEMA). *Soc. Psychiatry Psychiatr. Epidemiol.* **2016**, *51*, 1211–1223. [CrossRef] [PubMed]

17. Mennis, J.M.; Mason, M.; Light, J.; Rusby, J.; Westling, E.; Way, T.; Zharakis, N.; Flay, B. Does substance use moderate the association of neighborhood disadvantage with perceived stress and safety in the activity spaces of urban youth. *Drug Alcohol Depend.* **2016**, *165*, 288–292. [CrossRef] [PubMed]

18. Epstein, D.H.; Tyburski, M.; Craig, I.M.; Phillips, K.A.; Jobes, M.L.; Vahabzadeh, M.; Mezghanni, M.; Lin, J.-L.; Furr-Holden, C.D.M.; Preston, K.L. Real-time tracking of neighborhood surroundings and mood in urban drug misusers: Application of a new method to study behavior in its geographical context. *Drug Alcohol Depend.* **2014**, *134*, 22–29. [CrossRef]

19. Freisthler, B.; Lipperman-Kreda, S.; Bersamin, M.; Gruenewald, P.J. Tracking the when, where, and with whom of alcohol use: Integrating ecological momentary assessment and geospatial data to examine risk for alcohol-related problems. *Alcohol Res. Curr. Rev.* **2014**, *36*, 29–38.

20. Mcquoid, J.; Thrul, J.; Ling, P. A geographically explicit ecological momentary assessment (GEMA) mixed method for understanding substance use. *Soc. Sci. Med.* **2018**, *202*, 89–98. [CrossRef]

21. Mennis, J.; Mason, M.J.; Ambrus, A.; Way, T.; Henry, K. The spatial accuracy of geographic ecological momentary assessment (GEMA): Error and bias due to subject and environmental characteristics. *Drug Alcohol Depend.* **2017**, *178*, 188–193. [CrossRef]

22. Zandbergen, P.A.; Barbeau, S.J. Positional accuracy of assisted GPS data from high sensitivity GPS-enabled mobile phones. *J. Navig.* **2011**, *64*, 381–399. [CrossRef]

23. Watkins, K.L.; Regan, S.D.; Nguyen, N.; Businelle, M.S.; Kendzor, D.E.; Lam, C.; Balis, D.; Cuevas, A.G.; Cao, Y.; Reitzel, L.R. Advancing cessation research by integrating EMA and geospatial methodologies: Associations between tobacco retail outlets and real-time smoking urges during a quit attempt. *Nicot. Tob. Res.* **2014**, *16*, S93–S101. [CrossRef] [PubMed]

24. Birhrmann, K.; Ersboll, A.K. Estimating range of influence in case of missing spatial data: A simulation study on binary data. *Int. J. Health Geogr.* **2015**, *14*, 1. [CrossRef] [PubMed]

25. Reich, B.J.; Chang, H.H.; Strickland, M.J. Spatial health effects analysis with uncertain residential locations. *Stat. Methods Med. Res.* **2014**, *23*, 156–168. [CrossRef] [PubMed]

26. Oliver, M.N.; Matthews, K.A.; Siadaty, M.; Hauck, F.R.; Pickle, L.W. Geographic bias related to geocoding in epidemiologic studies. *Int. J. Health Geogr.* **2005**, *4*, 29. [CrossRef] [PubMed]

27. Zhang, Z.; Manjourides, J.; Cohen, T.; Hu, Y.; Jiang, Q. Spatial measurement errors in the field of spatial epidemiology. *Int. J. Health Geogr.* **2016**, *15*, 21. [CrossRef] [PubMed]

28. Pigott, T.D. A review of methods for missing data. *Educ. Res. Eval.* **2001**, *7*, 353–383. [CrossRef]

29. Peugh, J.L.; Enders, C.K. Missing data in educational research: A review of reporting practices and suggestions for improvement. *Rev. Educ. Res.* **2004**, *74*, 525–556. [CrossRef]

30. Graham, J.W. Missing data analysis: Making it work in the real world. *Ann. Rev. Psychol.* **2009**, *60*, 549–576. [CrossRef]

31. Little, R.J.A.; Rubin, D.B. *Statistical Analysis with Missing Data*, 2nd ed.; Wiley: London, UK, 2002.

32. Carpenter, J.; Kenward, M. *Multiple Imputation and its Application*; Wiley: London, UK, 2013.

33. Rezvan, P.H.; Lee, K.J.; Simpson, J.A. The rise of multiple imputation: A review of the reporting and implementation of the method in medical research. *BMC Med. Res. Methodol.* **2015**, *15*, 30. [CrossRef]

34. Henry, K.A.; Boscoe, F.P. Estimating the accuracy of geographical imputation. *Int. J. Health Geogr.* **2008**, *7*, 3. [CrossRef] [PubMed]

35. Goldberg, D.W. *A Geocoding Best Practices Guide*; The North American Association of Central Cancer Registries: Springfield, IL, USA, 2008.

36. Boscoe, F.P. The science and art of geocoding: Tips for improving match rates and handling unmatched cases in analysis. In *Geocoding Health Data*; Rushton, G., Armstrong, M.P., Gittler, J., Greene, B.R., Pavlik, C.E., West, M.M., Zimmerman, D.L., Eds.; CRC Press: New York, NY, USA, 2008; pp. 95–110.

37. Zimmerman, D.L. Statistical methods for incompletely and incorrectly geocoded cancer data. In *Geocoding Health Data*; Rushton, G., Armstrong, M.P., Gittler, J., Greene, B.R., Pavlik, C.E., West, M.M., Zimmerman, D.L., Eds.; CRC Press: New York, NY, USA, 2008; pp. 165–180.

38. Walter, S.R.; Rose, N. Random property allocation: A novel geographic imputation procedure based on a complete geocoded address file. *Spat. Spatio-Temporal Epidemiol.* **2013**, *6*, 7–16. [CrossRef]

39. Bocci, C.; Rocco, E. Estimates for geographical domains through geoadditive models in presence of incomplete geographical information. *Stat. Methods Appl.* **2014**, *23*, 283–305. [CrossRef]

40. Hibbert, J.D.; Liese, A.D.; Lawson, A.; Porter, D.E.; Puett, R.C.; Standiford, D.; Liu, L.; Dabelea, D. Evaluating geographic imputation approaches for zip code level data: An application to a study of pediatric diabetes. *Int. J. Health Geogr.* **2009**, *8*, 54. [CrossRef] [PubMed]

41. Curriero, F.C.; Kulldorff, M.; Boscoe, F.P.; Klassen, A.C. Using imputation to provide location information for nongeocoded addresses. *PLoS ONE* **2010**, *5*, e8998. [CrossRef]

42. Zhang, Y.; Yang, T.-C.; Matthews, S.A. Inferring censored geo-information with non-representative data. In *Machine Learning and Data Mining in Pattern Recognition*; Perner, P., Ed.; Springer: Basel, Switzerland, 2016; Volume 9729, pp. 229–235, ISBN 978-3-319-41919-0.

43. Meseck, K.; Jankowska, M.M.; Schipperijn, J.; Natarajan, L.; Godbole, S.; Carson, J.; Temoto, M.; Crist, K.; Kerr, J. Is missing geographic positioning system data in accelerometry studies a problem, and is imputation the solution? *Geospat. Health* **2016**, *11*, 403. [CrossRef] [PubMed]

44. Mason, M.J.; Mennis, J.; Light, J.; Rusby, J.; Westling, E.; Crewe, S.; Way, T.; Flay, B.; Zaharakis, N.M. Parents, peers, and places: Young urban adolescents' microsystems and substance use involvement. *J. Child Fam. Stud.* **2016**, *25*, 1441–1450. [CrossRef] [PubMed]

45. Mason, M.; Light, J.; Mennis, J.; Rusby, J.; Westling, E.; Way, T.; Zaharakis, N.; Flay, B. Neighborhood disorder, peer network health, and substance use among young urban adolescents. *Drug Alcohol Depend.* **2017**, *178*, 208–214. [CrossRef] [PubMed]

46. Moberg, D.P.; Hahn, L. The adolescent drug involvement scale. *J. Adolesc. Chem. Depend.* **1991**, *2*, 75–88. [CrossRef]

47. Ross, C.E.; Mirowsky, J. Neighborhood disadvantage, neighborhood disorder and health. *J. Health Sociol. Behav.* **2001**, *42*, 258–276. [CrossRef]

48. Rubin, D.B. Inference and missing data. *Biometrika* **1976**, *63*, 581–592. [CrossRef]

49. Andridge, R.R.; Little, R.J.A. A review of hot deck imputation for survey non-response. *Int. Stat. Rev.* **2010**, *78*, 40–64. [CrossRef] [PubMed]

50. Rudolph, A.E.; Bazzi, A.R.; Fish, S. Ethical considerations and potential threats to validity for three methods commonly used to collect geographic information in studies among people who use drugs. *Addict. Behav.* **2016**, *61*, 84–90. [CrossRef] [PubMed]

51. Rudolph, A.E.; Young, A.M.; Havens, J.R. Privacy, confidentiality, and safety considerations for conducting geographic momentary assessment studies among persons who use drugs and men who have sex with men. *J. Urban Health* **2018**. [CrossRef] [PubMed]

52. Mennis, J. Dasymetric spatiotemporal interpolation. *Prof. Geogr.* **2016**, *68*, 92–102. [CrossRef]

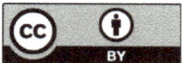

International Journal of
**Environmental Research
and Public Health**

MDPI

Article

Environmental, Individual and Personal Goal Influences on Older Adults' Walking in the Helsinki Metropolitan Area

Tiina E. Laatikainen [1],*, Mohammad Haybatollahi [2] and Marketta Kyttä [1]

[1]   Department of Built Environment, Aalto University, P.O. BOX. 14400, 00076 Aalto, Finland;
      marketta.kytta@aalto.fi
[2]   Department of Public Health, University of Helsinki, 00014 Helsinki, Finland;
      mohammad.haybatollahi@helsinki.fi
*   Correspondence: tiina.laatikainen@aalto.fi

Received: 13 November 2018; Accepted: 21 December 2018; Published: 26 December 2018

Abstract: Physical activity is a fundamental factor in healthy ageing, and the built environment has been linked to individual health outcomes. Understanding the linkages between older adult's walking and the built environment are key to designing supportive environments for active ageing. However, the variety of different spatial scales of human mobility has been largely overlooked in the environmental health research. This study used an online participatory mapping method and a novel modelling of individual activity spaces to study the associations between both the environmental and the individual features and older adults' walking in the environments where older adult's actually move around. Study participants ($n = 844$) aged 55+ who live in Helsinki Metropolitan Area, Finland reported their everyday errand points on a map and indicated which transport mode they used and how frequently they accessed the places. Respondents walking trips were drawn from the data and the direct and indirect effects of the personal, psychological as well as environmental features on older adults walking were examined. Respondents marked on average, six everyday errand points and walked for transport an average of 20 km per month. Residential density and the density of walkways, public transit stops, intersections and recreational sports places were significantly and positively associated with older adult's walking for transport. Transit stop density was found having the largest direct effect to older adults walking. Built environment had an independent effect on older adults walking regardless of individual demographic or psychological features. Education and personal goals related to physical activities had a direct positive, and income a direct negative, effect on walking. Gender and perceived health had an indirect effect on walking, which was realized through individuals' physical activity goals.

Keywords: walking; active travel; ageing; physical environment; personal projects; activity space; Public Participatory GIS (PPGIS)

---

1. Introduction

Extensive evidence exists that physical activity (PA) has notable health benefits for older adults [1–4]. In addition, maintaining mobility—one's ability to move around and take care of everyday activities—is a fundamental factor in healthy aging [5,6]. Research has also shown that active travel (AT), namely walking and cycling, has health benefits across population even after adjustment for other forms of PA [7]. In their recent review, Cerin and colleagues [8] found strong links between the neighborhood physical environment and older adults' AT. Thus, it is of prime importance to ensure that older adults can sustain mobility in their everyday environments.

According to the ecological models of health behavior [9,10] multiple levels of factors influence human health behavior, often including intrapersonal, interpersonal, organizational, community, physical environmental, and policy. These factors work together and influences interact across different levels, meaning that individuals with high motivation for sports might react differently to new bike lanes implemented to their neighborhood than those who are not very interested in sports living in the same area [11]. According to Sallis and Owen [11] studies with multilevel approach should explain health behaviors better than studies that focus only on single level. Despite this notion, previous research has concentrated mainly on identifying either individual or physical environmental factors related to PA in general or to some specific domain of PA in particular.

Research focusing on the associations between individual factors and PA have found a host of individual characteristics associated with older adults' PA [12–14]. Aside from the individual demographic factors, a few studies have examined the associations between PA and intrapersonal factors, such as motivation and self-efficacy [14–17]. Studies examining associations between individual goal setting and PA conclude that having specific health- and PA-related goals is an important component to increasing exercise and PA in older adults [18–20].

Besides studying actual health related goal setting, researchers have studied the interactions between general personal goals, health and PA [21–26]. Personal goals, often referred also as personal projects, are defined as intentions that describe motivational features behind people's actions or states people strive to achieve or avoid in the future [23,24,27,28]. Older adults' personal goals related to physical activity and cultural functions have been found associated with high exercise activity [23]. According to Little et al. [28] personal projects as analytical units are nested within a larger social ecological framework for personality and developmental science. The social ecological model by Little et al. [28] proposes, rather similarly to the ecological model of health behavior [11], that both personal features as well as environmental features have direct effects as well as indirect influences through personal projects to the outcome measures such as the physical well-being. A few studies have used the social ecological model or the concept of personal goals to explore what features support or hinder PA [22,25]. However, in their systematic review Notthoff and colleagues [14] concluded that studies examining associations between older adults' intrapersonal factors, such as motivational goals or self-efficacy, and PA are still rather scarce.

Research that focuses simply on the individual influences on PA have been criticized for failing to acknowledge the context where the behavior actually takes place [10,29]. However, the past decade has introduced a growing number of studies that examine the influences of the physical environment on PA [30,31]. Most studies have examined the associations between the neighborhood built and natural environments and health of older adults [32–36]. According to these studies, walkability, connectivity, density, mixed land-use, green and water environments, and closeness to home of everyday destinations are important characteristics of the environments that support healthy aging [6,32,37,38].

However, most of these studies focus simply on the physical environmental factors in the immediate home vicinity and their associations with PA by analyzing the built environment features around individuals' residences or neighborhoods that have been delineated through administrative units or residential buffers with varying radii and buffering methods [39]. Analyses of people's everyday mobility behavior and exposure outside their residential neighborhoods have been problematic, leading to flawed interpretations about the health impacts of physical environmental factors [39–41]. Also, according to Blacksher and Lovasi [42] there is a lack of research that recognizes that the effect of physical environment on health is subject to human perception.

In this paper we aim to address the gap in research that focuses on the multiple-level influences of health behaviors and examine how multiple levels of factors influence older adults AT. While some individual features, such as gender, motivation and particular PA-related goals [14,19], and on the other hand certain environmental features [8,43] have shown influencing PA among older adults, these features have not been widely studied simultaneously and context-sensitively according to the principals of ecological models [11]. While it is well acknowledged that environmental context can shape or constrain individual determinants of health behavior, there have not been many studies examining the multifaceted influences of the environment and the individual on PA. This is especially true for outside the administrative or residential neighborhoods, perhaps due to considerable methodological challenges [10].

Participatory mapping methods, such as Public Participation Geographic Information System (PPGIS), have offered convenient tools for previous studies investigating the active two-way person-environment relationship [44–47]. Localization of human experiences and behavioral patterns by advanced public participatory mapping tools attaches them to a specific physical environmental context [48]. Thus, the human behavior and experiences get geographic coordinates, which allows simultaneous GIS-based analysis of human behavior in relation to the physical environment [49]. These kinds of spatial studies on human health behavior has proven effective and the usage of GPS tracking or map-based questionnaires have provided a way to overcome the identified contextual challenges, and improved our understanding about the mechanisms that connect place to health [39,50].

In this study, we examined the individual and physical environmental features that influence older adults' AT within their everyday environments, including the environment also outside their immediate home vicinity. We examined the AT as older adults' walking for transport, given the known health benefits and popularity of this particular travel mode among older adults [6,8,51]. We examined the walking of older adults who live in the capital region of Helsinki, Finland and focused on defining how and which of the environmental and individual factors direct their walking.

Previous studies adopting the principles of ecological models have had methodological challenges developing and collecting measures of influences at multiple levels and capturing the complex interactions of individual and physical environmental characteristics [11]. In addition, previous studies on physical environment and health has mainly focused on neighborhood environments, overlooking people's mobility behavior in non-residential locations [39,40]. To overcome the identified challenges, we used an online participatory mapping method and a novel modelling of individual activity spaces in this study, which enabled us to study simultaneously and context-sensitively the associations between both the individual and the environmental features and older adults' walking in the environments where they actually move around.

2. Materials and Methods

2.1. Study Area

The Helsinki Metropolitan Area (HMA) consists of four independent city units, Espoo, Helsinki, Kauniainen and Vantaa. Helsinki is the capital of Finland and forms with its surrounding three cities the HMA region. Finland and its capital region is an interesting and topical case study site due to the rapid population ageing in the country. The share of Finnish people over 65 years old is currently 21.4 percent and is estimated to be 26.4 percent of the population by 2030 and 28.7 percent by 2050 [52]. The ageing phenomena in Helsinki is currently still moderate compared to the whole country. At the beginning of 2018 there were about 25 65-years-olds per 100 working age adults in Helsinki whereas the numbers were 36 per 100 in the whole country. However, the amount 65-years-olds has increased 46 percent in Helsinki during the last decade, whereas the amount general population has increased only 17 percent [53]. GDP per capita (PPS) in HMA was 52.021 € in 2015 [54] and the region is characterized with good public transit connections and accessibility [55]. The pedestrian environment in HMA is generally good. Most of the arterial, collector as well as local roads have separated sidewalks. Sidewalks in the central areas are separated from the bicycle lanes, but in suburban areas, sidewalks are mainly shared between pedestrians and bicyclists. Pedestrian crossings are frequent both in the central urban areas as well as in the suburban areas. Signalled crosswalks are also common, but signals do not show minutes for walking. During winter most of the walkways, including sidewalks, separate pedestrian-only streets, sidewalks shared between pedestrian and bicyclists and common trails are routinely plough and gritted excluding some forest trails and jogging routes.

2.2. Participatory Mapping Method

Data were collected using an online participatory mapping method, PPGIS, which combines internet maps with traditional questionnaires [49]. PPGIS methods were developed for the purposes of both research and participatory planning practice to collect spatial experiential knowledge and to engage non-experts to identify the spatial dimensions of the environment [49]. In our study, respondents used an online interface to mark their (1) everyday errand points (EEPs) on a map (Figure 1). In addition, the respondents indicated which (2) transport mode they used and how (3) frequently they accessed the EEPs. The respondents were asked to mark on a map their (4) home and answer questions related to (5) their personal characteristics, such as their sociodemographic background and perceived health as well as (6) personal psychological features, namely respondents' personal goals.

With this place-based mapping method, we were able to study older adults' travel behavior spatially and context-sensitively by asking respondents to pinpoint their everyday behavior on the map. The respondents' individual characteristics were studied simultaneously with the physical environment by asking them to describe their sociodemographic background and to evaluate the importance of a series of personal goals. Localization of human behavioral patterns by participatory mapping tools attaches them to specific physical environmental context [48]. This way human behavior and experiences receive geographic coordinates, which allows simultaneous GIS-based analysis of human behavior in relation to the physical environment (Figure 1).

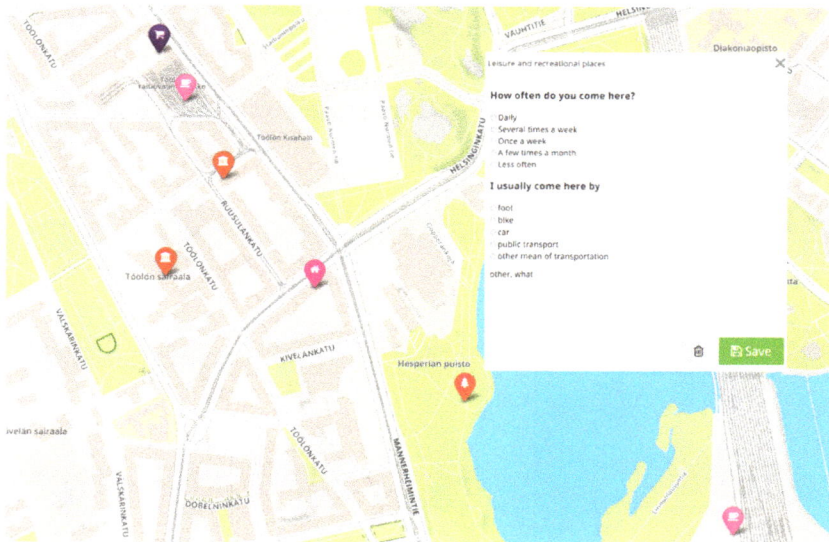

Figure 1. The online interface of the survey.

2.3. Home Range Model Capturing the Walking Behavior

Previous studies interested in the relationship between the built environment and human health, have mainly used static spatial units of analysis to capture the GIS-based physical environmental variables [56]. Administrative boundaries, postal code areas and census tracts are examples of static and simple spatial units of analysis to capture the environmental context. More developed spatial units of analysis are buffers, spherical or network, that are created around individual home locations of study participants [57,58]. All such approaches presume that individual health behavior is bound to static neighborhood boundaries or certain buffered distances around their home. These approaches have been criticized for being too static and not accounting for actual individual differences in mobility exterior to the place of residence since they tend to ignore individual's true spatio-temporal behavior [39,40,56,59,60]. Recently, researchers have proposed alternative modeling approaches that correspond more to individual activity patterns and are more adaptive in their boundaries and structure [56,60].

In this study we took a step forward from the static approaches for capturing the contextual effects related to older adults' active travel. Thus, we applied a dynamic model of home ranges developed by Hasanzadeh and colleagues [56]. The home range model is an individual-specific dynamic boundary method which take into account the individual-specific variations of home ranges, also referred to as activity spaces [56,60]. The model of home ranges is also parametric, meaning that it can be applied for different purposes and studies by specifying its parameters for each individual study purpose (more detailed description of the model parameters in [56]). The model uses customized minimum convex polygons created around individuals' home and everyday errand points to capture individuals' neighborhoods instead of plain static administrative boundaries or spherical buffers only around individuals' homes (Figure 2). In their recent study Laatikainen and colleagues [39] compared different neighborhood and activity space models to capture the physical environment. They found that novel activity space models such as the home range (HR) are in many cases more suitable approaches than static measures like buffers for measuring the physical environment and the activities of individuals and, thus, capturing individual environmental exposure. In their study Laatikainen et al. [39] found that walkability of individual home ranges was positively correlated with perceived wellbeing of older adults but warranted for more studies to investigate how the walkability of the home range is associated with AT. Thus, the home range model was applied in this study to capture the activity spaces of older adults and to study how the physical environment outside plain residential areas affect older adults walking. The home range (HR) was modelled for each respondent and the physical environment features within the HR's was calculated for each individual (Figure 2).

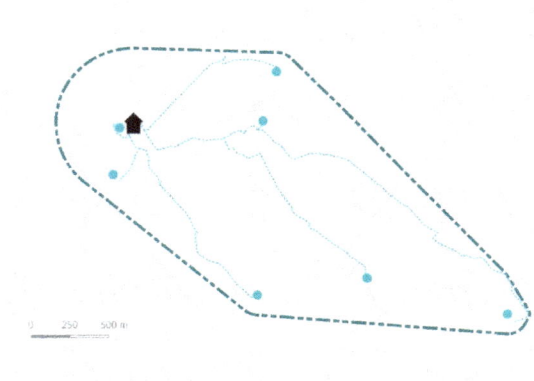

Figure 2. An example of an individual home range and active travel routes of a respondent.

2.4. Conceptual Framework and Hypotheses

Previous studies have examined the associations between both the individual and the environmental factors and PA, or more specifically the active travel behavior of older adults, concluding that multiple levels of factors affect the PA behaviour [8,11,14]. Following the principles of the ecological models of health behavior [11] and the social ecological model of Little [61] the conceptual framework for this study focuses on the impacts of the personal characteristics, environmental features and personal psychological features on AT of older adults (Figure 3). The framework illustrates the interactions among personal characteristics, different environmental features and personal goals on AT of older adults. The framework proposes that the personal characteristics, the environmental features as well as the psychological features, namely the personal goals, have direct effects, but that there are also indirect influences through personal psychological factors to the AT behavior of older adults. Thus, following the social ecological framework proposed by Little [61] we hypothesize that personal goals serve as mediating conduit through which different personal and environmental features influence the walking behavior of older adults (H4 and H5). In addition, we tested the direct modelling hypothesis by evaluating the direct relationship between the personal characteristics (H1), psychological features (H2) and environmental features (H3) and walking.

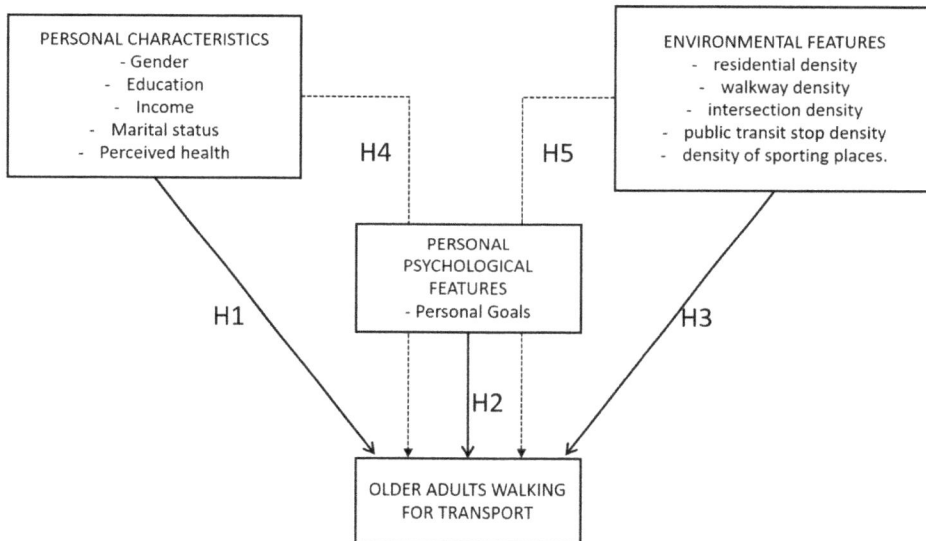

Figure 3. The conceptual framework.

2.5. Participants

A random sample of 5000 residents of the Helsinki Metropolitan Area (HMA) aged between 55 and 75 received an invitation letter by mail asking them to participate in an online mapping survey. A total of 1,139 full or partial responses were received, and after removing incomplete responses, 844 were taken for further analysis. Participants consisted of 447 women and 331 men with a mean age of 64.3 (SD = 5.52). The data showed general consistency on most sociodemographic variables within the study region (Table 1). The data was collected during early fall 2015. All subjects were informed about the study and its content in a letter inviting them to participate in the online survey. By participating in the survey all participants gave their consent for inclusion. The Research Ethics Committee of Aalto University approved the study protocol.

Table 1. The sociodemographic factors of respondents (*n* = 844).

Variable	Sample (%)	Statistics Finland (%) *
Gender		
Male	43	45
Female	57	55
Education [a]		
Basic education	12	40
Upper secondary education	42	33
Lower university degree	15	11
Higher university degree	31	17
Age		
55–64	52	55
65–74	48	45
Housing		
Apartment	59	70
Detached/row house	41	30
Retired	60	59
Income (median) [b]		
Ages 55–64	3501–4000	4001–4500
Ages 65–74	3001–3500	3001–3500

* The sample consists of Finnish people living in the capital area, aged 55–75, in 2015 (a and b exceptions).
[a] The reference sample consists of Finnish people living in the capital area, aged 55+, in 2014. [b] The reference sample consists of all Finnish people aged 55–75 in 2014.

2.6. Measures

Walking for transport. A dependent variable of walking was developed using the collected PPGIS data. The measure consisted of the EEP locations marked by participants with corresponding travel mode, frequency of visitation, and a network distance from place of residence to the location. In the survey respondents reported modes of traveling as walking, cycling, driving, or using public transit. Frequency of visitation was reported as daily, several times per week, several times per month, a few times per month, and less than monthly. Distances between home and visited places were calculated as the network distance between the home locations of each respondent and their EEPs (Figure 2). Each distance was weighted based on the frequency of visits per month (daily = 25, several times per week = 12, several times per month = 5, a few times per month = 3, less than monthly = 1). We excluded two days per week for the daily option to be equivalent to the weights of the home range model used in this study, where home is given a monthly visitation value of 30 [56]. Each calculated distance that was traveled by walking was categorized as walking and distances travelled by cycling, public transit or private car were omitted for this study. The final dependent variable was calculated as total monthly walking and is referred to walking hereafter.

Personal characteristics. To study the association between personal characteristics and walking, we analyzed respondents' individual demographic characteristics such as gender, education, income, marital status and perceived health. These particular variables were chosen because they have been linked to older adults PA behavior in previous research [14].

Personal goals. We analyzed respondents' personal goals in order to study the both the direct and indirect associations of older adults' intrapersonal psychological factors on walking. The personal goals were measured by means of 19 individualized states formulated based on previous extensive literature on older adults' personal goals [21,22,24,28,61–64]. In the survey, respondents were asked to rank the importance of the personal goals using a seven-point Likert scale that ranged from 0 (not important) to 6 (very important). The goals are listed hereafter in data analysis and Table 2.

Table 2. Explanatory factor analysis.

Items	Factors			
	1. PA and Sports	2. Caring for Others	3. Manage on One's Own	4. Culture and Social Affairs
Variance explained (%)	33	10	10	9
Everyday physical activities (e.g., walking, biking)	0.834			
Sports or dance hobby	0.682			
Maintaining health and functional capacity of the body	0.501		0.380	
Health and wellbeing of others		0.794		
Taking care of relatives		0.696		
Relationships		0.503		
Independent living, the preservation of an independent lifestyle			0.530	
Managing own financial issues and/or assets			0.505	
Maintaining memory capacities			0.486	
Cultural activities				0.627
Politics and social affairs			0.429	0.444
Social activities (i.e., clubs, voluntary work)				0.381

Note: Extraction Method: Principal Axis Factoring. Rotation Method: Promax with Kaiser Normalization.

Physical environment features. GIS-based variables were used to study the physical environment in relation to respondents' walking [6,57,65]. In their recent review Cerin and colleagues [8] concluded that older adults' AT was strongly positively associated with neighborhood walkability. Other previous studies have found PA in general and AT in particular positively associated with residential density, connectivity and density of destinations [6,31,66]. Instead of using the common walkability index [67], we calculated separate physical environment density measures to assess the walkability of the home ranges. This was due to high correlations between the measures of walkability index as well as between the walkability index and the size of the home range. Earlier studies have also highlighted the issues related to modifiable areal unit problem (MAUP) and to multicollinearity issues in the data [68,69]. In addition, using the land-use mix, an integral part of the walkability index, together with rather small spatial units has been found challenging also elsewhere [70]. Thus the following physical environment features were included in the study and calculated as follows:

Walkway density was assessed as the share of walkable streets within the HR. The walkway measure was calculated as the share of walkways in kilometers within the HR. The walkway dataset was drawn from Open Street Map (OSM) which is open geospatial data produced by a community of mappers. The dataset includes all streets that are meant only for walking but also streets that are shared for walking and bicycle as well as sidewalks that are along the side of a road. The data of OSM is fully open and licensed under the Open Data Commons Open Database License (ODbL) by the OpenStreetMap Foundation (OSMF).

Residential density was calculated as residential floor area divided by residential land use within each HR. The residential density measure was drawn from SeutuCD 2014, a regional dataset provided by Helsinki Region Environmental Services Authority HSY.

The connectivity was operationalized with two different measures: as the share of intersections of three or more road segments per individual home range [67] and as the share of public transit stops [8] within HR. The connectivity measures were drawn from the Digiroad 2017 dataset maintained by the Finnish Transport Agency.

The share of *sporting places* within HR was also calculated. The measure includes all sports facilities, recreation areas and hiking trails. The sporting places were drawn from the LIPAS dataset. LIPAS is developed by the Faculty of Sport and Health Sciences, University of Jyväskylä, in collaboration with the Ministry of Education and Culture, the Association of Finnish Local and Regional Authorities, various authorities of regional administration, municipalities, environmental administration, sports federations and other organisations, and the maintainers of sport facilities.

The physical environment variables were extracted and calculated using the ArcMap 10.5 program (Esri, Redlands, CA, USA). We created individual home ranges for each respondent as by the principles of the home range model [56]. Finally, we calculated all of the above listed physical environment variables within each individual home range.

2.7. Statistical Analysis

In order to investigate the structure underlying the intrapersonal psychological factors of the respondents, an explanatory factor analysis (EFA) with Promax rotation and Kaiser Normalization was conducted for 12 personal goal variables. Due to low correlations with other goal variables, seven personal goals were left out from the final EFA after careful examination of the correlation matrix. These were goals related to working, self-development, managing with diseases, religion, traveling, handcraft hobbies, and diet. After identifying the components, Anderson-Rubin factor scores were estimated for each participant.

Finally, the associations between walking and sociodemographic background characteristics, the physical environment variables, and goal factors were examined using ordinary least squares (OLS) regression. Direct, indirect, and total effect for mediation analysis were estimated using structural equation modeling without latent variable (or multiple regression) that allows the indirect (mediation) effect to be a product of the reduction of the total and direct effects of predictors on the outcome. The data for total walking, walkway and intersection density were positively skewed, thus we transferred these variables using square root transformation because the data contained zero values. The data were checked if they met the basic and specific assumptions of OLS regression analysis. The residuals were normally distributed, and the variability of the total walking was homoscedastic across the predictors. There were, however, high correlations between the physical environment measures, which indicated the existence of a multicollinearity issue if we used these variables together in a single model. Because only one physical environment measure was used in each model, the observed high correlation between the physical environment variables did not pose a multicollinearity issue to the results. IBM SPSS statistics 25 (IBM Corp, Armonk, NY, USA), Mplus version 7.3 (Program Copyright © 1998-2012 Muthén & Muthén) and statistics version 3.3.0 with R studio (RStudio: Integrated Development for R. RStudio, Inc., Boston, MA, USA) were used to perform the statistical analyses.

3. Results

The respondents (n = 788) marked, on average, six everyday errand points on the map in the survey and walked on average 20 kilometers per month (SD = 29.9). The descriptive statistics of all the measures used in the further analysis are presented in Table 3.

Table 3. The descriptive statistics of the variables used in the analysis.

Variable	n	Mean	SD
Total walking [a]	673	3.575	2.775
PA and Sports Goal Factor	693	14.685	3.094
Gender	693	0.431	0.495
Income	693	2.361	1.001
Education	693	2.631	1.045
Marital status	693	0.354	0.547
Perceived overall health	693	0.594	1.909
Walkway density [a]	693	22.318	17.067
Intersection density [a]	693	112.602	40.657
Public transit stop density	693	5.758	7.897
Residential density	693	1.203	3.548
Sporting places density	693	3.645	1.370

[a] Measure was transferred using square root transformation because the data contained zero values.

3.1. Older adults' Personal Goal Factors

An EFA was performed to study the personal goals and their effect on walking alongside the individual and environmental features. After carrying out the EFA analysis, four factors were extracted from the 12 personal goals that explain approximately 62% of the variance (Table 2). Each component was labeled according to their most representative personal goals. As reflected in Table 2, three goals contributed to the first factor. These goals dealt with PA, sports, and health and functional capacity. A high score in this component indicates that the respondent evaluated PA, health, and sports as important personal goals for them. We called this factor "PA and sports." Three goals related to the health of other people, relatives, and social relationships contributed to the second factor. A high score on this component indicates that the respondent evaluated others' health and wellbeing and social relationships as very important personal goals for them. This factor was named "caring for others." Three goals contributed to the third factor. These goals dealt with independent living and the preservation of an independent lifestyle, management of financial issues and/or assets, and maintaining memory capacities. Thus, we labeled the third factor as "manage on one's own". Finally, the last component was labeled "culture and social affairs" because the three goals contributing to this factor were cultural activities, politics, and social affairs and activities such as clubs and voluntary work. Factor loadings for all goal items were rather strong and well above 0.40, excluding social activities (i.e., clubs, voluntary work).

From the four factors, only the factor 1, the PA and sports, was found associated with walking ($\beta = 0.167$, $p < 0.001$). Thus, only the PA and sports goal factor was taken for further analysis.

3.2. Effects of Personal, Psychological and Environmental Features on Older Adults' Walking for Transport

We examined how personal, psychological and environmental features predicted walking behavior in older adults. We tested separate OLS regression models for each of the five density measures. Table 4 presents the standardized beta coefficients of walking predicted by environmental variables after controlling for PA and personal variables. As shown in Table 4, income has a significant negative and education has significant positive associations with walking in all of the five models, thus retaining H1 only partially, as gender, marital status and perceived health have no significant direct associations with walking. PA and sports-related personal goals has significant positive effect on walking, retaining H2 partially. The psychological factors associate positively with older adults' walking behavior (Table 3), but only those related to PA and sports as no other goal factors were found associating with walking for transport. As shown in Table 4, walkway density, intersection density, residential density, public transit stop density and density of sporting places have all significant positive associations with walking, thus retaining H3.

All of the five models resulted with alike outcomes. As shown by Table 4, income and education were found as the only personal characteristics having a direct effect on walking. In all five models, higher monthly income had a negative, but rather weak direct effect on walking, meaning that higher monthly income meant less walking to the everyday errand points. On contrary, higher education status had a positive yet also rather weak direct effect on walking, indicating that the higher the education status the more the respondent walked to access the EEP's (Table 4).

The studied psychological feature, the PA and sports goal factor, was found also having a direct effect on walking in each model, meaning that the higher score for PA and sports goals factor the person had the more they walked (Table 4). The environmental features, namely walkway density, intersection density, residential density, public transit stop density and the density of sporting places within the home range of each individual had all direct effect on walking and the direct effect of all the physical environmental features on walking was positive and quite large (Table 4 and Figure 4).

Table 4. The standardized model results for direct and total indirect effects of predictors on walking via PA and sports goal factor.

Predictors	Physical Environmental Features				
	Walkway Density	Intersection Density	Residential Density	Public Transit Stop Density	Sporting Places Density
	β	β	β	β	β
Gender [a]					
Direct effect [b]	0.002	0.002	−0.002	0.000	0.000
Total indirect effect [c]	−0.037 ***	−0.035 ***	−0.026 ***	−0.032 ***	−0.036 ***
Income					
Direct effect [b]	−0.097 *	−0.097 *	−0.080 *	−0.088 *	−0.107 *
Total indirect effect [c]	0.010	0.010	0.008	0.009	0.010
Education					
Direct effect [b]	0.100 *	0.105 **	0.075 *	0.089 *	0.112 **
Total indirect effect [c]	−0.010	−0.009	0.007	−0.008	−0.009
Marital Status					
Direct effect [b]	−0.059	−0.040	−0.044	−0.042	−0.055
Total indirect effect [c]	0.005	0.005	0.004	0.004	0.006
Perceived Health					
Direct effect [b]	−0.055	−0.054	−0.043	−0.049	−0.055
Total indirect effect [c]	0.047	0.045 ***	0.033 ***	0.040 ***	0.046 ***
Environmental features [d]					
Direct effect [b]	0.278 ***	0.092 *	0.720 ***	0.532 ***	0.135 **
Total indirect effect [c]	−0.001	0.000	0.003	0.003	−0.003
Personal Goal F1 (PA, sports)	0.175 ***	0.169 ***	0.124 ***	0.150 ***	0.171 ***
R-Square	0.125 ***	0.125 ***	0.126 ***	0.126 ***	0.125 ***
RMSEA	0.000	0.000	0.000	0.000	0.000
GFI	1.000	1.000	1.000	1.000	1.000
TLI	1.000	1.000	1.000	1.000	1.000

* $p < 0.05$, ** $p < 0.01$, *** $p < 0.001$, [a] reference category = woman, [b] The direct effect of predictor on outcome after controlling for mediator (PA). [c] The effect of predictor on outcome via mediator. [d] the regression coefficients for environmental measures are divided by columns. β = standardized beta coefficient. DV: Total walking. RMSEA (Root Mean Square Error of Approximation), GFI (Goodness of Fit Indices), TLI (Tucker-Lewis index).

3.2.1. Mediation Models

The indirect effects of personal as well as environmental variables on walking via PA and sport goal factor was examined using structural equation modeling. We tested five path models that all of them fitted the data perfectly (RMSEA = 0.00, CFI = 1.00, TLI = 1.00). Gender and perceived health were found having a significant indirect effect on walking through PA and sports goal factor in all of the five different models (Table 4 and Figure 4). Thus, the indirect effects of gender and perceived health are realized through PA and sports related personal goals retaining partially H4. The direct effect of gender on PA and sports goals varies very little model by model (from −0.210 to −0.211) and is negative, meaning that men, compared to women, had significantly less PA and sports related personal goal factor scores. The total indirect effect of gender on walking is significant and varies between −0.026 and −0.037 in the five different models (Figure 4), thus suggesting that the PA and sports goals mediate the effect on walking behavior between men and women.

The perceived health has a strong relationship with the PA and sports goals in all of the five models (0.268, $p < 0.001$) suggesting that older adults who perceive their overall health good report having PA and sports related personal goals. The total indirect effect of perceived health on walking is significant and varies between 0.033 and 0.0475 in the five different models (Figure 4), thus suggesting that personal goals related to PA and sports plays a mediating role in the relationship between perceived health and walking in older adults'.

As to the mediation analysis, we calculated the standardized estimation of direct, indirect and total effects of personal and environmental features on total walking with PA and sport goal factor as mediator. Figure 4 shows the results of significant direct and indirect paths. Walkway density, intersection density, residential density, public transit stop density and density of sporting places none have a significant effect on personal goals, thus rejecting the H5.

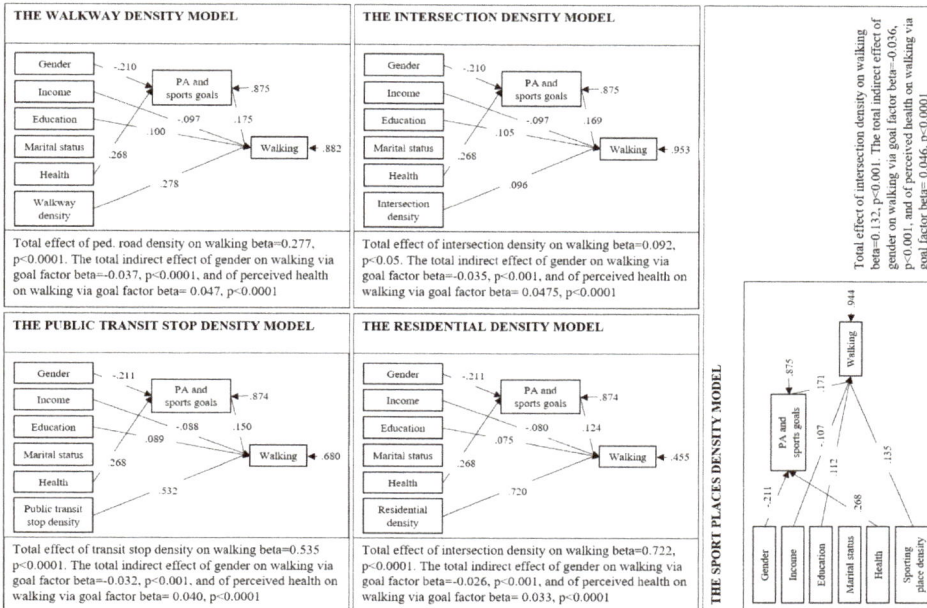

Figure 4. Significant paths with standardized Beta (β) for the five different theoretical models. The figure illustrates only the significant paths between different variables.

4. Discussion

The motivation for this study arose from the notions that research focusing on multiple-level influences on health behavior are still needed and that the health behavior of individuals is not bound to static neighborhood boundaries [11,40,71]. In addition, studies examining associations between older adults' psychological factors and PA is lacking [14]. While ecological models have raised interest among researchers, productive frameworks that focus context-sensitively and simultaneously on both the individual and the physical environment are still infrequent [9,42].

In this study, we examined the associations between the personal, psychological and the environmental features with older adults active travel behavior with a spatial approach that takes into account the various different spatial scales of human mobility. We aimed to determine which individual and environmental features explain walking for transport among older adults. We found that several physical environment features had significant and positive direct effects on older adults walking. The psychological features examined did not have a mediating role in the relationship between the physical environment and walking in older adults'. Thus, the physical environment had an independent effect on active mobility regardless of individual demographic or psychological features. Walkway density, residential density, connectivity, namely the density of public transit stops and intersections, and the density of recreational sport places within respondents' home ranges were significantly and positively associated with their walking for transport. Thus, the results suggest that the built environment plays a significant role in supporting walking of older adults, even for those not particularly interested in physical activities. From the physical environment features the residential and public transit stop density were found having largest direct effect to older adults walking. In the case of residential and public transit stop density their total effect to walking was clearly higher than the unexplained variance whereas the intersection and the sporting places density had rather small direct effect. However, all of these results support the previous findings about the independent effect of built environment to active travel of older adults [8,72]. Numerous studies have reported that well-connected, pedestrian friendly, and dense built environment influence positively mobility and physical activity of older adults [30]. However, in many of the previous studies, biased associations are possible because individuals who prefer an active lifestyle in general may seek to move around and live in areas of high walkability [73]. Our results add to the previous evidence by showing that the associations between built environment and walking behavior tend to exists even after controlling the motivational features behind people's actions. Thus, the physical environment can play strong role for older adults' walking behavior despite their personal interests and background.

Personal psychological features, namely the personal goals related to physical activity and sports, had a direct positive effect on walking, meaning that the higher the importance of physical activity and sports related goals were for the older adult the more they walked for transport. Based on the personal goals that the participants reported, we identified four goal factors. These factors included goals related to physical activity and sports, caring for others, managing on one's own, and culture and social affairs. Only physical activity and sports was significantly associated with active mobility and the other three factors had no significant association. These results are in line with previous research where respondents who reported having personal goals related to exercise were found four times more likely to have high exercise activity than those who did not report exercise-related goals [22].

The physical activity and sports goals had also a mediating effect on the relationship between gender as well as perceived health and walking. Thus, our results further strengthen the notion that psychological factors are associated with physical activity in older adults [14] and that personal characteristics have indirect influences through personal goals to the outcome measures [28]. Previous studies have concluded that personal goals are potential for studying and representing the volitional process people use in choosing their everyday behaviors and are central to motivation [21]. Our results suggest that strong interest toward physical activity and sports can affect the active mobility behavior of a person.

We found income and education having a direct effect on walking for transport in older adults. Income was negatively associated with walking, meaning that higher the income the less the respondent walked for transport. However, this finding is not a major public health concern firstly because the direct effect was small and individuals with higher income have been shown replacing the lower transport walking behavior with other forms of physical activity [74,75]. In contrast, the lower socio-economic status has been linked to less recreational walking among older adults [76], whereas King and colleagues [77] found the neighborhood income not being associated with active transport. Education had a direct positive effect on walking, meaning that higher the education level the more the older adults walked for transport. Similar results have been found in studies among the general population, where higher education was found positively associated with frequency of transport-related walking where leisure-time physical activities explained the higher frequencies [74]. Higher levels of walking for transport in higher education groups could be explained here by the attitude towards, and adoption of, an active lifestyle similarly as by Cerin and colleagues [67]. However, these results warrant for careful considerations on the importance of health and physical activity education interventions among older adults [78]. In contrast to these findings, Cerin and colleagues [75] found respondents with higher education reporting lower levels of within-neighbourhood and overall transport walking in Hong Kong elders.

The individual home range modeling approach enabled us to study the characteristics of the environment within those exact geographical areas where the respondents live in and report moving around [56]. A majority of studies use plain administrative units or spherical buffers as geographical units of analysis when conducting research on built environment effects on health, and thus are susceptible to the uncertain geographic context problem [55,70]. Many studies still to date examine individual health behavior out of context, disconnected from the physical environment where the behavior actually takes place, or focus merely on personal perceptions of neighborhood characteristics [23,43,79]. The spatial dimensions and modeling techniques related to studies on the contextual effects have been shown to have a clear effect on the outcomes of studies but these should be more carefully examined in future research [39,40,59]. The future studies should take into careful consideration also the modifiable areal unit problem (MAUP), the uncertain geographic context problem (UGCoP) as well as the ways to measure the walkability of the environment in different contexts [59,70,80,81].

We acknowledge that our study has several limitations. The PPGIS methodology could be seen as causing limitations for the studied population group, as those with poor computer literacy or no access to internet could be excluded from the study. However, Finns are technologically well-oriented, and age does not play a significant role in their use of public e-services [82]. In addition, the suitability of the PPGIS method for older adults has been studied, and the results showed its applicability to both older adults and a wider audience, including people with low mapping experience and poor computer literacy [83]. Our walking for transport measure could be seen vulnerable to the bias of self-reporting. However, in a study by Crutzen and Göritz [84] no significant associations between social desirability and self-reported physical activity in web-based research was found. Measuring the destination density in more detail could have added value to the study, but due to data limitations this was not possible. Future research should focus in more detail to the destination density and their quality related to walking for transport [8,32,66]. The cross-sectional nature of this study can be also seen a one of the limitations.

5. Conclusions

We studied the associations between the personal, psychological and the environmental features and older adults walking. We examined the direct effects of the personal, psychological as well as environmental features on older adults walking as well as the indirect influences of environmental and personal characteristics through psychological features, namely individuals' personal goals. Walkway density, residential density, connectivity, and the density of recreational sport places within respondents' home ranges had an independent effect on older adults walking for transport regardless of individual demographic or psychological features. Residential and public transit stop density were found having largest direct effect to older adults walking. Thus, the walkable, well-connected and destination rich environment may encourage the walking behavior even of those who are not very interest in physical activities. Personal goals related to physical activity and sports had also a direct positive effect on walking. Additionally, we found an indirect effect of gender as well as of perceived health on walking which was realized through individuals' physical activity and sports goals.

Future research should aim for longitudinal studies to more comprehensively examine causal relations and use other advanced data modeling among the studied variables, as suggested elsewhere [9]. According to our results and previous literature, we suggest that future studies on physical activity and health interventions should investigate simultaneously the personal and psychological as well as the physical environment features on human mobility with spatially bounded context-specific methods to be able to capture individuals' true exposure to environmental influences [30,39,59,85].

Author Contributions: Conceptualization, T.E.L., M.H. and M.K.; Data curation, T.E.L. and M.H.; Formal analysis, T.E.L. and M.H.; Funding acquisition, M.K.; Investigation, T.E.L.; Methodology, T.E.L.; Visualization, T.E.L.; Writing—original draft, T.E.L., M.H. and M.K.

Funding: This research was funded by Academy of Finland, grant number 13297753, and Opetus- ja Kulttuuriministeriö: ActivAGE project.

Acknowledgments: We would thank the anonymous reviewers for their invaluable contribution in reviewing the manuscript. We wish to thank our funders Academy of Finland and Finnish Education and Culture ministry. We would also like to thank Kamyar Hasanzadeh for his insightful comments to the manuscript and help applying the advanced home range model.

Conflicts of Interest: The authors declare no conflict of interest.

References

1. Chodzko-Zajko, W.J.; Proctor, D.N.; Fiatarone Singh, M.A.; Minson, C.T.; Nigg, C.R.; Salem, G.J.; Skinner, J.S. Exercise and physical activity for older adults. *Med. Sci. Sports Exerc.* **2009**, *41*, 1510–1530. [CrossRef] [PubMed]

2. Rantakokko, M.; Iwarsson, S.; Hirvensalo, M.; Leinonen, R.; Heikkinen, E.; Rantanen, T. Unmet physical activity need in old age. *J. Am. Geriatr. Soc.* **2010**, *58*, 707–712. [CrossRef] [PubMed]

3. Nelson, M.E.; Rejeski, W.J.; Blair, S.N.; Duncan, P.W.; Judge, J.O.; King, A.C.; Macera, C.A.; Castaneda-Sceppa, C. Physical activity and public health in older adults: Recommendation from the American College of Sports Medicine and the American Heart Association. *Med. Sci. Sports Exerc.* **2007**, *39*, 1435–1445. [CrossRef] [PubMed]

4. Hirvensalo, M.; Lampinen, P.; Rantanen, T. Physical exercise in old age: An eight-year follow-up study on involvement, motives, and obstacles among persons age 65–84. *J. Aging Phys. Act.* **1998**, *6*, 157–168. [CrossRef]

5. Rejeski, W.J.; Brubaker, P.H.; Goff, D.C.; Bearon, L.B.; McClelland, J.W.; Perri, M.G.; Ambrosius, W.T. Translating weight loss and physical activity programs into the community to preserve mobility in older, obese adults in poor cardiovascular health. *Arch. Intern. Med.* **2011**, *171*, 880–886. [CrossRef] [PubMed]

6. Winters, M.; Voss, C.; Ashe, M.C.; Gutteridge, K.; McKay, H.; Sims-Gould, J. Where do they go and how do they get there? Older adults' travel behaviour in a highly walkable environment. *Soc. Sci. Med.* **2015**, *133*, 304–312. [CrossRef] [PubMed]

7. Kelly, P.; Kahlmeier, S.; Götschi, T.; Orsini, N.; Richards, J.; Roberts, N.; Scarborough, P.; Foster, C. Systematic review and meta-analysis of reduction in all-cause mortality from walking and cycling and shape of dose response relationship. *Int. J. Behav. Nutr. Phys. Act.* **2014**, *11*, 132. [CrossRef]

8. Cerin, E.; Nathan, A.; van Cauwenberg, J.; Barnett, D.W.; Barnett, A. The neighbourhood physical environment and active travel in older adults: A systematic review and meta-analysis. *Int. J. Behav. Nutr. Phys. Act.* **2017**, *14*, 15. [CrossRef] [PubMed]

9. Bauman, A.E.; Reis, R.S.; Sallis, J.F.; Wells, J.C.; Loos, R.J.F.; Martin, B.W. Correlates of physical activity: Why are some people physically active and others not? *Lancet* **2012**, *380*, 258–271. [CrossRef]

10. Sallis, J.; Cervero, R.B.; Ascher, W.; Henderson, K.A.; Kraft, M.K.; Kerr, J. An ecological approach to creating active living communities. *Annu. Rev. Public Health* **2006**, *27*, 297–322. [CrossRef]

11. Sallis, J.F.; Owen, N. Ecological models of health behavior. In *Health Behavior: Theory, Research, and Practice*, 5th ed.; Glanz, K., Rimer, B.K., Viswanath, K., Eds.; Jossey-Bas: San Francisco, CA, USA, 2015; pp. 43–64.

12. Costello, E.; Kafchinski, M.; Vrazel, J.; Sullivan, P. Motivators, barriers, and beliefs regarding physical activity in an older adult population. *J. Geriatr. Phys. Ther.* **2011**, *34*, 138–147. [CrossRef] [PubMed]

13. McAuley, E.; Morris, K.S.; Motl, R.W.; Hu, L.; Konopack, J.F.; Elavsky, S. Long-term follow-up of physical activity behavior in older adults. *Health Psychol.* **2007**, *26*, 375. [CrossRef] [PubMed]

14. Notthoff, N.; Reisch, P.; Gerstorf, D. Individual Characteristics and Physical Activity in Older Adults: A Systematic Review. *Gerontology* **2017**, *63*, 443–459. [CrossRef] [PubMed]

15. Resnick, B.; Orwig, D.; Hawkes, W.; Shardell, M.; Golden, J.; Werner, M.; Zimmerman, S.; Magaziner, J. The Relationship Between Psychosocial State and Exercise Behavior of Older Women 2 Months after Hip Fracture. *Rehabil. Nurs.* **2012**, *32*, 139–149. [CrossRef]

16. Schüz, B.; Wurm, S.; Warner, L.M.; Wolff, J.K.; Schwarzer, R. Health motives and health behaviour self-regulation in older adults. *J. Behav. Med.* **2014**, *37*, 491–500. [CrossRef] [PubMed]

17. Umstattd, M.R.; Hallam, J. Older adults' exercise behavior: Roles of selected constructs of social-cognitive theory. *J. Aging Phys. Act.* **2007**, *15*, 206–218. [CrossRef] [PubMed]

18. Anderson-Bill, E.S.; Winett, R.A.; Wojcik, J.R.; Williams, D.M. Aging and the social cognitive determinants of physical activity behavior and behavior change: Evidence from the guide to health trial. *J. Aging Res.* **2011**, *2011*, 505928. [CrossRef] [PubMed]

19. Hall, K.S.; Crowley, G.M.; Bosworth, H.B.; Howard, T.A.; Morey, M.C. Individual progress toward self-selected goals among older adults enrolled in a physical activity counseling intervention. *J. Aging Phys. Act.* **2010**, *18*, 439–450. [CrossRef]

20. Teixeira, P.J.; Carraça, E.V.; Markland, D.; Silva, M.N.; Ryan, R.M. Exercise, physical activity, and self-determination theory: A systematic review. *Int. J. Behav. Nutr. Phys. Act.* **2012**, *9*, 78. [CrossRef]

21. Powell Lawton, M.; Moss, M.S.; Winter, L.; Hoffman, C. Motivation in later life: Personal projects and well-being. *Psychol. Aging* **2002**, *17*, 539–547. [CrossRef]

22. Saajanaho, M.; Viljanen, A.; Read, S.; Rantakokko, M.; Tsai, L.-T.; Kaprio, J.; Jylhä, M.; Rantanen, T. Older women's personal goals and exercise activity: An 8-year follow-up. *J. Aging Phys. Act.* **2014**, *22*, 386–392. [CrossRef] [PubMed]

23. Saajanaho, M.; Rantakokko, M.; Portegijs, E.; Törmäkangas, T.; Eronen, J.; Tsai, L.-T.; Jylhä, M.; Rantanen, T. Personal goals and changes in life-space mobility among older people. *Prev. Med.* **2015**, *81*, 163–167. [CrossRef] [PubMed]

24. Salmela-Aro, K.; Read, S.; Nurmi, J.-E.; Koskenvuo, M.; Kaprio, J.; Rantanen, T. Personal goals of older female twins genetic and environmental effects. *Eur. Psychol.* **2009**, *14*, 160–167. [CrossRef]

25. Ward Thompson, C.; Aspinall, P.A. Natural environments and their impact on activity, health, and quality of life. *Appl. Psychol. Health Well-Being* **2011**, *3*, 230–260. [CrossRef]

26. Roe, J.J.; Aspinall, P.A. Adolescents' Daily Activities and the Restorative Niches that Support Them. *Int. J. Environ. Res. Public Health* **2012**, *9*, 3227–3244. [CrossRef] [PubMed]

27. Little, B.R. Personal projects a rationale and method for investigation. *Environ. Behav.* **1983**, *15*, 273–309. [CrossRef]

28. Little, B.R.; Salmela-Aro, K.; Phillips, S.D. *Personal Project Pursuit: Goals, Action, and Human Flourishing*; Psychology Press: New York, NY, USA, 2017.

29. Kyttä, M. *Children in Outdoor Contexts. Affordances and Independent Mobility in the Assessment of Environmental Child Friendliness*; Helsinki University of Technology: Espoo, Finland, 2004.

30. Kerr, J.; Rosenberg, D.; Frank, L. The Role of the Built Environment in Healthy Aging: Community Design, Physical Activity, and Health among Older Adults. *J. Plan Lit.* **2012**, *27*, 43–60. [CrossRef]

31. Sallis, J.F.; Cerin, E.; Conway, T.L.; Adams, M.A.; Frank, L.D.; Pratt, M.; Salvo, D.; Schipperijn, J.; Smith, G.; Cain, K.L.; Davey, R. Physical activity in relation to urban environments in 14 cities worldwide: A cross-sectional study. *Lancet* **2016**, *387*, 2207–2217. [CrossRef]

32. Chudyk, A.M.; Winters, M.; Moniruzzaman, M.; Ashe, M.C.; Gould, J.S.; McKay, H. Destinations matter: The association between where older adults live and their travel behavior. *J. Transp. Health* **2015**, *2*, 50–57. [CrossRef] [PubMed]

33. Clarke, P.; Nieuwenhuijsen, E.R. Environments for healthy ageing: A. critical review. *Maturitas* **2009**, *64*, 14–19. [CrossRef]

34. Ottoni, C.A.; Sims-Gould, J.; Winters, M.; Heijnen, M.; McKay, H.A. "Benches become like porches": Built and social environment influences on older adults' experiences of mobility and well-being. *Soc. Sci. Med.* **2016**, *169*, 33–41. [CrossRef] [PubMed]

35. Keskinen, K.E.; Rantakokko, M.; Suomi, K.; Rantanen, T.; Portegijs, E. Nature as a facilitator for physical activity: Defining relationships between the objective and perceived environment and physical activity among community-dwelling older people. *Health Place* **2018**, *49*, 111–119. [CrossRef] [PubMed]

36. Yen, I.H.; Michael, Y.L.; Perdue, L. Neighborhood Environment in Studies of Health of Older Adults: A Systematic Review. *Am. J. Prev. Med.* **2009**, *37*, 455–463. [CrossRef] [PubMed]

37. Frank, L.; Kerr, J.; Rosenberg, D.; King, A. Healthy aging and where you live: Community design relationships with physical activity and body weight in older Americans. *J. Phys. Act. Health* **2010**, *7* (Suppl. S1), S82–S90. [CrossRef]

38. Sugiyama, T.; Ward Thompson, C. Older people's health, outdoor activity and supportiveness of neighbourhood environments. *Landsc. Urban Plan.* **2007**, *83*, 168–175. [CrossRef]

39. Laatikainen, T.E.; Hasanzadeh, K.; Kyttä, M. Capturing exposure in environmental health research: Challenges and opportunities of different activity space models. *Int. J. Health Geogr.* **2018**, *17*, 29. [CrossRef]

40. Kwan, M.-P. The Neighborhood Effect Averaging Problem (NEAP): An Elusive Confounder of the Neighborhood Effect. *Int. J. Environ. Res. Public Health* **2018**, *15*, 1841. [CrossRef]

41. Hasanzadeh, K.; Laatikainen, T.; Kyttä, M. A place-based model of local activity spaces: Individual place exposure and characteristics. *J. Geogr. Syst.* **2018**, *20*, 227. [CrossRef]
42. Blacksher, E.; Lovasi, G.S. Place-focused physical activity research, human agency, and social justice in public health: Taking agency seriously in studies of the built environment. *Health Place* **2012**, *18*, 172–179. [CrossRef] [PubMed]
43. Chaudhury, H.; Campo, M.; Michael, Y.; Mahmood, A. Neighbourhood environment and physical activity in older adults. *Soc. Sci. Med.* **2016**, *149*, 104–113. [CrossRef]
44. Brown, G.; Raymond, C.M. Methods for identifying land use conflict potential using participatory mapping. *Landsc. Urban Plan.* **2014**, *122*, 196–208. [CrossRef]
45. Brown, G.; Schebella, M.F.; Weber, D. Using participatory GIS to measure physical activity and urban park benefits. *Landsc. Urban Plan.* **2014**, *121*, 34–44. [CrossRef]
46. Kytta, A.M.; Broberg, A.K.; Kahila, M.H. Urban environment and children's active lifestyle: Softgis revealing children's behavioral patterns and meaningful places. *Am. J. Health Promot.* **2012**, *26*, e137–e148. [CrossRef] [PubMed]
47. Schmidt-Thome, K.; Wallin, S.; Laatikainen, T.; Kangasoja, J.; Kyttä, M. Exploring the use of PPGIS in self-organizing urban development: Case softGIS in Pacific Beach. *J. Commun. Inform.* **2014**, *10*, 131–144.
48. Kyttä, M.; Broberg, A.; Tzoulas, T.; Snabb, K. Towards contextually sensitive urban densification: Location-based softGIS knowledge revealing perceived residential environmental quality. *Landsc. Urban Plan.* **2013**, *113*, 30–46. [CrossRef]
49. Brown, G.; Kyttä, M. Key issues and research priorities for public participation GIS (PPGIS): A synthesis based on empirical research. *Appl. Geogr.* **2014**, *46*, 122–136. [CrossRef]
50. Kestens, Y.; Thierry, B.; Shareck, M.; Steinmetz-Wood, M.; Chaix, B. Integrating activity spaces in health research: Comparing the VERITAS activity space questionnaire with 7-day GPS tracking and prompted recall. *Spat. Spatio-Temporal Epidemiol.* **2018**, *25*, 1–9. [CrossRef]
51. Humpel, N.; Owen, N.; Iverson, D.; Leslie, E.; Bauman, A. Perceived environment attributes, residential location, and walking for particular purposes. *Am. J. Prev. Med.* **2004**, *26*, 119–125. [CrossRef] [PubMed]
52. Official Statistics of Finland. Population Projection. Available online: http://www.stat.fi/til/vaenn/index_en.html (accessed on 13 November 2018).
53. The Population Demographics. The Ageing in Helsinki. 2018. Available online: https://ikaantyneethelsingissa.fi/vaesto_rakenne (accessed on 4 December 2018).
54. Helsinkiregion.fi. Helsinki region. Facts about the Helsinki Region. Available online: https://www.helsinkiregion.fi/hs/en/city-information/ (accessed on 13 November 2018).
55. Laatikainen, T.; Tenkanen, H.; Kyttä, M.; Toivonen, T. Comparing conventional and PPGIS approaches in measuring equality of access to urban aquatic environments. *Landsc. Urban Plan.* **2015**, *144*. [CrossRef]
56. Hasanzadeh, K.; Broberg, A.; Kyttä, M. Where is my neighborhood? A dynamic individual-based definition of Home zones. *Appl. Geogr.* **2017**, *84*, 1–10. [CrossRef]
57. Broberg, A.; Salminen, S.; Kyttä, M. Physical environmental characteristics promoting independent and active transport to children's meaningful places. *Appl. Geogr.* **2013**, *38*, 43–52. [CrossRef]
58. Frank, L.; Fox, E.H.; Ulmer, J.M.; Chapman, J.E.; Kershaw, S.E.; Sallis, J.F.; Conway, T.L.; Cerin, E.; Cain, K.L.; Adams, M.A.; Smith, G.R. International comparison of observation-specific spatial buffers: Maximizing the ability to estimate physical activity. *Int. J. Health Geogr.* **2017**, *16*, 4. [CrossRef]
59. Zhao, P.; Kwan, M.-P.; Zhou, S. The Uncertain Geographic Context Problem in the Analysis of the Relationships between Obesity and the Built Environment in Guangzhou. *Int. J. Environ. Res. Public Health* **2018**, *15*, 308. [CrossRef] [PubMed]
60. Perchoux, C.; Chaix, B.; Brondeel, R.; Kestens, Y. Residential buffer, perceived neighborhood, and individual activity space: New refinements in the definition of exposure areas—The RECORD Cohort Study. *Health Place* **2016**, *40*, 116–122. [CrossRef] [PubMed]
61. Little, B.R. Opening space for project pursuit: Affordance, restoration and chills. *Innov. Approaches Res. Landsc. Health Open Space People Space* **2010**, *2*, 163–278.
62. Lapierre, S.; Bouffard, L.; Bastin, E. Motivational goal objects in later life. *Int. J. Aging Hum. Dev.* **1992**, *36*, 279–292. [CrossRef] [PubMed]

63. Saajanaho, M.; Viljanen, A.; Read, S.; Eronen, J.; Kaprio, J.; Jylhä, M.; Rantanen, T. Mobility limitation and changes in personal goals among older women. *J. Gerontol. Ser. B Psychol. Sci. Soc. Sci.* **2016**, *71*, 1–10. [CrossRef]

64. Saajanaho, M.; Rantakokko, M.; Portegijs, E.; Törmäkangas, T.; Eronen, J.; Tsai, L.-T.; Jylhä, M.; Rantanen, T. Life resources and personal goals in old age. *Eur. J. Ageing* **2016**, *13*, 195–208. [CrossRef]

65. Laatikainen, T.E.; Broberg, A.; Kyttä, M. The physical environment of positive places: Exploring differences between age groups. *Prev. Med.* **2017**, *95*, S85–S91. [CrossRef]

66. Glazier, R.H.; Creatore, M.I.; Weyman, J.T.; Fazli, G.; Matheson, F.I.; Gozdyra, P.; Moineddin, R.; Shriqui, V.K.; Booth, G.L. Density, Destinations or Both? A Comparison of Measures of Walkability in Relation to Transportation Behaviors, Obesity and Diabetes in Toronto, Canada. *PLoS ONE* **2014**, *9*, e85295. [CrossRef]

67. Frank, L.D.; Sallis, J.F.; Saelens, B.E.; Leary, L.; Cain, L.; Conway, T.L.; Hess, P.M. The development of a walkability index: Application to the neighborhood quality of life study. *Br. J. Sports Med.* **2010**, *44*, 924–933. [CrossRef]

68. Tribby, C.P.; Miller, H.J.; Brown, B.B.; Werner, C.M.; Smith, K.R. Assessing built environment walkability using activity-space summary measures. *J. Transp. Land Use* **2016**, *9*, 187. [CrossRef]

69. Clark, A.; Scott, D. Understanding the impact of the modifiable areal unit problem on the relationship between active travel and the built environment. *Urban Stud.* **2014**, *51*, 284–299. [CrossRef]

70. Stockton, J.C.; Duke-Williams, O.; Stamatakis, E.; Mindell, J.S.; Brunner, E.J.; Shelton, N.J. Development of a novel walkability index for London, United Kingdom: Cross-sectional application to the Whitehall II Study. *BMC Public Health* **2016**, *16*, 416. [CrossRef] [PubMed]

71. Sawyer, A.; Ucci, M.; Jones, R.; Smith, L.; Fisher, A. Simultaneous evaluation of physical and social environmental correlates of physical activity in adults: A systematic review. *SSM—Popul. Health* **2017**, *3*, 506–515. [CrossRef] [PubMed]

72. Ding, D.; Sallis, J.F.; Conway, T.L.; Saelens, B.E.; Frank, L.D.; Cain, K.L.; Slymen, D.J. Interactive effects of built environment and psychosocial attributes on physical activity: A test of ecological models. *Ann. Behav. Med.* **2012**, *44*, 365–374. [CrossRef] [PubMed]

73. McCormack, G.R.; Shiell, A. In search of causality: A systematic review of the relationship between the built environment and physical activity among adults. *Int. J. Behav. Nutr. Phys. Act.* **2011**, *8*, 125. [CrossRef]

74. Cerin, E.; Leslie, E.; Owen, N. Explaining socio-economic status differences in walking for transport: An ecological analysis of individual, social and environmental factors. *Soc. Sci. Med.* **2009**, *68*, 1013–1020. [CrossRef]

75. Cerin, E.; Sit, C.H.P.; Barnett, A.; Johnston, J.M.; Cheung, M.-C.; Chan, W.-M. Ageing in an ultra-dense metropolis: Perceived neighbourhood characteristics and utilitarian walking in Hong Kong elders. *Public Health Nutr.* **2014**, *17*, 225–232. [CrossRef]

76. Kamphuis, C.B.M.; van Lenthe, F.J.; Giskes, K.; Huisman, M.; Brug, J.; Mackenbach, J.P. Socioeconomic differences in lack of recreational walking among older adults: The role of neighbourhood and individual factors. *Int. J. Behav. Nutr. Phys. Act.* **2009**, *6*, 1. [CrossRef]

77. King, A.C.; Sallis, J.F.; Frank, L.D.; Saelens, B.E.; Cain, K.; Conway, T.L.; Chapman, J.E.; Ahn, D.K.; Kerr, J. Aging in neighborhoods differing in walkability and income: Associations with physical activity and obesity in older adults. *Soc. Sci. Med.* **2011**, *73*, 1525–1533. [CrossRef] [PubMed]

78. Van Der Bij, A.K.; Laurant, M.G.H.; Wensing, M. Effectiveness of physical activity interventions for older adults: A review. *Am. J. Prev. Med.* **2002**, *22*, 120–133. [CrossRef]

79. Rantakokko, M.; Iwarsson, S.; Kauppinen, M.; Leinonen, R.; Heikkinen, E.; Rantanen, T. Quality of life and barriers in the urban outdoor environment in old age. *J. Am. Geriatr. Soc.* **2010**, *58*, 2154–2159. [CrossRef] [PubMed]

80. Kwan, M.-P. The uncertain geographic context problem. *Ann. Assoc. Am. Geogr.* **2012**, *102*, 958–968. [CrossRef]

81. Koohsari, M.J.; Owen, N.; Cerin, E.; Giles-Corti, B.; Sugiyama, T. Walkability and walking for transport: Characterizing the built environment using space syntax. *Int. J. Behav. Nutr. Phys. Act.* **2016**, *13*, 121. [CrossRef] [PubMed]

82. Taipale, S. The use of e-government services and the Internet: The role of socio-demographic, economic and geographical predictors. *Telecomm. Policy* **2013**, *37*, 413–422. [CrossRef]

83. Gottwald, S.; Laatikainen, T.E.; Kyttä, M. Exploring the usability of PPGIS among older adults: Challenges and opportunities. *Int. J. Geogr. Inf. Sci.* **2016**, *30*, 2321–2338. [CrossRef]
84. Crutzen, R.; Göritz, A.S. Does social desirability compromise self-reports of physical activity in web-based research? *Int. J. Behav. Nutr. Phys. Act.* **2011**, *8*, 31. [CrossRef]
85. Haybatollahi, M.; Czepkiewicz, M.; Laatikainen, T.; Kyttä, M. Neighbourhood preferences, active travel behaviour, and built environment: An exploratory study. *Transp. Res. Part F Traffic Psychol. Behav.* **2015**, *29*, 57–69. [CrossRef]

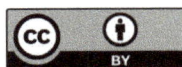

International Journal of
*Environmental Research
and Public Health*

MDPI

Article

Spatial Accessibility to Primary Healthcare Services by Multimodal Means of Travel: Synthesis and Case Study in the City of Calgary

Amritpal Kaur Khakh [1], Victoria Fast [1,*] and Rizwan Shahid [2]

[1] Department of Geography, University of Calgary, Calgary, AB T2N 1N4, Canada;
   amritpal.khakh@ucalgary.ca
[2] Primary Health Care, Alberta Health Services, Calgary, AB T2W 3N2, Canada; Rizwan.shahid@ahs.ca
* Correspondence: victoria.fast@ucalgary.ca; Tel.: +1-403-220-8353

Received: 28 November 2018; Accepted: 3 January 2019; Published: 9 January 2019

Abstract: Universal access to primary healthcare facilities is a driving goal of healthcare organizations. Despite Canada's universal access to primary healthcare status, spatial accessibility to healthcare facilities is still an issue of concern due to the non-uniform distribution of primary healthcare facilities and population over space—leading to spatial inequity in the healthcare sector. Spatial inequity is further magnified when health-related accessibility studies are analyzed on the assumption of universal car access. To overcome car-centric studies of healthcare access, this study compares different travel modes—driving, public transit, and walking—to simulate the multi-modal access to primary healthcare services in the City of Calgary, Canada. Improving on floating catchment area methods, spatial accessibility was calculated based on the Spatial Access Ratio method, which takes into consideration the provider-to-population status of the region. The analysis revealed that, in the City of Calgary, spatial accessibility to the primary healthcare services is the highest for the people with an access to a car, and is significantly lower with multimodal (bus transit and train) means despite being a large urban centre. The social inequity issue raised from this analysis can be resolved by improving the city's pedestrian infrastructure, public transportation, and construction of new clinics in regions of low accessibility.

Keywords: spatial accessibility; multimodal network; primary healthcare

---

1. Introduction

Internationally, access to primary healthcare services (e.g., family doctor) has long been widely accepted as one of the primary goals in fulfilling the health needs of individuals since these are often the first point of contact in the healthcare system; providing a wide range of services over time that focus on prevention and prognosis of diseases through early diagnosis, contrary to disease-oriented care [1–4]. Statistically, as of 2016, Canada has 2.6 physicians per 1000 people, which is significantly lower than the Organization for Economic Co-operation and Development (OECD) countries' average of 3.3 physicians per 1000 population [5]. Lower physician availability status in Canada, compared to the international standards, is escalated by uneven distribution of population and healthcare facilities over regions. As such, access to primary healthcare continues to be a pressing research and policy issue in Canada and globally.

Despite this, the term 'access' is still not well-defined [6–10]. The reason behind the ambiguity in defining healthcare access is that it is a multidimensional term. Access can be defined both as a noun, referring to the potential for healthcare use; and, a verb, referring to the interaction between the provider and the patient [3,11]. In order to better interpret access, it has been presented in terms of stages and dimensions. The two stages are 'potential' for healthcare and 'realized' service utilization, which correspond to the noun and verb definitions, respectively, of access [3].

The progression from potential to realized access can be impeded by the presence of a number of barriers. Penchansky and Thomas (1981) group the barriers according to five dimensions: availability, accessibility, affordability, acceptability, and accommodation. The last three aforementioned dimensions comprise the aspatial factors (independent of any geographic aspect), and refer to healthcare costs, cultural attributes and communication effectiveness, respectively. The first two dimensions (availability and accessibility) contain an inherent spatial component where the former refers to the capacity of the provider and the latter refers to the travel cost between the provider and the patient [12]. Commonly, in urban areas, where there is a provision of multiple provider service locations, availability and accessibility dimensions of access are considered in coherence. This union is referred to as 'spatial accessibility' [3].

Multiple methods, and combinations of methods, have been developed to derive an effective spatial accessibility measure, including traditional measures such as straight distance and supply-to-demand ratio [13,14], and advanced measures, such as two-step floating catchment area [15], three-step floating catchment area [10,16], and kernel density and enhanced variable two-step floating catchment area method (EV2SFCA and KD2SFCA) [14,17], with many others still actively under development by the research community. These measures of spatial accessibility have been extensively applied to detect non-uniform distribution of healthcare [10,16,18–22], and to optimize access to other services such as daycares, libraries, food stores, and district building energy plan [13,23,24]. Despite this growth in spatial accessibility methods, there is limited research spatial accessibility to primary healthcare by mode of transit.

When it comes to spatial access to primary healthcare, the assumption that all populations have access to a car which enables them to access the primary healthcare is highly generalized in the current measures. Car ownership is not universal. In fact, fewer people are getting their driver's license in the global south and north due to improved public and active transportation. A study led by the University of Michigan Transportation Research Institute showed that the number of young licensed drivers has decreased in half of the 15 countries they investigated, including Canada. Specifically, between the ages of 25 to 34, 92% percent of the people had a driver's license in 1999 and in 2009, this number dropped to 87% [25]. Further to this point, cities are encouraging citizens to employ greater use of active transportation networks, where an effective transition requires service and amenities that are accessible—by transit, and/or walking. To more accurately understand spatial access for non-drivers, it is crucial to measure the accessibility to primary healthcare facilities by alternative modes of travel.

Collectively, the distribution of facilities and the spatial networks of transportation are two significant determinants of spatial accessibility of primary healthcare facilities. Realizing the importance of adequate primary healthcare and mode of transportation, this research analyzes multimodal access to primary care in the City of Calgary, Canada. First, we explore current methods of measuring access, before settling on the spatial access ratio (SPAR) method. Then, spatial accessibility to the primary healthcare facilities in the city is analyzed, using SPAR, at the community level by simulating travel on walking, multimodal, and driving-oriented networks.

2. Data and Methods

2.1. Current Methods for Measuring Access

Over the last decades, various methods have been developed and applied to measuring spatial access. Guagliardo [3] has broadly grouped accessibility measures into four different categories: provider-to-population ratio, distance to the nearest provider, average distance to a group of providers, and gravity models. The first three metrics are easy to implement. With the advancement of Geographic Information Systems (GIS), access measures and conceptualizations have evolved to incorporate spatial measurement, a fundamental component in gravity models. The gravity models are considered to encompass the interaction between the provider and population more accurately than the methods in other three categories [26].

The common measure considered in spatial accessibility to primary healthcare facilities is Two Step Floating Catchment Area (2SFCA), a derivative of gravity models [17,21]. Similar to gravity models, these measures account for both supply (capacity of provider), demand (population needs) and the distance impedance components of spatial accessibility [16,18,27]. However, Luo and Wang [18] recognize two limitations to their 2SFCA methodology. Firstly, by considering a threshold travel time, it is concluded that 2SFCA provides a dichotomous measure (accessible/not accessible). In other words, the locations outside the catchment area are considered to have no access, whereas the resident catchment with service locations falling inside are considered to have full access to the services, due to the presence of artificially sharp catchment boundaries. Secondly, the distance decay within the catchment is not considered, it is assumed that all population locations within this area have an equal access to the primary care facility [18].

Attempts have been made to overcome the limitations of 2SFCA. One of the significant barriers recognized in access to healthcare is distance impedance between an individual's location and the primary healthcare facility. The distance impedance within the catchments of 2SFCA has been ignored which is usually not the case in the real world. As the distance increases, people tend to utilize the distant services less than the services available nearby [28]. The advanced catchment area methods have been synthesized where researchers have proposed putting weights within the catchment areas, incorporating continuous Gaussian distance decay, adjusting the catchment areas to meet different provider-to-provider ratio thresholds [29–31]. Even though efforts have been made to reflect distance decay measure and to adjust supply and demand in the Floating Catchment Area methods accurately, the applicability of these models is still limited due to inaccuracies which may have been introduced in the analysis by choosing arbitrary distance friction coefficient values [32].

The optimal way to infer an accurate distance coefficient value is to analyze the previous provider–patient interaction records, such as the time it takes the patient to access healthcare services. However, data on provider–patient interaction are not readily available which restricts the researchers to model the impedance by using the arbitrary friction values. Wan et al. [32] have proposed a measure, referred to as Spatial Access Ratio (SPAR) to overcome the uncertainty issues arising from previous accessibility measures. This measure is an advancement over the Enhanced 2SFCA method because it is less sensitive to distance impendence variable than the aforementioned methods. Ultimately, we chose to employ the SPAR method in this study.

Next, to more accurately understand spatial access for non-drivers, it is crucial to measure the spatial accessibility to primary healthcare by alternative modes of travel—considering walking and transit modes. Mao and Nekorchuk [33] have simulated the multimodal approach by specifying incremental catchment areas for different travel modes and obtaining the sum of the populations reached through different modes from healthcare facilities. However, this methodology has a limitation in the nature of the dataset used. To model travel by bus and car, the authors used the road network in simulating travel whereas the walkable mode of travel was not included in the multimodal analysis, concluding that doing so might have resulted in less heterogeneity in their results since people may prefer to access facilities in close proximity via the sidewalk or trail network.

In assessing walkability, it is often assumed that the roads selected to model pedestrian behavior are lined with sidewalks in a real setting. These results might lead to an overestimation of accessibility measures in regions where there is no proper sidewalk infrastructure. Iacono et al. [34] have pointed that the network specifications for walking are different than driving and are required to be presented at a finer scale due to different dimensions of the infrastructure. Using roads as a network for walking can result in loss of resolution since the road network cannot identify many of the shorter trips made by walking, and eventually, this results in uncertainty in the outputs [34]. Aimed towards bridging the gap between the travel networks used in access studies, this research focuses on measuring the access to primary healthcare in Calgary by considering appropriate network infrastructures. Specifically, sidewalks, trails and pathways were integrated into the analysis to model walking; bus routes and train network to model public transportation; and road networks to model driving.

2.2. Study Area

This study aimed to calculate the spatial accessibility of primary healthcare facilities by different travel modes in the city of Calgary in the province of Alberta, Canada. As of 2016, the City of Calgary had a total population of 1,239,220 (census subdivision), a land area of 5110 square kilometers, and a population density of 273 people per square km [35]. Administratively, there are 198 different communities (Figure 1) and 1594 dissemination areas (DA) in Calgary. Calgary also contains large urban parks and industrial regions that contain zero population. While the analysis was performed on all neighborhood types (see Figure 2), we show the areas with a hatched symbology to accurately reflect areas with no access versus areas with no population.

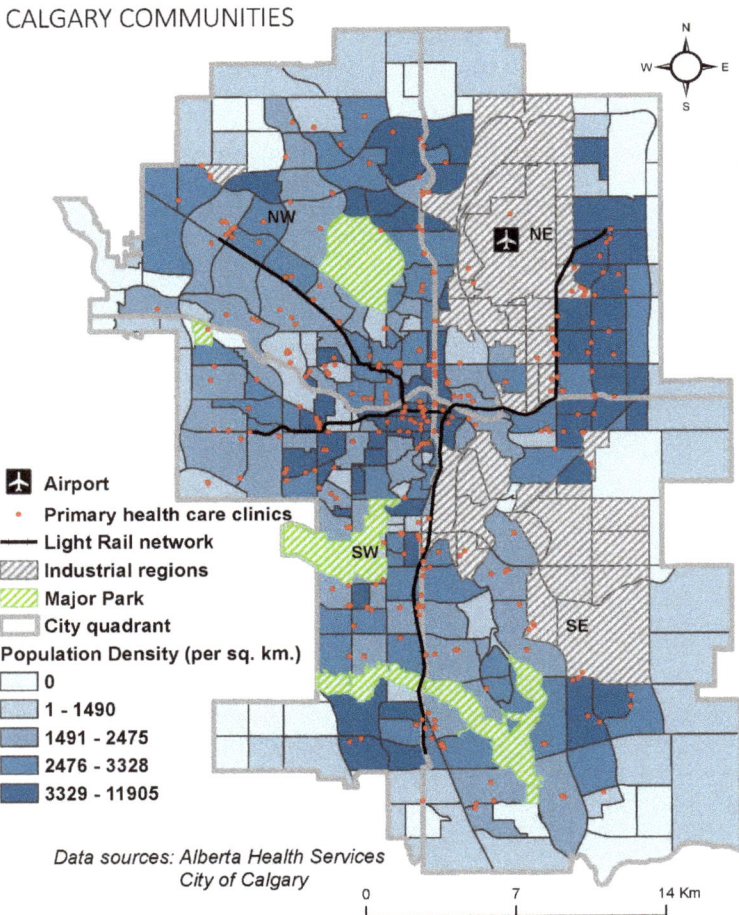

Figure 1. City of Calgary—Primary Healthcare Services by Community.

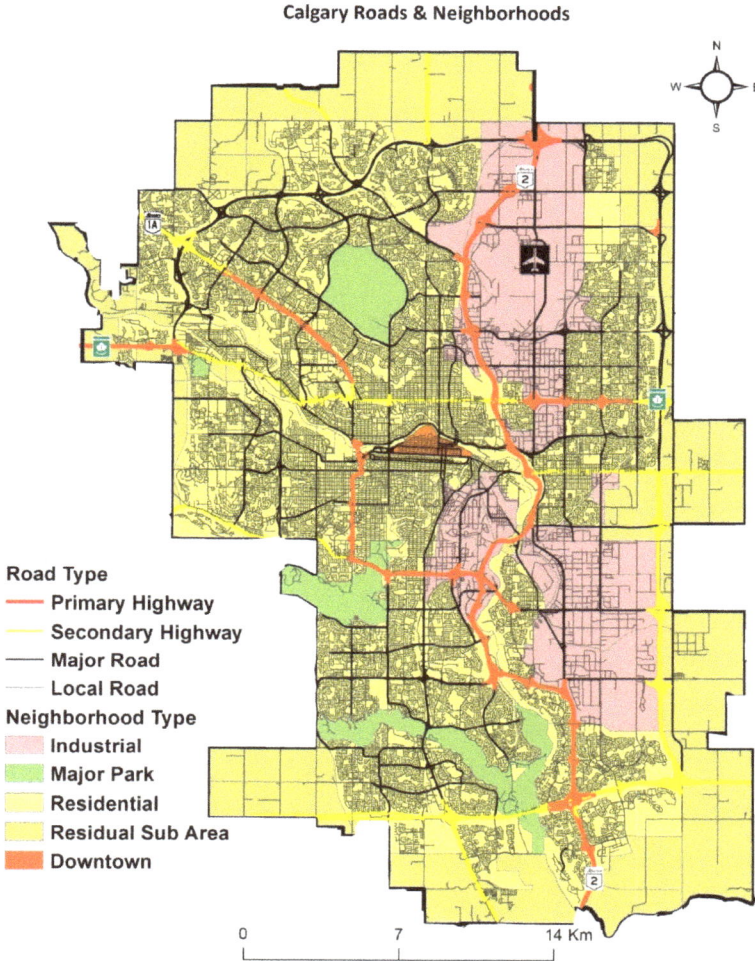

Figure 2. City of Calgary—Roads and Neighborhoods.

There is a physician shortage in Canada overall, and even more so in the province of Alberta and City of Calgary. In 2014, Statistics Canada reported that 14.9% of Canadians of age 12 and older did not have a regular family physician, whereas in Alberta, this percent increases to 19.9% [36] Within Alberta, 80.2% of people in the City of Calgary had an access to a family doctor as compared to 81.1% in the City of Edmonton. Furthermore, in Calgary, the cost of a standard hospital stay between 2015 and 2016 was calculated to be $8233, which is higher than the figures at national ($6098) and provincial ($8007) levels [37]. The lower than average access to a primary care physician in Alberta and specifically, in the City of Calgary, with high hospitalization cost leads to an extensive financial, mental, and physical toll on the population; emphasizing the importance of spatial accessibility to primary healthcare status in the city.

The analysis was performed at the dissemination area (DA) level as this is the smallest level of census division and consists of 400 to 700 people. This approach was taken to limit any inaccuracies resulting from loss of spatial resolution. On the other hand, the results are disseminated at the community level since, at this level, health statuses are derived based on various health parameters and city policies are set at community levels as people tend to associate themselves with the communities they are residing [38,39].

2.3. Data

The datasets used for this study are presented in Table 1. The clinic and sidewalk data were obtained directly from the source (the City of Calgary and Alberta Health Services respectively) and provide a snapshot of spatial accessibility at the time the analysis was performed. To make the sidewalk network more complete, the links between the sidewalks were generated by creating a buffer from the road intersections layer. This connected sidewalk data, along with trails and pathways were merged to model the walkable network. The walking speed was calculated as 4.8 km/h as per City of Calgary average walking speed standards [40,41]. While average walking speed does not consider different abilities, El-Geneidy el al. [42] compared different travel speeds used for walkability in literature and conclusively, proposed that the assumption of constant speed can be accepted to model travel by walking.

Table 1. Study data.

Dataset	Year	Source
Primary healthcare clinics	2017	Alberta Health Services
Calgary dissemination areas (DA)	2016	Statistics Canada
Population weighted centroids	2016	Statistics Canada
Calgary communities	2016	Open Calgary
Sidewalks and trails	2014	City of Calgary
Pathways	2016	Open Calgary
Road network	2016	City of Calgary
Road intersections	2016	City of Calgary
Bus routes and stops	2017	City of Calgary
Train lines (C-train) & Stations	2017	City of Calgary

The catchment radius for the methodology is 30 min, as this is most widely used in literature to measure spatial accessibility to primary healthcare facilities [18,31]. With the above considerations, the simple conversion of distance to time was calculated for sidewalks, trails, and pathways data to model walking. The bus routes and road network data was also converted from distance to time in ArcGIS with the following speed limit considerations for different roads in the City of Calgary (Table 2).

Table 2. Different road speed specifications.

Road Type	Speed (Km/h)
Collector	50
Major	65
Expressway	80
Alley	15

2.4. Building Spatial Network by Mode of Transportation

Each mode of travel was simulated in GIS platform through ESRI's ArcGIS (ESRI, Redlands, CA, USA) Network Analyst tool. The network analysis was performed on time instead of distance to facilitate comparison in results obtained by different modes of travel. Additionally, in past spatial accessibility studies, the catchment thresholds are also presented in time, specifically 30 min for the urban area [10,18,27,31]. For consistency, the same threshold time was set.

2.4.1. Building a Road Network

The first mode of travel in the analysis—access by driving—was simulated by travel along the roads, consisting of primary highway, secondary highway, major road, and local road (Figure 2).

The road-based analysis covers all car travel, including car ownership, taxis or newer shared mobility (i.e., Car2go) models. This dataset composed of end point connectivity between the road segments in the City, upon which topological relations were built as part of the road network analysis. Since the time attribute was required for the accessibility method to be applied, the conversion from distance to time was calculated with the speed limits specified in Table 2.

2.4.2. Building a Sidewalk Network

The sidewalk data obtained from the City of Calgary was not connected but rather, was presented in distinct gridded rectangular segments for each block. In order to create a functional walkable network, the following steps were completed: firstly, an 18-m radius buffer was created from the intersection point layer. The resulting buffer polygon was converted to line feature class and the lines were split at the points of intersections between the sidewalks and the line buffer. Finally, only those lines were retained which intersected with the road shapefile. This provided us with the crosswalks as the connections from one sidewalk block to another. One of the connections generated between sidewalks is presented in Figure 3. Eventually, the crosswalk and the sidewalk layers were merged together to create a walkable network. Considering the constant speed of travel (4.8 km/h), the simple conversion was performed to create walkable catchments based on travel time. This provided the second mode of travel in the analysis: accessibility by walking.

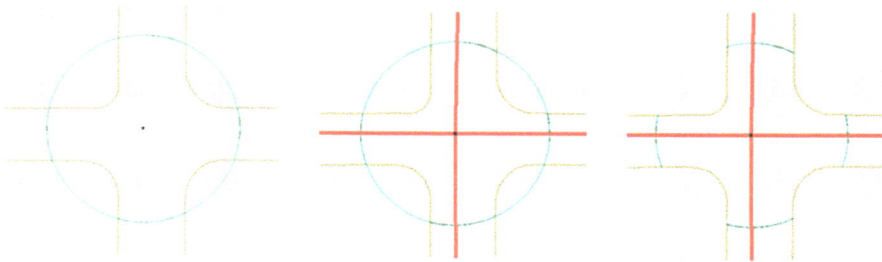

Figure 3. An illustration of analysis performed for crosswalk generation in ArcGIS (red lines = road network).

2.4.3. Building a Multimodal Network: Sidewalks Plus Bus Routes and Train Lines

The third mode of travel—accessibility by multimodal network—was created to simulate travel by public transit. The multimodal network was created by combining walkable network layer, bus routes (trip time was determined by calculating the time between the first and the last stop in the bus routes), bus stops as the link between the sidewalks and the bus routes, train lines, and train stations as a link between the sidewalks and the trains. The travel speed for bus routes were determined according to the speed specifications in Table 2. The bus routes were split at each bus stop to provide the entry and the exit points to buses from the sidewalks (Figure 4). Eventually all aforementioned layers were combined to build a functional multimodal network.

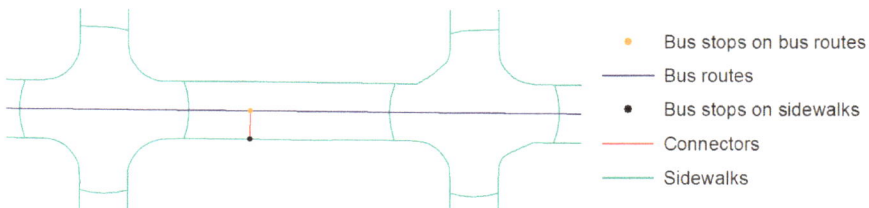

Figure 4. An illustration of connections between sidewalks and bus routes.

2.5. Spatial Accessibility Calculations by Different Modes of Travel

The spatial accessibility ratios were calculated based on the Spatial Access Ratio (SPAR) described in Section 2.1. This methodology was applied individually—by walking, multi-modal, and driving modes—to compare accessibility to the primary healthcare facilities by different modes of travel. We began by applying the distance impedance variant of the Two-Step Floating Catchment Area method: Enhanced Two-Step Floating Catchment Area (E2SFCA) [31]. We presented this advancement over 2SCFA to address its uniform access problem within the catchment area. Similar to 2SFCA, this method is applied in two steps (supply and demand models) with the addition of Gaussian weights to introduce distance decay within catchments.

Step 1 (supply model): A 30-min service area was generated around each primary care facility. The catchment was further divided into three travel subzones: the first zone between 0–10 min, second zone between 10–20 min, and third zone between 20–30 min. The population locations contained within each subzone were identified and the population at these locations was weighted according to the subzone it was contained within. Next, the Provider-to-Population ratio, Rj, of the primary care facility is calculated based on Luo and Qi's formula [31]:

$$R_j = \frac{S_j}{\sum_{k\in\{d_{kj}\leq D_r\}} P_k W_r}$$
$$= \frac{S_j}{\sum_{k\in\{d_{kj}\leq D_1\}} P_k W_1 + \sum_{k\in\{d_{kj}\leq D_2\}} P_k W_2 + \sum_{k\in\{d_{kj}\leq D_3\}} P_k W_3}$$

where

P_k refers to the population at the DA centroid location, k, falling within the catchment size j
S_j refers to number of general practitioners at the facility j
d_{kj} corresponds to the travel time between k and j
D_r is the rth travel time zone (where r = 1, 2 or 3)

Step 2 (demand model): From every population centroid location, all the primary care facility locations are identified within its 30-min service area in ArcGIS. The Provider-to-Population ratio, Rj, for the identified facility locations within the location are summed (Lu and Qi, 2009):

$$A_i^F = \sum_{j\in\{d_{ij}\in D_r\}} R_j W_r$$
$$= \sum_{j\in\{d_{ij}\in D_1\}} R_j W_1 + \sum_{j\in\{d_{ij}\in D_2\}} R_j W_2 + \sum_{j\in\{d_{ij}\in D_3\}} R_j W_3$$

where

A_i^F denotes the accessibility of population at location, i, to the facility
R_j corresponds to the weighted provider-to-population ratio (Step 1) that falls within the catchment size i
d_{ij} represents the travel time between i and j
W_r is the distance decay weight

The values of weights chosen for the three travel zones (1.00, 0.42 and 0.09 for W_1, W_2 and W_3 respectively) represent the sharper distance decay, which is prominent in the case of the presence of multiple service facilities, such as in the urban context. The rationality for these weights is based on the assumption that people tend to travel lesser distance in the presence of choice between the services [31]. Specifically, we use the sharper distance decay weights—W_1, W_2, and W_3 relating to the 0–10, 10–20, and 20–30 min range respectively—that Lou and Qi [31] establish for use in urban areas where there are more choices of facilities, rather than remote or rural areas where a slow distance decay is more realistic (people in rural areas travel further by necessity).

After applying the methodology of E2SFCA, the final step was to normalize the accessibility values as proposed by Wan et al. [43] to overcome the distance impedance uncertainty issues arising from previous accessibility measures. The SPAR values were calculated as a ratio between spatial accessibility index (that is, A_i^F at location, i) and the mean spatial accessibility of all population locations to derive normalized spatial accessibility indices. The SPAR methodology was applied in the GIS environment to analyze spatial accessibility to primary healthcare services by driving, walking, and multimodal (bus routes and train) means of travel from aforementioned networks. Quantile classification method was used to group the SPAR values with modifications to isolate the 0 values. Eventually, the shortage areas, exhibiting the 0 SPAR values, were identified and the population within the shortage areas was calculated by mode of travel.

2.6. Multiple Regression Analysis

Multiple regression analysis was performed using R to identify the relationship between accessibility indices by three modes of travel (SPAR values) and different social determinants of health, comprising of Pampalon Index (Table 3). The social determinants were comprised using the Pampalon Index (Table 3); a small area-based index used to reflect deprivation of relationships among individuals in workplace, community and family (social deprivation) and the deprivation of wealth, conveniences, and goods (material deprivation) [44,45].

Table 3. Pampalon index variables.

Variables
Proportion of the individuals separated, divorced, or widowed
Proportion of the persons living alone
Proportion of single-parent families
Proportion of persons without a high school diploma
Employment-population ratio
Average income

These determinants, at the DA level, were analyzed for correlation to reduce any redundancy in the results. Non-correlated independent variables were included in the multiple regression models for the results obtained from the three modes of travel. Since it is a spatial accessibility analysis, the regression models were subjected to measure spatial autocorrelation. To identify spatial autocorrelation in the SPAR values, Moran's I statistics were calculated for the accessibility values from three modes of travel. Due to the presence of spatial autocorrelation, spatial regression [46–48] was performed in R to account for spatial dependency, providing more accurate regression results.

For the spatial regression model, the predictor coefficients were obtained for the significant variables and their values were interpreted to deduce the link between the variables and the SPAR indices. The non-correlated variables for regression analysis were determined through correlation matrix analysis with a cut-off value of 0.70. The variables with the correlation values below 0.70 were retained in the regression analysis. Multiple regression analysis was performed on the selected independent variables with SPAR values as the dependent variable.

3. Results

A general comparison between spatial accessibility trends by driving, multimodal means, and walking illustrate that there are higher accessibility values estimated in the urban (core) region as compared to suburban regions by all modes of travel (Figure 5, a: road, b: multimodal, and c: walking). Additionally, the regions of high spatial accessibility are identified at the locations of the healthcare clinics for all analyses. In other words, the regions which were determined to have no accessibility were found to contain no healthcare facility in their proximity. A general comparison in travel by different modes revealed that spatial accessibility decreases when the mode of travel is changed from car to bus transit means, and reduced further by walking.

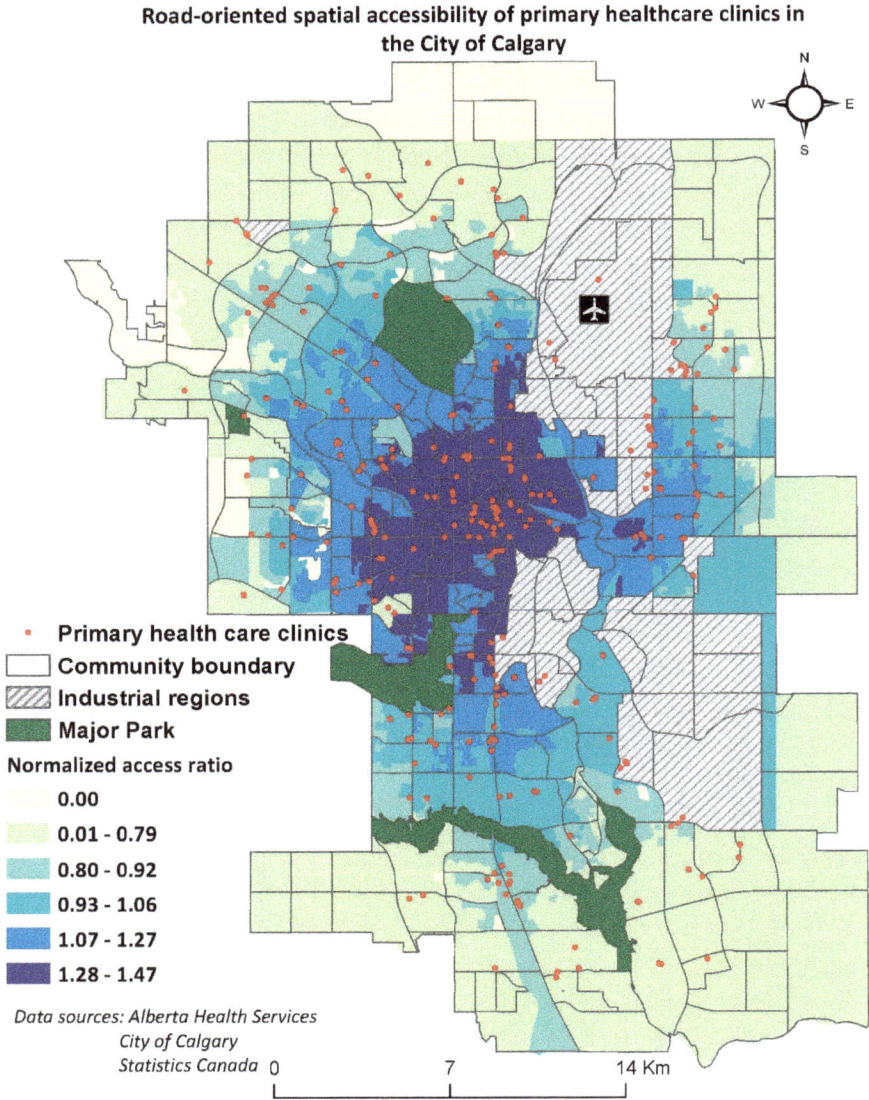

(a) Road-oriented spatial accessibility of primary healthcare clinics in the City of Calgary.

Figure 5. *Cont.*

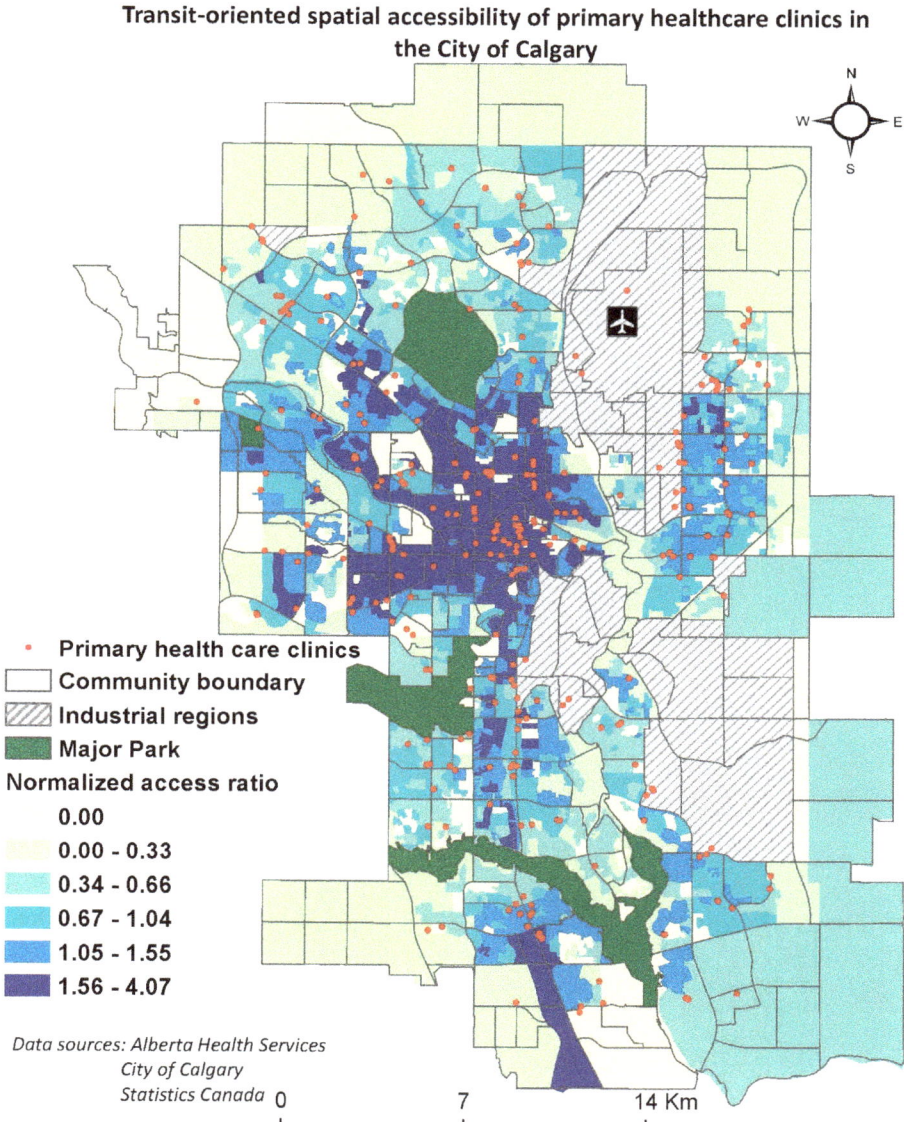

Transit-oriented spatial accessibility of primary healthcare clinics in the City of Calgary

(**b**) Transit-oriented spatial accessibility of primary healthcare clinics in the City of Calgary.

Figure 5. *Cont.*

Sidewalk spatial accessibility of primary healthcare clinics in the City of Calgary

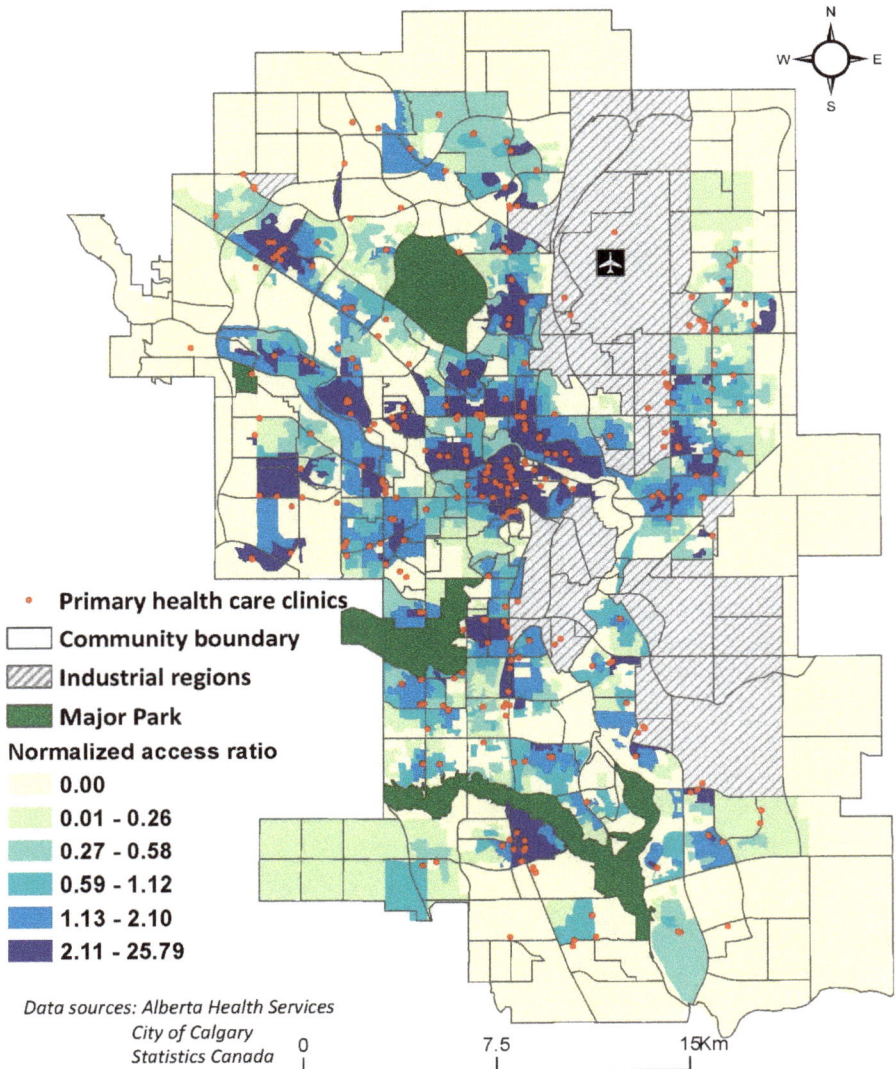

(c) Sidewalk-oriented spatial accessibility of primary healthcare clinics in the City of Calgary.

Figure 5. Spatial accessibility of the primary healthcare facilities in the City of Calgary by (**a**) driving, (**b**) multimodal means and (**c**) walking.

3.1. Accessibility by Driving

The greatest spatial accessibility to primary healthcare facilities in the City of Calgary was achieved by driving as compared to other modes of travel (Figure 5a). The initial inspection of the access status through this mode points out the decreasing trend in accessibility as one moves from the central to the peripheral regions of the city. According to this model, precisely 24 out of 1594 DAs, with the cumulative population of 30,090 (2.4% of the total population), had no spatial accessibility to primary healthcare facilities. Most of the DAs with no accessibility were found to be located in the Northwest region of the city.

3.2. Accessibility by Multimodal Means of Travel (Sidewalks, Bus Routes and Train Lines)

As compared to driving mode, spatial accessibility by multimodal means exhibits more intra-community variations over the City of Calgary (Figure 5b). Through this mode, the access status was observed to lie between the accessibility measured by driving and walking networks (Figure 5a,c). Specifically, less intra-community variations are observed than measured through walking and higher intra-community variations are identified than analysis performed on driving. For the multimodal means of travel, 151 out of 1594 DAs were identified with no access to healthcare, which were dispersed in different sections of Calgary of cumulative population of 137,745 (11.1% of total population).

3.3. Accessibility by Walking

The spatial accessibility to the primary healthcare facilities in the City by walking (Figure 5c), is substantially lower than that of driving or multimodal means. For this analysis, prominent intra-community variations in accessibility indices are observed. This implies that the access is not the same within the communities by walking, contradictory to the results obtained by other means. For this travel mode, 455 out of 1594 DAs were identified with no access to primary healthcare, which is home to 439,500 (35.5%) people in the city. Unlike access measured by driving mode, the regions with no accessibility can be found in all four quadrants of the city. Generally, regions with higher access are concentrated in the downtown section of the city.

3.4. Multiple Regression Analysis by Mode of Travel

The regression analysis for three modes of travel resulted in positively spatially auto-correlated residuals, implied by the high positive values of the Moran's I statistic (Table 4). This implies there is a spatial factor in determining the accessibility of primary healthcare facilities in the City of Calgary. This violated one of the assumptions of multiple regression. In other words, the residuals of the regression models should be independent of one another for the model to be considered valid. However, this was not the case in this research with positively auto-correlated residuals. Hence, the spatial regression analysis was performed to obtain regression results, while accounting for the spatial dependency of the nearby feature values.

Table 4. Spatial autocorrelation of residuals in DAs by different modes of travel.

Mode of Travel	Moran's I	*p*-Value
Walking	0.54	2.20×10^{-16}
Multimodal	0.46	2.20×10^{-16}
Car	0.49	2.20×10^{-16}

For the spatial regression analysis for travel by car, four variables were determined to be significant with less than 0.05 *p*-value: proportion of the individuals separated, divorced, or widowed; proportion of the persons living alone; average income; and proportion of single-parent families (Table 5).

Table 5. Relationship between significant variables and accessibility index for travel by car.

Coefficients	Estimate	Std. Error	z-Value	p-Value
1. Intercept	2.34×10^{-1}	1.58×10^{-2}	14.8425	$<2.20 \times 10^{-16}$
2. Proportion of the individuals separated, divorced, or widowed	-2.30×10^{-1}	8.22×10^{-2}	-2.7953	0.005186
3. Proportion of the persons living alone	4.18×10^{-1}	3.40×10^{-2}	12.2891	$<2.20 \times 10^{-16}$
4. Average income	3.34×10^{-7}	8.31×10^{-8}	4.0139	5.97×10^{-5}
5. Proportion of single-parent families	1.25×10^{-1}	5.54×10^{-2}	2.2541	0.024192
Rho: 0.66, LR test value: 1013.3, *p*-value: 2.22×10^{-1}				

AIC: -1370.7

Rho: Spatial autoregressive coefficient; LR: Lagrange Multiplier; AIC: Akaike Information Criterion.

The global spatial regression model (Table 6) reveals that there is an inverse relationship between the spatial accessibility and the proportion of the individuals separated, divorced, or widowed. In other words, the regions with high proportion of separated, divorced, or widowed individuals have lower accessibility to primary healthcare. On the other hand, the variables which were found to have a positive relationship with the increased SPAR were found to be proportion of the persons living alone, average income, and the proportion of single-parent families. Specifically, there seems to be a mismatch between the needs and resources for primary healthcare provisions. People with higher income tend to make use of healthcare facilities more as compared to low income individuals. The possible explanations for these trends are presented in discussion.

Table 6. Relationship between significant variables and accessibility index for travel by multimodal means.

Coefficients	Estimate	Std. Error	z-Value	p-Value
1. Intercept	1.46×10^{-1}	9.82×10^{-2}	1.4835	0.13793
2. Proportion of the individuals separated, divorced, or widowed	$-2.48 \times 10^{+0}$	2.72×10^{-1}	-9.1324	$<2 \times 10^{-16}$
3. Proportion of population living alone	$1.80 \times 10^{+0}$	1.24×10^{-1}	14.583	$<2 \times 10^{-16}$
4. Average income	5.76×10^{-7}	2.86×10^{-7}	2.0162	0.04378
5. Employment-population ratio	2.46×10^{-1}	1.37×10^{-1}	1.7973	0.07229
Rho: 0.55485, LR test value: 668.09, *p*-value: $<2.22 \times 10^{-16}$				

AIC: 2463.6

In regards to the multimodal means analysis, variables identified to be significant were proportion of the individuals separated, divorced, or widowed; proportion of population living alone; average income; and employment-population ratio. According to the SPAR model, there is a direct relationship between the SPAR values and these variables except for proportion of the individuals separated, divorced, or widowed. As the regions of high proportion of population living alone, high average income, and high employment-population ratio increases, the SPAR value increases. On the other hand, the regions with high proportion of the individuals separated, divorced, or widowed were found to have the low SPAR values as seen in the driving mode of travel analysis. Again, possible explanations are provided in discussion.

When the mode of travel is changed to walking, the spatial regression results are different from the other two analyses. In this case, the significant variables were calculated to be proportion of the individuals separated, divorced, or widowed and proportion of people living alone. The trend between the SPAR values and these two variables is similar as observed for the SPAR analysis in other two modes of travel scenarios. The regions with high proportion of people living alone and low proportion of the individuals separated, divorced, or widowed were found in high spatial access areas (Table 7). These trends are further discussed in the discussion section.

Table 7. Relationship between significant variables and accessibility index for travel by walking.

Coefficients	Estimate	Std. Error	z-Value	p-Value
1. Intercept	0.278341	0.077647	3.5847	0.000338
2. Proportion of the individuals separated, divorced, or widowed	−2.39588	0.671931	−3.5657	0.000363
3. Proportion of population living alone	2.06158	0.289785	7.1142	1.13×10^{-12}
Rho: 0.54755, LR test value: 608.09, p-value: $<2.22 \times 10^{-16}$				
AIC: 5595.9				

4. Discussion

4.1. Accessibility Status of the Primary Healthcare Facilities by Different Modes of Travel

In regard to spatial accessibility measured by all three different modes, the regions which were identified to have no spatial accessibility were found to contain no healthcare facilities in its vicinity. This implies that the spatial distribution of primary healthcare facilities is non-uniform and hence, points out the spatial disparity in terms of healthcare allocation in space. A general comparison for accessibility to primary healthcare facilities with different modes revealed that populations without access to a car have a significantly lower access ratio as compared to population who can drive (Table 8). It is evident that both the shortage area and population served increased in number in the following order of travel mode considered: walking, multimodal (bus routes and train), and car. This implies that if the population does not have access to an automobile and relies on bus transit/train for mobility, the accessibility index of the travel to the primary healthcare facilities decreases; comparatively larger areas of the City of Calgary are found to have no accessibility to primary healthcare facilities. As a result, a higher proportion of the population of the City of Calgary is not served by the healthcare systems equally due to the distance barrier posed from limited access by public transit and walking.

Table 8. Physician shortage area statistics.

Mode of Travel	Shortage Area (km²)	Population in the Shortage Areas	% of Total Population in Shortage Area
Driving	50.6	30,090	2.5%
Multimodal	140.9	137,745	11.1%
Walking	520.9	439,500	35.5%

Additionally, while comparing the results from different modes, it should be noted that the range of SPAR values differs among different modes. Specifically, the spatial accessibility range is lowest for the analysis by car travel (0.00–1.47). This analysis assumed that all of the population had access to a car, which resulted in the increasing ability to access the primary care overall. The small range implies that the assumption of universal access to a car smoothed the differences between the accessibility measures, resulting in the lower standard deviation (low variation in access in the City of Calgary). As the mode of travel is changed to multimodal (walking, bus routes, and train lines), the range increases (0.00–4.07). It can be deduced that more regional variability is identified with multi-modal network analysis as compared to the car analysis. This might have resulted from the kind of infrastructure in place that not all roads are bus routes, resulting in limiting choices of the primary healthcare facilities to the population to regions where bus service or the train lines are available. Another rationality behind this greater variation in access over space might be the unavailability of sidewalk infrastructure in non-core regions of the City of Calgary, resulting in limited access to the facilities. Further, the regional variability is highest for the walkability analysis (0.00–25.79). It is inferred that this would have resulted from the lower speed of pedestrians as compared to speeds in other travel models, concluding in higher spatial differences in the final output.

4.2. Relationship between Spatial Accessibility and Social Determinants of Health

The regression analysis between the accessibility index and the social determinants of health provided different results for each mode of travel. The aim of regression analysis was to detect any regions with low accessibility, where the vulnerable population is residing. There were two significant variables that were consistent among the three analyses: proportion of people living alone and proportion of the individuals separated, divorced, or widowed. This points out the mismatch between the needs and resources in primary healthcare provision. Specifically, it is important to determine the areas where there is a greater proportion of the individuals separated, divorced, or widowed, as these areas were found to have low access. Two key limitations were identified relating to the accuracy of travels speeds and actual car use, and employment status of the doctors. The same evaluation was used for all the features in travel networks; whereas, different elevation can result in travel at different speeds. Because of Calgary's location in the foothills of the Rocky Mountains, the elevation varies from one place to another. We also did not consider time delays at intersections, leading to variations in travel speeds. Since the analyses were conducted on the travel time, not considering the elevation and delay times at intersections might not have truly captured the real-time spatial accessibility status of primary care in the city of Calgary. We also did not consider the status of access to a car through ownership, compared to new approaches to mobility such as car sharing, which in future studies, could be analyzed and paired with the access results. Another limitation is that the number of Full-Time Equivalent physicians, service hours, and days of clinics' workings were not considered in the analysis. This information is crucial in determining whether the facility is capable of providing services. Ignoring these variables in the analysis might lead to inaccurate results regarding the availability of primary care in the city. There is also a lack of consideration of the general public's perception on their accessibility status to primary healthcare facilities in this analysis. Qualitative data on the public's perception of access and quantitative determination of access as performed in this analysis can be compared to obtain a holistic view of spatial accessibility to primary healthcare facilities in the City of Calgary.

Regardless of the limitations, it is important to consider the findings of this study to advocate for access for all populations regardless of socio-economic factors, such as access to a vehicle. The underlying purpose of this research was to examine the current situation of primary healthcare status in regards to clinic location, the population ability to access them, and the mode of travel used to travel to the healthcare services. An important next step would be to consider these factors to target future services to areas with the lowest (and in some cases nonexistent) access.

5. Conclusions

This research points out one of the biggest gaps in healthcare accessibility studies to date. The problem persists as most of the studies are conducted on the assumption of universal access to car. Specifically, in urban areas, a major proportion of people rely exclusively on public transportation for travel; serving as the motivation of this research. Specifically, we compared the effectiveness of different modes of travel in regard to accessibility to the primary healthcare facilities in the City of Calgary. People with access to a car were found to have the highest level of spatial accessibility to primary healthcare facilities in the city, with only 2.5% of the population in the shortage area. On the other hand, limited access was found for people relying on public transportation for accessing healthcare (11.1% of the population) and the lowest access was identified when the mode of travel was changed to walking only—over one third of the population (35.5%) reside in the shortage area. In other words, the social disparity in access to healthcare facilities was identified to be 14 times higher for people without access to a car. The regression analysis showed that the low-income regions corresponded to high access values. These were consistent with the previous research pointing out that people residing in low-income neighborhoods tend to utilize more healthcare services. Other variables were not consistent throughout different modes of travel analysis.

It is concluded that in the City of Calgary more primary healthcare facilities are required to be located in under-served areas or the pedestrian, or public transportation infrastructure needs to be improved—or ideally both. This study is important as it advocates for access without financial, environmental and ethical barriers as no person should have limited access to health due to not having an access to a private vehicle as everyone has an equal right to proper healthcare access. It can be deduced from the accessibility outputs that large portions of the City of Calgary have a low walking and public transit access. An effective solution to this problem might be to lessen the zoning restriction in certain communities to accommodate more primary healthcare facilities in the City of Calgary. Alternatively, walkability can be improved overall if the pedestrian infrastructure is enhanced in the City of Calgary. These changes are expected to improve the overall access to primary healthcare.

Author Contributions: Conceptualization, A.K.K. & V.F.; Methodology, A.K.K., V.F. & R.S.; Software, A.K.K., V.F. & R.S.; Validation, A.K.K., V.F. & R.S.; Formal Analysis, A.K.K., V.F. & R.S.; Investigation, A.K.K., V.F. & R.S.; Resources, A.K.K., V.F. & R.S.; Data Curation, A.K.K., V.F. & R.S.; Writing-Original Draft Preparation, A.K.K.; Writing-Review & Editing, A.K.K., V.F. & R.S.; Visualization, A.K.K., V.F. & R.S.; Supervision, V.F. & R.S.; Project Administration, V.F.

Funding: This research received no external funding.

Conflicts of Interest: The authors declare no conflict of interest.

References

1. UN General Assembly. *Universal Declaration of Human Rights*; UN General Assembly: New York, NY, USA, 1948.
2. Grad, F.P. The Preamble of the Constitution of the World Health Organization. *Bull. World Health Organ.* **2002**, *80*, 981.
3. Guagliardo, M.F. Spatial Accessibility of Primary Care: Concepts, Methods and Challenges. *Int. J. Health Geogr.* **2004**, *3*, 3. [CrossRef] [PubMed]
4. Starfield, B.; Shi, L.; Macinko, J. Contribution of Primary Care to Health Systems and Health. *Milbank Q.* **2005**, *83*, 457–502. [CrossRef] [PubMed]
5. Canadian Medical Association. Basic Physician Facts. Available online: https://www.cma.ca/En/Pages/basic-physician-facts.aspx (accessed on 10 November 2017).
6. Aday, L.A.; Andersen, R.M. Equity of Access to Medical Care: A Conceptual and Empirical Overview. *Med. Care* **1981**, *19*, 4–27. [CrossRef] [PubMed]
7. Ansari, Z. A Review of Literature on Access to Primary Health Care. *Aust. J. Prim. Health* **2007**, *13*, 80–95. [CrossRef]
8. Penchansky, R.; Thomas, J.W. The Concept of Access: Definition and Relationship to Consumer Satisfaction. *Med. Care* **1981**, *19*, 127–140. [CrossRef] [PubMed]
9. Rogers, A.; Flowers, J.; Pencheon, D. Improving Access Needs a Whole Systems Approach. *BMJ* **1999**, *319*, 866–867. [CrossRef]
10. Shah, T.I.; Bell, S.; Wilson, K. Spatial Accessibility to Health Care Services: Identifying under-Serviced Neighbourhoods in Canadian Urban Areas. *PLoS ONE* **2016**, *11*, 1–22. [CrossRef]
11. McGrail, M.R. Spatial Accessibility of Primary Health Care Utilising the Two Step Floating Catchment Area Method: An Assessment of Recent Improvements. *Int. J. Health Geogr.* **2012**, *11*, 50. [CrossRef]
12. Khan, A.A. An Integrated Approach to Measuring Potential Spatial Access to Health Care Services. *Socioecon. Plan. Sci.* **1992**, *26*, 275–287. [CrossRef]
13. Guo, Y.; Chan, C.H.; Yip, P.S.F. Spatial Variation in Accessibility of Libraries in Hong Kong. *Libr. Inf. Sci. Res.* **2017**, *39*, 319–329. [CrossRef]
14. Cheng, G.; Zeng, X.; Duan, L.; Lu, X.; Sun, H.; Jiang, T.; Li, Y. Spatial Difference Analysis for Accessibility to High Level Hospitals Based on Travel Time in Shenzhen, China. *Habitat Int.* **2016**, *53*, 485–494. [CrossRef]
15. Ma, L.; Luo, N.; Wan, T.; Hu, C.; Peng, M. An Improved Healthcare Accessibility Measure Considering the Temporal Dimension and Population Demand of Different Ages. *Int. J. Environ. Res. Public Health* **2018**, *15*, 2421. [CrossRef] [PubMed]
16. Chu, H.J.; Lin, B.C.; Yu, M.R.; Chan, T.C. Minimizing Spatial Variability of Healthcare Spatial Accessibility—The Case of a Dengue Fever Outbreak. *Int. J. Environ. Res. Public Health* **2016**, *13*, 1235. [CrossRef] [PubMed]
17. Ni, J.; Wang, J.; Rui, Y.; Qian, T.; Wang, J. An Enhanced Variable Two-Step Floating Catchment Area Method for Measuring Spatial Accessibility to Residential Care Facilities in Nanjing. *Int. J. Environ. Res. Public Health* **2015**, *12*, 14490–14504. [CrossRef] [PubMed]

18. Luo, W.; Wang, F. Measures of Spatial Accessibility to Health Care in a GIS Environment: Synthesis and a Case Study in the Chicago Region. *Environ. Plan. B Plan. Des.* **2003**, *30*, 865–884. [CrossRef]
19. Yang, D.H.; Goerge, R.; Mullner, R. Comparing GIS-Based Methods of Measuring Spatial Accessibility to Health Services. *J. Med. Syst.* **2006**, *30*, 23–32. [CrossRef]
20. Khakh, A.K.; Fast, V. Measuring Spatial Accessibility of Healthcare Services in Calgary. *J. Transp. Health* **2017**, *7*, S13–S14. [CrossRef]
21. Luo, J.; Chen, G.; Li, C.; Xia, B.; Sun, X.; Chen, S. Use of an E2SFCA Method to Measure and Analyse Spatial Accessibility to Medical Services for Elderly People in Wuhan, China. *Int. J. Environ. Res. Public Health* **2018**, *15*, 1503. [CrossRef]
22. Pan, X.; Kwan, M.-P.; Yang, L.; Zhou, S.; Zuo, Z.; Wan, B.; Pan, X.; Kwan, M.-P.; Yang, L.; Zhou, S.; et al. Evaluating the Accessibility of Healthcare Facilities Using an Integrated Catchment Area Approach. *Int. J. Environ. Res. Public Health* **2018**, *15*, 2051. [CrossRef]
23. Fransen, K.; Neutens, T.; De Maeyer, P.; Deruyter, G. A Commuter-Based Two-Step Floating Catchment Area Method for Measuring Spatial Accessibility of Daycare Centers. *Health Place* **2015**, *32*, 65–73. [CrossRef] [PubMed]
24. Yu, D.; Tan, H.; Ruan, Y. An Improved Two-Step Floating Catchment Area Method for Supporting District Building Energy Planning: A Case Study of Yongding County City, China. *Appl. Energy* **2012**, *95*, 156–163. [CrossRef]
25. Sivak, M.; Schoettle, B. Recent Changes in the Age Composition of Drivers in 15 Countries. *Traffic Inj. Prev.* **2012**, *13*, 126–132. [CrossRef] [PubMed]
26. Khan, A.A.; Bhardwaj, S.M. Access to Health Care. A Conceptual Framework and Its Relevance to Health Care Planning. *Eval. Health Prof.* **1994**, *17*, 60–76. [CrossRef] [PubMed]
27. Wang, F.; Luo, W. Assessing Spatial and Nonspatial Factors for Healthcare Access: Towards an Integrated Approach to Defining Health Professional Shortage Areas. *Health Place* **2005**, *11*, 131–146. [CrossRef] [PubMed]
28. Wing, P.; Reynolds, C. The Availability of Physician Services: A Geographic Analysis. *Health Serv. Res.* **1988**, *23*, 649–667. [PubMed]
29. Delamater, P.L. Spatial Accessibility in Suboptimally Configured Health Care Systems: A Modified Two-Step Floating Catchment Area (M2SFCA) Metric. *Health Place* **2013**, *24*, 30–43. [CrossRef]
30. Luo, W.; Whippo, T. Variable Catchment Sizes for the Two-Step Floating Catchment Area (2SFCA) Method. *Health Place* **2012**, *18*, 789–795. [CrossRef]
31. Luo, W.; Qi, Y. An Enhanced Two-Step Floating Catchment Area (E2SFCA) Method for Measuring Spatial Accessibility to Primary Care Physicians. *Health Place* **2009**, *15*, 1100–1107. [CrossRef]
32. Wan, N.; Zhan, F.B.; Zou, B.; Chow, E. A Relative Spatial Access Assessment Approach for Analyzing Potential Spatial Access to Colorectal Cancer Services in Texas. *Appl. Geogr.* **2012**, *32*, 291–299. [CrossRef]
33. Mao, L.; Nekorchuk, D. Measuring Spatial Accessibility to Healthcare for Populations with Multiple Transportation Modes. *Health Place* **2013**, *24*, 115–122. [CrossRef] [PubMed]
34. Iacono, M.; Krizek, K.J.; El-Geneidy, A. Measuring Non-Motorized Accessibility: Issues, Alternatives, and Execution. *J. Transp. Geogr.* **2010**, *18*, 133–140. [CrossRef]
35. Statistics Canada. Census Profile. Catalogue No 98-316-X2016001. Geography: Calgary [Census Metropolitan Area], Alberta [Province]. Available online: http://www12.statcan.gc.ca/census-recensement/2016/dp-pd/prof/index.cfm?Lang=E (accessed on 7 November 2017).
36. Statistics Canada. A Profile of Persons with Disabilities among Canadians Aged 15 Years or Older. 2012. Available online: http://www.statcan.gc.ca/pub/89-654-x/89-654-x2015001-eng.pdf (accessed on 7 November 2017).
37. Canadian Institute for Health Information. Hospital Stays in Canada. Available online: https://www.cihi.ca/en/hospital-stays-in-canada (accessed on 8 November 2017).
38. Riger, S.; Lavrakas, P.J. Community Ties: Patterns of Attachment and Social Interaction in Urban Neighborhoods. *Am. J. Community Psychol.* **1981**, *9*, 55–66. [CrossRef]
39. Gauvin, L.; Robitaille, É.; Riva, M.; McLaren, L.; Dassa, C.; Potvin, L. Conceptualizing and Operationalizing Neighbourhoods. *Can. J. Public Health* **2007**, *98*, 518–526.
40. Saghapour, T.; Moridpour, S.; Thompson, R.G. Modeling Access to Public Transport in Urban Areas. *J. Adv. Transp.* **2016**, *50*, 1785–1801. [CrossRef]

41. Saghapour, T.; Moridpour, S.; Thompson, R.G. Estimating Walking Access Levels Incorporating Distance Thresholds of Built Environment Features. *Int. J. Sustain. Transp.* **2018**, 1–14. [CrossRef]

42. El-Geneidy, A.M.; Levinson, D.M. *Access to Destinations: Development of Accessibility Measures*; Minnesota Department of Transportation: St. Paul, MN, USA, 2006.

43. Wan, N.; Zou, B.; Sternberg, T. A Three-Step Floating Catchment Area Method for Analyzing Spatial Access to Health Services. *Int. J. Geogr. Inf. Sci.* **2012**, *26*, 1073–1089. [CrossRef]

44. Pampalon, R.; Hamsel, D.; Gamache, P.; Philibert, M.; Raymond, G.; Simpson, A. An Area Based Material and Social Deprivation Index for Public Health in Quebec and Canada. *Can. J. Public Health* **2012**, *103*, S17–S22.

45. Alberta Health Services. *Pampalon Deprivation Index: User Guide for Alberta*; Alberta Health Services: Edmonton, AB, Canada, 2016; pp. 1–27.

46. Wong, M.S.; Ho, H.C.; Yang, L.; Shi, W.; Yang, J.; Chan, T.C. Spatial Variability of Excess Mortality during Prolonged Dust Events in a High-Density City: A Time-Stratified Spatial Regression Approach. *Int. J. Health Geogr.* **2017**, *16*, 1–14. [CrossRef]

47. Mahara, G.; Wang, C.; Yang, K.; Chen, S.; Guo, J.; Gao, Q.; Wang, W.; Wang, Q.; Guo, X. The Association between Environmental Factors and Scarlet Fever Incidence in Beijing Region: Using Gis and Spatial Regression Models. *Int. J. Environ. Res. Public Health* **2016**, *13*, 1083. [CrossRef]

48. Mobley, L.R.; Kuo, T.M.; Urato, M.; Subramanian, S. Community Contextual Predictors of Endoscopic Colorectal Cancer Screening in the USA: Spatial Multilevel Regression Analysis. *Int. J. Health Geogr.* **2010**, *9*, 1–11. [CrossRef] [PubMed]

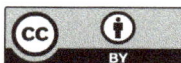

International Journal of
*Environmental Research
and Public Health*

MDPI

Article

Roles of Different Transport Modes in the Spatial Spread of the 2009 Influenza A(H1N1) Pandemic in Mainland China

Jun Cai [1,2], Bo Xu [1,2], Karen Kie Yan Chan [1,2], Xueying Zhang [3], Bing Zhang [4], Ziyue Chen [5] and Bing Xu [1,2,*]

[1]   Ministry of Education Key Laboratory for Earth System Modeling, Department of Earth System Science, Tsinghua University, Beijing 100084, China; cai-j12@mails.tsinghua.edu.cn (J.C.); xu-b15@mails.tsinghua.edu.cn (B.X.); cqe15@mails.tsinghua.edu.cn (K.K.Y.C.)
[2]   Joint Center for Global Change Studies, Beijing 100875, China
[3]   Department of Environmental Medicine and Public Health, Icahn School of Medicine at Mount Sinai, New York, NY 10029, USA; xueying.zhang@mssm.edu
[4]   School of Public Health (Shenzhen), Sun Yat-sen University, Shenzhen 518107, China; zhangbing4502431@outlook.com
[5]   State Key Laboratory of Remote Sensing Science, College of Global Change and Earth System Science, Beijing Normal University, Beijing 100875, China; zychen@bnu.edu.cn
*   Correspondence: bingxu@tsinghua.edu.cn; Tel.: +86-010-6279-0189

Received: 29 November 2018; Accepted: 9 January 2019; Published: 14 January 2019

Abstract: There is increasing concern about another influenza pandemic in China. However, the understanding of the roles of transport modes in the 2009 influenza A(H1N1) pandemic spread across mainland China is limited. Herein, we collected 127,797 laboratory-confirmed cases of influenza A(H1N1)pdm09 in mainland China from May 2009 to April 2010. Arrival days and peak days were calculated for all 340 prefectures to characterize the dissemination patterns of the pandemic. We first evaluated the effects of airports and railway stations on arrival days and peak days, and then we applied quantile regressions to quantify the relationships between arrival days and air, rail, and road travel. Our results showed that early arrival of the virus was not associated with an early incidence peak. Airports and railway stations in prefectures significantly advanced arrival days but had no significant impact on peak days. The pandemic spread across mainland China from the southeast to the northwest in two phases that were split at approximately 1 August 2009. Both air and road travel played a significant role in accelerating the spread during phases I and II, but rail travel was only significant during phase II. In conclusion, in addition to air and road travel, rail travel also played a significant role in accelerating influenza A(H1N1)pdm09 spread between prefectures. Establishing a multiscale mobility network that considers the competitive advantage of rail travel for mid to long distances is essential for understanding the influenza pandemic transmission in China.

Keywords: China; 2009 influenza A(H1N1) pandemic; transport modes; rail travel; spatial spread; quantile regression

1. Introduction

Four influenza pandemics occurred at intervals of several decades during the past 100 years, the most recent of which occurred in 2009 and was caused by influenza A(H1N1)pdm09 virus [1]. Cases of human infection with influenza A(H1N1)pdm09 virus were first identified in the United States (US) and Mexico in early April 2009 [2]. The rapid global spread of the virus led the World Health Organization (WHO) to raise the influenza pandemic alert level to the highest phase six on 11 June 2009 [3]. On 10 August 2010, the WHO announced that the world had moved into the post-pandemic period [4]. As of 1 August 2010, laboratory-confirmed cases of influenza A(H1N1)pdm09 including over 18,449 deaths had been reported from more than 214 countries or regions worldwide [5]. The actual fatality of the pandemic could be much higher; it was estimated to have caused between 100,000 and 400,000 deaths globally in the first 12 months of the pandemic [6].

Prior to the emergence of influenza A(H1N1)pdm09 virus, a number of studies had assessed the role of air travel in the spread of pandemic and seasonal influenza viruses at global and regional scales [7–12]. It is recognized that the global spread of pandemic influenza is largely associated with international air travel, especially during the introduction period. Therefore, following initial detection of influenza A(H1N1)pdm09 virus in North America, numerous studies employed statistical and mathematical models that incorporated air transportation data to explain its global dissemination [13–20]. A multiscale mobility network comprised of long-range airline traffic and short-scale local commutes was also used to approximate the spreading scenarios at a global scale [21,22]. However, controversy remains over whether short-distance commutes or long-range air travel has more influence on regional influenza spread in the US [11,23]. On the one hand, short-distance commutes have been identified as a major driver of between-state influenza spread [12,23,24]; on the other hand, long-range air travel has also been connected to inter-regional spread [10]. Thus, to improve our understanding of the drivers of spread, it is essential to examine the roles of different transport modes in influenza transmission at a regional scale.

Most previous investigations concentrated on the effects of transport modes on influenza spread in the US. However, few studies examined transport modes in a similarly sized country with a much larger population, such as China. In the US, the vast majority of people travel by automobile for shorter distances and by airplane for longer distances. Trains accounted for only 0.74% of passenger-miles traveled in the US in 2009 [25]. In contrast, railway is a common and principal mode for intermediate and long-range travel between cities in mainland China [26]. For example, 5.12% (77.1–86.9%, after removal of the short-distance traffic volume) of the total passengers in mainland China in 2009 were handled by trains [27]. Consequently, models based on human mobility patterns in the US such as the global epidemic and mobility (GLEaM) model [28] may not be suitable for mainland China. Furthermore, the multiscale mobility network used by the GLEaM model does not contain any commuting data from mainland China [21]. Due to the unique transportation system, it is necessary to investigate the roles of different transport modes in the spatial spread of influenza in mainland China. The increased disease surveillance and data availability in the context of the 2009 influenza A(H1N1) pandemic [24] provides a unique opportunity to conduct such an investigation.

After the first confirmed case of influenza A(H1N1)pdm09 that was imported into mainland China on 10 May 2009 [29], the virus spread rapidly. By 5 July 2009, 1040 cumulative confirmed cases—including 758 imported cases and 282 autochthonous cases—were reported in 24 provinces across mainland China [30]. The rapid transmission and substantial impact of the disease on the public health system caused great concern [31]. A few scholars explored the effects of transport modes on spatial transmission at different geographical scales in mainland China. Xiao et al. [32] analyzed the spatiotemporal transmission of influenza A(H1N1)pdm09 via road traffic between counties and towns within Changsha city, and their results showed that inter-county bus stations played an important role in epidemic diffusion. Fang et al. [33] used survival analysis to analyze the impact of travel-related risk factors on the inter-county invasion of influenza A(H1N1)pdm09 in mainland China, and they found that counties close to airports and intersected by highways rather than railways were significantly associated with earlier virus presence. Their findings of an insignificant influence of rail travel on influenza A(H1N1)pdm09 spread may have been due to the county level at which their study was conducted. In contrast, other research suggested that rail travel played an important role in influenza A(H1N1)pdm09 spread across mainland China, including a reported transmission of the virus on a train [34]. Moreover, in the hybrid model developed by Weng and Ni [35] to evaluate the containment and mitigation strategies of influenza A(H1N1)pdm09 in mainland China, trains and airlines were transportation modes for travel between prefecture-level cities, which indicated they were responsible for the large-scale spread of the virus. In response to the conflicting results regarding the effects of different transport modes on influenza transmission, particularly air and rail travel, we examined their roles in the spread of influenza A(H1N1)pdm09 in mainland China at the prefecture level.

In this study, we characterized the spatial variability in arrival and peak times of influenza A(H1N1)pdm09 transmission across the 340 affected prefectures in mainland China based on daily laboratory-confirmed infections from 10 May 2009 to 30 April 2010. We first evaluated the effects of airports and high-ranking railway stations on arrival time and peak time. To quantify the roles of different transport modes in the two spread phases of the pandemic, we fitted quantile regression models to assess the relationships between various quantiles of arrival timing and passenger traffic via air, rail, and road in 115 prefectures with data for all three transport modes.

2. Materials and Methods

2.1. Epidemiological Data

We obtained data from all influenza A(H1N1)pdm09 cases reported to the China Information System for Disease Control and Prevention (CISDCP) from 10 May 2009, when the first confirmed case was reported, to 30 April 2010. These were all classified as suspected and laboratory-confirmed cases. For more details about CISDCP and case definitions, refer to [33]. We only used the laboratory-confirmed cases in our analyses. Case information included but was not limited to case classification, gender, birth date, onset date, diagnosis date, occupation, residential address, work address, and hospital admission address. The residential address of each case was geocoded into latitude and longitude coordinates with the Google Geocoding API [36]. The resulting geographic coordinates were examined at the county level to ensure geocoding quality. The spatiotemporal distribution of the cases is shown in Figure 1.

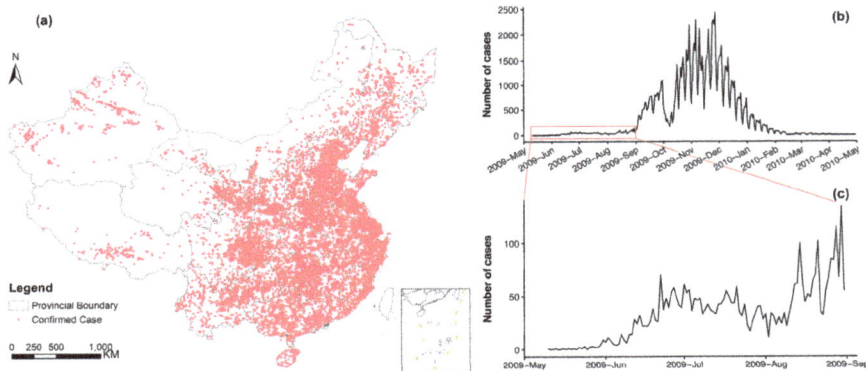

Figure 1. The spatial and temporal distribution of all 127,797 laboratory-confirmed influenza A(H1N1)pdm09 cases reported to the China Information System for Disease Control and Prevention in mainland China from 10 May 2009 to 30 April 2010: (**a**) spatial distribution of geocoded residential addresses; (**b**) the daily epidemic curve from 10 May 2009 to 30 April 2010; (**c**) the enlarged daily epidemic curve from 10 May 2009 to 31 August 2009.

2.2. Passenger Volume Data

Mainland China is comprised of 31 provinces that are further divided into 341 administrative prefectures. The passenger volumes of air, rail, road, and boat travel for each prefecture in 2009 were obtained from the 2010 China City Statistical Yearbook [37]. Because the data were only available for 281 prefecture-level cities, we supplemented passenger volume data for the remaining prefectures by individually looking up the 2009 statistical bulletins on national economic and social development.

Finally, of all 340 affected prefectures, 334 (98.2%) had passenger volumes for at least one type of transport mode. Here, only air, rail, and road passenger volumes were included in our analyses, given that boat passenger volumes had the smallest proportion of total passenger volumes (0.7%) and explained the least variance in arrival days defined below (3.2%). The availability of air, rail, and road transport varied across 334 prefectures. All three transport modes were available in 115 (33.8%) prefectures; air and road transport were both available in 20 (5.9%) prefectures, while rail and road transport were both available in 140 (41.2%) prefectures. The automobile was the only transport mode for the remaining 59 (17.3%) prefectures.

2.3. Definitions of Arrival Day and Peak Day

A daily epidemic curve of newly confirmed cases for each prefecture was generated based on the diagnosis date using the R package incidence [38]. To characterize the inter-prefecture spread of influenza A(H1N1)pdm09 in mainland China, two measures—arrival day and peak day—were derived from the epidemic curve. As defined in [16], arrival day for a given prefecture was defined as the number of days from 10 May 2009 (the date of the first country case) to the date of the first case in each prefecture. Likewise, peak day was defined as the number of days from 10 May 2009 to the date with the highest incidence (Figure 2).

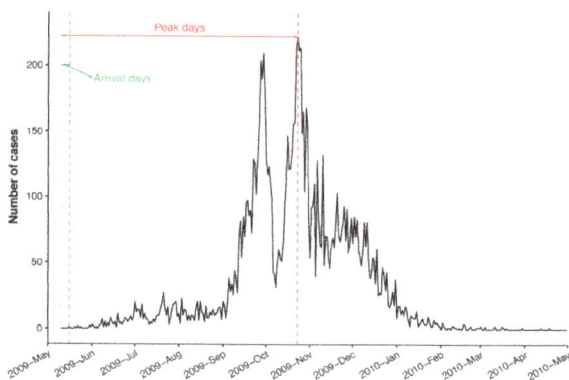

Figure 2. Illustration of arrival days and peak days using the daily epidemic curve of confirmed cases in Beijing. The gray, green, and red vertical dashed lines represent, respectively, the date of the first case in mainland China (10 May 2009), the date of the first case in Beijing (16 May 2009), and the date with the highest incidence in Beijing (23 October 2009).

2.4. Comparisons of Arrival Days and Peak Days between Prefectures with and without Transport Hubs

The presence of railway stations is a better proxy of passenger volume than being intersected by railways because there are prefectures that are intersected by railways but do not have railway stations (e.g., Luzhou, a city located in Sichuan province). Hence, we compiled a list of all the airports and railway stations in mainland China at the end of 2009 and identified their locations on the map. The National Railway Administration of China manages railway stations according to their status level, which is determined by the daily arrival, departure, and transfer passenger volume (DPV) as well as by their geographical conditions. Status levels are classified as principal (DPV > 60,000), first-rank (DPV = 15,000–60,000), second-rank (DPV = 5000–15,000), third-rank (DPV = 2000–5000), fourth-rank, or fifth-rank passenger stations. To ensure that prefectures were exposed to intensive railway transportation, only principal, first-, and second-class railway stations were used to indicate exposure in our analyses. All 340 prefectures were assigned to "with airport" or "without airport" categories and "with railway station" or "without railway station" categories based on whether there was an airport or railway station inside the prefecture (Figure 3a,b). To evaluate the respective effects of the presence of airports and railway stations on the inter-prefecture invasion of influenza A(H1N1)pdm09, we used the Mann-Whitney U test at the 95% confidence level to examine whether prefectures with and without a particular transport hub showed a significant difference in arrival day. The same test was also applied to peak day.

The spatial stratified heterogeneity (SSH) of arrival day is realized by the Heihe-Tengchong line (hereafter referred to as the Hu line [39]) (Figure 3c). To measure the degree of the stratified heterogeneity [40], we stratified 340 prefectures based on the relative positions of their administrative centers and the Hu line. Then, the SSH q-statistic for the stratified arrival days was calculated, and the significance of the stratified heterogeneity was also tested with a significance level of 0.05 using the R package geodetector [41]. Using the same procedure, we also assessed the assumption that there is SSH in peak days stratified by the Hukun Railway (Figure 3d). Furthermore, to detect the determinant power of transport hubs to the SSH of arrival day, the q-statistic and corresponding p value were also calculated for the airports and railway stations factors, respectively. The same analysis was also applied to peak day.

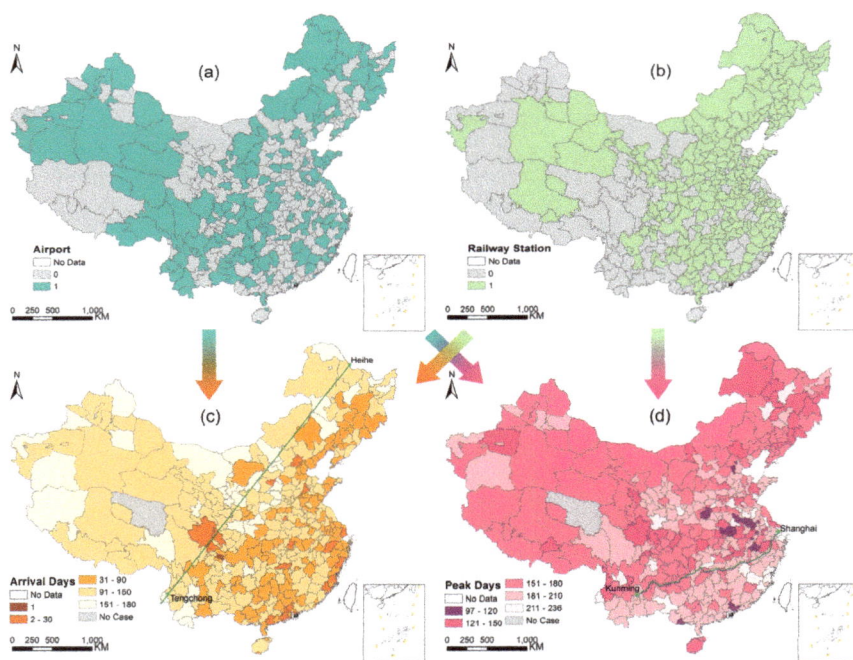

Figure 3. The presence/absence (1/0) of (**a**) airports and (**b**) railway stations in prefectures, and the distributions of (**c**) arrival days and (**d**) peak days for prefectures. The green line in (**c**) indicates the Heihe-Tengchong (Hu) line, and the one in (**d**) indicates the Hukun Railway that connects Shanghai and Kunming. The arrows illustrate that arrival days (or peak days) between prefectures with and without airports (or railway stations) are compared using the Mann-Whitney U test, and their spatial heterogeneity stratified by airports (or railway stations) are detected using q-statistic test.

2.5. Quantile Regression of Arrival Days on Passenger Volumes

Because there was large variance in passenger volumes across prefectures, log transformations were conducted on the air, rail, and road passenger volume data to shrink their scales. We performed Pearson's correlation analysis to identify the associations between log-transformed passenger volumes and arrival days for each transport mode.

To examine the roles of transport modes in shaping the two peaks of the bimodal distribution of arrival days (Figures 4 and 5a), we applied quantile regression to fit specified percentiles of arrival days. Quantile regression, introduced by Koenker and Bassett [42], is distribution agnostic and capable of modeling the entire distribution of the response. In contrast, standard ordinary least squares regression only models the mean of the response. To consider the effect of prefectural locations on the spatial spread of influenza A(H1N1)pdm09, latitudes and longitudes of their administrative centers were also included as covariates. We therefore fitted the following multivariate quantile regression model to assess the associations between different quantiles of arrival days and passenger volumes for multiple transport modes in the 115 prefectures where data on all three transport modes were available:

$$Q_\tau(y_i) = \beta_0(\tau) + \beta_1(\tau)Lat_i + \beta_2(\tau)Lng_i + \beta_3(\tau)\log(PAir_i)$$
$$+\beta_4(\tau)\log(PRail_i) + \beta_5(\tau)\log(PRoad_i), \tag{1}$$

where y_i is the arrival day in prefecture i ($i = 1,\ldots,115$), τ is the quantile level, and $Q_\tau(y_i)$ is the corresponding conditional quantile of arrival days. $\beta_0(\tau)$ denotes the intercept for quantile level τ. Lat_i and Lng_i are the latitude and longitude coordinates of the administrative center in prefecture i. $\log(PAir_i)$, $\log(PRail_i)$, and $\log(PRoad_i)$ are the log-transformed air, rail, and road passenger volumes (10,000 persons) in prefecture i, respectively, and $\beta_1(\tau),\ldots,\beta_5(\tau)$ are the corresponding regression coefficients for quantile level τ.

We separately fitted the quantile regression models for the quantile levels $\tau = 0.25, 0.50$, and 0.75. To fully describe the bimodal distribution of arrival days, quantile process regressions for uniformly spaced values of τ in the interval $(0, 1)$ with an increment of 0.05 were also fitted. The 95% confidence intervals (CIs) for coefficient estimates were calculated using the default "rank" method [43].

The quantile regression was implemented using R package quantreg [44]. All data analyses were performed in R version 3.5.1 [45].

3. Results

3.1. Summary of Influenza A(H1N1)pdm09 Infections in Mainland China

The first case of influenza A(H1N1)pdm09 in mainland China was confirmed on 10 May 2009 as a Chinese student returning from the United States to Neijiang city, Sichuan province [29]. On 29 May 2009, the first secondary case of influenza A(H1N1)pdm09 in mainland China was confirmed in Guangzhou city, Guangdong province [46]. Also in Guangzhou, the first untraceable autochthonous case of influenza A(H1N1)pdm09 in mainland China was confirmed on 11 June 2009 [47]. As shown in Figure 1c, the number of confirmed cases increased slowly from May 2009 to the end of August 2009 with a small uplift around late June. Starting in September 2009, when the new school term began, the number of confirmed cases increased substantially but decreased sharply during the eight-day National Day holiday (1–8 October 2009). The number of confirmed cases then rebounded at the end of the holiday period and peaked by the end of November 2009 (Figure 1b). By the end of April 2010, a total of 127,797 confirmed cases of influenza A(H1N1)pdm09, including 806 deaths, had been reported to the Chinese Center for Disease Control and Prevention from 340 of all 341 prefectures; only Yushu, a less populated prefecture in Qinghai province, reported no cases (Figure 3c).

3.2. Effects of Airports and Railway Stations on Influenza A(H1N1)pdm09 Inter-Prefecture Spread and Peak

The arrival days and peak days for the 340 affected prefectures are summarized in Table 1. The arrival days for the 340 affected prefectures ranged from 1–180 days (median: 119 days, interquartile range (IQR): 61–136 days), while peak days distributed in a narrower range of 97–236 days (median: 179 days, IQR: 163–198 days). Both the maps of arrival days (Figure 3c) and peak days (Figure 3d) showed apparent SSH; most prefectures with earlier arrival days were located in the southeast of the Hu line ($q = 0.143, p < 0.001$), whereas prefectures with relatively late peak times were generally located below the Hukun Railway ($q = 0.091, p = 0.002$). Using a Pearson's correlation coefficient test, no significant correlation between arrival day and peak day was found ($r = -0.08$, $p = 0.13$).

The distributions of arrival days and peak days by transport hub presence are shown in Figure 4. The plots of arrival days show a bimodal distribution with two peaks. The first peak of arrival days occurred around 40 days, while the second peak of arrival days occurred around 125 days. The distribution of arrival days was different between prefectures with and without transport hubs. Specifically, the two peaks were of similar intensity for prefectures with a transport hub, whereas the second peak of arrival days was greater than the first for prefectures without a transport hub. The plots of peak days have a less distinctive double-peak feature. The first smaller peak occurred around 125 days, and the second larger peak occurred around 175 days—before the end of November 2009. There was no apparent difference in the distribution of peak days between prefectures with and without airports. However, the distribution of peak days changed less abruptly for prefectures without railway stations than with.

Table 1. Summary statistics of arrival days and peak days for 340 affected prefectures in mainland China.

Category		Arrival Day [a]					Peak Day				
		Min	Q1	Median	Q3	Max	Min	Q1	Median	Q3	Max
All (340)		1	61	119	136	180	97	163	179	198	236
Airport	With (155)	4	41	106	134	180	113	162	180	196	228
	Without (185)	1	75	120	136	175	97	164	179	199	236
Railway station	With (234)	1	53	111	129	175	97	163	179	196	236
	Without (106)	17	93	128	140	180	117	164	181	199	236

[a] Arrival day and peak day are calculated as starting from 10 May 2009, the date of the first confirmed case reported in mainland China.

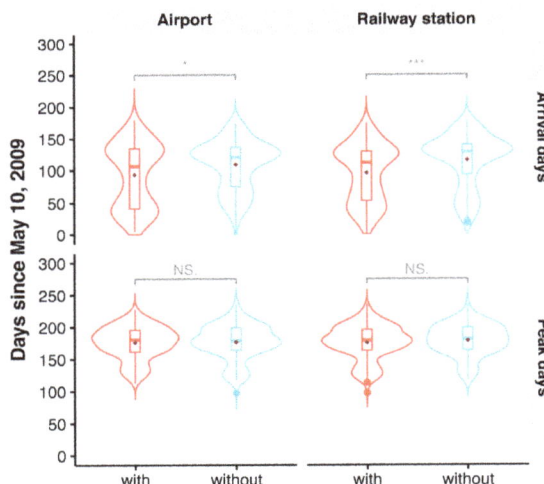

Figure 4. Violin plots of arrival days and peak days between prefectures with (in red) and without (in cyan) airports (or railway stations). Box plots are embedded into violin plots to add summary statistics. The dark red points represent the mean arrival days (or peak days). * $p < 0.05$; *** $p < 0.001$; NS., not significant for comparing arrival days (or peak days) between prefectures with and without transport hubs using a Mann-Whitney U test.

Among the 340 affected prefectures, 155 (45.6%) prefectures with airports were generally affected earlier than the other 185 (54.4%) prefectures without airports (median arrival days: 106 days versus 120 days; Mann-Whitney U test, $p = 0.005$, see Figure 4). In contrast, no statistically significant difference in peak day between these two groups was found (median: 180 days versus 179 days; Mann-Whitney U test, $p = 0.87$, see Figure 4). The railway station results were similar to the airport results. There was a statistically significant difference in arrival day between the 234 (68.8%) prefectures with railway stations and the 106 (31.2%) prefectures without (median: 111 days versus 128 days; Mann-Whitney U test, $p < 0.001$, see Figure 4). By contrast, no statistically significant difference in peak day was detected between these two groups (median: 179 days versus 181 days; Mann-Whitney U test, $p = 0.42$, see Figure 4). The SSH q-statistic showed consistent results with the Mann-Whitney U test. There was significant stratified heterogeneity in arrival day for both stratifications of airports ($q = 0.031$, $p = 0.001$) and railway stations ($q = 0.042$, $p = 0.002$), whereas no significant stratified heterogeneity in peak day was detected for the stratifications of airports ($q = 0.000$, $p = 0.897$) or railway stations ($q = 0.003$, $p = 0.817$). The difference in median arrival day between prefectures with and without transport hubs was ~2 weeks (120 days versus 106 days for airport; 128 days versus 111 days for railway station). Additionally, there was approximately a one week lag in median arrival day when comparing the corresponding analysis of railway stations with airports (111 days versus 106 days for prefectures with transport hubs; 128 days versus 120 days for prefectures without transport hubs). By comparison, the median peak was around 180 days irrespective of the presence of transport hubs in the prefectures (Table 1).

3.3. Roles of Transport Modes in Inter-Prefecture Spread of Influenza A(H1N1)pdm09

The correlations between arrival days and log-transformed passenger volumes by transport modes are presented in Table 2. For each transport mode, log-transformed passenger volumes were negatively correlated with arrival days across prefecture groups, but the relationships were significant in all prefecture groups except for the 20 prefectures with only air and road transport ($r = -0.32$, $p = 0.17$ for air travel; $r = -0.34$, $p = 0.14$ for road travel).

Table 2. Pearson correlation coefficients between arrival days and log-transformed passenger volumes by transport modes in 334 prefectures.

Transport Modes (No. of Prefectures)	log(*PAir*)	log(*PRail*)	log(*PRoad*)
Air + Rail + Road (115)	−0.58 ***	−0.47 ***	−0.60 ***
Air + Road (20)	−0.32	-	−0.34
Rail + Road (140)	-	−0.17 *	−0.25 **
Road (59)	-	-	−0.54 ***

Note: log(*PAir*), log(*PRail*), and log(*PRoad*) are the log-transformed air, rail, and road passenger volumes (10,000 persons) in each prefecture. * Correlation coefficient is significant at the 0.05 level (2-tailed), ** for 0.01, and *** for 0.001. All values are rounded to two decimal places.

As previously shown in Figure 4, mainland China experienced two distinct phases of inter-prefecture spread of influenza A(H1N1)pdm09. To examine the roles of different transport modes in these two spread phases, we focused our analyses on the 115 prefectures where all three transport modes were available. As shown in Figure 5a, the distribution of arrival days in 115 prefectures was bimodal with two peaks at approximately 40 (20 June 2009) and 125 (15 September 2009) days. The respective peaks coincided with a small uplift (Figure 1c) and a sharp increase (Figure 1b) in the daily influenza A(H1N1)pdm09 incidence in mainland China. These two phases (I and II) with peaks at the 0.25 and 0.75 quantiles of arrival days were split by the 0.50 quantile (80 days since 10 May 2009, i.e., approximately 1 August 2009) (Figure 5a). The associations between the 0.25, 0.50, and 0.75 quantiles of arrival days and passenger volumes for the different transport modes in 115 prefectures are presented in Table 3. Irrespective of the quantile level τ, latitude coordinates for affected prefectures were significantly positively associated with arrival day, whereas longitude coordinates were significantly negatively related to arrival day. After adjusting for the geographic locations of prefectures, both air and road passenger volumes in log-scale were significantly negatively associated with arrival day for $\tau = 0.25$, 0.50, and 0.75. By contrast, log-transformed rail passenger volumes were also negatively associated with arrival day across the three quantile levels; however, the association was significant only for $\tau = 0.75$ (regression coefficient = -5.42, 95% CI: -16.80, -0.45). As indicated by the pseudo R^2, the quantile regression model for $\tau = 0.50$ explained the most variance in arrival days (45%).

Table 3. Multivariate quantile regression showing the associations between the 0.25, 0.50, and 0.75 quantiles of arrival days and passenger volumes of three transport modes in 115 prefectures.

Variables [a]	$\tau = 0.25$	$\tau = 0.50$	$\tau = 0.75$
Intercept	274.08 (222.13, 344.09) [b]	295.84 (201.19, 381.45)	256.25 (189.21, 457.03)
Lat	1.95 (1.30, 3.69)	1.78 (1.36, 3.34)	2.29 (1.00, 4.06)
Lng	-1.38 (-1.83, -0.46)	-1.15 (-2.22, -0.55)	-0.80 (-2.33, -0.33)
log(*PAir*)	-7.23 (-10.75, -0.38)	-9.54 (-15.13, -4.81)	-12.10 (-14.90, -6.12)
log(*PRail*)	-1.99 (-12.41, 0.97)	-6.18 (-14.41, 1.99)	-5.42 (-16.80, -0.45)
log(*PRoad*)	-9.04 (-15.52, -3.05)	-7.58 (-15.41, -1.37)	-6.73 (-15.35, -0.23)
R^2 [c]	0.33	0.45	0.41

[a] *Lat* and *Lng* are prefectural latitude and longitude coordinates. log(*PAir*), log(*PRail*), and log(*PRoad*) are the log-transformed air, rail, and road passenger volumes (10,000 persons) in each prefecture. [b] All regression coefficients are rounded to two decimal places. Numbers in parentheses are 95% confidence intervals. [c] Pseudo R^2 are reported for quantile regression.

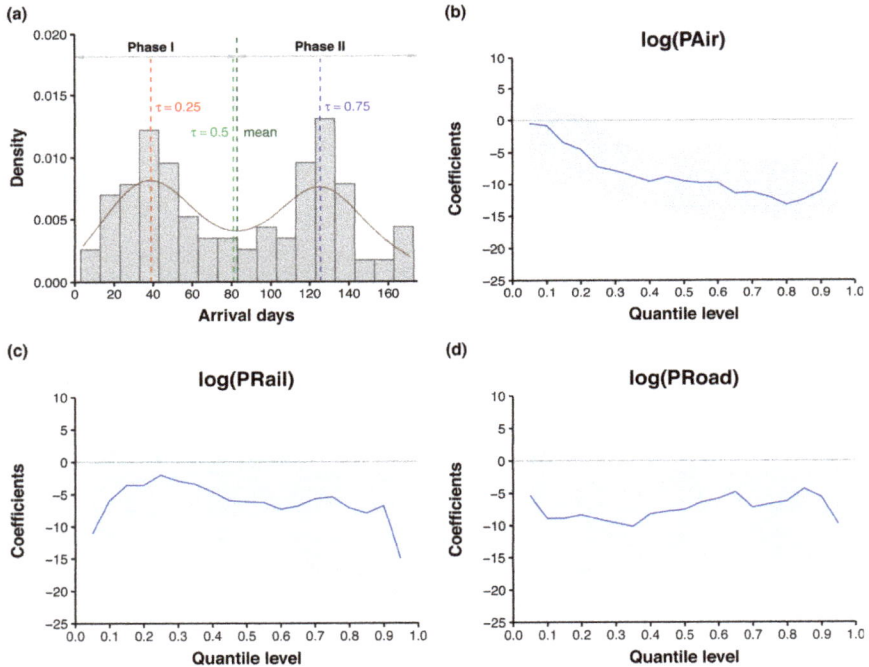

Figure 5. Quantile process regression of arrival days in 115 prefectures. In (**a**) the density plot of arrival days, the red, green, and blue vertical lines indicate, respectively, the $\tau = 0.25$, 0.50, and 0.75 quantiles of arrival days, whereas the dark green vertical line indicates the mean arrival days. In quantile process plots for log-transformed air (**b**), rail (**c**), and road (**d**) passenger volumes, the blue curves and shaded areas represent the quantile regression coefficients and 95% confidence intervals.

The quantile process plots of the three transport modes shown in Figure 5 further demonstrate the change in quantile regression coefficients and 95% CIs as a function of quantile level τ. As τ increases, the regression coefficient of log-transformed air passenger volume decreases, whereas the regression coefficient of log-transformed rail passenger volume increases slightly before $\tau = 0.25$, then decreases. Yet, the regression coefficient of log-transformed road passenger volume is constant prior to $\tau = 0.4$, then increases slightly with the increase of τ. We further observed that the negative associations between log-transformed air passenger volume and the lower quantiles of arrival day appear to be insignificant because the upper confidence limits are greater than 0 for quantile levels less than 0.25. Likewise, log-transformed rail passenger volumes significantly negatively affected ≥ 0.70 quantiles of arrival days.

4. Discussion

To understand the roles of different transport modes in the spread of the 2009 influenza A(H1N1) pandemic between prefectures across mainland China, this work used arrival day and peak day to characterize the pandemic spread and evaluated the influence of travel-related factors on it. During the entire invasion period of the virus, road travel consistently played a significant role. Rail travel played an insignificant role during phase I but significantly affected the inter-prefecture spread during phase II. The role of air travel became more important as the virus spread.

4.1. Two Phases and Direction of Influenza A(H1N1)pdm09 Spread between Prefectures

While a pronounced double-wave feature in the daily epidemic curve was barely noticeable prior to the National Day holiday, the remarkably bimodal distribution of arrival days suggests that the inter-prefecture spread of influenza A(H1N1)pdm09 across mainland China had two distinct phases that were split at approximately 1 August 2009. Interestingly, the phase I of spatial spread coincided with the early containment phase of the 2009 pandemic when an individual case-based surveillance was implemented until mid-July 2009 [48]. Our results suggest that containment measures successfully suppressed the increase in influenza A(H1N1)pdm09 incidence during phase I but failed to restrict its spatial expansion. Consequently, individual case-based surveillance was terminated by mid-August 2009 [48], which made the inter-prefecture of influenza A(H1N1)pdm09 easier during phase II. Additionally, according to the associations between school openings and influenza A(H1N1)pdm09 transmission found in the US [49,50], school openings in early September 2009 may have also contributed to the second peak of influenza A(H1N1)pdm09 spread between prefectures.

Quantile regression analyses showed that the arrival time of influenza A(H1N1)pdm09 in an individual prefecture was always significantly negatively and positively associated with prefectural longitudes and latitudes, respectively, regardless of spread phase. These results suggest that the virus generally spread from the southeast to the northwest of mainland China, which confirms previous findings [33]. The observed direction of spatial spread reflected the fact that, during the early containment phase, a large proportion of international-travel related cases were imported into mainland China via international airports in eastern coastal cities, particularly those in Guangdong and Fujian provinces [33,48]. From there, the infection was disseminated to the other parts of mainland China. This fact was also partially responsible for the earlier presence of influenza A(H1N1)pdm09 in prefectures located in the southeast of the Hu line. Another factor strongly related to this phenomenon was the obvious spatial heterogeneity of the population distribution stratified by the Hu line. In the southeast of the Hu line, 93.9% of the population in 2015 live in 42.8% of the area, and the population density is 314.9 people/km^2, 20.5 times that of the other side [51]. As a result, significant stratified heterogeneity of arrival day was detected for the stratification of the Hu line, whose determinant power was as much as 14.9%.

4.2. Impact of Transport Hubs on Arrival Day and Peak Day

The lack of significant correlation between arrival day and peak day among the 340 affected prefectures indicates that the early arrival of influenza A(H1N1)pdm09 was not associated with early peak incidence as one might expect. Specifically, the peaks in prefectures above the Hukun Railway were concentrated before the end of November 2009, which was approximately two months earlier than the typical peak of seasonal influenza epidemics in Northern China (January–February) [52]. This is because, as a novel virus to which humans have little immunity, influenza A(H1N1)pdm09 is associated with high mortality and can spread more quickly than mild seasonal influenza epidemics [12]. It is interesting to note that the apparent difference in peak time of the influenza pandemic was delineated by the Hukun Railway rather than 27° N, which was suggested by Yu et al. [52] for identifying epidemiological regions characterized by distinct influenza seasonality in China. This discrepancy may be because Yu et al. conducted their analysis at the province level by aggregating sentinel hospital-based influenza surveillance data. This emphasizes the need to characterize the influenza seasonal patterns in China at the prefecture level.

The presence of airports or high-ranking railway stations in prefectures significantly advanced arrival day but had no evident impact on peak day. This finding is also confirmed by the SSH q-statistic test; 3.1% and 4.2% of the SSH of arrival day were attributed to airports and railway stations. On the contrary, the almost zero determinant powers of both airports ($q = 0.000$) and railway stations ($q = 0.003$) to peak day suggest that the spatial heterogeneity of peak day was not associated with the presence of transport hubs. A possible explanation for this difference might be that, because airports and railway stations are suitable proxy variables for air and rail travel, the arrival of passengers increased the probability of transmitting influenza A(H1N1)pdm09. However, once these prefectures were affected, peak of transmission within a prefecture was more likely to be determined by local environmental factors such as humidity and temperature [52–54]. More specifically, experimental studies indicate that aerosol transmission of influenza A(H1N1)pdm09 is sensitive to temperature and humidity [55]. Our previous analyses also suggested that absolute humidity was the dominant meteorological factor associated with spatial spread of influenza A(H1N1)pdm09 across mainland China [56]. Furthermore, prefectures with airports or high-ranking railway stations generally have high population density and greater mobility. Therefore, the approximate two week lag in arrival day between prefectures with and without transport hubs suggests that influenza A(H1N1)pdm09 might spread rapidly and hierarchically among populous cities and then to less populated areas across mainland China, which may resemble the spatial spread patterns previously described for seasonal flu in the US [12]. This proposed pattern is supported by a study on human travel patterns in mainland China, which also suggested that a pandemic emerging in more developed areas might be expected to spread more rapidly [57]. In addition to timing, a recent study indicated that urbanization and humidity have strong influences over the epidemic intensity of influenza [58].

4.3. Roles of Transport Modes in Inter-Prefecture Spread of Influenza A(H1N1)pdm09

The negative quantile regression coefficients of air and rail passenger volume on arrival day supported our hypothesis that air and rail travel accelerated the inter-prefecture spread of influenza A(H1N1)pdm09 across mainland China. The most interesting finding was that both air and road travel played a significant role in accelerating influenza A(H1N1)pdm09 spread between prefectures across phases I and II, whereas the coefficient for rail travel was only significant during phase II. This finding could be explained by the fact that after entering mainland China, numerous international travel-related cases continued to travel back to their hometowns by air and road. Thus, the role of rail travel was not apparent during phase I. Meanwhile, students returned to school at the start of the new term in early September 2009, and increased student mobility led to the increase in influenza A(H1N1)pdm09 transmission at that time. In particular, college students mostly undertook trans-city travel, for which railway is the dominant transport mode in mainland China [26]. Thus, the role of rail travel became more important during phase II. To our knowledge, the dynamic effects of transport modes on influenza A(H1N1)pdm09 spread only were reported for road traffic in a local study conducted in Changsha city [32].

Regarding the roles of air and road travel in the spatial spread of influenza A(H1N1)pdm09 across mainland China, our results are consistent with [33]. However, it should also be noted that our findings on the role of rail travel is contrary to that of Fang et al. [33], who found an insignificant association between counties intersected by railways and virus arrival. Despite the different transport-related variables and statistical methods used, this inconsistency may be mainly attributed to the difference in spatial scales of investigation. Our study was conducted at the prefecture level, whereas theirs were carried out at the county level. As noted by Dai and Jin [26], transport modes have different competing advantages for different distances, and railway is the dominant mode for intermediate and long-range travel between cities in mainland China. Therefore, the distance between counties is too short to examine the role of rail travel in the spatial spread of influenza A(H1N1)pdm09. Instead, assessing roles of different transport modes at the prefecture level is appropriate because it can avoid two situations—the coarse data available at the provincial level would inadequately describe the spatial spread of the pandemic, and the insufficient number of cases at the county level would result in unreliable epidemic curves that are used to derive the spatial patterns of pandemic spread. Furthermore, the difference in spatial scales of investigation may also partially explain the controversy between Viboud et al. [12] and Brownstein et al. [10] regarding the drivers of seasonal influenza spread in the US. It can therefore be suggested that influenza propagation is driven by different transport modes at different spatial scales; while air travel plays a role in long-range dissemination across regions, between-state or even between-city spread is driven by short-distance commutes.

4.4. Limitations and Prospect

Our study had several limitations. First, due to resource limitations in case identification and outbreak investigation, the reporting criteria for case-based surveillance changed from individual cases regardless of clinical severity to hospitalized cases by mid-August 2009 [48]. Arrival days after mid-August 2009 tended to be biased because mild and asymptomatic patients might not have sought hospital care. The underreported cases during the later stage of the pandemic, particularly the large drop in case number due to the National Day holiday, may also have influenced peak day estimation. Moreover, annual passenger traffic data available for 2009 were used to examine the roles of transport modes in the inter-prefecture invasion of influenza A(H1N1)pdm09 for May–November 2009. Using monthly transportation data from the invasion period, or even data corresponding to the quantiles of interest for arrival day, could improve model performance. Finally, although regression coefficients for the different transport modes can be directly compared based on their magnitudes, we were unable to draw a definite conclusion about the relative importance of different transport modes for accelerating the inter-prefecture spread of influenza A(H1N1)pdm09.

To address such a challenge, a multiscale mobility network based on human mobility patterns in China needs to be established. The mobility network should be comprised not only of long-range airline and short-distance road traffic flows but also of intermediate and long-range rail travel flows. Additionally, sophisticated mathematical models with considerations given to administrative hierarchy of population and human travel rules should also be developed to better simulate the spread of pandemic influenza across China. The hybrid model combining meta-population and agent-based models proposed by Weng and Ni [35] seems to be a direction worth exploring further in future research.

5. Conclusions

We conclude that, in addition to air and road travel, rail travel also played a significant role in accelerating the inter-prefecture spread of influenza A(H1N1)pdm09 across mainland China. Our study provides evidence that the role of different transport modes in the spatial spread of influenza should be evaluated at the appropriate spatial scale. Our findings suggest that establishing a multiscale mobility network that considers the unique competitive advantage of rail travel for mid to long distances is essential to understanding pandemic influenza spread and to informing control strategies for future pandemics in China.

Data Accessibility: The data and analysis code for this study have been made publicly available under MIT license at the GitHub repository, https://github.com/caijun/H1N1Transport.

Author Contributions: Conceptualization, J.C. and B.X. (Bing Xu); methodology, J.C., B.X. (Bo Xu) and K.K.Y.C.; formal analysis, J.C.; data curation, J.C. and B.X. (Bo Xu); writing—original draft preparation, J.C.; writing—review and editing, J.C., B.X. (Bo Xu), K.K.Y.C., X.Z., B.Z. and Z.C.; visualization, J.C.; funding acquisition, B.X. (Bing Xu).

Funding: This research was funded by National Key Research and Development Program of China (2016YFA0600104), National Natural Science Foundation of China (81673234), Beijing Natural Science Foundation (Beijing Science Foundation for Distinguished Young Scholars), China Association for Science and Technology Youth Talent Lift Project.

Acknowledgments: J.C. is grateful to Huaiyu Tian for his thorough and constructive comments that helped to improve the manuscript.

Conflicts of Interest: The authors declare no conflict of interest. The funders had no role in the design of the study; in the collection, analyses, or interpretation of data; in the writing of the manuscript, or in the decision to publish the results.

References

1. Past Pandemics. Available online: http://www.euro.who.int/en/health-topics/communicable-diseases/influenza/pandemic-influenza/past-pandemics (accessed on 10 October 2018).

2. Novel Swine-Origin Influenza A (H1N1) Virus Investigation Team, Emergence of a Novel Swine-Origin Influenza A (H1N1) Virus in Humans. *N. Engl. J. Med.* **2009**, *360*, 2605–2615. [CrossRef] [PubMed]

3. World Now at the Start of 2009 Influenza Pandemic. Available online: http://www.who.int/mediacentre/news/statements/2009/h1n1_pandemic_phase6_20090611/en/ (accessed on 20 December 2016).

4. H1N1 in Post-Pandemic Period. Available online: http://www.who.int/mediacentre/news/statements/2010/h1n1_vpc_20100810/en/ (accessed on 20 December 2016).

5. Pandemic (H1N1) 2009—Update 112. Available online: http://www.who.int/csr/don/2010_08_06/en/ (accessed on 19 December 2016).

6. Dawood, F.S.; Iuliano, A.D.; Reed, C.; Meltzer, M.I.; Shay, D.K.; Cheng, P.-Y.; Bandaranayake, D.; Breiman, R.F.; Brooks, W.A.; Buchy, P.; et al. Estimated global mortality associated with the first 12 months of 2009 pandemic influenza A H1N1 virus circulation: A modelling study. *Lancet Infect. Dis.* **2012**, *12*, 687–695. [CrossRef]

7. Colizza, V.; Barrat, A.; Barthélemy, M.; Vespignani, A. The role of the airline transportation network in the prediction and predictability of global epidemics. *Proc. Natl. Acad. Sci. USA* **2006**, *103*, 2015–2020. [CrossRef] [PubMed]

8. Grais, R.; Hugh Ellis, J.; Glass, G. Assessing the impact of airline travel on the geographic spread of pandemic influenza. *Eur. J. Epidemiol.* **2003**, *18*, 1065–1072. [CrossRef] [PubMed]

9. Grais, R.F.; Ellis, J.H.; Kress, A.; Glass, G.E. Modeling the Spread of Annual Influenza Epidemics in the U.S.: The Potential Role of Air Travel. *Health Care Manag. Sci.* **2004**, *7*, 127–134. [CrossRef] [PubMed]

10. Brownstein, J.S.; Wolfe, C.J.; Mandl, K.D. Empirical Evidence for the Effect of Airline Travel on Inter-Regional Influenza Spread in the United States. *PLoS Med.* **2006**, *3*, e401. [CrossRef] [PubMed]

11. Viboud, C.; Miller, M.A.; Grenfell, B.T.; Bjørnstad, O.N.; Simonsen, L. Air Travel and the Spread of Influenza: Important Caveats. *PLoS Med.* **2006**, *3*, e503. [CrossRef]

12. Viboud, C.; Bjørnstad, O.N.; Smith, D.L.; Simonsen, L.; Miller, M.A.; Grenfell, B.T. Synchrony, Waves, and Spatial Hierarchies in the Spread of Influenza. *Science* **2006**, *312*, 447–451. [CrossRef]

13. Khan, K.; Arino, J.; Hu, W.; Raposo, P.; Sears, J.; Calderon, F.; Heidebrecht, C.; Macdonald, M.; Liauw, J.; Chan, A.; et al. Spread of a Novel Influenza A (H1N1) Virus via Global Airline Transportation. *N. Engl. J. Med.* **2009**, *361*, 212–214. [CrossRef]

14. Hosseini, P.; Sokolow, S.H.; Vandegrift, K.J.; Kilpatrick, A.M.; Daszak, P. Predictive Power of Air Travel and Socio-Economic Data for Early Pandemic Spread. *PLoS ONE* **2010**, *5*, e12763. [CrossRef]

15. Jiang, Z.; Bai, J.; Cai, J.; Li, R.; Jin, Z.; Xu, B. Characterization of the Global Spatio-temporal Transmission of the 2009 Pandemic H1N1 Influenza. *J. Geo-Inf. Sci.* **2012**, *14*, 794–799. [CrossRef]

16. Brockmann, D.; Helbing, D. The Hidden Geometry of Complex, Network-Driven Contagion Phenomena. *Science* **2013**, *342*, 1337–1342. [CrossRef] [PubMed]

17. Wang, L.; Wu, J.T. Characterizing the dynamics underlying global spread of epidemics. *Nat. Commun.* **2018**, *9*, 218. [CrossRef] [PubMed]

18. Xu, B.; Jin, Z.; Jiang, Z.; Guo, J.; Timberlake, M.; Ma, X. Climatological and Geographical Impacts on the Global Pandemic of Influenza A (H1N1) 2009. In *Global Urban Monitoring and Assessment through Earth Observation*; CRC Press: Boca Raton, FL, USA, 2014; pp. 233–248.

19. Chang, C.; Cao, C.; Wang, Q.; Chen, Y.; Cao, Z.; Zhang, H.; Dong, L.; Zhao, J.; Xu, M.; Gao, M.; et al. The novel H1N1 Influenza A global airline transmission and early warning without travel containments. *Chin. Sci. Bull.* **2010**, *55*, 3030–3036. [CrossRef]

20. Kenah, E.; Chao, D.L.; Matrajt, L.; Halloran, M.E.; Longini, I.M., Jr. The Global Transmission and Control of Influenza. *PLoS ONE* **2011**, *6*, e19515. [CrossRef] [PubMed]

21. Balcan, D.; Colizza, V.; Gonçalves, B.; Hu, H.; Ramasco, J.J.; Vespignani, A. Multiscale mobility networks and the spatial spreading of infectious diseases. *Proc. Natl. Acad. Sci. USA* **2009**, *106*, 21484–21489. [CrossRef]

22. Tizzoni, M.; Bajardi, P.; Poletto, C.; Ramasco, J.; Balcan, D.; Goncalves, B.; Perra, N.; Colizza, V.; Vespignani, A. Real-time numerical forecast of global epidemic spreading: Case study of 2009 A/H1N1pdm. *BMC Med.* **2012**, *10*, 165. [CrossRef]

23. Charu, V.; Zeger, S.; Gog, J.; Bjørnstad, O.N.; Kissler, S.; Simonsen, L.; Grenfell, B.T.; Viboud, C. Human mobility and the spatial transmission of influenza in the United States. *PLoS Comput. Biol.* **2017**, *13*, e1005382. [CrossRef]

24. Gog, J.R.; Ballesteros, S.; Viboud, C.; Simonsen, L.; Bjornstad, O.N.; Shaman, J.; Chao, D.L.; Khan, F.; Grenfell, B.T. Spatial Transmission of 2009 Pandemic Influenza in the US. *PLoS Comput. Biol.* **2014**, *10*, e1003635. [CrossRef]

25. National Transportation Statistics 2011. Available online: https://www.bts.gov/archive/publications/national_transportation_statistics/2011/index (accessed on 20 September 2018).

26. Dai, T.; Jin, F. Spatial interaction and network structure evolvement of cities in terms of China's rail passenger flows. *Chin. Geogr. Sci.* **2008**, *18*, 206–213. [CrossRef]

27. Ministry of Transport of China. *China Transport Statistical Yearbook 2010*; China Communications Press: Beijing, China, 2010; p. 283.

28. Broeck, W.V.D.; Gioannini, C.; Gonçalves, B.; Quaggiotto, M.; Colizza, V.; Vespignani, A. The GLEaMviz computational tool, a publicly available software to explore realistic epidemic spreading scenarios at the global scale. *BMC Infect. Dis.* **2011**, *11*, 37. [CrossRef]

29. Cao, B.; Li, X.; Shu, Y.; Jiang, N.; Chen, S.; Xu, X.; Wang, C. Clinical and Epidemiologic Characteristics of 3 Early Cases of Influenza A Pandemic (H1N1) 2009 Virus Infection, People's Republic of China, 2009. *Emerg. Infect. Dis. J.* **2009**, *15*, 1418.

30. News Release Conference On Prevention and Control of Influenza A(H1N1). Available online: http://www.scio.gov.cn/xwfbh/gbwxwfbh/xwfbh/wsb/Document/358894/358894.htm (accessed on 10 September 2018).

31. Liang, W.; Feng, L.; Xu, C.; Xiang, N.; Zhang, Y.; Shu, Y.; Wang, H.; Luo, H.; Yu, H.; Liang, X.; et al. Response to the first wave of pandemic (H1N1) 2009: Experiences and lessons learnt from China. *Public Health* **2012**, *126*, 427–436. [CrossRef] [PubMed]

32. Xiao, H.; Tian, H.; Zhao, J.; Zhang, X.; Li, Y.; Liu, Y.; Liu, R.; Chen, T. Influenza A (H1N1) transmission by road traffic between cities and towns. *Chin. Sci. Bull.* **2011**, *56*, 2613–2620. [CrossRef]

33. Fang, L.-Q.; Wang, L.-P.; de Vlas, S.J.; Liang, S.; Tong, S.-L.; Li, Y.-L.; Li, Y.-P.; Qian, Q.; Yang, H.; Zhou, M.-G.; et al. Distribution and Risk Factors of 2009 Pandemic Influenza A (H1N1) in Mainland China. *Am. J. Epidemiol.* **2012**, *175*, 890–897. [CrossRef] [PubMed]

34. Cui, F.; Luo, H.; Zhou, L.; Yin, D.; Zheng, C.; Wang, D.; Gong, J.; Fang, G.; He, J.; McFarland, J.; et al. Transmission of Pandemic Influenza A (H1N1) Virus in a Train in China. *J. Epidemiol.* **2011**, *21*, 271–277. [CrossRef] [PubMed]

35. Weng, W.; Ni, S. Evaluation of containment and mitigation strategies for an influenza A pandemic in China. *Simulation* **2015**, *91*, 407–416. [CrossRef]

36. Google Geocoding API. Available online: https://developers.google.com/maps/documentation/geocoding/intro (accessed on 20 December 2013).

37. Organization of Urban Socio-Economic Survey, National Bureau of Statistics of China. *China City Statistical Yearbook 2010*; China Statistics Press: Beijing, China, 2010; p. 283.

38. Kamvar, Z.N.; Cai, J.; Schumacher, J.; Jombart, T. Epidemic curves made easy using the R package incidence. *F1000Research* **2019**. Manuscript submitted for publication.

39. Hu, H. The Distribution of Population in China, With Statistics and Maps. *Acta Geogr. Sin.* **1935**, *2*, 33–74.

40. Wang, J.-F.; Zhang, T.-L.; Fu, B.-J. A measure of spatial stratified heterogeneity. *Ecol. Ind.* **2016**, *67*, 250–256. [CrossRef]

41. Geodetector: Stratified Heterogeneity Measure, Dominant Driving Force Detection, Interaction Relationship Investigation. Available online: https://CRAN.R-project.org/package=geodetector (accessed on 2 January 2019).

42. Koenker, R.; Bassett, G. Regression Quantiles. *Econometrica* **1978**, *46*, 33–50. [CrossRef]

43. Koenker, R. Confidence Intervals for Regression Quantiles. In *Asymptotic Statistics*; Mandl, P., Hušková, M., Eds.; Physica-Verlag HD: Heidelberg, Germany, 1994; pp. 349–359.

44. Quantreg: Quantile Regression. Available online: https://CRAN.R-project.org/package=quantreg (accessed on 10 October 2018).

45. R Core Team. *R: A Language and Environment for Statistical Computing*; R Foundation for Statistical Computing: Vienna, Austria, 2018.

46. Confirmation of the First Secondary Case of Influenza A(H1N1) in Mainland China. Available online: http://www.gov.cn/govweb/jrzg/2009-05/29/content_1327042.htm (accessed on 10 September 2018).

47. Cowling, B.J.; Lau, L.L.H.; Wu, P.; Wong, H.W.C.; Fang, V.J.; Riley, S.; Nishiura, H. Entry screening to delay local transmission of 2009 pandemic influenza A (H1N1). *BMC Infect. Dis.* **2010**, *10*, 82. [CrossRef] [PubMed]

48. Yu, H.; Cauchemez, S.; Donnelly, C.A.; Zhou, L.; Feng, L.; Xiang, N.; Zheng, J.; Ye, M.; Huai, Y.; Liao, Q. Transmission dynamics, border entry screening, and school holidays during the 2009 influenza A (H1N1) pandemic, China. *Emerg. Infect. Dis.* **2012**, *18*, 758. [CrossRef] [PubMed]

49. Huang, K.E.; Lipsitch, M.; Shaman, J.; Goldstein, E. The US 2009 A(H1N1) Influenza Epidemic: Quantifying the Impact of School Openings on the Reproductive Number. *Epidemiology* **2014**, *25*, 203. [CrossRef] [PubMed]

50. Chao, D.L.; Halloran, M.E.; Longini, I.M. School opening dates predict pandemic influenza A(H1N1) outbreaks in the United States. *J. Infect. Dis.* **2010**, *202*, 877–880. [CrossRef] [PubMed]

51. Li, M.; He, B.; Guo, R.; Li, Y.; Chen, Y.; Fan, Y. Study on Population Distribution Pattern at the County Level of China. *Sustainability* **2018**, *10*, 3598. [CrossRef]

52. Yu, H.; Alonso, W.J.; Feng, L.; Tan, Y.; Shu, Y.; Yang, W.; Viboud, C. Characterization of Regional Influenza Seasonality Patterns in China and Implications for Vaccination Strategies: Spatio-Temporal Modeling of Surveillance Data. *PLoS Med.* **2013**, *10*, e1001552. [CrossRef]

53. Alonso, W.J.; Viboud, C.; Simonsen, L.; Hirano, E.W.; Daufenbach, L.Z.; Miller, M.A. Seasonality of Influenza in Brazil: A Traveling Wave from the Amazon to the Subtropics. *Am. J. Epidemiol.* **2007**, *165*, 1434–1442. [CrossRef]

54. Chowell, G.; Towers, S.; Viboud, C.; Fuentes, R.; Sotomayor, V.; Simonsen, L.; Miller, M.; Lima, M.; Villarroel, C.; Chiu, M.; et al. The influence of climatic conditions on the transmission dynamics of the 2009 A/H1N1 influenza pandemic in Chile. *BMC Infect. Dis.* **2012**, *12*, 298. [CrossRef]

55. Steel, J.; Palese, P.; Lowen, A.C. Transmission of a 2009 Pandemic Influenza Virus Shows a Sensitivity to Temperature and Humidity Similar to That of an H3N2 Seasonal Strain. *J. Virol.* **2011**, *85*, 1400–1402. [CrossRef]

56. Zhao, X.; Cai, J.; Feng, D.; Bai, Y.; Xu, B. Meteorological influence on the 2009 influenza A (H1N1) pandemic in mainland China. *Environ. Earth Sci.* **2016**, *75*, 1–9. [CrossRef]

57. Garske, T.; Yu, H.; Peng, Z.; Ye, M.; Zhou, H.; Cheng, X.; Wu, J.; Ferguson, N. Travel Patterns in China. *PLoS ONE* **2011**, *6*, e16364. [CrossRef]

58. Dalziel, B.D.; Kissler, S.; Gog, J.R.; Viboud, C.; Bjørnstad, O.N.; Metcalf, C.J.E.; Grenfell, B.T. Urbanization and humidity shape the intensity of influenza epidemics in U.S. cities. *Science* **2018**, *362*, 75. [CrossRef] [PubMed]

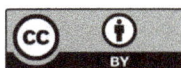

International Journal of
*Environmental Research
and Public Health*

MDPI

Article

Association Between the Activity Space Exposure to Parks in Childhood and Adolescence and Cognitive Aging in Later Life

Mark P.C. Cherrie [1,*], Niamh K. Shortt [1], Catharine Ward Thompson [2], Ian J. Deary [3] and Jamie R. Pearce [1]

[1] Centre for Research on Environment, Society and Health (CRESH), University of Edinburgh, Edinburgh EH8 9XP, UK; Niamh.Shortt@ed.ac.uk (N.K.S.); jamie.pearce@ed.ac.uk (J.R.P.)
[2] OPENspace Research Centre, University of Edinburgh, Edinburgh EH3 9DF, UK; c.ward-thompson@ed.ac.uk
[3] Centre for Cognitive Ageing and Cognitive Epidemiology, Department of Psychology, University of Edinburgh, Edinburgh EH3 9DF, UK; iand@exseed.ed.ac.uk
* Correspondence: mark.cherrie@ed.ac.uk; Tel.: +44-131-650-2800

Received: 25 January 2019; Accepted: 17 February 2019; Published: 21 February 2019

Abstract: The exposure to green space in early life may support better cognitive aging in later life. However, this exposure is usually measured using the residential location alone. This disregards the exposure to green spaces in places frequented during daily activities (i.e., the 'activity space'). Overlooking the multiple locations visited by an individual over the course of a day is likely to result in poor estimation of the environmental exposure and therefore exacerbates the contextual uncertainty. A child's activity space is influenced by factors including age, sex, and the parental perception of the neighborhood. This paper develops indices of park availability based on individuals' activity spaces (home, school, and the optimal route to school). These measures are used to examine whether park availability in childhood is related to cognitive change much later in life. Multi-level linear models, including random effects for schools, were used to test the association between park availability during childhood and adolescence and cognitive aging (age 70 to 76) in the Lothian Birth Cohort 1936 participants (N = 281). To test for the effect modification, these models were stratified by sex and road traffic accident (RTA) density. Park availability during adolescence was associated with better cognitive aging at a concurrently low RTA density ($\beta = 0.98$, 95% CI: 0.36 to 1.60), but not when the RTA density was higher ($\beta = 0.22$, 95% CI: -0.07 to 0.51). Green space exposure during early life may be important for optimal cognitive aging; this should be evidenced using activity space-based measures within a life-course perspective.

Keywords: green space; road traffic accidents; cognitive aging; activity space; life-course perspectives; environmental exposures

---

1. Introduction

The neighborhood environment during early life may be important for mental health [1] and cognitive aging [2], given that this is a period of heightened brain plasticity in childhood [3] and behavioral development in adolescence [4] (see Figure 1 in [5]). Green space may play a role in cognitive development, with several studies finding an association between higher exposure to green spaces and better childhood academic performance [6–8] and social, emotional, and behavioral outcomes [9]. Evidence for the association between green space and improved cognitive development being mediated through lower air pollution has been presented [8,10], although other distinctive benefits to cognitive health have been proposed. Green space may have a positive effect on a child's cognitive development by providing a space for physical activity [11] and by moderating the impact of life stress and adversity [12], as well as indirectly through reduced stress in the child's caregiver [13]. Both increased physical activity and reduced stress could increase educational involvement and attainment throughout life and could, therefore, boost cognitive reserve; this, in theory, could create a buffer against a future decline in cognitive function in later life [14].

A number of studies have also found a greater availability of green space in adulthood to be associated with higher cognitive function [15]. Only one study has been longitudinal, spanning 14 years in later life and using a baseline measure of the green space contact (daily vs. rarely gardening) [16]. Given the difficulty of continuously measuring contact with the natural environment throughout life, there is a lack of evidence on whether the green space can have lifelong effects on cognitive aging. We previously created a measure of the lifelong exposure to green space (park availability) from childhood to later adulthood in areas across the Edinburgh region of Scotland. Using this measure, we found that the higher childhood residential-based park availability was associated with a slower rate of decline in cognitive function from age 70 to 76, conditional on the sustained availability in adulthood [2]. Whilst this life-course research was an important advance in terms of understanding how environmental circumstances in childhood can have lifelong implications for health, the approach relied on simplistic residential-based measures of green space exposure, based solely on the participants' residential location. Exposure based on residential location can be prone to misclassification bias, due to the movement of people outside of their neighborhood for work, school, or recreation [17,18]. Areas where people travel to and from during their daily activities are termed the 'activity space'. One previous study investigated the association between activity space greenness and the cognitive development in children and found that a higher level of greenness surrounding the school, home, and on the child's route to school was associated with a greater improvement in the 12-month working memory and attentiveness [8].

This paper seeks to combine the approaches of these two studies [2,8] by using an activity space measure of the green space in the same life-course model of cognitive aging published previously [2]. In doing so, the paper simultaneously addresses key aspects of contextual uncertainty that have threatened to undermine the robustness of studies examining the connections between health and places. Firstly, we developed a measure of exposure that moved beyond simple residential estimates by also using information on the availability of green space (identified as the area of public parks within a buffer zone) nearby the school and the route to school. This more sophisticated measure of the exposure was then used in a life-course model as a predictor of the cognitive aging in later life [2].

The conceptual model shows that the childhood activity space can be defined by geographic locations around the home, primary and secondary school, recreation spaces, and the routes between these areas. The movement around these locations is influenced by demographic characteristics (e.g., age) and the parental perceptions of space (e.g., safety). Activity spaces for childhood life stages (e.g., infancy) determine the exposure to urban green space (e.g., public parks), which can influence healthy cognitive aging, after accounting for green space access in later life and socioeconomic status.

While we may assume a certain spatial extent of mobility around certain points of interest (i.e., home and school), the actual movement is influenced by factors such as age, sex, and the parental perception of traffic safety [19]. We, therefore, hypothesized that being female [20], of a lower age, and living in an area with a higher number of Road Traffic Accidents (RTAs) (as a proxy for the parental perception of traffic safety [19]), would limit the activity space, reduce the exposure to green space, and attenuate associations with cognitive aging in later life. To test these hypotheses, we divided the estimates of the exposure to public parks into childhood (age 4–11) and adolescence (age 11–18) categories and used these as the primary predictors in a multi-level regression model. Our first aim was to determine whether the availability of public parks in childhood and adolescence was associated with cognitive aging later in life. Our second aim was to determine whether these associations were modified by the sex of the participant or by RTA levels in early life activity spaces. The conceptual model is detailed in Figure 1.

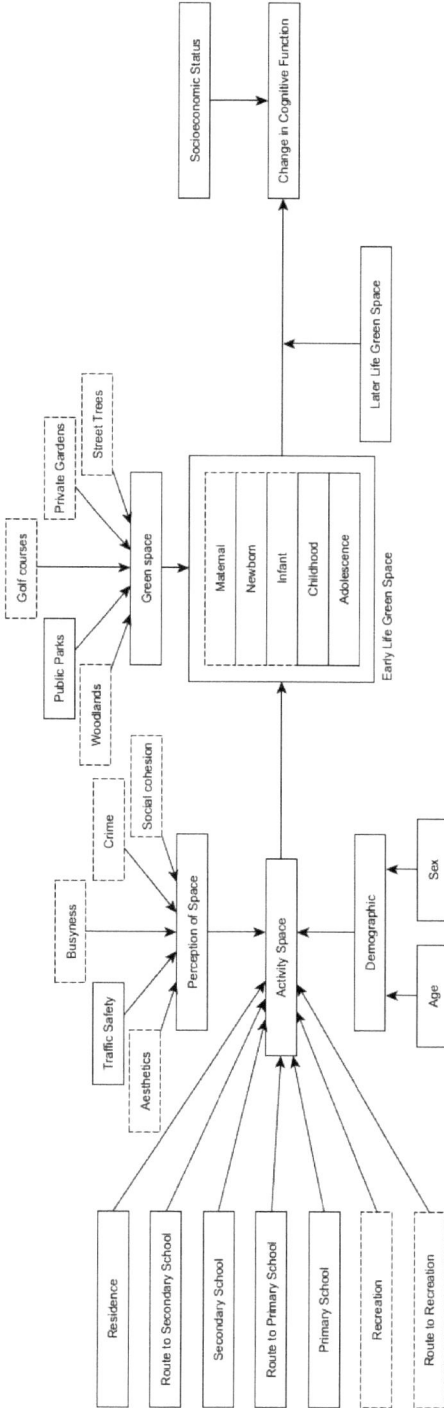

Figure 1. The conceptual model of the relationship between early life green space and cognitive aging in later life. The continuous lined boxes: Measured in the current study. The dotted lined boxes: Unmeasured in the current study.

2. Materials and Methods

2.1. Study Design and Setting

The Lothian Birth 1936 (LBC1936), based within and around the British city of Edinburgh, follows a subgroup of community-dwelling older people, most of whom took a test of their general intelligence in 1947 (at age 11) as part of the Scottish Mental Survey 1947 (SMS1947; N = 70,805). The cohort participants were re-contacted between 2004 and 2007 if they were identified from the Community Health Index (GP-registered individuals) and/or through media adverts; from 2318 responses, 1091 were eligible for wave 1 data collection, at a mean age of 70 years [21–23]. The interviews were held at the Wellcome Trust Clinical Research Facility at the Western General Hospital in Edinburgh. To assess residential movement throughout life, the participants were asked to complete a decade-based "life grid" questionnaire (see Supplementary Materials Figure S1) at a mean age of 78 (July 2014–April 2015). The life grid questionnaire technique minimizes recall bias by encouraging the participant to input global and local events as memory prompts [24]. Participants in the LBC1936 at age 78 (N = 704) were requested to provide a residential address for each decade from the 1930s onwards. The completion of the life grid questionnaire was 84% (N = 593/704).

2.2. Measures of the Green Space and Road Traffic Accidents

The "Civic Survey and Plan for the City & Royal Burgh of Edinburgh" was published in 1949 and includes surveys of population, education, recreation, housing, green space, and traffic from the 1940s, as well as a number of associated maps of these data [25]. We digitized the area of public parks using Map 9 as our measure of childhood green space for the LBC1936 [24]. We also digitized a public park measure from adulthood (1969; the participant mean age of the LBC1936 participants was 33) using data collected by the Town Planning Department, Edinburgh [26]. Further details on these data and the strengths and limitations are presented elsewhere [24]. The road traffic accident point locations were available from 1937 and 1946 in Map 13 [25] and were georeferenced using ArcGIS. Kernel Density Estimation (KDE) was used to create a continuous surface based on the locations of RTAs. The KDE divides the area containing RTAs into 100 by 100 m cells, then provides a proximity-weighted (a 1500 m search radius was used as the hypothesized upper-end distance that a child might walk, i.e., a 30-min walking distance) estimate of the density of accidents per km^2.

2.3. Linking the Measures of Parks and the Road Traffic Accident Density to the LBC1936

The participants were eligible for the current analysis if they had an Edinburgh-based address from 1936–1952 (N = 311) and at least one address during adulthood (N = 281). The locations they resided in for the longest duration between 1936 and 1952 were used as their home location so that each participant had only one childhood home address. The locations of primary and secondary schools in Edinburgh were identified from the survey of Abercrombie and Plumstead (1949) and were georeferenced, which we linked to the name of the school that the participant attended. We simulated an optimal route to school based on contemporary Google Maps (2017) walking directions using the "ggmap" package in R 3.3.2. To estimate the public park availability, we created a buffer (1000 m) surrounding the participant's home, primary school, and secondary school. The intersection between the buffer and the public parks determined the availability (i.e., the area of the parks within the buffer as a percentage of the total buffer area). We created a buffer surrounding the route to school and the availability of public parks was assessed by the intersection, as above. Where the route and the home or school buffer overlapped, the overlap was discounted, to avoid overestimation. The road traffic accident density was estimated by using the values from the density surface at the home and school points.

2.4. Childhood and Adolescence Activity Space-Derived Green Space and Road Traffic Accident Density

In summary, we gained eight measures of the environment for each participant, including the public park availability for the home, primary school, and secondary school, the route from the home to the primary school, the route from the home to the secondary school, and the RTA density around the home, primary school, and secondary school.

From these measures, we built two public park indices: The childhood index (age 4–11), which consisted of the park availability at the home, primary school, and on the route to primary school; and the adolescence index (age 11–18), which consisted of the park availability at the home, secondary school, and on the route to secondary school. We weighted each variable in the index by the hypothesized average daylight hours (12 h) spent in each home (3 h), school (8 h), and on the route to school (1 h), as defined in a previous study [8]. In a sensitivity analysis, we created the childhood and adolescence indices for the following activity space buffers: Large (home: 1500 m, school: 1500 m, route: 300 m) and small (home: 500 m, school: 500 m, route: 100 m). The largest buffer size (1500 m) was determined by data on the typical distances traveled to city parks in the survey conducted in 1969, which found that approximately 90% of the 500 people surveyed traveled up to 1.6 km to reach public parks within the city [26].

Road traffic accident indices were constructed by applying the same temporal weighting as above so that we had RTA indices for childhood and adolescence to match with the public park indices. These indices were categorized as high and low by the median. All georeferencing was undertaken using ArcMap 10.1 GIS software (ESRI, Redlands, CA, USA) and the geoprocessing was undertaken in R 3.3.2 (R Foundation for Statistical Computing, Vienna, Austria).

2.5. Outcome: Change in Cognitive Function

Age-standardized test scores for the Moray House Test no. 12 (MHT) were used as the measure of cognitive function at the mean ages of 70 and 76 [27]. This is the same test that participants had taken in the Scottish Mental Survey 1947 at the mean age of 11 years old. The MHT contains 71 items on a range of mental tasks (e.g., following directions, reasoning, arithmetic) and had a maximum score of 76. It is a paper-and-pencil test and there is a time limit of 45 min. The concurrent validity in childhood is shown by a correlation of about 0.8, with an individually-administered Terman-Merrill revision of the Stanford Binet test [27]. The MHT has concurrent validity in older age, as seen by a high correlation with the Wechsler tests of intelligence [28]. The change from age 70 to age 76 in cognitive function was determined by calculating the standardized residuals, which were predicted using a linear regression model with the latter time point as the dependent variable and the earlier time point as the independent variable. This change score was interpreted as the deviation from what was expected, given the prior test scores, so that a positive coefficient was a better than expected change and a negative coefficient was a worse than expected change.

2.6. Covariates

The relationship between park availability and cognitive function could be affected by socioeconomic status [29]. Therefore, in the models, we used the father's Occupational Social Class (OSC) as a covariate to represent the childhood socioeconomic status. This variable was created by classifying the father's occupation into one of the following categories: I: "Professional", II: "Managerial and technical occupations", IIIN: Skilled occupations, non-manual", IIIM: "Skilled occupations, manual", IV: "Partly skilled occupations", and V: "Unskilled occupations". This was then dichotomized into professional-managerial (I, II) and skilled, partly skilled, unskilled (IIIN, IIIM, IV, V) categories. We also used the questionnaire response on the number of people per room in the childhood home, asked at age 70, to further account for the childhood socioeconomic status. For the socioeconomic status during adulthood, we used the participant's OSC coded in the same way. We also used several variables relating to behavior (i.e., childhood smoking, adulthood smoking, and adulthood alcohol consumption), which are often associated with socioeconomically patterned geographical variables [30], proposed to be on the pathway between environmental variables and cognitive health [5]. Further details on the operationalization of covariates are provided elsewhere [2]. The percentage of missing information for covariates and outcomes was low (≤6%) and was assumed to be missing at random. We used multiple imputation by chained equations, using the "mice" R package with selected auxiliary variables known to be associated with the outcome and covariates, to create 20 complete datasets [2]. The results presented are the pooled estimates from these datasets.

2.7. Statistical Analysis

We developed multi-level linear regression models, clustering participants within their schools, to account for the structure of the data. We used the participant's primary or secondary school as a random effect. It was previously found that the relationship between the childhood park availability and later adulthood cognitive function is modified by the adulthood park availability [2], with this model being the best fitting out of a number of other candidate life-course models (Supplementary Materials Figure S2). Therefore, we used the participants' home addresses from 1953–1989 (i.e., the mean of the park availability surrounding each home location) to create a multiplicative interaction variable (with the buffer size corresponding to the early life variable). These interaction variables were used as fixed effect predictors. A linear model was constructed, with the change in cognitive function from age 70 to age 76 as the dependent variable. We present the results adjusted for sex, childhood covariates (i.e., the father's OSC, people per room in the childhood home, and childhood smoking), and adulthood covariates (adulthood OSC, alcohol consumption, and smoking status). We ran the models for the full cohort and then stratified by sex and road traffic accident density. In a sensitivity analysis, we used the Bonferroni adjustment for multiple comparisons. The statistical significance was set at $p < 0.05$. All statistical analyses were conducted using the 'lme4' package in R 3.3.2.

3. Results

The distribution of the LBC1936 analysis sample for selected characteristics is presented in Table 1. There were slightly more men, more participants who had fathers in a "skilled, partly skilled or unskilled" OSC, and approximately equal proportions of the participants in a "professional-managerial" or "skilled, partly skilled or unskilled" OSC. The most common qualification was attained from high school ("O-level or equivalent" (47%)), followed by "No qualification" (15%). In comparison to the full sample of LBC1936 participants who supplied their residential address history (N = 592), the analysis sample (N = 281) had a higher number of participants in lower socioeconomic status and lower educational attainment categories (Supplementary Materials Table S1).

Table 1. Selected characteristics for the LBC1936 sample (N = 281).

Characteristic	Mean ($\pm$SD); N (%)
Sex	
Female	134 (48)
Father's Occupational Social Class	
Professional-managerial (I/II)	62 (22)
Skilled, partly skilled, unskilled (III/IV/V)	203 (72)
Missing	16 (6)
Participant's Occupational Social Class	
Professional-managerial (I/II)	151 (54)
Skilled, partly skilled, unskilled (III/IV/V)	127 (45)
Missing	3 (1)
Public parks (%)	
Childhood Index	8.6 $\pm$ 7.3
Adolescence Index	9.1 $\pm$ 6.9
Road traffic accident density (per km^2)	
Childhood Index	6.9 $\pm$ 3.6
Adolescence Index	14.5 $\pm$ 5.2
Change in cognitive function from age 70 to age 76 on Moray House Test	1.01 $\pm$ 0.95
Missing	0

Notes: For continuous variables, the mean is presented with the standard deviation. For categorical variables, the number is presented with the percentage in brackets. The percentages may not add to 100 due to rounding.

A slightly larger availability of parks was found during adolescence (9.1% ± 6.9) compared to childhood (8.6 ± 7.3) (Table 1). The road traffic accident density was much higher during adolescence (14.5 km^2 ± 5.2) compared with childhood (6.9 km^2 ± 3.6), due to secondary schools being close to the main thoroughfares through the city and primary schools being located in local, more residential, areas spread around the city (Figure 2). The road traffic accident density was concentrated in the center and North East (in the port of Leith), whereas public parks were more equally spaced, but with the greatest area close to the center due to the largest park in Edinburgh being located there.

The availability of parks during adolescence was associated with better cognitive aging (β = 0.27, 95% CI: 0.00 to 0.55) to a greater extent, compared with the childhood availability of parks (β = 0.22, 95% CI: −0.07 to 0.51) (Table 2). The marginal effects of the park availability during childhood and adolescence, conditional on the availability of adulthood parks, is presented in Figure 3. This shows that the coefficient for the park availability during adolescence becomes increasingly positive (better cognitive aging) with an increasing adulthood park availability. The associations were slightly higher in the females compared to the males; males had a coefficient of 0.21 (95% CI: −0.20 to 0.62) and females had a coefficient of 0.33 (95% CI: −0.07 to 0.72), however, the female coefficient was not notably higher (Table 2). The park availability during adolescence had strong associations with better cognitive aging in participants with a lower RTA density (β = 0.98, 95% CI: 0.36 to 1.60); this was not the case when the RTA density was higher (β = 0.08, 95% CI: −0.29 to 0.45) (Table 2). In the sensitivity analysis with smaller and larger sized buffers, the childhood and the adolescent park availability were not associated with cognitive aging (Supplementary Materials Table S2). In our case, applying a multiple testing correction would have meant that our main finding, i.e., adolescent park availability with a low RTA density, occurred by chance.

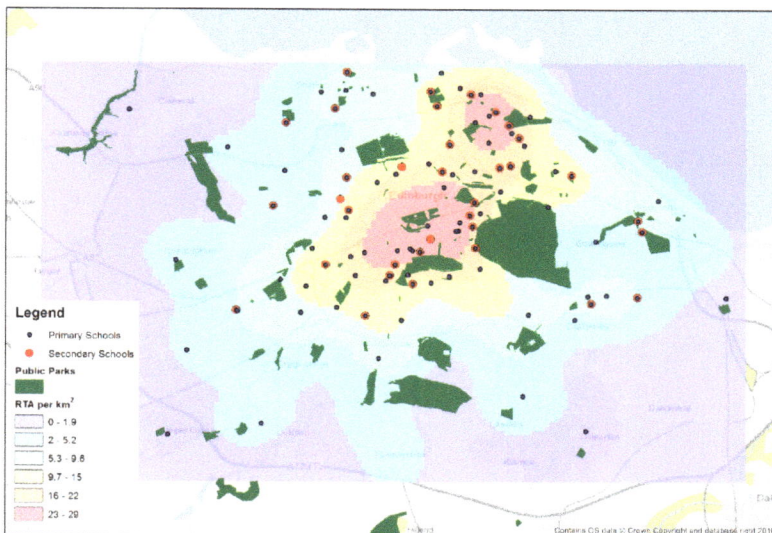

Figure 2. Public parks (1949) and the road traffic accident density (1937/1946) in Edinburgh, UK, in relation to primary and secondary schools.

This shows the marginal effects of the childhood park availability on cognitive change from age 70 to 76, conditional on the percentage of parks in adulthood. This shows that the childhood/adolescent park availability had an increasingly positive/advantageous association with the cognitive change from age 70 to 76 years, as the person's adulthood park availability increased.

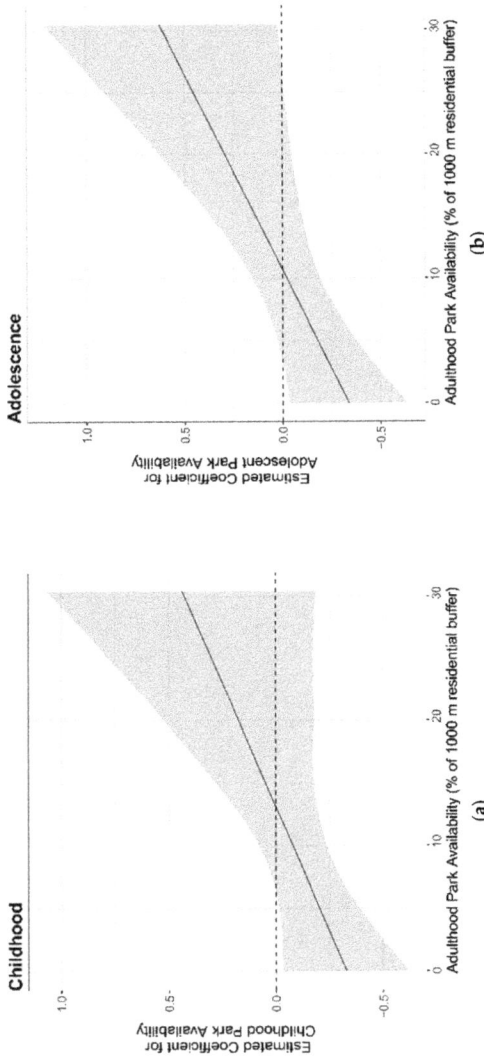

Figure 3. The marginal effects of the activity space park availability on cognitive change from age 70–76, by age period: (**a**) Childhood (age 4–11); (**b**) Adolescence (age 11–18).

Table 2. The life-course analysis on childhood (age 4–11) and adolescent (age 11–18) park availability and cognitive change in later life.

Life-course Park Availability [a]	Change in Cognitive Function from Age 70 to Age 76 [b]				
	All [c]	Males [d]	Females [d]	Low Traffic Accident Density [c]	High Traffic Accident Density [c]
Childhood Activity Space * Adulthood Residence	0.22 (−0.07 to 0.51) [0.1475]	0.13 (−0.32 to 0.57) [0.5764]	0.33 (−0.07 to 0.73) [0.1016]	0.52 (−0.08 to 1.13) [0.0877]	0.14 (−0.27 to 0.54) [0.5054]
Adolescent Activity Space * Adulthood Residence	0.27 (0.00 to 0.55) [0.0496]	0.21 (−0.20 to 0.62) [0.3100]	0.33 (−0.07 to 0.72) [0.1022]	0.98 (0.36 to 1.60) [0.0022]	0.08 (−0.29 to 0.45) [0.6677]

[a] The park availability is determined using the % of the area within a 1000 m buffer surrounding the home and school and a 200 m buffer surrounding the route to school. [b] Odds Ratio (95% CI) [p-value]. [c] Adjusted for the sex, father's occupational social class, people per room in the childhood home, childhood smoking, adulthood OSC, alcohol consumption, and smoking status. [d] Adjusted for the father's occupational social class, people per room in the childhood home, childhood smoking, adulthood OSC, alcohol consumption, and smoking status. * Interaction term.

4. Discussion

4.1. Principal Findings

The current study has used a novel approach of utilizing information on the home, school, and optimal route to school to estimate the park availability in early life and investigate the associations with cognitive aging in later life. Our current work builds on previous literature on everyday time-space interactions and their relation to experiences over the life-course [31]. A key novelty of this study is the integration of early life activity space-based measures within a life course framework, which addresses two important concerns identified in the literature on contextual uncertainty [18]. Public park availability for the adolescent activity space (home, school, route to secondary school) was positively associated with better cognitive aging in later life, especially for those living in low RTA density areas. This is in addition to residence-only models found in this sample previously [2]. Crucially, these associations were shown to be more robust to the adjustment of socioeconomic and behavioral variables than in the model using residence-only exposure, which did not hold after adjustment ($\beta = 0.26$, 95% CI: -0.06 to 0.57) [2]. This shows that the variation in the effect size of the association between green space and cognitive aging is partly dependent on how the geographical exposure is specified and operationalized, which is an example of the uncertain geographic context problem (UGCP) [17]. Recent work has emphasized the salience of the UGCP in the study of the built environment in general and green space in particular, on obesity [32,33]. Further work is required to investigate statistical and theory-driven strategies to determine an optimal measurement of activity spaces, which are specific to certain exposures and outcome relationships.

4.2. Relation to Other Studies

The greater independence of mobility during adolescence may explain why the adolescent park availability seemed to be more important for cognitive aging than in childhood (i.e., the exposure estimates were more accurate). A potential mechanism behind this finding is that parks affect behavioral development in adolescence [34]. A recent study found that aggressiveness in adolescents was reduced with greater greenness within 1000 m from the home; the difference between the highest and lowest greenness exposures within the study equated to roughly 2–2.5 years of behavioral maturation [34]. We found that the results were non-significant with smaller (500 m) and larger (1500 m) sized buffers. In residence-only models previously, both 1000 m and 1500 m buffers were significant [2]. This indicates that activity space-based measures of green space are more sensitive to buffer sizes. We found support for a modification of the effect between park availability and cognitive aging by the RTA density. This could be explained by the activity space, and therefore the exposure to parks, being reduced for participants with a higher road traffic accident density. Both perceptions of road safety [35] and road safety features (i.e., more traffic lights) [36] were associated with a greater likelihood of walking and cycling, although this was limited to girls only.

4.3. Strengths and Weaknesses

We have been able to test for an association between the green space availability in early life and cognitive aging between childhood and later life, after the adjustment for childhood and adulthood covariates, due to the rich longitudinal information collected on the participants from the LBC1936. Our use of a publicly accessible measure of green space was a strength, in that public parks would have provided opportunities for physical activity and stress reduction during childhood, arguably more so than ambient greenness that includes street trees, for example [37]; however, we acknowledge that other green spaces (e.g., golf courses) may have been used and may have benefited the participants. Our work is unique, in that we are attempting to recreate the activity spaces of the children in the 1940s. The landscape available to children has changed appreciably since then; no doubt a much higher percentage of children were undertaking unaccompanied travel in the 1940s compared with today. Estimates of such independent travel to school from 1971 and 1990 show that, in 1971, 80% of seven and eight-year-olds (data unavailable for older age groups) traveled to school without adult supervision, compared with only 9% in 1990 [38]. During this time, the volume of road traffic doubled but fatal accidents involving children halved [38]. Therefore, a child's activity space in the 1940s would have been less constrained and more influenced by factors such as the RTA density than today. The activity space indices created in our current study are useful and valid for exploring a more complete exposure to green space in early life than those focused solely on the area around the home.

However, there were limitations to the study. We have focused on childhood and adolescence but the park availability during pregnancy and in infancy may be equally as important; these aspects were not measured in the current study. For the residential information, we were limited by the retrospective data collection of childhood residential information, which is prone to recall bias. Due to the sample criteria (e.g., living in Edinburgh throughout life), the sample may have suffered from selection bias, although we have previously shown that this Edinburgh 'life-course' sample does not deviate substantially from the full sample on key characteristics [1]. For the two time periods of interest (childhood and adolescence), we only had two locations to determine the activity space indices. These indices were limited by the simple estimation of the time spent in each location (based on a typical weekday), which doesn't account for weekend days or holidays when the exposure to the green space surrounding the home would arguably be much more important than the exposure surrounding the school [39]. The optimal routes, in particular, may be prone to error, as it is impossible to know how precisely they represent the actual route taken by the participant, which might have varied day-to-day [40]. We are also limited by the use of the contemporary road networks in estimating the movement in the city during the 1950s. However, there were very limited changes to the urban infrastructure in Edinburgh compared to other cities (e.g., Glasgow's introduction of inner-city motorways), due to greater local support for conserving the city's architectural heritage and the smaller scale of any slum clearance projects. An important determinant of the route is the mode of transport, which was assumed to be walking, as this would have been more likely during the 1940s; however, we are unable to discount that this may have drawn associations towards the null, as argued elsewhere [41]. Finally, when analyzing geographic-based exposures, there is debate as to whether a correction for multiple testing should be applied when using multiple buffers.

4.4. Study Implications

The access to nearby green space at an adolescent age near home, school, and between the two, may be an important factor for cognitive wellbeing that remains apparent into old age. We found this association in a generation who would have had considerably greater freedom to roam at that age than the current adolescents do. The road characteristics (i.e., the frequency of traffic accidents) also influenced the degree to which this benefit was found.

These findings are particularly relevant today, as children are spending more time indoors [42] and the activity spaces of children and adolescents, especially girls, are increasingly constrained, both spatially and socially (i.e., adult supervised) [20]. Unstructured play and exploration can deliver the benefits of green space for young people [43]; however, this relies on the design of urban environments that are safe, both structurally and as perceived. A recent systematic review found some evidence for interventions on road traffic safety being associated with reduced injuries, casualties, and collisions involving school children [44]. Policymakers should look to implement similar interventions and work with researchers using data on salutogenic areas (e.g., parks and green walking and cycling infrastructure) to promote safe and healthy spaces and routes through the city.

Future research should address the challenge of incorporating activity space-based exposure over the life-course. In addition to age, sex, and co-existing environmental variables, future studies should investigate socioeconomic modifiers of lifetime activity space extent. The main challenge is to determine ways to gather and process the relevant data. In historical cohorts, additional questions on the places frequented for recreation, e.g., the locations of friends and family [45], could be added to life grid questionnaires (although care would have to be taken to avoid respondent fatigue).

In contemporary cohorts, a series of GPS collections could also be taken longitudinally using GPS loggers, as in the Adolescent Health and Development in Context study [46], or perhaps less intrusively via smartphone apps [47]. The information from the apps could be processed using algorithms to determine local activity spaces [48], providing data on where the participants move in relation to the set buffer zones and how the optimal routes compare to the actual routes taken [49].

5. Conclusions

Utilizing information on everyday locations supplementary to the home to determine the public park availability in early life has reinforced previous associations with cognitive aging. Factors such as road traffic accidents seem to be important in determining the size of an adolescent's activity space and their propensity to spend time in natural environments, which may ultimately promote or inhibit their successful cognitive aging later in life. Our study has demonstrated the value of integrating activity space measures into life-course analyses, which is an important priority for researchers concerned with the connections between health and place.

Supplementary Materials: The following are available online at http://www.mdpi.com/1660-4601/16/4/632/s1, Figure S1: Example of life grid questionnaire; Figure S2: Life-course Model Selection; Table S1: Comparison between LBC1936 analysis sample and residential life course sample; Table S2: Relationship between childhood and adolescent activity space park availability and cognitive change in later life, by buffer size.

Author Contributions: J.R.P., C.W.T., I.J.D., and N.K.S. conceived and designed the experiments; C.W.T., J.R.P., I.J.D., N.K.S., and M.P.C.C. performed the experiments; M.P.C.C. analyzed the data; J.R.P., C.W.T., I.J.D., N.K.S., and M.P.C.C. wrote the paper.

Funding: This project is part of the three-year Mobility, Mood and Place (MMP) research project (2013–2016), supported by Research Councils UK under the Lifelong Health and Wellbeing Cross-Council Programme [grant reference number EP/K037404/1] and funded by the Engineering and Physical Sciences Research Council (EPSRC), the Economic and Social Research Council (ESRC) and in collaboration with the Arts & Humanities Research Council (AHRC). The LBC1936 is supported by Age UK (Disconnected Mind programme grant). The LBC1936 work was undertaken in The University of Edinburgh Centre for Cognitive Ageing and Cognitive Epidemiology, part of the cross council Lifelong Health and Wellbeing Initiative (MR/K026992/1); funding from the UK Biotechnology and Biological Sciences Research Council (BBSRC) and the UK Medical Research Council (MRC) is gratefully acknowledged. JP and NS were also supported by the European Research Council [ERC-2010-StG grant 263501]. The APC was funded by the University of Edinburgh.

Acknowledgments: The support of the CRESH team for their helpful editorial input. We would also like to thank Caroline Lancaster, Catherine Tisch, and Eric Grosso for their assistance in geocoding the participant addresses.

Conflicts of Interest: The authors declare no conflict of interest.

References

1. Pearce, J.; Cherrie, M.; Shortt, N.; Deary, I.; Ward Thompson, C. Life course of place: A longitudinal study of mental health and place. *Trans. Inst. Br. Geogr.* **2018**. [CrossRef]
2. Cherrie, M.P.C.; Shortt, N.K.; Mitchell, R.J.; Taylor, A.M.; Redmond, P.; Thompson, C.W.; Starr, J.M.; Deary, I.J.; Pearce, J.R. Green space and cognitive ageing: A retrospective life course analysis in the Lothian Birth Cohort 1936. *Soc. Sci. Med. (1982)* **2018**, *196*, 56–65. [CrossRef] [PubMed]
3. Gale, C.R.; O'Callaghan, F.J.; Godfrey, K.M.; Law, C.M.; Martyn, C.N. Critical periods of brain growth and cognitive function in children. *Brain* **2004**, *127*, 321–329. [CrossRef] [PubMed]
4. Casey, B.J.; Getz, S.; Galvan, A. The adolescent brain. *Dev. Rev.* **2008**, *28*, 62–77. [CrossRef] [PubMed]
5. Anstey, K.J. Optimizing cognitive development over the life course and preventing cognitive decline: Introducing the Cognitive Health Environment Life Course Model (CHELM). *Int. J. Behav. Dev.* **2014**, *38*, 1–10. [CrossRef]
6. Wu, C.D.; McNeely, E.; Cedeno-Laurent, J.G.; Pan, W.C.; Adamkiewicz, G.; Dominici, F.; Lung, S.C.C.; Su, H.J.; Spengler, J.D. Linking Student Performance in Massachusetts Elementary Schools with the "Greenness" of School Surroundings Using Remote Sensing. *PLoS ONE* **2014**, *9*, e108548. [CrossRef]
7. Matsuoka, R.H. Student performance and high school landscapes: Examining the links. *Landsc. Urban Plan.* **2010**, *97*, 273–282. [CrossRef]

8. Dadvand, P.; Nieuwenhuijsen, M.J.; Esnaola, M.; Forns, J.; Basagana, X.; Alvarez-Pedrerol, M.; Rivas, I.; Lopez-Vicente, M.; De Castro Pascual, M.; Su, J.; et al. Green spaces and cognitive development in primary schoolchildren. *Proc. Natl. Acad. Sci. USA* **2015**, *112*, 7937–7942. [CrossRef]

9. Richardson, E.A.; Pearce, J.; Shortt, N.K.; Mitchell, R. The role of public and private natural space in children's social, emotional and behavioural development in Scotland: A longitudinal study. *Environ. Res.* **2017**, *158*, 729–736. [CrossRef]

10. Sunyer, J.; Esnaola, M.; Alvarez-Pedrerol, M.; Forns, J.; Rivas, I.; Lopez-Vicente, M.; Suades-Gonzalez, E.; Foraster, M.; Garcia-Esteban, R.; Basagana, X.; et al. Association between Traffic-Related Air Pollution in Schools and Cognitive Development in Primary School Children: A Prospective Cohort Study. *PLoS Med.* **2015**, *12*. [CrossRef]

11. Tomporowski, P.D.; Davis, C.L.; Miller, P.H.; Naglieri, J.A. Exercise and Children's Intelligence, Cognition, and Academic Achievement. *Educ. Psychol. Rev.* **2008**, *20*, 111–131. [CrossRef]

12. Wells, N.M.; Evans, G.W. Nearby Nature: A Buffer of Life Stress among Rural Children. *Environ. Behav.* **2003**, *35*, 311–330. [CrossRef]

13. Ramchandani, P.; Psychogiou, L. Paternal psychiatric disorders and children's psychosocial development. *Lancet* **2009**, *374*, 646–653. [CrossRef]

14. Lenehan, M.E.; Summers, M.J.; Saunders, N.L.; Summers, J.J.; Vickers, J.C. Relationship between education and age-related cognitive decline: A review of recent research. *Psychogeriatrics* **2015**, *15*, 154–162. [CrossRef] [PubMed]

15. De Keijzer, C.; Gascon, M.; Nieuwenhuijsen, M.J.; Dadvand, P. Long-Term Green Space Exposure and Cognition Across the Life Course: A Systematic Review. *Curr. Environ. Health Rep.* **2016**, *3*, 468–477. [CrossRef]

16. McCallum, J.; Simons, L.A.; Simons, J.; Friedlander, Y. Delaying dementia and nursing home placement: The Dubbo study of elderly Australians over a 14-year follow-up. *Ann. N. Y. Acad. Sci.* **2007**, *1114*, 121–129. [CrossRef]

17. Kwan, M.-P. The Uncertain Geographic Context Problem. *Ann. Assoc. Am. Geogr.* **2012**, *102*, 958–968. [CrossRef]

18. Pearce, J.R. Complexity and Uncertainty in Geography of Health Research: Incorporating Life-Course Perspectives. *Ann. Am. Assoc. Geogr.* **2018**, 1–8. [CrossRef]

19. Villanueva, K.; Giles-Corti, B.; Bulsara, M.; McCormack, G.R.; Timperio, A.; Middleton, N.; Beesley, B.; Trapp, G. How far do children travel from their homes? Exploring children's activity spaces in their neighborhood. *Health Place* **2012**, *18*, 263–273. [CrossRef]

20. Mackett, R.; Brown, B.; Gong, Y.; Kitazawa, K.; Paskins, J. Children's independent movement in the local environment. *Built Environ.* **2007**, *33*. [CrossRef]

21. Deary, I.J.; Gow, A.J.; Taylor, M.D.; Corley, J.; Brett, C.; Wilson, V.; Campbell, H.; Whalley, L.J.; Visscher, P.M.; Porteous, D.J.; et al. The Lothian Birth Cohort 1936: A study to examine influences on cognitive ageing from age 11 to age 70 and beyond. *BMC Geriatr.* **2007**, *7*, 28. [CrossRef] [PubMed]

22. Taylor, A.M.; Pattie, A.; Deary, I.J. Cohort Profile Update: The Lothian Birth Cohorts of 1921 and 1936. *Int. J. Epidemiol.* **2018**. [CrossRef] [PubMed]

23. Deary, I.J.; Gow, A.J.; Pattie, A.; Starr, J.M. Cohort profile: The Lothian Birth Cohorts of 1921 and 1936. *Int. J. Epidemiol.* **2012**, *41*, 1576–1584. [CrossRef] [PubMed]

24. Pearce, J.; Shortt, N.; Rind, E.; Mitchell, R. Life Course, Green Space and Health: Incorporating Place into Life Course Epidemiology. *Int. J. Environ. Res. Public Health* **2016**, *13*, 331. [CrossRef] [PubMed]

25. Abercrombie, P.; Plumstead, D.; Council, E.T. *A Civic Survey and Plan for the City & Royal Burgh of Edinburgh*; Oliver and Boyd: Edinburgh, UK, 1949.

26. Town Planning Department Edinburgh. *Open Space Plan for Edinburgh*; Town Planning Department Edinburgh: Edinburgh, UK, 1969.

27. SCRE. *The Trend of Scottish Intelligence*; University of London Press: London, UK, 1949.

28. Deary, I.J.; Johnson, W.; Starr, J.M. Are Processing Speed Tasks Biomarkers of Cognitive Aging? *Psychol. Aging* **2010**, *25*, 219–228. [CrossRef]

29. McEachan, R.R.C.; Prady, S.L.; Smith, G.; Fairley, L.; Cabieses, B.; Gidlow, C.; Wright, J.; Dadvand, P.; van Gent, D.; Nieuwenhuijsen, M.J. The association between green space and depressive symptoms in pregnant women: Moderating roles of socioeconomic status and physical activity. *J. Epidemiol. Commun. Health* **2016**, *70*, 253–259. [CrossRef]

30. Baumann, M.; Spitz, E.; Guillemin, F.; Ravaud, J.-F.; Choquet, M.; Falissard, B. Associations of social and material deprivation with tobacco, alcohol, and psychotropic drug use, and gender: A population-based study. *Int. J. Health Geogr.* **2007**, *6*. [CrossRef]

31. Helen, J.; Rachel, P.; Colin, P. Multiple Scales of Time–Space and Lifecourse. *Environ. Plan. A Econ. Space* **2011**, *43*, 519–524. [CrossRef]

32. Zhao, P.X.; Kwan, M.P.; Zhou, S.H. The Uncertain Geographic Context Problem in the Analysis of the Relationships between Obesity and the Built Environment in Guangzhou. *Int. J. Environ. Res. Public Health* **2018**, *15*, 308. [CrossRef]

33. Klompmaker, J.O.; Hoek, G.; Bloemsma, L.D.; Gehring, U.; Strak, M.; Wijga, A.H.; van den Brink, C.; Brunekreef, B.; Lebret, E.; Janssen, N.A.H. Green space definition affects associations of green space with overweight and physical activity. *Environ. Res.* **2018**, *160*, 531–540. [CrossRef]

34. Younan, D.; Tuvblad, C.; Li, L.; Wu, J.; Lurmann, F.; Franklin, M.; Berhane, K.; McConnell, R.; Wu, A.H.; Baker, L.A.; et al. Environmental Determinants of Aggression in Adolescents: Role of Urban Neighborhood Greenspace. *J. Am. Acad. Child. Adolesc. Psychiatry* **2016**, *55*, 591–601. [CrossRef] [PubMed]

35. Alison, C.; Jo, S.; Karen, C.; Louise, B.; Sarah, G.; David, C. How Do Perceptions of Local Neighborhood Relate to Adolescents' Walking and Cycling? *Am. J. Health Promot.* **2005**, *20*, 139–147. [CrossRef]

36. Carver, A.; Timperio, A.F.; Crawford, D.A. Neighborhood road environments and physical activity among youth: The CLAN study. *J. Urban Health* **2008**, *85*, 532–544. [CrossRef] [PubMed]

37. Cohen, D.A.; McKenzie, T.L.; Sehgal, A.; Williamson, S.; Golinelli, D.; Lurie, N. Contribution of public parks to physical activity. *Am. J. Public Health* **2007**, *97*, 509–514. [CrossRef] [PubMed]

38. Hillman, M.; Adams, J.; Whitelegg, J. *One False Move*; Policy Studies Institute: London, UK, 1990.

39. Lachowycz, K.; Jones, A.P.; Page, A.S.; Wheeler, B.W.; Cooper, A.R. What can global positioning systems tell us about the contribution of different types of urban greenspace to children's physical activity? *Health Place* **2012**, *18*. [CrossRef]

40. Harrison, F.; Burgoine, T.; Corder, K.; van Sluijs, E.M.; Jones, A. How well do modelled routes to school record the environments children are exposed to?: A cross-sectional comparison of GIS-modelled and GPS-measured routes to school. *Int. J. Health Geogr.* **2014**, *13*, 5. [CrossRef]

41. Burgoine, T.; Jones, A.P.; Namenek Brouwer, R.J.; Benjamin Neelon, S.E. Associations between BMI and home, school and route environmental exposures estimated using GPS and GIS: Do we see evidence of selective daily mobility bias in children? *Int. J. Health Geogr.* **2015**, *14*, 8. [CrossRef]

42. Arundell, L.; Fletcher, E.; Salmon, J.; Veitch, J.; Hinkley, T. A systematic review of the prevalence of sedentary behavior during the after-school period among children aged 5–18 years. *Int. J. Behav. Nutr. Phys. Act.* **2016**, *13*, 93. [CrossRef]

43. Travlou, P. Wild Adventure Space for Young People. In *Open Space: People Space*; Routledge: London, UK, 2007.

44. Audrey, S.; Batista-Ferrer, H. Healthy urban environments for children and young people: A systematic review of intervention studies. *Health Place* **2015**, *36*, 97–117. [CrossRef]

45. Chambers, T.; Pearson, A.L.; Kawachi, I.; Rzotkiewicz, Z.; Stanley, J.; Smith, M.; Barr, M.; Ni Mhurchu, C.; Signal, L. Kids in space: Measuring children's residential neighborhoods and other destinations using activity space GPS and wearable camera data. *Soc. Sci. Med. (1982)* **2017**, *193*, 41–50. [CrossRef]

46. Browning, C.; Calder, C.; Cooksey, E.; Mei-Po, K. Adolescent Health and Development in Context. Available online: http://sociology.osu.edu/browning-adolescent-health-and-development-context (accessed on 15 February 2019).

47. York Cornwell, E.; Cagney, K.A. Aging in Activity Space: Results From Smartphone-Based GPS-Tracking of Urban Seniors. *J. Gerontol. Ser. Bpsychol. Sci. Soc. Sci.* **2017**, *72*, 864–875. [CrossRef] [PubMed]

48. Wei, Q.; She, J.; Zhang, S.; Ma, J. Using Individual GPS Trajectories to Explore Foodscape Exposure: A Case Study in Beijing Metropolitan Area. *Int. J. Environ. Res. Public Health* **2018**, *15*, 405. [CrossRef]

49. Evenson, K.R.; Furberg, R.D. Moves app: A digital diary to track physical activity and location. *Br. J. Sports Med.* **2016**. [CrossRef]

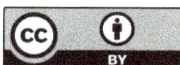

MDPI

St. Alban-Anlage 66

4052 Basel

Switzerland

Tel. +41 61 683 77 34

Fax +41 61 302 89 18

www.mdpi.com

International Journal of Environmental Research and Public Health Editorial Office

E-mail: ijerph@mdpi.com

www.mdpi.com/journal/ijerph

www.ingramcontent.com/pod-product-compliance
Lightning Source LLC
Chambersburg PA
CBHW051709210326
41597CB00032B/5414